Non-Neoplastic Disorders of Bone Marrow

ATLAS OF NONTUMOR PATHOLOGY

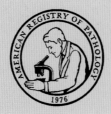 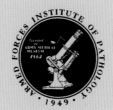

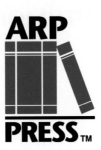

ARP
PRESS™

Editorial & Production Manager: Mirlinda Q. Caton
Production Editor: Dian S. Thomas
Editorial Assistant: Melanie J. De Boer
Editorial Assistant: Magdalena Silva
Copyeditor: Audrey Kahn

ATLAS OF NONTUMOR PATHOLOGY

First Series
Fascicle 6

Non-Neoplastic Disorders of Bone Marrow

Kathryn Foucar, MD

David S. Viswanatha, MD

Carla S. Wilson, MD, PhD

Published by the
American Registry of Pathology
Washington, DC
in collaboration with the
Armed Forces Institute of Pathology
Washington, DC

2008

ATLAS OF NONTUMOR PATHOLOGY

Available from the American Registry of Pathology
Armed Forces Institute of Pathology
Washington, DC 20306-6000
www.afip.org
ISBN: 1-933477-04-0
978-1-933477-04-6

INTRODUCTION TO SERIES

This is the sixth Fascicle of the Atlas of Nontumor Pathology, a complementary series to the Armed Forces Institute of Pathology (AFIP) Atlas of Tumor Pathology, first published in 1949.

For several years, various individuals in the pathology community have suggested the formation of a new series of monographs concentrating on this particular area. In 1998, an Editorial Board was appointed and outstanding authors chosen shortly thereafter.

The purpose of the atlas is to provide surgical pathologists with ready expert reference material most helpful in their daily practice. The lesions described relate principally to medical non-neoplastic conditions. Many of these lesions represent complex entities and, when appropriate, we have included contributions from internists, radiologists, and surgeons. This has led to some increase in the size of the monographs, but the emphasis remains on diagnosis by the surgical pathologist.

Previously, the Fascicles have been available on CD-ROM format as well as in print. In order to provide the widest possible advantages of both modalities, we have formatted the print Fascicle on the World Wide Web. Use of the Internet allows cross-indexing within the Fascicles as well as linkage to PubMed.

Our goal is to continue to provide expert information at the lowest possible cost. Therefore, marked reductions in pricing are available to residents and fellows as well as to pathology faculty and other staff members purchasing the Fascicles on a subscription basis.

We believe that the Atlas of Nontumor Pathology will serve as an outstanding reference for surgical pathologists as well as an important contribution to the literature of other medical specialties.

Donald West King, MD
William A. Gardner, MD
Leslie H. Sobin, MD
J. Thomas Stocker, MD
Bernard Wagner, MD

PREFACE AND ACKNOWLEDGEMENTS

This Fascicle on non-neoplastic disorders is devoted to the assessment of bone marrow in pediatric and adult patients. Although the emphasis is clearly on the successful diagnosis of non-neoplastic bone marrow disorders, neoplastic processes are briefly highlighted in discussions of differential diagnostic considerations.

The early chapters focus on hematopoiesis, bone marrow topobiology, indications for bone marrow examination, and the utility of specific types of bone marrow specimens in diagnostic assessment. It is challenging to focus on bone marrow findings in non-neoplastic disorders because of the critical role of peripheral blood smear findings in establishing a diagnosis in many non-neoplastic hematologic conditions. Consequently, chapter 3 focuses almost exclusively on a clinical/peripheral blood approach to non-neoplastic hematologic disorders. In addition, blood findings are integrated with the bone marrow pathology in each chapter.

Lineage-based non-neoplastic erythroid, myeloid, megakaryocytic, and lymphoid disorders are discussed as well as bone marrow findings in patients with systemic, nonhematologic disorders. A standardized format is used to the best extent possible for each chapter, with an emphasis on categorizing disorders based on patient age, constitutional versus acquired conditions, and pathogenetic mechanism. Because of this combined lineage-based and disease-based approach, there is some unavoidable overlap of content between chapters. Cross referencing refers the reader to the specific chapter with the most comprehensive discussion.

Several individuals at the University of New Mexico Health Sciences Center deserve acknowledgment for their major contributions to the completion of this project. Linda Borgman was invaluable in all aspects of manuscript preparation and support, while Michael Grady provided instrumental support with the images. Pamela Flores was the technical assistant for the bone marrow procedure images. The authors would also like to acknowledge Drs. Richard Brunning and Russell Brynes for their helpful reviews of this book. Colleagues, fellows, and residents in the Department of Pathology have provided invaluable support by submitting cases to us for photography. In addition, pathologists throughout the country provided slides on unique bone marrow disorders; these individuals are acknowledged in the figure legends. Two such pathologists, Drs. Cordelia Sever and Steve Kroft, warrant special recognition for the large number of exemplary cases that they kindly shared with us. Similarly, Parvin Izadi, MT (ASCP)SH provided many pediatric bone marrow specimens for photography.

Finally, overall support for this undertaking was provided by the Department of Pathology, University of New Mexico Health Sciences Center, under the strong leadership of Dr. Mary Lipscomb.

Kathryn Foucar, MD

David S. Viswanatha, MD

Carla S. Wilson, MD, PhD

Department of Pathology, University of New Mexico Health Sciences Center

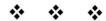

As co-authors, Drs. Viswanatha and Wilson would like to recognize the remarkable dedication, effort and oversight of Dr. Foucar in the realization of this book. She was responsible for writing a majority of the chapters, and single-handedly undertook the overwhelming task of photography. Her breadth of knowledge, experience, and influence as a teacher, mentor, and friend was a source of inspiration to us during the completion of our respective sections, and persists in our careers today.

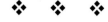

DEDICATIONS

To Elliott, Jim, and Charlie Foucar

Kathy Foucar, MD

For Anne, Adrianna, and Cara

David S. Viswanatha, MD

To Corey, Matthew, and Stephen Tancik

Carla S. Wilson, MD, PhD

CONTENTS

1 NORMAL ANATOMY AND HISTOLOGY OF BONE MARROW

FETAL HEMATOPOIESIS

In the developing embryo and fetus, hematopoiesis is first detected in the yolk sac and sequentially in the dorsal aorta (aorta-gonad-mesonephros), liver, spleen, and finally the bone marrow. In the yolk sac, hematopoiesis occurs in the 2nd and 3rd embryonic weeks and is characterized by the sequential formation of waves of hematopoietic progenitor cells with limited reconstitution capacity (2,8). This site is restricted to the exclusive production of nucleated erythroid cells within blood islands; these primitive nucleated erythrocytes are the first circulating cells of the developing embryo (2,4,6,8). The earliest multilineage hematopoietic precursor cells are found in the embryonic dorsal aorta (aorta-gonad-mesonephros/para-aortic splanchnopleura) (1,2,4,8). Specialized adhesion molecules produced by stromal cells within both the yolk sac and dorsal aorta promote hematopoiesis and angiogenesis (5). Indeed, a common in utero precursor cell for hematopoietic and endothelial cells has been proposed and termed the hemangioblast (3,8).

Stem cell migration to the fetal liver results in hepatic hematopoiesis by about 6 weeks of gestation, followed shortly thereafter (at about 7 weeks of gestation) by seeding of the fetal spleen (1,6,7). Hematopoiesis is detected in fetal bone marrow by 14 weeks of gestation, and bone marrow is the primary site of hematopoiesis throughout the rest of gestation. The vertebral column is the most active site of fetal bone marrow hematopoiesis followed by femur, pelvis, fibula/tibia, and humerus (7).

HEMATOPOIESIS

Stem Cells

The production of all hematolymphoid lineages within the bone marrow is achieved by the coordinated interaction of hematopoietic stem cells, the bone marrow microenvironment, and various stimulatory and inhibitory regulatory factors. This tightly regulated process involves self-renewal of hematopoietic stem cells and the production of lineage-committed progenitor cells; the latter undergo a cascade of differentiation resulting in the diverse mature hematolymphoid elements that are released into the blood (15,28).

The hematopoietic specificity of bone marrow–derived stem cells has been challenged, and a "plasticity" of these stem cells has been postulated (18). Although controversial, some evidence suggests that bone marrow–derived stem cells may be induced to give rise to various nonhematolymphoid lineages such as muscle, cartilage, and nerve (18). The recent detection of a second category of stem cell, the mesenchymal stem cell, has prompted reconsideration of this hypothesis. Consequently, current investigators propose that mesenchymal stem cells are the progenitors of nonhematopoietic lineages, not the hematopoietic stem cells (13,21,22). These mesenchymal stem cells are a normal constituent of the bone marrow microenvironment and give rise to mesenchymal bone marrow stromal constituents including fibroblasts, adipose cells, endothelial cells, osteoblasts/osteocytes, and chondroblasts/chondrocytes (33).

Hematopoietic stem cells are not specifically identifiable by the traditional morphologic review of bone marrow aspirate smears, although a resemblance to small lymphoid cells is suggested. Instead, stem cells are defined by functional properties or immunophenotypic profile. Hematopoietic stem cells are capable of both self-renewal and multilineage differentiation, a proposed unique property of asymetric cell division which results in one new stem cell and one daughter cell capable of differentiation (12,16). Immunophenotypic features of hematopoietic stem cells include expression of CD34, c-kit, and Thy1, while both CD38 and specific lineage markers are typically absent (18,20,27,28,35). Expression of CD34, other adhesion molecules, and chemokine and cytokine receptors is linked to the localization (homing) of hematopoietic stem cells in highly specific bone marrow microenvironment niches (33).

The homing of hematopoietic stem cells and progenitor cells is regulated by cytokines, chemokines, and adhesion molecules (14,24,30). Stromal cells provide survival and regulatory signals by direct contact with stem/progenitor cells within a microenvironmental niche (24). Hematopoietic stem cells localize to the endosteal region of bone marrow; key signaling interactions between hematopoietic stem cells and subendosteal osteoblasts account for this unique localization (12a,16,23,26,30,33). Recent studies suggest a major role for osteoblasts in supporting hematopoiesis and regulating the size of the hematopoietic stem cell pool (12a,16,30,33). The selective paratrabecular localization of immature granulocytic cells can be appreciated by morphologic and immunohistochemical assessment. In contrast, both lineage-committed progenitor cells and terminally-differentiated cells tend to localize to central regions of the medullary cavity (29).

The transition from the undifferentiated status of hematopoietic stem cells to committed lineage-specific differentiation is characterized by the regulation of expression of lineage-specific genes (27). The expression of these lineage-specific genes allows the committed progenitor cells to respond to stimuli generated from bone marrow microenvironment elements, ultimately resulting in the production of various mature progeny (27). Lineage commitment is associated with the loss of the self-renewal capability.

Bone Marrow Microenvironment

The functional unit of hematopoiesis, the bone marrow microenvironment, includes the capillary-venous sinus, the surrounding extracellular matrix, and stromal elements. This is a highly organized, three-dimensional matrix composed of structural scaffolding produced by bone marrow stromal cells (fibroblasts, macrophages, endothelial cells, adipocytes, and reticular cells). The extracellular matrix includes regulatory factors as well as fibronectin, collagen, laminin, and various proteoglycans (25,29,33). Interactions with the bone marrow microenvironment determine the fate of hematopoietic stem cells, since all aspects of he-

matopoietic stem cell activity are influenced by these bone marrow microenvironment niches (16,19,24,30,33,36). T cells within the bone marrow microenvironment play a key role in hematopoietic regulation by stimulating various target cells to produce either stimulatory or inhibitory regulatory factors. Similarly, monocytes/macrophages within the microenvironment produce many cytokines such as interleukin (IL)1, IL6, granulocyte colony-stimulating factor (G-CSF), and monocyte–colony-stimulating factor (M-CSF), all of which interact directly with hematopoietic stem cells and progenitor cells (19). These regulatory factors may be secreted into the extracellular matrix or remain cell surface associated (11,33).

Regulatory Factors

Numerous cytokines play a critical role in hematopoiesis (Table 1-1). The majority of these cytokines are produced within the bone marrow microenvironment by T cells, macrophages, osteoblasts, and various other mesenchymal stromal cells (33,34). By binding to specific membrane receptors on target cells, these cytokines initiate a cascade of intracellular genetic events that promote proliferation and maturation (9). Steady state hematopoiesis is maintained by both stimulatory and inhibitory regulatory factor production as listed in Table 1-1. Some cytokines act on the earliest hematopoietic stem cells, while others control the proliferation and maturation of lineage-committed progenitor cells.

Stem cell factor (SCF) is a prototypic early acting cytokine that is critical not only for sustaining hematopoiesis but also for stem cell migration and adhesiveness (10). In addition to its action on hematopoietic stem cells through interaction with its cognate receptor c-kit, SCF is also critical for mast cell proliferation, maturation, and survival, accounting for its alternate name of mast cell growth factor. Other early acting cytokines include FLT3 (FMS-like tyrosine kinase 3) ligand and IL1, IL3, IL6, and IL11. Granulocyte-monocyte–colony-stimulating factor (GM-CSF) is also a multilineage cytokine whose major action is on granulocytic and erythroid colony forming units in cell culture assays. Prototypic late-acting cytokines include G-CSF, erythropoietin, and thrombopoietin, which stimulate lineage-committed progenitor

Table 1-1
HEMATOPOIETIC REGULATORY GROWTH FACTORS[a]

Regulatory Factor	Comments
Early Acting Cytokines; Multilineage, Pleiotropic or Synergistic Growth Factors	
Stem cell factor	Ligand for c-kit receptor In receptor tyrosine kinase superfamily Many other names: kit ligand, steel factor, mast cell growth factor Influences stem cell migration, adhesiveness, proliferation Required to support hematopoiesis Synergistic with other regulatory factors
Granulocyte/monocyte colony-stimulating factor (GM-CSF)	Multilineage cytokine Promotes cell survival by suppressing apoptosis
Interleukins (IL) 1, 3, 4, 6, 7, 11, 12	Multilineage (including B and T cells) cytokines Synergistic with other interleukins; IL-6 critical for plasma cell production
IL3	Multi-CSF, multilineage cytokine Promotes cell survival by suppressing apoptosis
FLK2/FLT3 (FMS-like tyrosine kinase 3) ligand	Multilineage growth factor in receptor tyrosine kinase superfamily
Lineage-Specific Cytokines	
Granulocyte colony-stimulating factor (G-CSF)	Proliferation, maturation of neutrophilic lineage
Monocyte colony-stimulating factor (M-CSF)	Proliferation, maturation of monocytic/macrophage lineage
IL5	Promotes eosinophil, basophil production
Erythropoietin	Proliferation, maturation of erythroid lineage
Thrombopoietin	Proliferation, maturation of megakaryocytic lineage
Inhibitory Factors	
Transforming growth factor-beta (TGF-β)	Mediates other negative regulatory factors
Interferon-alpha (IFN-α)	Nonlineage-specific inhibitory protein
Tumor necrosis factor-alpha (TNF-α)	Nonlineage-specific inhibitory protein
Macrophage inflammatory protein-1alpha (MIP1α)	Antagonizes positive regulatory factors
Lactoferrin, transferrin	Myeloid inhibitory proteins; suppress GM-CSF production by monocytes and T cells

[a]Data from references: 9, 10, 17, 25, 31, 32, and 34.

cells to produce neutrophils, erythrocytes, and megakaryocytes, respectively.

By integrating the various stimulatory cytokines with the stages of hematopoiesis, the production of various lineages can be illustrated schematically (fig. 1-1). An artistic rendition of hematopoiesis with the architectural localization of specific lineages and stromal elements is presented in figure 1-2.

LINEAGE DEVELOPMENT

Granulocytic Cells

The production of mature granulocytic elements from hematopoietic stem cells is an exquisitely regulated process that is controlled by abundant transcription factors. These regulate the expression of numerous genes, including those encoding for growth factors, growth factor receptors, adhesion molecules, and various enzymes (54,59,65). Early transcriptional regulation of myelopoiesis involves SPI-1/PU.1, RUNX1, and core binding factor gene expression (42,68). G-CSF is the dominant regulatory factor influencing committed progenitor cell differentiation into neutrophils (43). Terminal granulocytic differentiation also is the result of a highly coordinated transcription program which promotes complete differentiation into neutrophils, with the subsequent acquisition of responsiveness to activating infection-mediated stimuli (64). Homeostasis is maintained by inhibitors of granulocytic proliferation such as lactoferrin and transferrin (Table 1-1) (62).

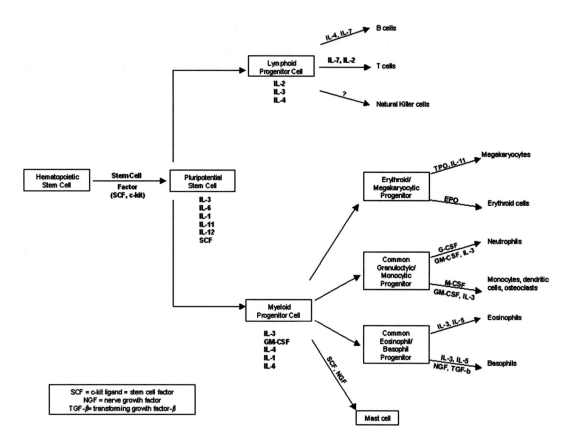

Figure 1-1
SCHEMATIC OF HEMATOPOIESIS

Schematic of hematopoiesis with stimulatory cytokines showing progression from pluripotential hematopoietic stem cell to broad lymphoid and myeloid lineages. Further differentiation results in the production of normal lymphoid and hematopoietic lineages as well as osteoclasts and dendritic cells. (IL = interleukin; CSF = colony-stimulating factor; EPO = erythropoietin; TPO = thrombopoietin.)

The earliest recognizable myeloid cell is the myeloblast. The myeloblast is characterized by a blastic nucleus with dispersed chromatin and variably prominent nucleoli; the cytoplasm is generally moderate in amount and either agranular or only minimally granular (Table 1-2; figs. 1-3–1-5). Myeloblasts are infrequent in normal bone marrow and can be highlighted by the presence of patchy cytoplasmic myeloperoxidase positivity (fig. 1-6). Granulocytic lineage elements express various myeloid-specific antigens including CD13 and CD33; myeloblasts can be distinguished from more mature granulocytic elements by expression of CD34 and human leukocyte antigen (HLA)-DR (fig. 1-7).

Another immunophenotypic "marker" of immaturity is CD117 (c-kit receptor) expression, which is evident on immature granulocytic and monocytic cells. However, CD117 is also present on immature lymphoid and erythroid cells and mature mast cells, while CD34 is expressed on the earliest progenitor cells of multiple lineages, including lymphoid precursors (44). Despite a characteristic immunophenotypic profile, myeloblasts are best enumerated by morphologic assessment. Both CD34 and HLA-DR expression diminish in conjunction with the morphologic features of maturation, which include the successive condensation of nuclear chromatin in conjunction with the simultaneous acquisition of first, primary, and later, secondary and gelatinous granules within the cytoplasm (fig. 1-8) (46).

Although maturation is a biologic continuum, by convention, maturing granulocytic cells are designated as promyelocytes, neutrophilic myelocytes, neutrophilic metamyelocytes, band

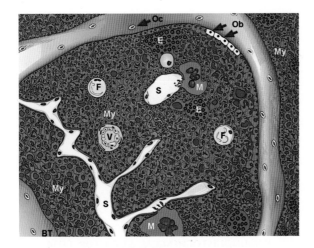

Figure 1-2
NORMAL BONE MARROW

Artistic rendition of normal bone marrow with key architectural features highlighted. (S = sinus; E = erythroid colonies; BT = bony trabeculae; My = immature myeloid, paratrabecular, perivascular; V = vessel; Oc = osteocyte; F = fat cell; Ob = osteoblast; M = platelet-shedding megakaryocyte.)

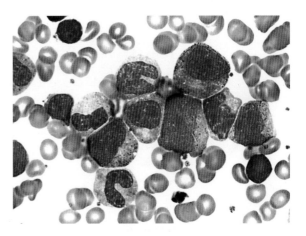

Figure 1-3
STAGES OF NEUTROPHILIC MATURATION

The stages of myeloid maturation, including myeloblast (center), promyelocytes, myelocytes, and bands showing progression from immature to mature granulocytic cells, are seen in a bone marrow aspirate (Wright stain).

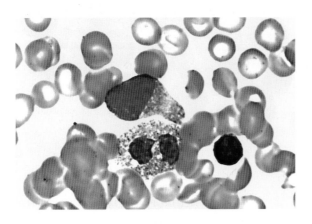

Figure 1-4
MYELOBLAST WITH AGRANULAR CYTOPLASM

A myeloblast with agranular cytoplasm and a large immature nucleus in a bone marrow aspirate (Wright stain).

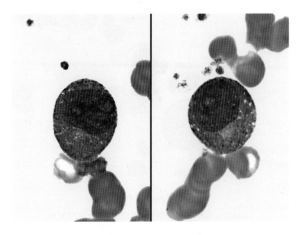

Figure 1-5
MYELOBLAST AND EARLY PROMYELOCYTE

This composite shows two late myeloblasts, early neutrophilic promyelocytes with eccentric nuclei, and the early appearance of primary granules (bone marrow aspirate; Wright stain).

neutrophils, and segmented neutrophils (Table 1-2; fig. 1-9) (38,50). Myeloblasts typically account for less than 3 percent of the total cells in a differential cell count, while the successive stages are progressively more abundant, with band and mature segmented neutrophils the most numerous. Immature granulocytic cells are localized to paratrabecular and perivascular regions of the hematopoietic cavity, while more mature granulocytic cells are more centrally situated in the maturation storage compartment; here, cells are available for rapid release into the circulation (fig. 1-10). These normal localization niches can be highlighted by immunohistochemical staining for myeloperoxidase, which tends to be more intense in the primary granule-rich, immature granulocytic cells (figs. 1-11, 1-12). Neutrophil mobilization is stimulated by a variety of factors including CXC chemokines

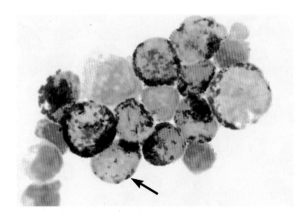

Figure 1-6
MYELOPEROXIDASE CYTOCHEMICAL STAIN

Granular myeloperoxidase positivity (MPO) in the cytoplasm of myeloblasts (arrow) and maturing myeloid cells (bone marrow aspirate).

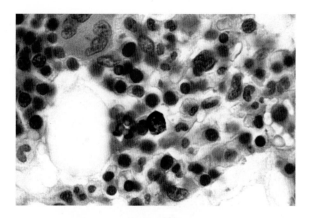

Figure 1-7
IMMUNOHISTOCHEMICAL STAIN FOR CD34

Immunohistochemical stain for CD34 shows a rare positive cell in normal elderly adult bone marrow.

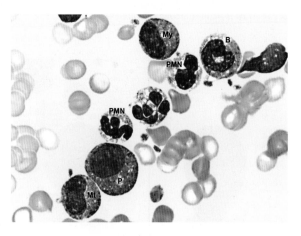

Figure 1-8
STAGES OF NEUTROPHILIC MATURATION

Progressive nuclear maturation from the round eccentric nucleus of a promyelocyte (P) (lower left) through the myelocyte (My), metamyelocyte (Mt), band (B), and segmented neutrophil (PMN) (bone marrow aspirate smear; Wright stain).

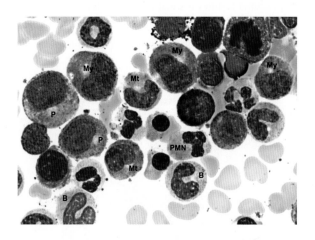

Figure 1-9
STAGES OF NEUTROPHILIC MATURATION

The stages of neutrophilic maturation in a bone marrow aspirate include early promyelocyte (P), neutrophilic myelocyte (My), neutrophilic metamyelocyte (Mt), band neutrophil (B), and segmented neutrophil (PMN). The progression from basophilic to eosinophilic cytoplasm and the acquisition of first, primary, and then, secondary granules in conjunction with gradual and progressive nuclear segmentation and condensation of the nuclear chromatin are evident (Wright stain).

which are systemic inflammatory mediators (40). Chemokine-mediated neutrophil mobilization is caused by the modulation of adhesion molecule expression (40).

In addition to myeloperoxidase, primary granules also contain lysozyme, defensins, elastase, and acid hydrolases, along with other constituents (39,46). These primary (azurophilic) granules are acquired at the myeloblast/promyelocyte stage of maturation and play a key role in defense from microbial invasion and in phagocytosis (fig. 1-13).

Secondary granules are first evident at the early neutrophilic myelocyte stage of maturation; these granules contain lactoferrin, leukocyte alkaline phosphatase, vitamin B_{12}-binding proteins, lysozyme, and other constituents (fig. 1-14) (46). These fine granules impart a pink, subtly granular appearance to the cytoplasm of

Table 1-2
GRANULOPOIESIS[a]

Stage of Maturation	Morphology	Cytochemical/Immunophenotypic Properties
Myeloblast	High nuclear to cytoplasmic ratio Blastic, dispersed chromatin Agranular, minimally granular cytoplasm	Myeloperoxidase + or – Most myeloblasts are CD34+, HLA-DR+, and coexpress myeloid+ lineage antigen such as CD33
Promyelocyte	Eccentric nucleus with prominent para-nuclear hof (pale zone) Sparse, concentrated azurophilic granules	Myeloperoxidase + Typically CD34 –, HLA-DR –, and myeloid antigen + (e.g., CD33, CD13)
Neutrophilic myelocyte	Round nucleus with condensed chromatin Moderate to abundant secondary (specific) granules which give the cytoplasm a finely granular pink appearance	Myeloperoxidase +, leukocyte alkaline phosphatase + Myeloid antigen + (CD34 –, HLA-DR –)
Neutrophilic metamyelo-cyte	Indented nucleus, condensed chromatin Cytoplasm packed with granules with predominance of secondary granules	Myeloperoxidase +, leukocyte alkaline phosphatase + Myeloid antigen + (CD34-, HLA-DR-)
Band neutro-phil	Horseshoe-shaped mature nucleus lacking discrete indentations Cytoplasm packed with granules with predominance of secondary granules; gelatinous granules also present	Myeloperoxidase +, leukocyte alkaline phosphatase + Myeloid antigen + (CD34 – HLA-DR –)
Neutrophil	3-5 discrete nuclear lobes Highly condensed chromatin Cytoplasm packed with granules with predominance of secondary granules; gelatinous granules also present	Myeloperoxidase+, leukocyte alkaline phosphatase + Myeloid antigen + (CD34 –, HLA-DR –)

[a]Data from references 39, 46, and 62.

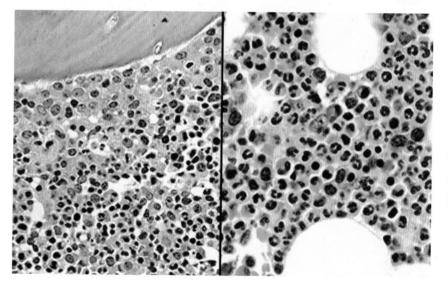

Figure 1-10

LOCALIZATION OF NEUTROPHILIC CELLS

This composite shows the para-trabecular localization of immature myeloid elements (left), while more mature granulocytic cells are concentrated in central intra-medullary areas (right) (hematoxylin and eosin [H&E] stain).

neutrophilic myelocytes, and persist throughout the subsequent maturation to neutrophils (figs. 1-15, 1-16). Upon release, these granule constituents appear to play a key role in neutrophil adhesion (46).

The least well-recognized and most poorly understood type of neutrophil granule is the gelatinase (tertiary) granule, which lacks both myeloperoxidase and lactoferrin, but contains gelatinase, acetyltransferase, and lysozyme

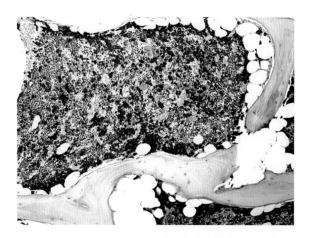

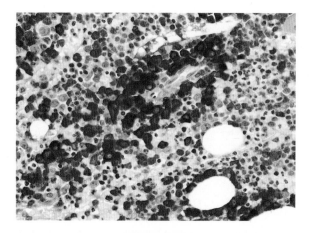

Figure 1-11

IMMUNOHISTOCHEMISTRY FOR MYELOPEROXIDASE

MPO stain of a bone marrow core biopsy section highlights the tendency for the bright positive immature myeloid elements to reside adjacent to bony trabeculae.

Figure 1-12

IMMUNOCYTOCHEMISTRY FOR MYELOPEROXIDASE

Brightly MPO-positive immature myeloid cells demonstrate a normal perivascular distribution in this bone marrow core biopsy section.

Figure 1-13

COMPOSITE OF PROMYELOCYTES

Primary granule formation begins in this prominent paranuclear hof. The eccentric nucleus typifies a neutrophilic promyelocyte (bone marrow aspirate; Wright stain).

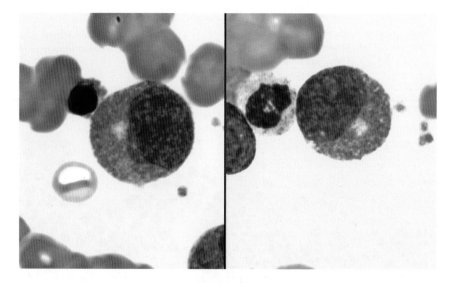

(39,46,49a,62). Maturation stages from neutrophilic myelocyte, neutrophilic metamyelocyte, band neutrophil, to segmented neutrophil are characterized by terminal cytoplasmic maturation and gradual nuclear condensation and segmentation (figs. 1-17, 1-18).

The granulopoietic cycle within the bone marrow takes 10 to 14 days, but can be accelerated by pharmacologic doses of recombinant cytokines, either G-CSF or GM-CSF (62). Daily production rates for neutrophils exceed 2 x 10^9/kg, and neutrophils circulate only briefly in the peripheral blood before migrating into tissues (61). The blood component of neutrophils includes both circulating and marginated pools of relatively equal size (figs. 1-19, 1-20). Marginated neutrophils are attached to endothelial cells, an initial step in tissue migration. Neutrophils, largely via release of granule contents, play a major role in host defense from microbial, especially bacterial, infections, in conjunction with other cytotoxic and phagocytic functions. In addition to the "procytokines" listed above, neutrophil homeostasis is maintained by the coordinated interaction of inhibitory factors such as lactoferrin (62).

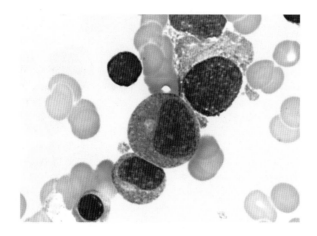

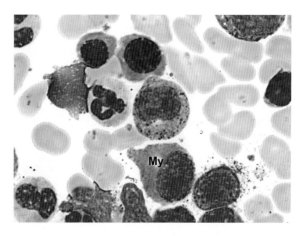

Figure 1-14
NEUTROPHILIC MYELOCYTE

Secondary granule formation begins in the Golgi region highlighted by the paranuclear hof in this early neutrophilic myelocyte (bone marrow aspirate; Wright stain).

Figure 1-15
NEUTROPHILIC MYELOCYTE

Mature neutrophilic myelocyte (My) has pinkish cytoplasm characterized by dispersed secondary granules (bone marrow aspirate; Wright stain).

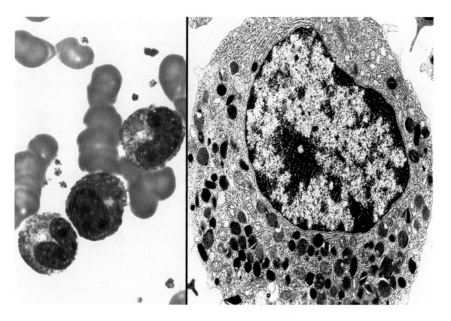

Figure 1-16
NEUTROPHILIC MATURATION

Left: Composite of a neutrophilic myelocyte (center), neutrophilic metamyelocyte (top), and band neutrophil (bottom) in a bone marrow aspirate smear shows the progression of maturation changes of the nucleus and cytoplasm.

Right: Electron micrograph of a myelocyte shows primary and secondary granules (bone marrow aspirate; Wright stain).

Monocytic and Dendritic Cells

Monocytes/macrophages and various types of dendritic cells share a common progenitor cell with granulocytes (65). Monocytes and related dendritic cells play a pivotal role in host defense from microbial pathogens, wound healing, angiogenesis, hematopoiesis, and various inflammatory reactions (49). Although ubiquitous in all organs, macrophages/histiocytes and dendritic cells are generally inconspicuous in normal tissues due to their sparse numbers

and typical, isolated individual cell distribution. Both GM-CSF and M-CSF play major roles in the induction of monocyte/macrophage production within the bone marrow (49).

Dendritic cells are related to monocytes/macrophages and play a key role in the innate immune response (56,63). Evidence suggests that these unique antigen-presenting cells may be derived from either myeloid or lymphoid progenitor cells (55,57,67). Dendritic cells are responsible for T-cell activation in the generation of a

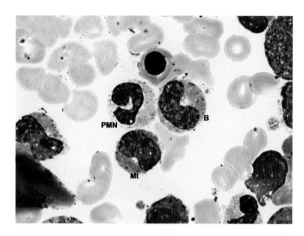

Figure 1-17
LATE STAGES OF NEUTROPHILIC MATURATION

The neutrophilic metamyelocyte (Mt), band neutrophil (B), and segmented neutrophil (PMN) evident in the center of this bone marrow aspirate smear highlight the nuclear and cytoplasmic features of maturation (Wright stain).

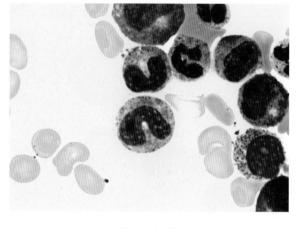

Figure 1-18
BAND NEUTROPHIL

Band neutrophils are characterized by a horseshoe-shaped nucleus without evidence of early constriction or segmentation. Two band neutrophils in the center of the slide can be compared to the adjacent segmented neutrophil (bone marrow aspirate; Wright stain).

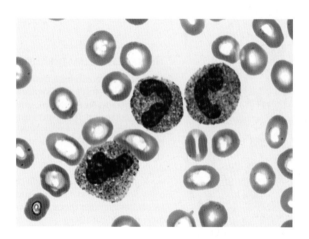

Figure 1-19
BAND AND MATURE NEUTROPHILS

Band and mature neutrophils circulate in the peripheral blood (patient on granulocytic colony-stimulating factor [G-CSF]; Wright stain.)

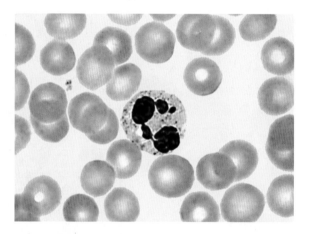

Figure 1-20
MATURE SEGMENTED NEUTROPHIL

A segmented neutrophil with a Barr body in the peripheral blood of a normal female (Wright stain).

primary immune response (67). Dendritic cells are defined more by their functional activities than by specific morphologic features, although immunophenotypic subsets are well described (55,56). Normal ranges for absolute dendritic cell counts in blood specimens from healthy adults are very low: 40/µL or less (47).

Circulating monocytes are identified by their morphologic features, which include large size, reniform or folded nuclei, and abundant pale gray cytoplasm with sparse fine granules (fig. 1-21). Although monocytic leukemias may be composed of monoblasts and promonocytes, neither monoblasts nor promonocytes are typically evident in normal bone marrow. Morphologically defined from studies of related leukemias, prototypic monoblasts have round to oval nuclei with dispersed, blastic nuclear chromatin (fig. 1-22). The cytoplasm is characteristically abundant and pale blue, with either

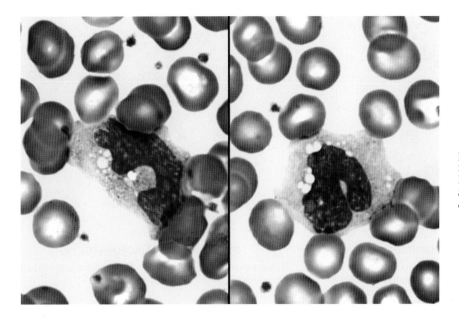

Figure 1-21
MONOCYTES

This peripheral blood composite shows mature circulating monocytes with abundant, vacuolated, slate blue-gray cytoplasm and a reniform/folded nuclear configuration (Wright stain).

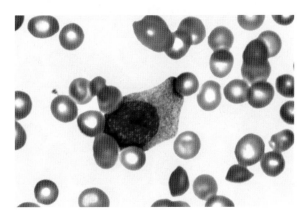

Figure 1-22
LEUKEMIC MONOBLAST

A leukemic monoblast has voluminous, slate blue-gray, finely granular cytoplasm and an immature round nucleus (Wright stain).

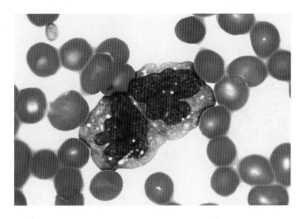

Figure 1-23
LEUKEMIC PROMONOCYTES

Leukemic promonocytes have abundant cytoplasm and folded, immature nuclei (Wright stain).

agranular or subtle, finely granular cytoplasm. Promonocytes are slightly more mature and demonstrate a folded nuclear configuration with a typically prominent nucleolus and fairly dispersed nuclear chromatin (fig. 1-23). The cytoplasm of promonocytes is abundant and similar to that of monoblasts.

Mature monocytes comprise less than 5 percent of the total cells in normal bone marrow, and are morphologically similar to their blood counterpart cells (fig. 1-21). Once monocytes migrate from the peripheral blood to tissue, matu-

ration to macrophages/histiocytes occurs. Fixed tissue macrophages have round nuclei, variably prominent nucleoli, and abundant cytoplasm which frequently contains ingested cellular elements (figs. 1-24, 1-25). Macrophages are readily apparent on bone marrow aspirate smears and are concentrated within particles. In normal bone marrow, macrophages are generally less obvious, unless they contain ingested material from cell turnover, i.e., tingible body type (fig. 1-26).

Diffuse cytoplasmic positivity for alpha-naphthyl butyrate and alpha-naphthyl acetate

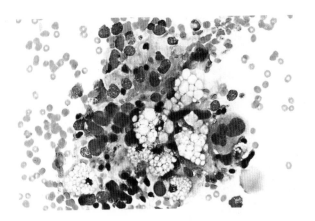

Figure 1-24
BONE MARROW MACROPHAGES

Several bone marrow macrophages as well as fat cells are evident in the center of this hypocellular bone marrow aspirate smear following induction chemotherapy (Wright stain).

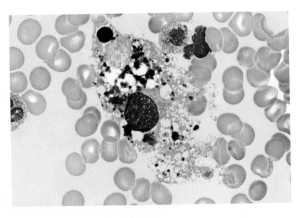

Figure 1-25
BONE MARROW MACROPHAGE

Bone marrow macrophage shows abundant iron and an ingested orthochromic normoblast nucleus.

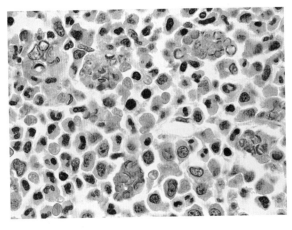

Figure 1-26
MACROPHAGES INGESTING NUCLEAR DEBRIS

Hypercellular bone marrow core biopsy shows dispersed macrophages (histiocytes) containing ingested nuclear debris (H&E stain).

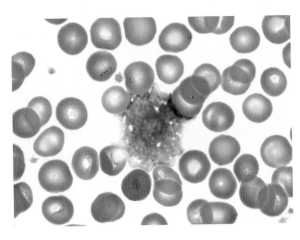

Figure 1-27
NONSPECIFIC ESTERASE CYTOCHEMICAL STAIN

Cytochemical staining for nonspecific esterase (alpha-naphthol butyrate) shows diffuse positivity in the monocyte.

esterase (so-called nonspecific esterases) can be demonstrated by cytochemical stains in all monocyte stages (fig. 1-27). Immunohistochemical markers most commonly used to highlight monocytes/macrophages include lysozyme, CD68 (KP1 or PG-M1 epitopes), and CD163. These immunohistochemical markers have good sensitivity but variable specificity for monocytic differentiation (fig. 1-28) (41,52,58). The unique immunophenotype of the dendritic cells varies by the specific cell type, and differences in phenotype are based on derivation from either myeloid or lymphoid progenitor cells (55,57). Dendritic cells are infrequent in bone marrow, and immunohistochemical techniques (a profile consisting of CD68-, CD123-, and CD43-positive, myeloperoxidase-negative cells) are generally required for cell identification (fig. 1-29) (56).

The bone marrow is the primary site of monocyte/macrophage/dendritic cell production; the primary growth factor mediators of monocyte production include M-CSF, GM-CSF, and IL3. Monocytic production within bone marrow is

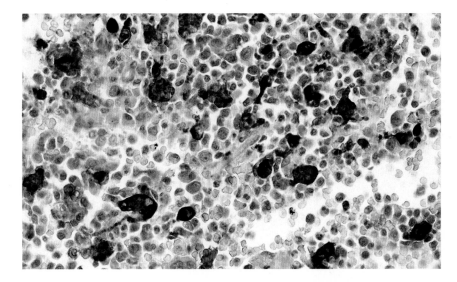

Figure 1-28
**IMMUNOHISTOCHEMICAL
STAIN FOR CD68**
CD68 immunohistochemical
stain highlights increased benign
macrophages in a bone marrow
core biopsy.

Figure 1-29
**IMMUNOHISTOCHEMICAL
STAIN FOR CD1A
AND S-100 PROTEIN**
This composite shows rare
CD1a-positive cells (left) and
slightly more numerous S-100
protein–positive cells (right) in a
normal bone marrow core biopsy
from 1-year-old female.

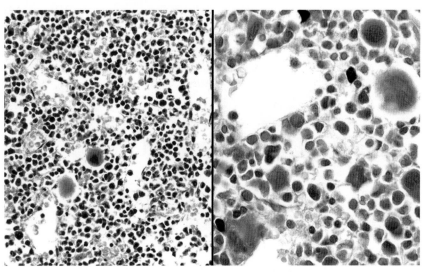

estimated to take about 2 to 3 days. The cells are directly released into the circulation and do not constitute a bone marrow reserve compartment (66). Monocytes circulate in the blood for 8 to 12 hours. Like neutrophils, monocytes within blood may be either circulating or marginated (66). In addition to bone marrow macrophages and dendritic cells, osteoclasts represent another monocyte lineage–derived cell that is crucial for bone resorption and remodeling (discussed later in this chapter).

Other Granulocytic Cells

Other types of granulocytic cells noted in blood and bone marrow include eosinophils, basophils, and, in bone marrow only, mast cells.

Although poorly understood, a hybrid eosinophil/basophil precursor cell has been postulated, while mast cells appear to be derived as a separate lineage (45). IL3 and IL5 drive eosinophil production; IL3 also plays a major role in basophil and mast cell production, in conjunction with other factors (45). For example, SCF (mast cell growth factor) is a critical factor in the induction of mast cell production (45,60).

The distinctive granules of each of these three granulocytic cell types allows for easy identification of eosinophils, basophils, and mast cells on bone marrow aspirate smears or in blood, although mast cells do not typically circulate in normal subjects. On bone marrow aspirate smears, both eosinophilic myelocytes

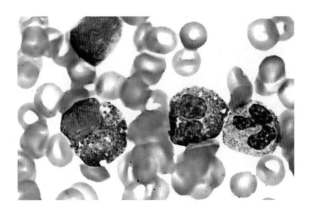

Figure 1-30
EOSINOPHILIC MYELOCYTE
Bone marrow aspirate smear contains an eosinophilic myelocyte (left), mature eosinophil (center), and segmented neutrophil (right) (Wright stain).

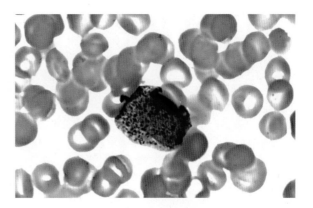

Figure 1-31
BASOPHILIC MYELOCYTE
A basophilic myelocyte in a bone marrow aspirate smear (Wright stain).

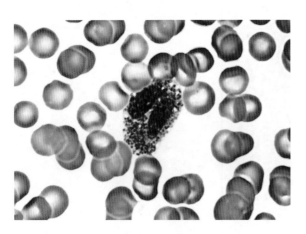

Figure 1-32
EOSINOPHIL
A mature bilobed eosinophil in a peripheral blood smear (Wright stain).

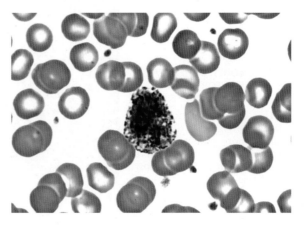

Figure 1-33
BASOPHIL
A mature segmented basophil in a peripheral blood smear (Wright stain).

and basophilic myelocytes may be evident (figs. 1-30, 1-31). Eosinophil granules are large and refractile, and contain major basic protein, eosinophil peroxidase, eosinophil cationic protein, and other factors (51). Eosinophils typically have bilobed nuclei (fig. 1-32). Eosinophil degranulation ameliorates immediate hypersensitivity reactions, and the granules are also effective antihelminthic agents (51). In addition, eosinophils produce SCF (c-kit ligand/mast cell growth factor), a property that may be linked to the close interaction between eosinophils and mast cells (48).

Both basophils and mast cells are effectors of the allergic response and immediate hypersensitivity reactions largely via mediator-stimulated granule release; the granules of each of these cells have similar contents, notably histamine and heparin (37,45). Both cell types are present in low numbers in bone marrow. Mature basophils have segmented nuclei, which may be obscured by the prominent coarse, purple-black cytoplasmic granules (fig. 1-33). In contrast, mast cells exhibit round to oval nuclei, and the cytoplasmic granules are smaller than basophil granules and are more purplish in color.

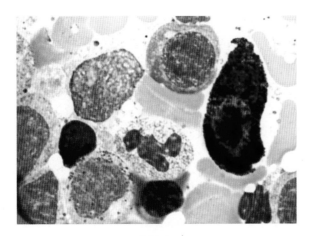

Figure 1-34
ELONGATED MAST CELL

A darkly staining, elongated, purple mast cell is present in a bone marrow aspirate smear. Granules partially obscure the nucleus (Wright stain).

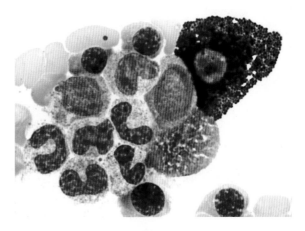

Figure 1-35
MAST CELL

The mast cell (upper right) in a bone marrow aspirate smear has an oval configuration and a small round mature nucleus (Wright stain).

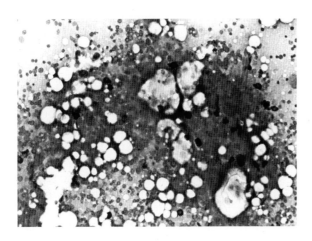

Figure 1-36
INCREASED MAST CELLS

A bone marrow particle has increased and individually dispersed dark purple-black mast cells (bone marrow aspirate; Wright stain).

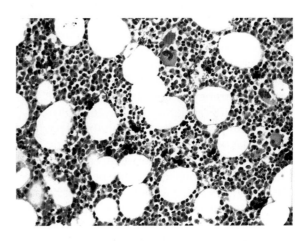

Figure 1-37
IMMUNOHISTOCHEMICAL STAIN FOR TRYPTASE

The tryptase stain highlights increased dispersed mast cells in a bone marrow core biopsy.

Similar to basophils, mast cell granules may overlay the nucleus, often obscuring it. Mast cells may be round, elongate, or even spindle shaped on bone marrow aspirate smears and core biopsy sections (figs. 1-34, 1-35). In normal bone marrow aspirate specimens, mast cells are concentrated within the stroma of bone marrow particles (fig. 1-36). They are more difficult to appreciate on core biopsy sections and are best identified by immunohistochemical assessment with either tryptase or CD117, which highlights the dispersed and perivascular distribution of these cells in normal bone marrow core biopsy sections (fig. 1-37) (37,45,53).

Erythroid Cells

Similar to other lineages, the production of erythroid elements is a highly regulated process in which committed progenitor cells differentiate along the erythroid lineage pathway under the control of cytokines, growth factors, and signals from the bone marrow microenvironment (72,76,77). These signals are transduced to

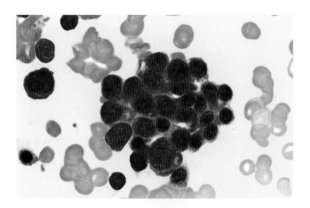

Figure 1-38
ERYTHROID CELLS

A clump of erythroid cells are at various stages of maturation in a bone marrow aspirate smear.

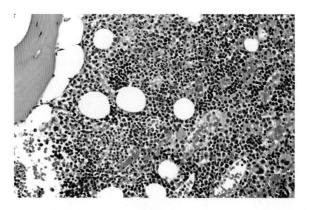

Figure 1-39
ERYTHROID HYPERPLASIA

Bone marrow core biopsy section shows erythroid hyperplasia. Distinct dark erythroid colonies are evident (H&E stain).

nuclear transcription factors which orchestrate the gene expression profile that directs progenitor cells to mature and differentiate along the erythroid pathway. *GATA1* and *SPI-1/PU.1* encode the key nuclear transcription factors required for erythropoiesis; *GATA1* is also required for megakaryocyte, eosinophil, basophil, and mast cell differentiation (69,71,76,77,80).

A common megakaryocytic/erythroid progenitor cell has been proposed, and cross reactivity to stimulatory cytokines between erythroid and megakaryocyte precursors has been described (70,74,79). As noted earlier, a variety of broadly acting growth factors/cytokines influences hematopoietic stem cells and very early erythroid progenitor cells, while erythropoietin is the dominant lineage-specific regulatory factor acting on committed progenitor cells, erythroblasts, and other immature erythroid elements to influence erythrocyte production and maturation. Indeed, erythropoietin is an obligatory growth factor for erythropoiesis, and controls both survival and proliferation of erythroid cells (72,77). Recent studies indicate the erythropoietin binds to a receptor that activates *JAK2*, initiating the downstream signaling pathways resulting in phosphorylation and activation of *GATA1* (81).

Erythropoiesis occurs in discrete colonies within the hematopoietic cavity, and can be highlighted by immunohistochemical assessment (figs. 1-38–1-41). A macrophage is frequently identified within these erythroid colonies, suggesting a specific bone marrow mi-croenvironmental localization of erythropoiesis, similar to other hematopoietic lineages (figs. 1-42, 1-43) (75). Recent studies confirm that the macrophage surface glycoprotein, CD163, is an erythroblast adhesion receptor (70a). The earliest recognizable erythroid precursor is the erythroblast (pronormoblast), which is characterized by a large round nucleus with dispersed chromatin and variably prominent nucleoli, as well as moderate amounts of deeply basophilic, agranular cytoplasm (figs. 1-44, 1-45).

Erythroid lineage maturation is characterized by a progressive decrease in nuclear size, progressive nuclear condensation with ultimate extrusion, and the simultaneous gradual production of hemoglobin within the cytoplasm. Erythrocyte maturation is largely dedicated to producing hemoglobin for its major function of oxygen delivery to tissues (80). The various proportions of basophilic, RNA-rich cytoplasm and hemoglobin account for the transition from deeply basophilic to polychromatophilic, and ultimately, to the deep red cytoplasm of mature erythrocytes.

The stages of maturation are designated as erythroblast (pronormoblast), basophilic normoblast, polychromatophilic normoblast, orthochromic normoblast, reticulocyte, and mature red blood cell (RBC) (figs. 1-46–1-49). It takes 5 to 7 days for erythrocyte production and maturation within the bone marrow, and mature RBCs are released into the blood as they are produced. Recent reports suggest that angiogenic factors produced by erythroid elements may

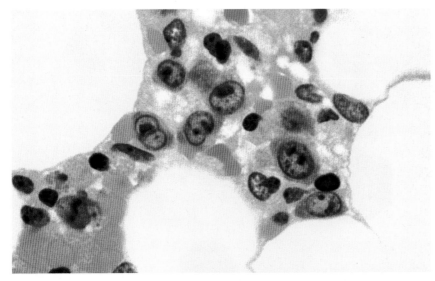

Figure 1-40
ERYTHROBLASTS

Normal erythroblasts with elongated oblong nucleoli, which frequently attach to the peripheral nuclear membrane, are evident in this bone marrow core biopsy section (H&E stain).

Figure 1-41
IMMUNOHISTOCHEMICAL STAIN FOR HEMOGLOBIN A

Prominent hemoglobin A (HgbA)-positive erythroid colonies are evident in this bone marrow core biopsy specimen from a patient with erythroid hyperplasia.

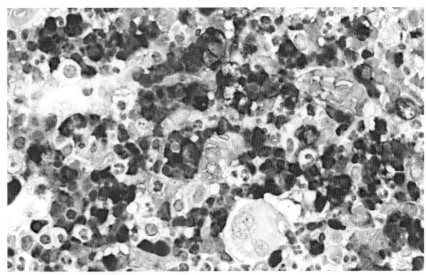

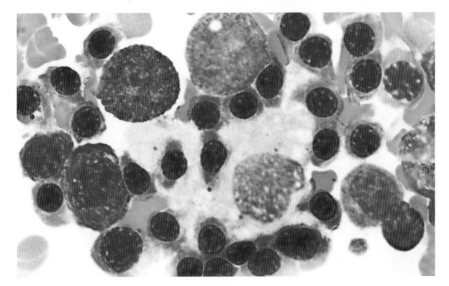

Figure 1-42
ERYTHROID COLONY WITH CENTRAL MACROPHAGE

Bone marrow aspirate smear shows an erythroid colony with a central macrophage (Wright stain).

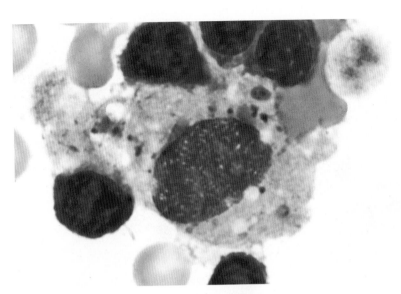

Figure 1-43
NORMOBLASTS
SURROUNDING MACROPHAGE

A macrophage is partially surrounded by basophilic normoblasts (bone marrow aspirate smear; Wright stain).

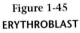

Figure 1-44
ERYTHROBLAST

An erythroblast has deeply basophilic cytoplasm and a round nuclear contour (bone marrow aspirate smear; Wright stain).

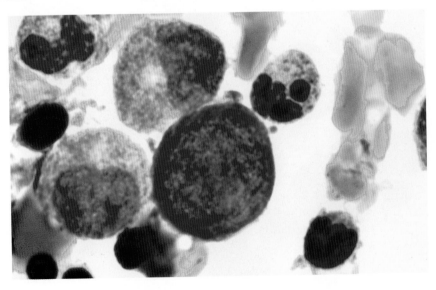

Figure 1-45
ERYTHROBLAST

An erythroblast with an immature nuclear chromatin configuration, nucleoli, and abundant deeply basophilic cytoplasm (bone marrow aspirate smear; Wright stain).

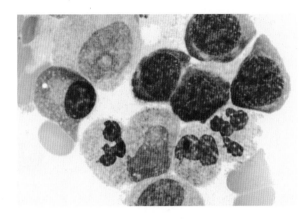

Figure 1-46
BASOPHILIC NORMOBLASTS

A collection of basophilic normoblasts is seen in a bone marrow aspirate smear (top). A plasma cell (left) with an eccentric nucleus, paranuclear hof (Golgi region), and "clockface" nuclear chromatin can be distinguished from the basophilic normoblasts (Wright stain).

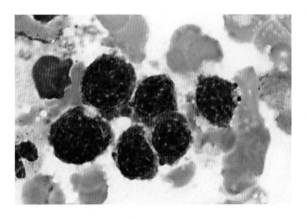

Figure 1-47
MATURING BASOPHILIC NORMOBLASTS

These maturing basophilic normoblasts have more condensed nuclear chromatin than illustrated in figure 1-46 (bone marrow aspirate; Wright stain).

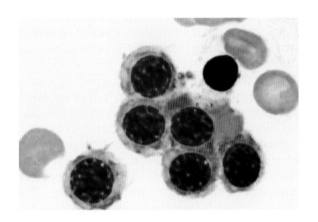

Figure 1-48
POLYCHROMATOPHILIC NORMOBLASTS

A collection of polychromatophilic normoblasts shows evidence of early hemoglobin production within the cytoplasm. Note extruded orthochrome nucleus (top right) (bone marrow aspirate; Wright stain).

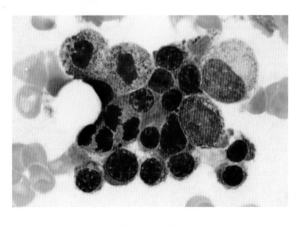

Figure 1-49
STAGES OF ERYTHROID MATURATION

Progressive erythroid maturation is evident in this collection of precursor cells consisting primarily of early and late orthochromic and polychromatophilic normoblasts (bone marrow aspirate; Wright stain).

facilitate macrophage-centered colony formation and the migration of newly formed RBCs into the peripheral circulation (78).

Complex protein sorting occurs during the extrusion of the pyknotic nucleus at the end of the orthochromic erythroblast stage of maturation (73). During this enucleation process, the plasma membrane and cytoskeleton are in a state of dynamic reorganization (73). The pyknotic nucleus is surrounded by a plasma membrane and then extruded, while the resulting reticulocyte retains its own plasma membrane (fig. 1-50) (73,77). The extruded nucleus is ingested by nearby macrophages (figs. 1-51, 1-52). Normal RBC count and hemoglobin and hematocrit levels are maintained by the appropriate balance between RBC production and destruction; erythrocyte daily production is approximately 3 x 10^9/kg (77).

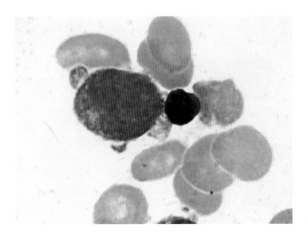

Figure 1-50
EXTRUDED ERYTHROID NUCLEUS

A reticulocyte is adjacent to an extruded nucleus, along with an erythroblast (Wright stain).

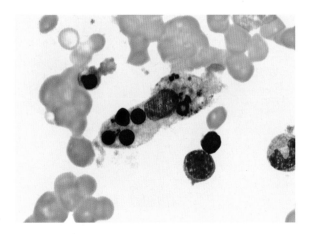

Figure 1-52
MACROPHAGE-CONTAINING INGESTED NUCLEI

A macrophage contains four ingested orthochrome nuclei (bone marrow aspirate; Wright stain).

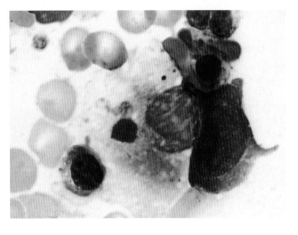

Figure 1-51
MACROPHAGE-CONTAINING ERYTHROID NUCLEUS

A macrophage contains an ingested orthochrome nucleus (bone marrow aspirate; Wright stain).

Megakaryocytes

As with all the components of hematopoiesis, megakaryopoiesis is highly regulated and localized to distinct bone marrow microenvironmental niches. Transcription factors play a critical role in megakaryopoiesis and are encoded by *GATA1, FOG1, NF-E2, FLI1,* and *RUNX1* (91). A common bipotential precursor for the megakaryocytic and erythroid lineages has been proposed (85). In addition to multilineage early-acting cytokines, thrombopoietin is an obligatory lineage-specific growth factor indirectly driving platelet production (88,89,96). The binding of thrombopoietin to its ligand (c-Mpl) activates *JAK2*, which in turn initiates a cascade of events that promote megakaryocyte proliferation and differentiation (94). Although thrombopoietin binding does not directly influence platelet release from megakaryocyte cytoplasm, it does augment megakaryocyte number, polyploidization (see below), and cytoplasmic maturation (94).

Unlike erythropoietin, which is produced in response to decreased oxygen delivery to tissues, evidence suggests that thrombopoietin is produced by the liver at a stable rate. The plasma thrombopoietin level is regulated by platelet mass, since platelets have thrombopoietin receptors. Thus, a decrease in platelet count results in an increased plasma thrombopoietin level, consequently stimulating megakaryopoiesis within the bone marrow (84). Conversely, plasma thrombopoietin levels should decline in association with high platelet counts, thus reducing platelet production.

The most immature megakaryocytic elements may not be readily identifiable on morphologic review, although they are well-characterized in tissue culture systems and by immunophenotypic assessment (Table 1-3) (90,93). The proposed stages of megakaryocyte maturation include the megakaryoblast, promegakaryocyte, and platelet-shedding megakaryocyte (figs. 1-53–1-58). Unlike other lineages, except at the earliest progenitor cell stages, megakaryocyte

Table 1-3
MEGAKARYOCYTE PRODUCTION AND MATURATION[a]

Stage of Maturation	Morphology	Cytochemical/Immunophenotypic Properties
Megakaryoblast	Difficult to recognize by morphology alone, but tends to be large blast with a high nuclear to cytoplasmic ratio, basophilic cytoplasm, and variable cytoplasmic blebbing	Platelet peroxidase evident by immuno-electron microscopic techniques Variable CD34 expression Expression of lineage-specific antigens such as CD41, CD42b, CD61, and Mpl1
Promegakaryocyte	Spectrum of large cells with various degrees of nuclear lobulation Progressive increase in overall size, variable cytoplasmic granules	Loss of CD34 but retention of the full complement of megakaryocyte-associated antigens
Platelet-shedding megakaryocyte	Large multilobulated megakaryocytes with highly condensed nuclear chromatin reside adjacent to bone marrow sinuses Voluminous amounts of cytoplasm with abundant cytoplasmic granules	Expression of some megakaryocyte-associated antigens such as CD31, CD41, vWF increases with maturation

[a]Data from references 84, 86, 90, 92, and 96.

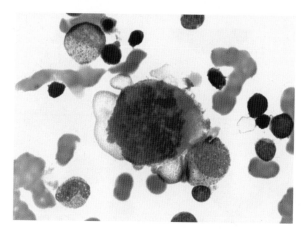

Figure 1-53
IMMATURE MEGAKARYOCYTE

An immature megakaryocyte with prominent cytoplasmic blebbing (bone marrow aspirate; Wright stain).

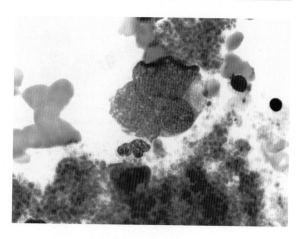

Figure 1-54
IMMATURE MEGAKARYOCYTE AND PLATELET CLUMP

An immature megakaryocyte with a high nuclear to cytoplasmic ratio adjacent to large platelet clumps (bone marrow aspirate; Wright stain).

proliferation is not associated with cell division; instead, megakaryocyte maturation is characterized by the progressive doubling of nuclear material, with the multilobulation of a single nucleus, termed endomitosis (82,87,91a, 94,95,97). Consequently, overall megakaryocyte size increases with maturation secondary to increases in nuclear size as well as even more substantial increases in the amount of cytoplasm (94). Increased size in conjunction with the striking nuclear lobulation renders megakaryocytes readily identifiable on both aspirate smears and biopsy sections (figs. 1-59, 1-60). Megakaryocytes are concentrated within

particles in bone marrow aspirate smears, while they are typically individually dispersed in clot and core biopsy sections (figs. 1-61, 1-62).

Megakaryopoiesis occurs on the adventitial surface of the bone marrow capillary venous sinus, and platelets are directly shed into the peripheral circulation from megakaryocyte projections (figs. 1-63–1-65) (83,92). In tissue culture systems, platelets are derived from numerous elongated proplatelet processes, but in vivo mechanisms of platelet production are not well understood (93). Both the hematoxylin and eosin (H&E) stain and immunohistochemical techniques highlight megakaryocyte number

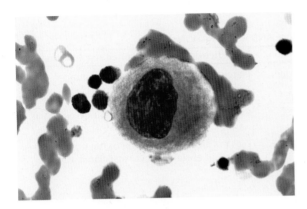

Figure 1-55
MATURING MEGAKARYOCYTE

Early to middle maturation stage megakaryocyte with round nucleus and abundant cytoplasm (bone marrow aspirate; Wright stain).

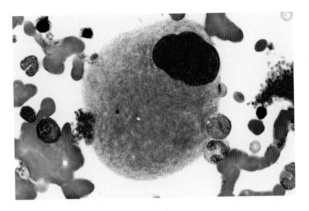

Figure 1-56
MATURING MEGAKARYOCYTE

Further megakaryocyte maturation is characterized by eccentric localization and voluminous amounts of cytoplasm (bone marrow aspirate; Wright stain).

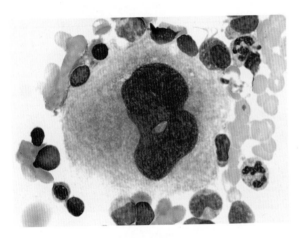

Figure 1-57
ENDOMITOSIS OF MEGAKARYOCYTE

Endomitosis, characterized by nuclear lobulation without segmentation, is apparent in this maturing megakaryocyte (bone marrow aspirate; Wright stain).

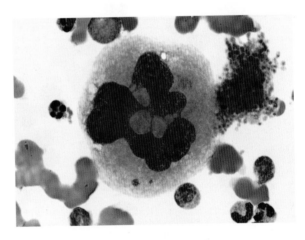

Figure 1-58
MATURE MEGAKARYOCYTE

Prominent nuclear lobulation with interconnected lobules is evident in this mature megakaryocyte with an adherent large platelet clump (bone marrow aspirate; Wright stain).

and distribution on core biopsy sections (fig. 1-66). The final states of megakaryocyte maturation are characterized by the maturation of the cytosol so that platelets can be produced by the shedding of the cytoplasm (83,97). After all platelets are released, the senescent megakaryocyte, consisting of a nucleus surrounded by minimal cytoplasm, undergoes apoptosis with subsequent phagocytosis by macrophages (fig. 1-67) (83). Under homeostatic conditions, platelet production rates are approximately 2 x 10^9/kg/day, but this can increase substantially in response to decreased platelet survival times as occurs in immune-mediated disorders and microvascular angiopathies (84).

Lymphoid and Natural Killer Cells

The bone marrow is the site of origin of B, T, and natural killer (NK) precursor cells from progeny of the hematopoietic stem cells that give rise to both hematopoietic and lymphoid lineages (100). While immature T cells migrate to the thymus for maturation, the bone marrow is the site of B-cell development (107,108).

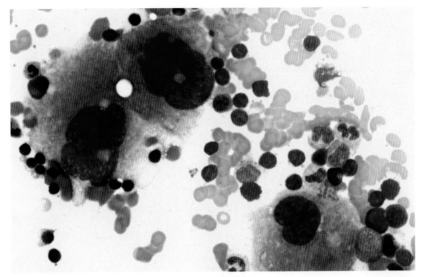

Figure 1-59
STAGES OF MEGAKARYOCYTE MATURATION

Several megakaryocytes at various stages of maturation are evident in this bone marrow aspirate smear (Wright stain).

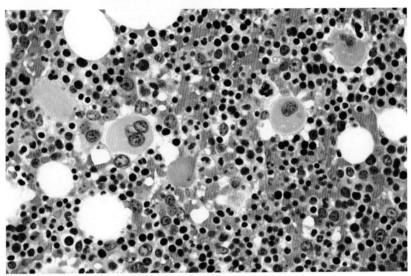

Figure 1-60
MEGAKARYOCYTES IN CLOT SECTION

Megakaryocytes are individually dispersed in this bone marrow clot section (H&E stain).

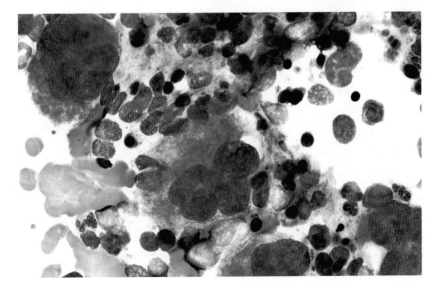

Figure 1-61
MEGAKARYOCYTES WITHIN BONE MARROW PARTICLES

Megakaryocytes are concentrated within bone marrow particles in this case of megakaryocytic hyperplasia (bone marrow aspirate; Wright stain).

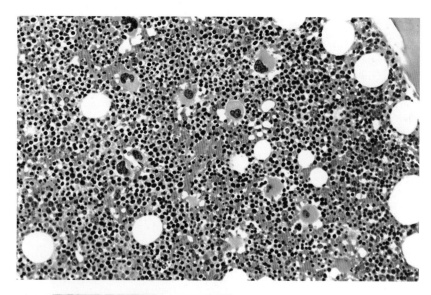

Figure 1-62
MEGAKARYOCYTES
IN CORE BIOPSY

This bone marrow core biopsy shows individually distributed megakaryocytes. Although megakaryocytes reside adjacent to bone marrow sinuses, this is often not readily apparent on core biopsy sections (H&E stain).

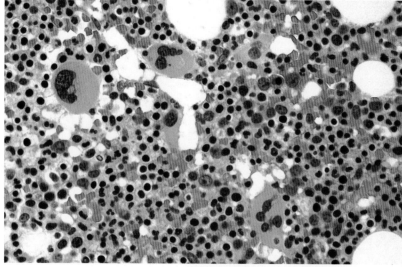

Figure 1-63
PERISINUSOIDAL
MEGAKARYOCYTES

Perisinusoidal and intrasinusoidal localization of megakaryocytes is evident in this bone marrow biopsy from an adult patient (H&E stain).

Figure 1-64
PERISINUSOIDAL
MEGAKARYOCYTES

Perisinusoidal localization of megakaryocytes is highlighted at high magnification of this bone marrow core biopsy section (H&E stain).

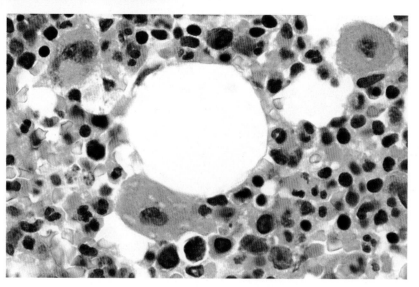

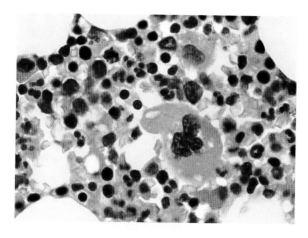

Figure 1-65

PROJECTION OF MEGAKARYOCYTE CYTOPLASM INTO SINUS

The megakaryocyte cytoplasm projects into the sinus lumen in this bone marrow core biopsy section from an adult patient. Platelets shed directly from this cytoplasmic projection into the circulation (H&E stain).

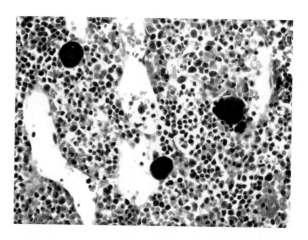

Figure 1-66

IMMUNOHISTOCHEMICAL STAIN FOR CD42B

Perisinusoidal localization of megakaryocytes is highlighted by immunoperoxidase stain for CD42b (bone marrow core biopsy).

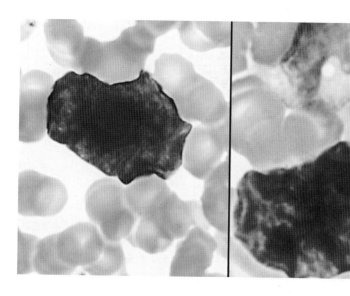

Figure 1-67

MEGAKARYOCYTE NUCLEI IN BLOOD

This composite shows circulating mature megakaryocyte nuclei, a finding that is typical in newborns but can be seen in patients of all ages (peripheral blood; Wright stain).

Plasma cells are derived from terminally differentiated B cells (109). In adults, mature B, T, and NK cells circulate in the blood, while more immature-appearing lymphoid cells may be evident on blood smears from infants and young children (fig. 1-68).

Aside from plasma cells, the lineage and stage of maturation of lymphoid cells within the bone marrow are optimally determined by immunophenotypic and molecular techniques (figs. 1-69–1-71) (101). Immature benign B lymphoid cells, termed hematogones, may be abundant in specimens from pediatric patients. These benign B-cell precursors are the predominant lymphoid population in bone marrow specimens from preterm neonates (106). Hematogones exhibit distinctive morphologic and immunophenotypic features (figs. 1-72–1-74). The nuclear chromatin is highly condensed in contrast to the finely dispersed chromatin of a typical blast. By flow cytometric immunophenotyping, a spectrum of maturation from immature to mature B cells is typical in bone marrow specimens containing abundant hematogones (see chapter 8) (103).

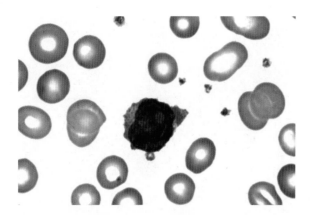

Figure 1-68
IMMATURE LYMPHOID CELL IN BLOOD

An immature lymphoid cell with dispersed chromatin and an irregular nuclear configuration is evident in the peripheral blood of a normal infant (Wright stain).

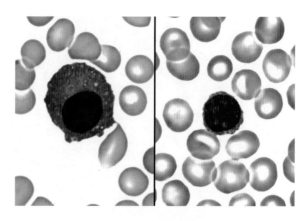

Figure 1-69
PLASMA CELL AND LYMPHOCYTE

A normal plasma cell (left) is compared to a normal mature lymphocyte (right) (bone marrow aspirate, left; peripheral blood, right; Wright stain).

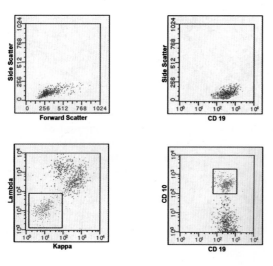

Figure 1-70
FLOW CYTOMETRY OF LYMPHOCYTES

By gating the lymphocyte population by forward and side scatter properties, an admixture of mature polyclonal B cells and surface immunoglobulin-negative, CD10-positive hematogones is evident in a normal bone marrow aspirate (multicolor flow cytometry).

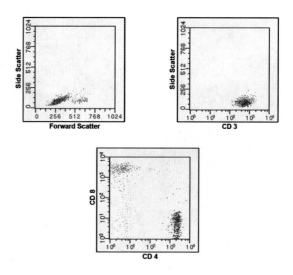

Figure 1-71
FLOW CYTOMETRY OF LYMPHOCYTES

By gating the lymphocyte population by forward and side scatter properties, normal helper (CD4) and cytotoxic/suppressor (CD8) populations of CD3-positive T cells are identified in normal bone marrow (multicolor flow cytometry).

Except in specimens with abundant hematogones, T cells predominate in normal bone marrow and exhibit a patchy, partially perivascular distribution (fig. 1-75). Mature B cells are less numerous than T cells and are randomly distributed and dispersed, individually or in small clusters (figs. 1-76, 1-77).

Mature plasma cells have distinctive morphologic features that include eccentric nuclei with a "clockface" chromatin pattern, a prominent paranuclear hof, and abundant basophilic cytoplasm that may contain immunoglobulin vacuoles (fig. 1-78). Plasma cells are infrequent in bone marrow, comprising less than 5 percent of the total cells; the relative proportion of both plasma cells and lymphocytes is substantially increased in conditions with reduced hematopoietic elements, while absolute increases in plasma

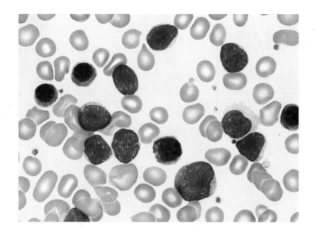

Figure 1-72
BONE MARROW HEMATOGONES

Numerous benign lymphoid cells with homogeneous condensed nuclear chromatin (hematogones) are evident in this bone marrow aspirate smear from a young child (Wright stain).

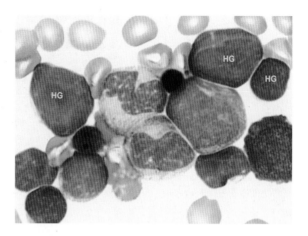

Figure 1-73
BONE MARROW HEMATOGONES

Nuclei of hematogones are medium sized to large, have homogeneous condensed chromatin, and range from round to irregular (top right) (Wright stain).

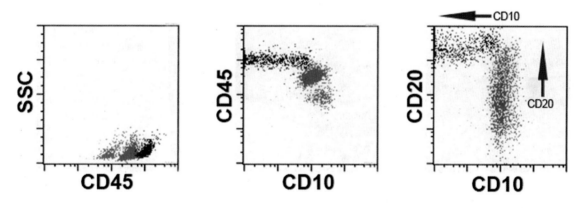

Figure 1-74
FLOW CYTOMETRY OF HEMATOGONES

Multicolor flow cytometry highlights the progressive maturation of hematogones as reflected by a spectrum of CD45, CD10, and CD20 expression consistent with ongoing maturation.

cells occur in infectious and inflammatory conditions (fig. 1-79). On core biopsy sections, normal plasma cells exhibit a propensity for a perivascular localization, which can be highlighted by immunohistochemical staining for CD138 (figs. 1-80, 1-81). Benign plasma cells have a polytypic kappa to lambda light chain ratio (102).

The least frequent lymphoid cell in blood and bone marrow is the true NK cell, initially recognized by its functional properties and subsequently defined by its immunophenotypic profile (98,105). True NK cells are surface CD3-negative, CD56-positive, CD16-positive lymphoid cells and are critical components of the innate immune system because they produce immunoregulatory cytokines. True NK cells also mediate cytotoxicity against target cells that lack matching major histocompatibility complex (MHC) ligands (98,104,110). Cells exhibiting this immunophenotypic and functional profile have the morphologic characteristics of large granular lymphocytes, although cytotoxic T cells (surface CD3 and CD8 positive) also share this morphology (fig. 1-82).

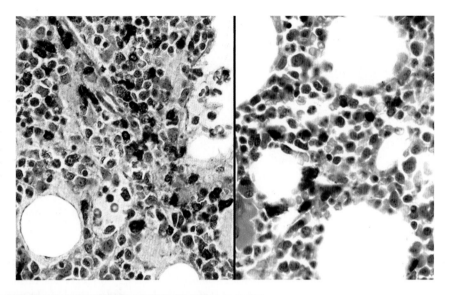

Figure 1-75

IMMUNOHISTOCHEMICAL STAIN FOR CD3

The perivascular (left) and patchy interstitial (right) distribution of T cells is evident on the bone marrow core biopsy from an adult.

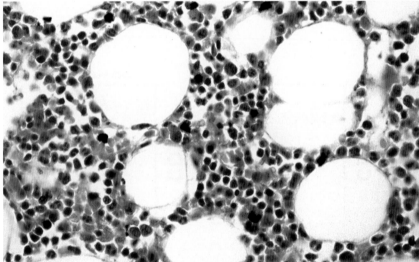

Figure 1-76

IMMUNOHISTOCHEMICAL STAIN FOR CD20

Scant, dispersed individual B cells are evident in this bone marrow core biopsy specimen from a young adult.

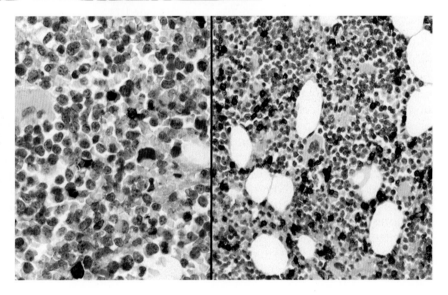

Figure 1-77

IMMUNOHISTOCHEMICAL STAIN FOR CD3 AND CD20

This composite of a bone marrow clot section from a premature infant with increased hematogones shows a side-by-side comparison of the number of CD3-positive T cells (left) and the number of CD20-positive B cells (right). Because of the increased numbers of hematogones, B cells are more numerous than T cells (immunoperoxidase stain for CD3 and CD20). (Courtesy of Dr. L. Rimsza, Tuscon, AZ.)

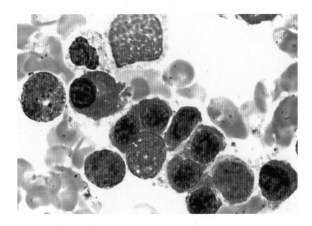

Figure 1-78
PLASMA CELL AND ERYTHROID CELLS

A plasma cell with an eccentric round nucleus, "clockface" chromatin, and abundant basophilic cytoplasm with a paranuclear hof (top) is adjacent to erythroid cells (Wright stain).

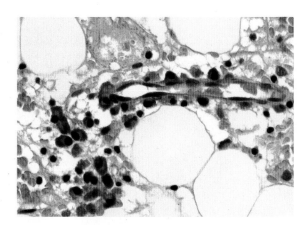

Figure 1-79
PERIVASCULAR PLASMA CELLS

A hypocellular bone marrow aspirate shows a relative increase in plasma cells (H&E stain).

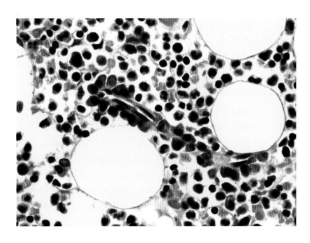

Figure 1-80
PERIVASCULAR PLASMA CELLS

The perivascular distribution of the plasma cells is highlighted (bone marrow core biopsy; H&E stain).

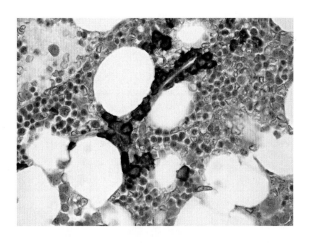

Figure 1-81
IMMUNOHISTOCHEMICAL STAIN FOR CD138

CD138 highlights perivascular plasma cells (bone marrow core biopsy).

The cytoplasmic granules of large granular lymphocytes (either true NK or cytotoxic T cells) contain perforin and granzymes; these granules can be highlighted immunohistochemically with antibodies directed against granzyme and T-cell intracellular antigen 1 (TIA-1) (fig. 1-83). The release of perforin and granzyme is a major mechanism by which pathogen-containing cells or tumor cells are killed (99). Increased numbers of NK cells may be evident in the blood and bone marrow during acute infectious processes, notably viral infections, as well as in response to inflammatory conditions or neoplasms (see chapter 8). In general, however, NK cells with a large granular lymphocyte morphology are inconspicuous in both bone marrow aspirate and core biopsy specimens. Immunophenotypic assessment is the optimal modality to delineate this lineage in bone marrow, and either flow cytometric immunophenotyping or immunohistochemical assessment can be utilized (fig. 1-84).

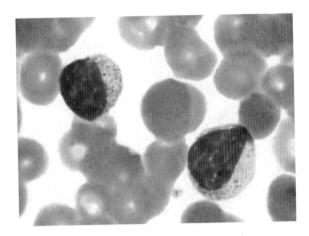

Figure 1-82
LARGE GRANULAR LYMPHOCYTES

True natural killer cells with the morphologic features of large granular lymphocytes are evident in this peripheral blood smear. The lineage was confirmed by flow cytometry (Wright stain).

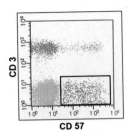
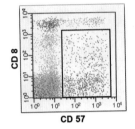
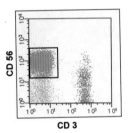

Figure 1-84
FLOW CYTOMETRY OF NATURAL KILLER CELLS

True natural killer cells (boxes) can be delineated by multicolor flow cytometry. These cells typically express CD56 but are negative for CD3, while cytotoxic/suppressor T cells are typically CD3, CD57, and CD8 positive.

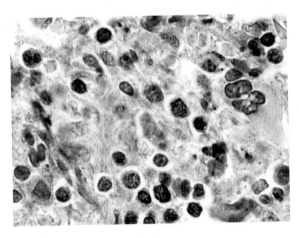

Figure 1-83
IMMUNOHISTOCHEMICAL STAIN FOR TIA-1

The TIA-1 immunohistochemical stain highlights cytoplasmic granules in a bone marrow core biopsy with increased large granular lymphocytes.

Bone

Bone is essential for the support of hematopoiesis. Dense cortical bone provides the outer support and structure for all bones containing a medullary cavity. This cavity is traversed by a network of fine trabecular bone, which provides the framework for the vascular and stromal meshwork that constitutes the bone marrow microenvironment (fig. 1-85). Three cell types are associated with bony trabeculae: osteoblasts, osteoclasts, and osteocytes.

Age-related variations in bony trabeculae are prominent. In neonates and young infants, ossification of bony trabeculae is often incomplete, while in older children and adults, bony trabeculae are normally well ossified (figs. 1-86–1-89). In children, these intramedullary bony trabeculae show active bone remodeling and are lined by osteoblasts with intermittent osteoclasts (figs. 1-90–1-93). In normal bone remodeling, bone resorption by osteoclasts is coordinated with bone formation by osteoblasts. Osteoblasts assemble to form new bone in the lacunar spaces vacated by osteoclasts, a process called coupling (111). In contrast, bone marrow specimens from elderly patients do not show evidence of active remodeling and, in fact, often show thinning of the bony trabeculae, which may be linked to declining hematopoietic cellularity.

Osteoblasts are stromal-derived cells which produce the bony substrate. Recent evidence suggests that osteoblasts play a major role in both hematopoietic stem cell localization to the endosteum of bony trabeculae and in the regulation of early hematopoiesis (see earlier

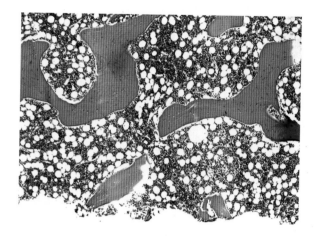

Figure 1-85
BONY TRABECULAE, 16-YEAR-OLD MALE

Normal bony trabeculae from 16-year-old male (bone marrow core biopsy; H&E stain).

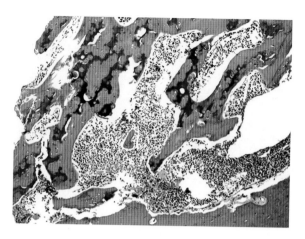

Figure 1-86
BONY TRABECULAE, NEWBORN

Bone marrow from a newborn shows incomplete ossification of bony trabeculae (H&E stain).

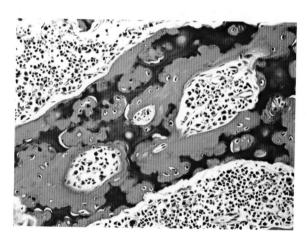

Figure 1-87
BONY TRABECULAE, NEWBORN

High-power view of bony trabeculae from a newborn bone marrow shows irregular areas of incomplete ossification, which is physiologic for this age (H&E stain).

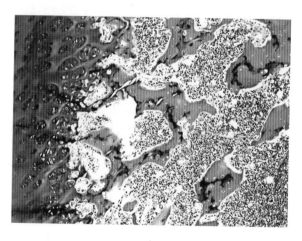

Figure 1-88
BONY TRABECULAE, 21-MONTH-OLD CHILD

Progressive, yet incomplete, maturation of bony trabeculae is evident in a bone marrow core biopsy from 21-month-old child (H&E stain).

section) (112,119,121). In addition, circulating osteoblast-lineage cells have been noted in normal control subjects; these circulating osteoblast-lineage cells are much more abundant during physiologic prepubertal growth (113).

Osteoclasts resorb bone and are derived from a common monocytic/macrophage/dendritic progenitor cell (114–117). Two essential cytokines are linked to osteoclastogenesis: M-CSF and RANKL (receptor activator of nuclear factor–kappa B ligand), which is also called TRANCE (tumor-necrosis factor-related activa-tion-induced cytokine) (115,117,120). Both human and murine studies indicate that immature dendritic cells (mouse) or blood monocytic cells (human) differentiate into osteoclasts in the presence of M-CSF and RANKL (115,118,120). Osteoclasts can be identified on both bone marrow aspirate smears and core biopsy sections. These multinucleated cells can be distinguished from megakaryocytes by their round discrete nuclei, coarse cytoplasmic "bone sand" in mature cells, and paratrabecular localization often within scalloped spaces (figs. 1-94, 1-95).

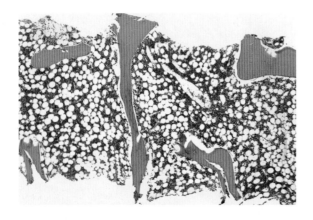

Figure 1-89
BONY TRABECULAE, 43-YEAR-OLD FEMALE
Mature bony trabeculae in a 43-year-old woman (bone marrow core biopsy; H&E stain).

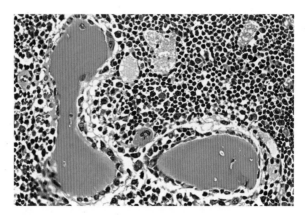

Figure 1-90
BONY TRABECULAE, 9-MONTH-OLD BABY
Osteoblast rimming of bony trabeculae in 9-month-old infant (bone marrow core biopsy; H&E stain).

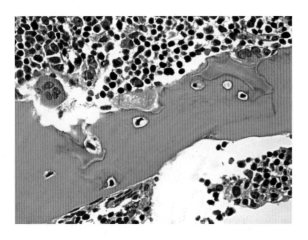

Figure 1-91
**MULTINUCLEATED OSTEOCLAST
ADJACENT TO BONY TRABECULAE**
Multinucleated osteoclasts are within resorption lacunae in normal bony trabeculae from a 9-month-old infant. Osteocytes are within the lacunar spaces (bone marrow core biopsy; H&E stain).

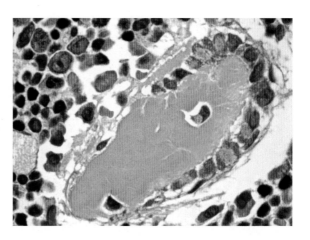

Figure 1-92
OSTEOBLASTS RIMMING BONY TRABECULAE
Individual osteoblasts surround the bony trabeculae in a 9-month-old infant (bone marrow core biopsy; H&E stain).

Osteoblasts have single nuclei and, because these nuclei are markedly eccentric, resemble enlarged plasma cells on bone marrow aspirate and imprint smears. Osteoblasts also contain a cytoplasmic pale area (hof) which, unlike plasma cells, is separated from the nucleus (fig. 1-96). If active bone remodeling is in progress, osteoblasts rim bony trabeculae in a single file. In older patients, osteoblasts and osteoclasts are typically not evident, unless bone remodeling has been initiated by some pathologic process (fig. 1-97).

Osteocytes, like osteoblasts, are stromal cell derived. They reside within the lacunar spaces of bony trabeculae (fig. 1-98). Loss of osteocytes from the lacunar spaces is a feature of necrotic bone (figs. 1-99, 1-100).

AGE-RELATED NORMAL
BONE MARROW HISTOLOGY

The salient age-related variations in bone marrow specimens from normal subjects are highlighted in Table 1-4. In general, bone marrow cellularity declines with age, but there are fairly wide ranges in normal cellularity for each age group.

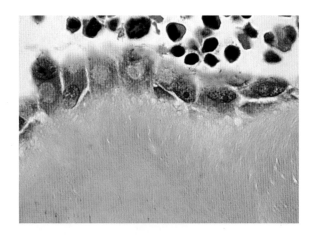

Figure 1-93
OSTEOBLASTS RIMMING BONY TRABECULAE

A prominent cytoplasmic hof is evident in osteoblasts rimming bony trabeculae in 9-month-old infant (bone marrow core biopsy; H&E stain).

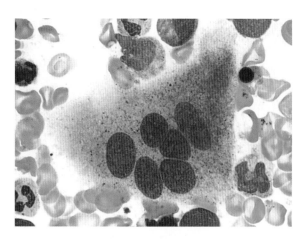

Figure 1-94
OSTEOCLAST

Multinucleated osteoclast with "bone sand" is seen in a bone marrow aspirate.

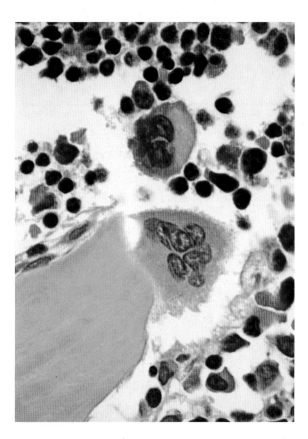

Figure 1-95
OSTEOCLAST AND MEGAKARYOCYTE

An osteoclast (bottom) and a megakaryocyte (top) are compared (bone marrow core biopsy; H&E stain).

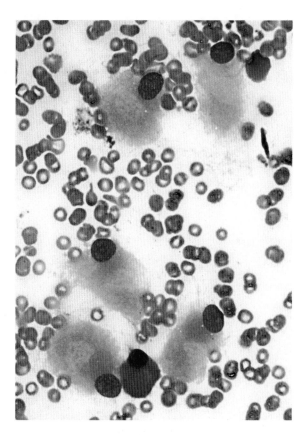

Figure 1-96
OSTEOBLASTS

Multiple osteoblasts with markedly eccentric nuclei are present in a bone marrow aspirate smear. Compare with the nuclear and cytoplasmic features of the plasma cell (bottom center) (Wright stain).

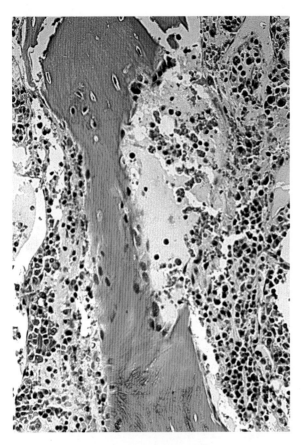

Figure 1-97
PATHOLOGIC BONY CHANGES

Pathologic bone resorption and remodeling are evident in a bone marrow smear from 46-year-old woman (H&E stain).

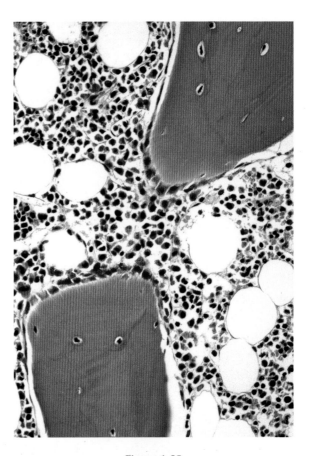

Figure 1-98
OSTEOCYTES WITHIN BONY TRABECULAE

Osteocytes are within normal bony trabeculae in a bone marrow specimen from 13-year-old girl. Note the osteoblast rimming, which is normal for the age of the patient (H&E stain).

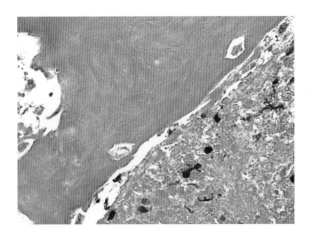

Figure 1-99
NECROTIC BONE

Necrotic bone with loss of osteocytes is present in a massively necrotic core biopsy specimen (H&E stain).

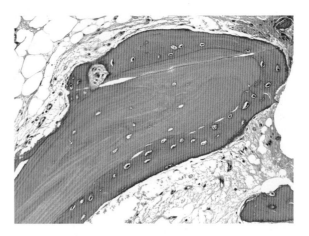

Figure 1-100
NECROTIC BONE

A layer of viable new bone forms over dead bone (H&E stain).

Table 1-4

AGE-RELATED NORMAL HISTOLOGY OF BONE MARROW[a]

Patient Age	Cellularity	Bony Trabeculae	Cellular Composition
Newborn	Up to 100%, but may be lower	Very active bone remodeling and incomplete ossification of cortical bone	Blasts up to 5% Predominance of myeloid cells except in cases in which hematogones are numerous; myeloid to erythroid ratio of ~ 4:1 Lymphoid cells, notably hematogones, may be numerous
Infant	Variable, up to 100%, but may be lower	Very active bone remodeling and incomplete ossification of cortical bone	Blasts up to 5% Predominance of myeloid elements; myeloid to erythroid ratio: ~ 5-10:1 Erythroid elements markedly reduced during physiologic nadir Lymphoid cells, notably hematogones, may be abundant (up to 50% of cells)
Child	60-80%	Active bone remodeling	Blasts up to 5 percent, but usually lower Myeloid elements predominate; myeloid to erythroid ratio: ~ 3:1 Lymphocytes, notably hematogones, may be abundant
Young adult	50-70%	Bone remodeling may be evident, especially in young males	Blasts generally <5% Myeloid elements predominate; myeloid to erythroid ratio: ~ 3:1 Lymphocytes generally inconspicuous, but may range up to 20%
Adult	40-60%	Bone remodeling absent Osteoclasts and osteoblasts inconspicuous Bony trabeculae may be thinned (osteopenic), especially in females	Blasts generally <3% Myeloid elements predominate; myeloid to erythroid ratio: ~ 3-4:1 Lymphocytes usually inconspicuous, but may range up to 20%
Elderly	25-40%	Bone remodeling absent Osteoblasts and osteoclasts inconspicuous Bony trabeculae may be thinned (osteopenic), especially in females	Blasts <3% Myeloid elements predominate; myeloid to erythroid ratio: ~ 3-4:1 Mild dysplastic features may be noted Lymphocytes are generally inconspicuous, but may range up to 20%, especially if hematopoiesis is reduced. Lipogranulomas and lymphoid aggregates may be present

[a]Data from references 122 through 129; see Appendix for additional normal range information.

Significant declines in overall cellularity do not typically occur until old age (figs. 1-101, 1-102) (126,128). Although normal neonates and infants may exhibit 100 percent bone marrow cellularity, it is more often in the range of 80 percent (fig. 1-103) (126). Active bone remodeling is an expected feature in bone marrow specimens from growing patients, while this finding often reflects a pathologic process in adults.

Significant age-related variations in the cellular composition of bone marrow include the prominent lymphocytosis due to hematogones that is typical in infants and young children, the decline in erythropoiesis that characterizes the physiologic nadir in early infancy, and the mild decline in erythropoiesis in elderly patients (122,128,129). Controversy exists as to whether the mild anemia that is common in elderly patients is the result of physiologic factors such as declining bone marrow cellularity and decreased

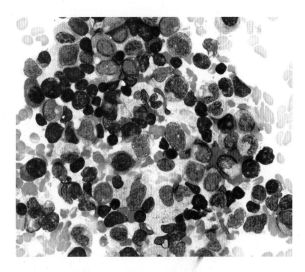

Figure 1-101

BONE MARROW ASPIRATE, 11-MONTH-OLD INFANT

A cellular bone marrow particle without apparent fat from an 11-month-old infant (Wright stain).

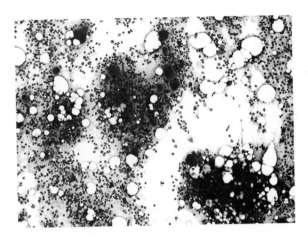

Figure 1-102
BONE MARROW ASPIRATE, ADULT
Bone marrow aspirate smear from an adult shows fat admixed with hematopoietic elements (Wright stain).

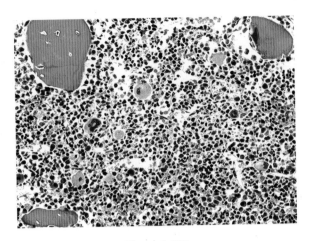

Figure 1-103
BONE MARROW CORE BIOPSY, 1-YEAR-OLD
Bone marrow core biopsy from a 1-year-old shows 100 percent cellularity (H&E stain).

levels of progenitor cells or a pathologic process that has yet to be elucidated (123). Reduced erythropoietin levels have been documented in elderly patients in limited studies (123). Likewise, age-related decreases in neutrophil function, lymphopoiesis, and lymphocyte function have been described (123).

REFERENCES

Fetal Hematopoiesis

1. Giebel B, Corbeil D, Beckmann J, et al. Segregation of lipid raft markers including CD133 in polarized human hematopoietic stem and progenitor cells. Blood 2004;104:2332-8.
2. Hadland BK, Huppert SS, Kanungo J, et al. A requirement for Notch1 distinguishes 2 phases of definitive hematopoiesis during development. Blood 2004;104:3097-105.
3. Kennedy M, D'Souza SL, Lynch-Kattman M, Schwantz S, Keller G. Development of the hemangioblast defines the onset of hematopoiesis in human ES cell differentiation cultures. Blood 2007;109;2679-87.
4. Marshall CJ, Thrasher AJ. The embryonic origins of human haematopoiesis. Br J Haematol 2001;112:838-50.
5. Ohneda O, Ohneda K, Arai F, et al. ALCAM (CD166): its role in hematopoietic and endothelial development. Blood 2001;98:2134-42.
6. Traver D, Miyamoto T, Christensen J, Iwasaki-Arai J, Akashi K, Weissman IL. Fetal liver myelopoiesis occurs through distinct, prospectively isolatable progenitor subsets. Blood 2001;98:627-35.
7. Wilpshaar J, Joekes EC, Lim FT, et al. Magnetic resonance imaging of fetal bone marrow for quantitative definition of the human fetal stem cell compartment. Blood 2002;100:451-7.
8. Zambidis ET, Peault B, Park TS, Bunz F, Civin CI. Hematopoietic differentiation of human embryonic stem cells progresses through sequential hematoendothelial, primitive, and definitive stages resembling human yolk sac development. Blood 2005;106:860-70.

Hematopoiesis: Stem Cells, Microenvironment, and Regulatory Factors

9. Abbas AK, Lichtman AH. Cytokines. In: Cellular and molecular immunology, 5th ed. Philadelphia: WB Saunders; 2003:243-73.
10. Broudy VC. Stem cell factor and hematopoiesis. Blood 1997;90:1345-64.
11. Burger JA, Spoo A, Dwenger A, Burger M, Behringer D. CXCR4 chemokine receptors (CD184) and alpha4beta1 integrins mediate spontaneous migration of human CD34+ progenitors and acute myeloid leukaemia cells beneath marrow stromal cells (pseudoemperipolesis). Br J Haematol 2003;122:579-89.

12. Clarke MF. Chronic myelogenous leukemia—identifying the hydra's heads. N Engl J Med 2004;351:634-6.

12a. Dao MA, Creer MH, Nolta JA, Verfaillie CM. Biology of umbilical cord blood progenitors in bone marrow niches. Blood 2007;110:74-81.

13. Dazzi F, Ramasamy R, Glennie S, Jones SP, Roberts I. The role of mesenchymal stem cells in haemopoiesis. Blood Rev 2006;20:161-71.

14. Fukuda S, Broxmeyer HE, Pelus LM. Flt3 ligand and the Flt3 receptor regulate hematopoietic cell migration by modulating the SDF-1alpha(CXCL12)/CXCR4 axis. Blood 2005;105:3117-26.

15. Furukawa Y, Kikuchi J, Nakamura M, Iwase S, Yamada H, Matsuda M. Lineage-specific regulation of cell cycle control gene expression during haematopoietic cell differentiation. Br J Haematol 2000;110:663-73.

16. Giebel B, Zhang T, Beckmann J, et al. Primitive human hematopoietic cells give rise to differentially specified daughter cells upon their initial cell division. Blood 2006;107:2146-52.

17. Guthridge MA, Barry EF, Felquer FA, et al. The phosphoserine-585-dependent pathway of the GM-CSF/IL-3/IL-5 receptors mediates hematopoietic cell survival through activation of NF-kappaB and induction of bcl-2. Blood 2004;103:820-7.

18. Herzog EL, Chai L, Krause DS. Plasticity of marrow-derived stem cells. Blood 2003;102:3483-93.

19. Iwata M, Awaya N, Graf L, Kahl C, Torok-Storb B. Human marrow stromal cells activate monocytes to secrete osteopontin, which down-regulates Notch1 gene expression in CD34+ cells. Blood 2004;103:4496-502.

20. Jamieson CH, Ailles LE, Dylla SJ, et al. Granulocyte-macrophage progenitors as candidate leukemic stem cells in blast-crisis CML. N Engl J Med 2004;351:657-67.

21. Kucia M, Reca R, Jala VR, Dawn B, Ratajczak J, Ratajczak MZ. Bone marrow as a home of heterogenous populations of nonhematopoietic stem cells. Leukemia 2005;19:1118-27.

22. Lakshmipathy U, Verfaillie C. Stem cell plasticity. Blood Rev 2005;19:29-38.

23. Lapidot T, Dar A, Kollet O. How do stem cells find their way home? Blood 2005;106:1901-10.

24. Laurence AD. Location, movement and survival: the role of chemokines in haematopoiesis and malignancy. Br J Haematol 2006;132:255-67.

25. Majka M, Janowska-Wieczorek A, Ratajczak J, et al. Numerous growth factors, cytokines, and chemokines are secreted by human CD34(+) cells, myeloblasts, erythroblasts, and megakaryoblasts and regulate normal hematopoiesis in an autocrine/paracrine manner. Blood 2001;97:3075-85.

26. Moore KA, Lemischka IR. "Tie-ing" down the hematopoietic niche. Cell 2004;118:139-40.

27. Muller-Sieburg CE, Cho RH, Karlsson L, Huang JF, Sieburg HB. Myeloid-biased hematopoietic stem cells have extensive self-renewal capacity but generate diminished lymphoid progeny with impaired IL-7 responsiveness. Blood 2004;103:4111-8.

28. Muller-Sieburg CE, Cho RH, Thoman M, Adkins B, Sieburg HB. Deterministic regulation of hematopoietic stem cell self-renewal and differentiation. Blood 2002;100:1302-9.

29. Nilsson SK, Johnston HM, Coverdale JA. Spatial localization of transplanted hemopoietic stem cells: inferences for the localization of stem cell niches. Blood 2001;97:2293-9.

30. Nilsson SK, Johnston HM, Whitty GA, et al. Osteopontin, a key component of the hematopoietic stem cell niche and regulator of primitive hematopoietic progenitor cells. Blood 2005;106:1232-9.

31. Skubitz K. Neutrophilic leukocytes. In: Greer JP, Foerster J, Lukens J, et al., eds. Wintrobe's clinical hematology, 11th ed. Philadelphia: Lippincott Williams & Wilkins; 2004:267-310.

32. Slater NJ, Yamaguchi M, Rothwell DG, Baker P, Heyworth CM, Chopra R. The human granulocyte/macrophage colony-stimulating factor receptor alpha2 isoform influences haemopoietic lineage commitment and divergence. Br J Haematol 2003;122:150-8.

33. Taichman RS. Blood and bone: two tissues whose fates are intertwined to create the hematopoietic stem-cell niche. Blood 2005;105:2631-9.

34. Thomas D, Vadas M, Lopez A. Regulation of haematopoiesis by growth factors—emerging insights and therapies. Expert Opin Biol Ther 2004;4:869-79.

35. Whiting KA, McGuckin CP, Wertheim D, Pearce D, Pettengell R. Three-dimensional analysis of CD34 sialomucin distribution on cord blood and bone marrow. Br J Haematol 2003;122:771-7.

36. Wilson A, Trumpp A. Bone-marrow haematopoietic-stem-cell niches. Nat Rev Immunol 2006;6:93-106.

Granulocytic, Monocytic, and Dendritic Cells

37. Befus A, Denburg J. Basophilic leukocytes: mast cells and basophils. In: Greer JP, Foerster J, Lukens J, et al, eds. Wintrobe's clinical hematology, 11th ed. Philadelphia: Lippincott Williams & Wilkins; 2004:335-48.

38. Bjerregaard MD, Jurlander J, Klausen P, Borregaard N, Cowland JB. The in vivo profile of transcription factors during neutrophil differentiation in human bone marrow. Blood 2003;101:4322-32.

39. Borregaard N, Sehested M, Nielsen BS, Sengelov H, Kjedsen L. Biosynthesis of granule proteins in normal human bone marrow cells. Gelatinase is a marker of terminal neutrophil differentiation. Blood 1995;85:812-7.

40. Burdon PC, Martin C, Rankin SM. The CXC chemokine MIP-2 stimulates neutrophil mobilization from the rat bone marrow in a CD49d-dependent manner. Blood 2005;105:2543-48.

41. Chang CC, Eshoa C, Kampalath B, Shidham VB, Perkins S. Immunophenotypic profile of myeloid cells in granulocytic sarcoma by immunohistochemistry. Correlation with blast differentiation in bone marrow. Am J Clin Pathol 2000;114:807-11.

42. de Bruijn MF, Speck NA. Core-binding factors in hematopoiesis and immune function. Oncogene 2004;23:4238-48.

43. Ebihara Y, Xu MJ, Manabe A, et al. Exclusive expression of G-CSF receptor on myeloid progenitors in bone marrow CD34+ cells. Br J Haematol 2000;109:153-61.

44. Escribano L, Ocqueteau M, Almeida J, Orfao A, San Miguel JF. Expression of the c-kit (CD117) molecule in normal and malignant hematopoiesis. Leuk Lymphoma 1998;30:459-66.

45. Falcone FH, Haas H, Gibbs BF. The human basophil: a new appreciation of its role in immune responses. Blood 2000;96:4028-38.

46. Gullberg U, Andersson E, Garwicz D, Lindmark A, Olsson I. Biosynthesis, processing and sorting of neutrophil proteins: insight into neutrophil granule development. Eur J Haematol 1997;58:137-53.

47. Haller Hasskamp J, Zapas JL, Elias EG. Dendritic cell counts in the peripheral blood of healthy adults. Am J Hematol 2005;78:314-5.

48. Hartman M, Piliponsky AM, Temkin V, Levi-Schaffer F. Human peripheral blood eosinophils express stem cell factor. Blood 2001;97:1086-91.

49. Hashimoto S, Suzuki T, Dong HY, Yamazaki N, Matsushima K. Serial analysis of gene expression in human monocytes and macrophages. Blood 1999;94:837-44.

49a. Jacobsen LC, Theilgaard-Monch K, Christensen EI, Borregaard N. Arginase 1 is expressed in myelocytes/metamyelocytes and localized in gelatinase granules of human neutrophils. Blood 2007;109:3084-7.

50. Kierszenbaum AL. Blood and hematopoiesis. In: Histology and cell biology: an introduction to pathology. Philadelphia: Mosby; 2002:147-75.

51. Lacy P, Becker A, Moqbel R. The human eosinophil. In: Greer JP, Foerster J, Lukens J, et al, eds. Wintrobe's clinical hematology, 11th ed. Philadelphia: Lippincott Williams & Wilkins; 2004:311-33.

52. Lau SK, Chu PG, Weiss LM. CD163: a specific marker of macrophages in paraffin-embedded tissue samples. Am J Clin Pathol 2004;122:794-801.

53. Li WV, Kapadia SB, Sonmez-Alpan E, et al. Immunohistochemical characterization of mast cell disease in paraffin sections using tryptase, CD68, myeloperoxidase, lysozyme, and CD20 antibodies. Mod Pathol 1996;9:982-8.

54. Lian Z, Wang L, Yamaga S, et al. Genomic and proteomic analysis of the myeloid differentiation program. Blood 2001;98:513-24.

55. Lipscomb MF, Masten BJ. Dendritic cells: immune regulators in health and disease. Physiol Rev 2002;82:97-130.

56. MacDonald KP, Munster DJ, Clark GJ, Dzionek A, Schmitz J, Hart DN. Characterization of human blood dendritic cell subsets. Blood 2002;100:4512-20.

57. Manz MG, Traver D, Miyamoto T, et al. Dendritic cell potentials of early lymphoid and myeloid progenitors. Blood 2001;97:3333-41.

58. Menasce LP, Banerjee SS, Beckett E, Harris M. Extra-medullary myeloid tumour (granulocytic sarcoma) is often misdiagnosed: a study of 26 cases. Histopathology 1999;34:391-8.

59. Nakajima H, Ihle JN. Granulocyte colony-stimulating factor regulates myeloid differentiation through CCAAT/enhancer-binding protein epsilon. Blood 2001;98:897-905.

60. Shelburne CP, McCoy ME, Piekorz R, et al. Stat5 expression is critical for mast cell development and survival. Blood 2003;102:1290-7.

61. Sievers EL, Dale DC. Non-malignant neutropenia. Blood Rev 1996;10:95-100.

62. Skubitz K. Neutrophilic leukocytes. In: Greer JP, Foerster J, Lukens J, et al, eds. Wintrobe's clinical hematology, 11th ed. Philadelphia: Lippincott Williams & Wilkins; 2004:267-310.

63. Sun CM, Fiette L, Tanguy M, Leclerc C, Lo-Man R. Ontogeny and innate properties of neonatal dendritic cells. Blood 2003;102:585-91.

64. Theilgaard-Monch K, Jacobsen LC, Borup R, et al. The transcriptional program of terminal granulocytic differentiation. Blood 2005;105:1785-96.

65. Ward AC, Loeb DM, Soede-Bobok AA, Touw TP, Friedman AD. Regulation of granulopoiesis by transcription factors and cytokine signals. Leukemia 2000;14:973-90.

66. Weinberg J. Mononuclear phagocytes. In: Greer JP, Foerster J, Lukens J, et al, eds. Wintrobe's clinical hematology, 11th ed. Philadelphia: Lippincott Williams & Wilkins; 2004:349-86.

67. Wilson HL, O'Neill HC. Identification of differentially expressed genes representing dendritic cell precursors and their progeny. Blood 2003;102:1661-9.

68. Zhu J, Emerson SG. Hematopoietic cytokines, transcription factors and lineage commitment. Oncogene 2002;21:3295-313.

Erythroid Cells

69. Back J, Dierich A, Bronn C, Kastner P, Chan S. PU.1 determines the self-renewal capacity of erythroid progenitor cells. Blood 2004;103:3615-23.

70. Debili N, Coulombel L, Croisille L, et al. Characterization of a bipotent erythro-megakaryocytic progenitor in human bone marrow. Blood 1996;88:1284-96.

70a. Fabriek BO, Polfliet MM, Vloet RP, et al. The macrophage CD163 surface glycoprotein is an erythroblast adhesion receptor. Blood 2007;109:5223-9.

71. Fujiwara Y, Chang AN, Williams AM, Orkin SH. Functional overlap of GATA-1 and GATA-2 in primitive hematopoietic development. Blood 2004;103:583-5.

72. Gabrilove J. Overview: erythropoiesis, anemia, and the impact of erythropoietin. Semin Hematol 2000;37(Suppl 6):1-3.

73. Lee JC, Gimm JA, Lo AJ, et al. Mechanism of protein sorting during erythroblast enucleation: role of cytoskeletal connectivity. Blood 2004;103:1912-9.

74. Liu W, Wang M, Tang DC, Ding I, Rodgers GP. Thrombopoietin has a differentiative effect on late-stage human erythropoiesis. Br J Haematol 1999;105:459-69.

75. Nilsson SK, Johnston HM, Coverdale JA. Spatial localization of transplanted hemopoietic stem cells: inferences for the localization of stem cell niches. Blood 2001;97:2293-9.

76. Suzuki N, Suwabe N, Ohneda O, et al. Identification and characterization of 2 types of erythroid progenitors that express GATA-1 at distinct levels. Blood 2003;102:3575-83.

77. Testa U. Apoptotic mechanisms in the control of erythropoiesis. Leukemia 2004;18:1176-99.

78. Tordjman R, Delaire S, Plouet J, et al. Erythroblasts are a source of angiogenic factors. Blood 2001;97:1968-74.

79. Vannucchi AM, Paoletti F, Linari S, et al. Identification and characterization of a bipotent (erythroid and megakaryocytic) cell precursor from the spleen of phenylhydrazine-treated mice. Blood 2000;95:2559-68.

80. Welch JJ, Watts JA, Vakoc CR, et al. Global regulation of erythroid gene expression by transcription factor GATA-1. Blood 2004;104:3136-47.

81. Zhao W, Kitidis C, Fleming MD, Lodish HF, Ghoffari S. Erythropoietin stimulates phosphorylation and activation of GATA-1 via the PI3-kinase/AKT signaling pathway. Blood 2006;107:907-15.

Megakaryoctyes

82. Casella I, Feccia T, Chelucci C, et al. Autocrine-paracrine VEGF loops potentiate the maturation of megakaryocytic precursors through Flt1 receptor. Blood 2003;101:1316-23.

83. De Botton S, Sabri S, Daugas E, et al. Platelet formation is the consequence of caspase activation within megakaryocytes. Blood 2002;100:1310-7.

84. Drachman JG. Inherited thrombocytopenia: when a low platelet count does not mean ITP. Blood 2004;103:390-8.

85. Elagib KE, Racke FK, Mogass M, Khetawat R, Delehanty LL, Goldfarb AN. RUNX1 and GATA-1 coexpression and cooperation in megakaryocytic differentiation. Blood 2003;101:4333-41.

86. Foucar K. Reactive and neoplastic disorders of megakaryocytes. In: Bone marrow pathology. Chicago: ASCP Press; 2001:324-43.

87. Geddis AE, Kaushansky K. Megakaryocytes express functional Aurora-B kinase in endomitosis. Blood 2004;104:1017-24.

88. Kirito K, Fox N, Kaushansky K. Thrombopoietin stimulates Hoxb4 expression: an explanation for the favorable effects of TPO on hematopoietic stem cells. Blood 2003;102:3172-8.

89. Kirito K, Osawa M, Morita H, et al. A functional role of Stat3 in in vivo megakaryopoiesis. Blood 2002;99:3220-7.

90. Long MW. Megakaryocyte differentiation events. Semin Hematol 1998;35:192-9.

91. Lorsbach RB. Megakaryoblastic disorders in children. Am J Clin Pathol 2004;122(Suppl):S33-46.

91a. Muntean AG, Pang L, Poncz M, Dowdy SF, Blobel GA, Crispino JD. Cyclin D–Cdk4 is regulated by GATA-1 and required for megakaryocyte growth and polyploidization. Blood 2007;109:5199-207.

92. Nilsson SK, Johnston HM, Coverdale JA. Spatial localization of transplanted hemopoietic stem cells: inferences for the localization of stem cell niches. Blood 2001;97:2293-9.

93. Patel SR, Richardson JL, Schulze H, et al. Differential roles of microtubule assembly and sliding in proplatelet formation by megakaryocytes. Blood 2005;106:4076-85.

94. Raslova H, Baccini V, Loussaief L, et al. Mammalian target of rapamycin (mTOR) regulates both proliferation of megakaryocyte progenitors and late stages of megakaryocyte differentiation. Blood 2006;107:2303-10.

95. Raslova H, Roy L, Vourc'h C, et al. Megakaryocyte polyploidization is associated with a functional gene amplification. Blood 2003;101:541-4.

96. Sato T, Ono M, Fujita H, et al. Development of a liquid culture system for megakaryocyte terminal differentiation: fibrinogen promotes megakaryocytopoiesis but not thrombopoiesis. Br J Haematol 2003;121:315-23.

97. Zhang Y, Nagata Y, Yu G, et al. Aberrant quantity and localization of Aurora-B/AIM-1 and survivin during megakaryocyte polyploidization and the consequences of Aurora-B/AIM-1-deregulated expression. Blood 2004;103:3717-26.

Lymphoid and Natural Killer Cells

98. Farag SS, Caligiuri MA. Human natural killer cell development and biology. Blood Rev 2006;20:123-37.

99. Grossman WJ, Verbsky JW, Tollefsen BL, Kemper C, Atkinson JP, Ley TJ. Differential expression of granzymes A and B in human cytotoxic lymphocyte subsets and T regulatory cells. Blood 2004;104:2840-8.

100. Haddad R, Guardiola P, Izac B, et al. Molecular characterization of early human T/NK and B-lymphoid progenitor cells in umbilical cord blood. Blood 2004;104:3918-26.

101. Lucio P, Parreira A, van den Beemd MW, et al. Flow cytometric analysis of normal B cell differentiation: a frame of reference for the detection of minimal residual disease in precursor-B-ALL. Leukemia 1999;13:419-27.

102. Markey GM, Connolly N, Morris TC, Kettle P, Foster H. Plasma cell subtypes in bone marrow biopsies from patients without plasma cell dyscrasia. Br J Haematol 2001;114:958-9.

103. McKenna RW, Washington LT, Aquino DB, Picker LJ, Kroft SH. Immunophenotypic analysis of hematogones (B-lymphocyte precursors) in 662 consecutive bone marrow specimens by 4-color flow cytometry. Blood 2001;98:2498-507.

104. Mirandola P, Ponti C, Gobbi G, et al. Activated human NK and CD8+ T cells express both TNF-related apoptosis-inducing ligand (TRAIL) and TRAIL receptors but are resistant to TRAIL-mediated cytotoxicity. Blood 2004;104:2418-24.

105. Perez SA, Sotiropoulou PA, Gkika DG, et al. A novel myeloid-like NK cell progenitor in human umbilical cord blood. Blood 2003;101:3444-50.

106. Rimsza LM, Douglas VK, Tighe P, et al. Benign B-cell precursors (hematogones) are the predominant lymphoid population in the bone marrow of preterm infants. Biol Neonate 2004;86:247-53.

107. Rossi MI, Yokota T, Medina KL, et al. B lymphopoiesis is active throughout human life, but there are developmental age-related changes. Blood 2003;101:576-84.

108. Schonland SO, Zimmer JK, Lopez-Benitez CM, et al. Homeostatic control of T-cell generation in neonates. Blood 2003;102:1428-34.

109. Tarte K, Zhan F, De Vos J, Klein B, Shaughnessy J Jr. Gene expression profiling of plasma cells and plasmablasts: toward a better understanding of the late stages of B-cell differentiation. Blood 2003;102:592-600.

110. Trotta R, Parihar R, Yu J, et al. Differential expression of SHIP1 in CD56bright and CD56dim NK cells provides a molecular basis for distinct functional responses to monokine costimulation. Blood 2005;105:3011-8.

Bone

111. Canalis E. The fate of circulating osteoblasts. N Engl J Med 2005;352:2014-6.

112. Dazzi F, Ramasamy R, Glennie S, Jones SP, Roberts I. The role of mesenchymal stem cells in haemopoiesis. Blood Rev 2006;20:161-71.

113. Eghbali-Fatourechi GZ, Lamsam J, Fraser D, Nagel D, Riggs BL, Khosla S. Circulating osteoblast-lineage cells in humans. N Engl J Med 2005;352:1959-66.

114. Lean JM, Fuller K, Chambers TJ. FLT3 ligand can substitute for macrophage colony-stimulating factor in support of osteoclast differentiation and function. Blood 2001;98:2707-13.

115. Lee J, Kim K, Kim JH, et al. Id helix-loop-helix proteins negatively regulate TRANCE-mediated osteoclast differentiation. Blood 2006;107:2686-93.

116. Massey HM, Flanagan AM. Human osteoclasts derive from CD14-positive monocytes. Br J Haematol 1999;106:167-70.

117. Miyamoto T, Ohneda O, Arai F, et al. Bifurcation of osteoclasts and dendritic cells from common progenitors. Blood 2001;98:2544-54.

118. Rivollier A, Mazzorana M, Tebib J, et al. Immature dendritic cell transdifferentiation into osteoclasts: a novel pathway sustained by the rheumatoid arthritis microenvironment. Blood 2004;104:4029-37.

119. Taichman RS. Blood and bone: two tissues whose fates are intertwined to create the hematopoietic stem-cell niche. Blood 2005;105:2631-9.

120. Zauli G, Rimondi E, Nicolin V, Melloni E, Celeghini C, Secchiero P. TNF-related apoptosis-inducing ligand (TRAIL) blocks osteoclastic differentiation induced by RANKL plus M-CSF. Blood 2004;104:2044-50.

121. Zhu J, Emerson SG. A new bone to pick: osteoblasts and the haematopoietic stem-cell niche. Bioessays 2004;26:595-9.

Age-Related Normal Bone Marrow Histology

122. Bain BJ. The bone marrow aspirate of healthy subjects. Br J Haematol 1996;94:206-9.

123. Berkahn L, Keating A. Hematopoiesis in the elderly. Hematology 2004;9:159-63.

124. Cotelingam JD. Bone marrow biopsy: interpretive guidelines for the surgical pathologist. Adv Anat Pathol 2003;10:8-26.

125. den Ottolander GJ. The bone marrow aspirate of healthy subjects. Br J Haematol 1996;95:574-5.

126. Friebert SE, Shepardson LB, Shurin SB, Rosenthal GE, Rosenthal NS. Pediatric bone marrow cellularity: are we expecting too much? J Pediatr Hematol Oncol 1998;20:439-43.

127. Girodon F, Favre B, Carli PM, et al. Minor dysplastic changes are frequently observed in the bone marrow aspirate in elderly patients without haematological disease. Clin Lab Haematol 2001;23:297-300.

128. Hartsock RJ, Smith EB, Petty CS. Normal variations with aging of the amount of hematopoietic tissue in bone marrow from the anterior iliac crest. a study made from 177 cases of sudden death examined by necropsy. Am J Clin Pathol 1965;43:326-31.

129. Rosse C, Kraemer MJ, Dillon TL, McFarland R, Smith NJ. Bone marrow cell populations of normal infants; the predominance of lymphocytes. J Lab Clin Med 1977;89:1225-40.

PROCUREMENT AND INTERPRETATION OF THE BONE MARROW SPECIMEN

INDICATIONS FOR BONE MARROW BIOPSY

Examination of the bone marrow is a straightforward if not trivial procedure, very commonly performed in the investigation of both non-neoplastic and neoplastic diseases. Although hematologic disorders most often precipitate bone marrow evaluation, many nonhematologic pathologic processes can also be detected in the bone marrow, or are associated with characteristic bone marrow abnormalities. The ability to readily sample the bone marrow with relatively minimal risk to the patient provides an accessible source for procuring diagnostic biopsy tissue, as well as the means to effectively monitor subsequent disease changes or treatment responses.

The clinical indications for bone marrow sampling are quite broad (Table 2-1), but are based upon some common principles (5,8,10). These most often include the assessment of quantitative bone marrow abnormalities (i.e., alterations in overall production of one or more hematopoietic or lymphoid cell lineages) as evidenced by the presence of peripheral blood cytopenias or cytoses. Similarly, bone marrow biopsy may be sought to address the finding of a qualitative atypia of hematopoietic cell maturation, or to identify abnormal cellular infiltrates and stromal or bone changes. The bone marrow may also be sampled to obtain material for more specific investigations, such as viral and microbial culture studies, cell marker studies (e.g., by flow cytometry), cytogenetic studies, or specialized metabolic or biochemical assays. In many patients with primary bone marrow disorders or certain chronic disease conditions, the bone marrow can be sequentially studied to detect residual disease or possible disease progression. While it is evident that many bone marrow assessments are undertaken to evaluate for primary or secondary (metastatic) malignancies, many are obtained to investigate constitutional or acquired non-neoplastic disorders.

PROCUREMENT, QUALITY CONSIDERATIONS, AND INTERPRETATION OF THE BONE MARROW SPECIMEN

Key Components for Optimal Bone Marrow Assessment

For some benign hematologic disorders, such as iron deficiency anemia, a convincing diagnosis can be established with a complete blood count (CBC), peripheral smear slide morphology, and appropriate laboratory tests, without the requirement for bone marrow sampling. In more complex diagnostic situations (Table 2-1), however, morphologic study of the bone marrow becomes necessary, with the peripheral

---

Table 2-1

INDICATIONS FOR BONE MARROW BIOPSY

Abnormal peripheral blood findings not reconciled by clinical and laboratory investigations (e.g., unexplained cytopenias or cytoses, circulating blast cells, qualitative maturational or distinct cytologic abnormalities of blood cells); distinguish between primary bone marrow production deficit versus increased destruction of circulating blood cell elements

Primary diagnostic evaluation of hematolymphoid neoplasms (e.g., acute leukemias, chronic myeloproliferative disorders, myelodysplasias, non-Hodgkin and Hodgkin lymphomas, myeloma)

Pathologic staging of neoplasms (e.g., non-Hodgkin and Hodgkin lymphomas, sarcomas, carcinomas)

Evaluation of suspected congenital hematologic disorders (e.g., constitutional anemias)

Site for infectious disease assessment (e.g., patients with fever of unknown origin, or those in whom blood or other tissue sampling has been uninformative)

Monitoring of minimal residual disease status following institution of therapy for leukemias, lymphomas, some solid tumors (e.g., sarcomas)

Assessment of bone marrow iron stores and distribution

Evaluation for metabolic storage disorders

Documentation of bone changes suspected by radiologic or biochemical studies; assessment of metabolic bone disorders

blood count and smear review providing critical and complementary information to help define the nature of the bone marrow pathology. The diagnostic morphologist interpreting a bone marrow biopsy should ideally have several components at hand: pertinent clinical, laboratory, and radiologic findings; concurrent CBC results (with white blood cell differential count) and an accompanying peripheral blood smear; bone marrow aspirate slides; biopsy touch imprint preparations; aspirate clot sections; and core (trephine) biopsy sections (1,4,6,8,10).

Biopsy Sites and Potential Procedural Complications

The posterior iliac crest is by far the most common site for obtaining bone marrow tissue. This anatomic location is usually representative of active hematopoiesis, including age-related changes, seen elsewhere in the body. If the iliac crest sites are inaccessible or do not provide diagnostic material, sternal aspiration may be considered by the experienced operator.

In most instances, procurement of bone marrow aspirate and biopsy tissue is straightforward and results in only temporary discomfort at the procedural site; administration of local anesthetic is sufficient, and deep conscious sedation or general anesthesia are not typically required (7,12). Serious complications can occur, however, including excessive local bleeding, hematoma formation, neurologic trauma, or laceration of substernal, intraabdominal, or retroperitoneal tissues (2,3,13). These complications are rare (less than 0.1 percent) and related to technical inexperience or patient-specific factors. Hemorrhagic sequelae can clearly be exacerbated by the presence of a preexisting primary bleeding disorder, anticoagulant use, or underlying hematologic disease. The inability to optimally position or prepare the patient (due to physical disability, local skin infection, or other factors) or the particular character of the patient (e.g., a morbidly obese individual) may create substantial difficulties in establishing correct landmarks for proper bone marrow biopsy and thus increase the risk of adverse events. In such cases, an alternate biopsy site should be considered or the procedure should be performed by an individual with extensive experience in these problematic scenarios. In seemingly intractable situations, the use of computerized tomography (CT)-guided bone marrow biopsy has been proposed to more safely guide bone marrow sampling (9,11).

Sampling and Preparation of Bone Marrow Aspirate and Core Biopsy

The initial aspirate material for morphology can be applied to glass slides by two main methods (17). One technique is the "particle crush" preparation. In this approach, particulate bone marrow is dropped onto the center of one slide and gently overlaid with a second slide, causing the cells to spread out by surface tension forces. The two slides are then quickly and carefully drawn apart and the resultant "crush" preparation on the initial slide is air-dried and stained with Wright-Giemsa or a related hematologic stain (fig. 2-1A). Alternatively, a droplet of particulate bone marrow can be applied to one end of a glass slide, then pushed or spread with another slide in a continuous motion similar to a peripheral blood smear preparation (fig. 2-1B,C). The latter air-dried and stained "direct smear" preparation is illustrated in figure 2-1D.

Particle crush slides are usually excellent for cytologic examination and also provide details of diverse cell types found both in and around the aspirated bone marrow particles. In addition, a general impression of hematopoietic bone marrow cellularity can be obtained from these particles. Some features are obscured in crush preparations due to uneven distribution, cellular disruption, and differential staining effects. In contrast to particle crush preparations, direct smears typically generate a uniform spread of hematopoietic cells, and excess staining or crush artifact is often minimized. Nonetheless, cell types often associated with or near intact particles (e.g., small lymphocytes, mast cells, megakaryocytes) may not be as well represented in a direct smear slide. Ideally, it is preferable to derive information from both types of aspirate preparation.

The bone marrow core or trephine biopsy should be obtained at least 1 cm away from the site of aspiration in order to minimize the presence of aspiration artifact (i.e., the replacement of the intertrabecular bone marrow space by peripheral blood due to core sampling of the aspiration needle track). Although a separate

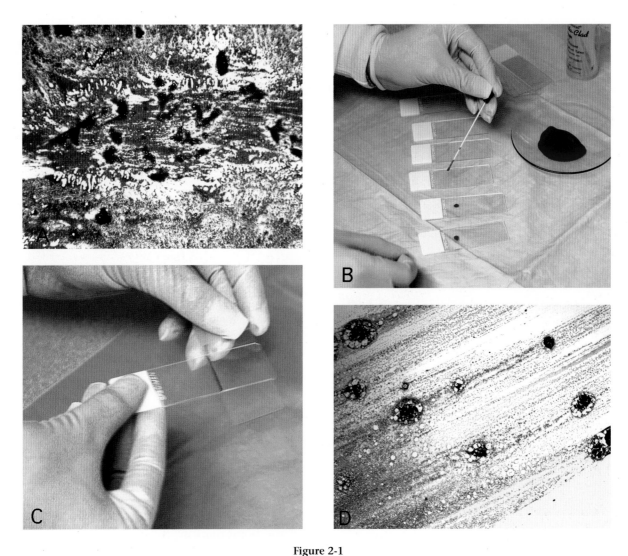

Figure 2-1

PREPARATION OF BONE MARROW ASPIRATE

A: A Wright-Giemsa–stained particle crush slide preparation of a bone marrow aspirate shows the centrally distributed particles and the dense spread of cells between them. Cytologic details are best preserved at the edges of these more densely cellular areas. The particle crush is useful for detailed cytologic examination and enumeration of cellular composition. In addition, certain cellular infiltrates, such as lymphocytes, may be observed surrounding the particles (Wright stain).

B,C: The method used to make a direct (or push) smear preparation of a bone marrow aspirate is illustrated. (Courtesy of Pamela Flores, Albuquerque, NM.)

D: On the stained direct smear slide, the distribution of particles is toward one edge of the slide. Direct smears are useful for obtaining a more even spread of particulate cells for fine cytologic evaluation, and often minimizes crush artifact (bone marrow aspirate; Wright stain).

skin incision is not needed, the operator will need to apply pressure with the trephine biopsy needle to move the skin and soft tissue to a different area over the iliac crest. Alternatively, the core biopsy can be sampled before the bone marrow aspirate is taken, in order to completely obviate the possibility of aspiration artifact. The extracted bone marrow core biopsy appears reddish brown (fig. 2-2, top); an excessive length of gray-white cartilaginous material signifies inadequate sampling of the medullary space.

Immediately following the release of the bone core fragment from the biopsy needle, several air-dried touch preparations (or imprints) of the tissue should be made on glass slides (fig. 2-2, bottom). The core biopsy is then placed in

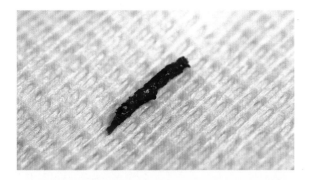

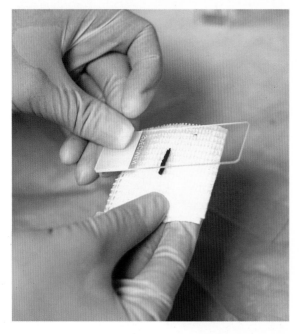

Figure 2-2

**BONE MARROW CORE BIOPSY
AND TOUCH PREPARATION**

Top: An excellent core biopsy extracted from the trephine needle appears reddish brown, indicating the presence of hematopoietic cells. Excessive pale-appearing cartilage or periosteal tissue is not evident.

Bottom: The procedure for making bone marrow biopsy touch preparations or imprints is shown. (Courtesy of Pamela Flores, Albuquerque, NM.)

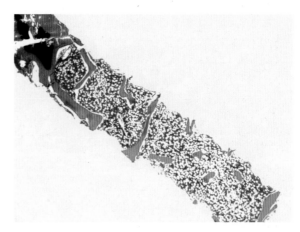

Figure 2-3

BONE MARROW CORE BIOPSY

A decalcified, fixed, hematoxylin and eosin (H&E)-stained thin section of a bone marrow core biopsy is of adequate interpretive length and high quality for complete evaluation. Excessive periosteal tissue or cartilage is not present. Low magnification examination is critical for assessing the biopsy quality, as well as for determining overall cellularity, presence of abnormal infiltrates, and character of the bone trabeculae.

tissue fixative and decalcified prior to routine histologic processing and paraffin embedding. Although mercury-based fixatives, such as B5, are commonly employed, these reagents are now less in favor owing to safety concerns. Alternative methods, including the use of 10 percent zinc formalin (or azide zinc formalin [AZF]), along with rapid microwave tissue processing, can reduce the time and potential toxicity of a bone marrow core biopsy preparation associated with more traditional fixatives (15). For best morphologic interpretation, hematoxylin and eosin (H&E)-stained core biopsy sections should be relatively thin (3 to 4 µm) (fig. 2-3).

In general, unilateral bone marrow core biopsies are usually sufficient to assess most disorders of the bone marrow. Bilateral sampling of the iliac crest sites, in conjunction with step sections of paraffin-embedded biopsies, has been advocated for bone marrow staging (for lymphoma or metastases), in order to increase the likelihood of detecting abnormalities that are typically present in a nonuniform distribution (14).

Adequacy and Quality Considerations

The quality of a bone marrow aspirate is based on the presence of adequate particles containing hematopoietic precursor cells and other cells of interest. The degree of cellular preservation is, therefore, a critical aspect of aspirate smear quality, since an acceptable technical sample with enough particulate bone marrow may be essentially uninterpretable if the manual slide preparation and staining are poor. The skill of the laboratory technologist is paramount in this process. The bone marrow core biopsy should be

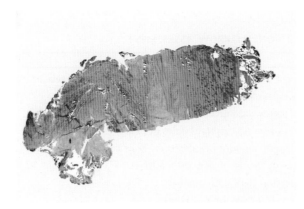

Figure 2-4

INADEQUATE BONE MARROW CORE BIOPSY

A technically poor quality bone marrow core biopsy is illustrated. Although of apparently adequate length, this biopsy is composed of mostly periosteal connective tissue, with only a miniscule amount of hematopoietic marrow at one end (H&E stain).

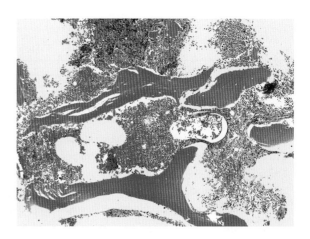

Figure 2-5

BONE MARROW CORE BIOPSY WITH ASPIRATION ARTIFACT

Excessive red blood cell replacement of the intertrabecular bone marrow space renders this specimen uninterpretable. This type of artifact is produced by trephine needle sampling through the area or track of a previous bone marrow aspiration attempt. This problem can be avoided by either placing the core biopsy needle at a site away from the aspiration track or procuring the biopsy prior to the aspiration attempt (H&E stain).

of sufficient length, preferably at least 1 cm, and should not include a substantial proportion of cartilaginous or periosteal connective tissue (fig. 2-4). As indicated, the presence of aspiration artifact (fig. 2-5) can completely obscure core biopsy histology and thus represents another aspect of quality evaluation.

A bone marrow aspiration attempt may result in a "dry tap" or may be excessively diluted by peripheral blood; these respective hypocellular (aparticulate) or hemodilute samples substantially compromise the ability to perform accurate cytomorphologic assessment. Although hemodilute specimens may still be acceptable for certain nonquantitative studies (e.g., cell marker analyses to determine if specific cell types are present or absent), the reviewing diagnostician must rely on features of the core biopsy histology and touch imprint cytology to compensate in part for the lack of a high quality aspirate. The touch imprint is particularly useful in this instance as a substitute for the aspirate (fig. 2-6); however, imprint preparations are often thicker, less uniform, and subject to staining artifacts, with somewhat poorer resolution of cytologic details in contrast to well-made aspirate smears. Cell-poor aspirations are encountered most frequently in the setting of bone marrow fibrosis or at the extremes of bone marrow cellularity (i.e., very hypocellular and markedly hypercellular or "packed" bone marrows). When special

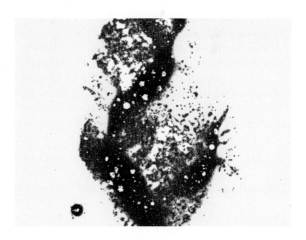

Figure 2-6

BONE MARROW CORE BIOPSY TOUCH PREPARATION

A typical core biopsy imprint preparation is stained with Wright-Giemsa. The touch preparation is often of lesser cytologic quality than an adequate and well-stained aspirate smear. In instances in which a satisfactory aspirate is not available, the touch imprint can substitute for cytologic evaluation.

studies such as flow cytometry or cytogenetics are clinically required in the setting of a dry-tap aspiration, one or preferably two biopsy cores of good length should be obtained and the cells disaggregated for these analyses (16).

Table 2-2

ELEMENTS OF QUALITY ASSURANCE IN BONE MARROW ASSESSMENT

Procedural	Interpretive
Clinical indication and relevant history	Concurrent CBC[a] with differential and peripheral smear present
Date and time	Adequate aspirate particles versus hemodilute or dry tap
Aspirate site	Aspirate smear stain quality and presence of artifacts
Aspirate quality: adequate, dry tap, clotted sample, etc.	Sufficient unstained aspirate slides or biopsy touch imprints
Extra aspirate samples drawn for special studies	Biopsy length; amount of subcortical bone or cartilage
Biopsy site, unilateral vs. bilateral	Presence and degree of aspiration artifact
Touch imprints made	Biopsy section H&E stain quality
Special use of biopsies (e.g., cultures, disaggregation for special studies as required)	Biopsy levels for staging procedures

[a]CBC = complete blood count; H&E = hematoxylin and eosin.

Table 2-3

COMMON CAUSES OF ARTIFACT OR POOR QUALITY IN BONE MARROW SAMPLE PREPARATIONS

Cause	Interpretive Problem
Excessive pressure with smear preparation, overly thick aspirate smears, or overstaining of aspirate slides	Obscuration of cytologic details due to disrupted cells or hyperchromatic stain artifact
Poor Wright-Giemsa stain composition	Poor tinctorial quality for cytologic study; unable to assess maturational abnormalities and may be difficult to distinguish some types of cells
Extensive hemodilution of aspirate	Inability to determine accurate bone marrow cell counts
Aspirate for morphology drawn into heparinized sample tube	Extensive effects on morphology; inability to assess fine cytologic details
Aspiration artifact in core biopsy sample	Inadequate evaluation of bone marrow space elements (may make biopsy assessment impossible if extensive)
Crushed or "accordion" type core biopsy	Elimination of bone marrow elements or crush artifacts precluding adequate morphologic biopsy study
Decalcification issues	Underdecalcification causes "chatter" effect in tissue sectioning and poor quality sections Overdecalcification leads to poor preservation of cytologic details in biopsy and can compromise robustness of special stains or immunohistochemistry
Thick sections of core biopsy or clot section	Poor cytologic details due to superimposition of cells, and/or excessive H&E[a] stain uptake
Inadequate core biopsy length or subcortical sampling	Insufficient cellular bone marrow for adequate biopsy evaluation

[a]H&E = hematoxylin and eosin.

The morphologist interpreting bone marrow aspirate and biopsy specimens should use a formal system to document the adequacy and quality in each case, including, at a minimum, the following parameters: sufficiency of particulate bone marrow (successful aspirate versus a dry tap); presence of sample clotting; aspirate slide and stain quality; interpretable core biopsy length (noting amount of excessive subcortical bone and cartilage if problematic); presence of aspiration artifact or core biopsy processing abnormalities; and quality of H&E-stained sections. Tracking these parameters serves not only as a log of quality for a given specimen, but also informs the clinician, pathologist, and laboratory technologist about recurrent technical issues of concern. These key features are summarized in Table 2-2, whereas Table 2-3 and figure 2-7 detail the common causes and examples of artifacts or poor quality bone marrow specimen preparations.

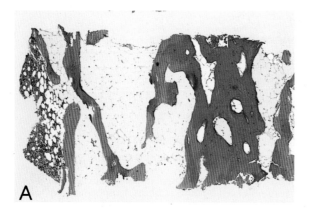

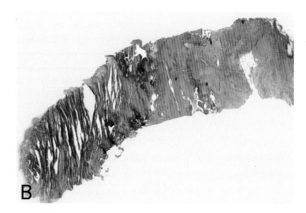

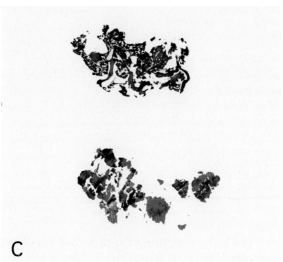

Figure 2-7

SUBOPTIMAL BONE MARROW CORE BIOPSY SPECIMENS

A: Hypocellularity in the subcortical region of the bone marrow biopsy can be observed in aplastic bone marrow, but also as a common change in older individuals. In the latter situation, a short core length may only encompass the region of adipocyte replacement, rendering the evaluation ineffective.

B: An "accordion" type of abnormality in which the bone trabeculae have been compacted together results in obliteration of the evaluable marrow space. This artifact is produced by excessive force when ejecting the core biopsy from the trephine needle.

C: This is a core biopsy of inadequate length. This type of poor quality specimen is almost of no value for specific clinical diagnostic indications (e.g., assessment for malignant infiltrates). (A–C: H&E stain).

Microscopic Interpretation of the Bone Marrow Aspirate and Biopsy: Qualitative and Quantitative Aspects

Despite some degree of individual idiosyncrasy in morphologically evaluating bone marrow specimens, the fundamental diagnostic approach is governed by a logical, systematic integration of a number of qualitative and quantitative parameters (18–22). These features are detailed in Table 2-4 and briefly summarized here. Clearly, in the course of nearly every bone marrow examination, knowledge of age-related normal range values for peripheral blood indices and bone marrow cell differential counts is required. Similarly, an understanding of changes in additional important variables, including bone marrow cellularity, the granulocyte to erythrocyte (G:E) ratio, the normal range of marrow lymphocytes and plasma cells, the presence of reticulin fibrosis, and the character of

the bone trabeculae, among others, is critical. A tabulation of generalized normal values for blood and bone marrow as well as variations of major bone marrow constituents with age are denoted in the Appendix.

The integration of concurrent CBC, white blood cell differential, and peripheral smear findings is of great relevance in fully correlating pathologic bone marrow changes with the clinical presentation. Changes in the number and/or cytologic appearance of circulating blood cellular components and the presence of abnormal circulating cells inform the morphologist about the possible differential diagnostic considerations to be expected in the bone marrow.

The bone marrow aspirate and core biopsy are thoroughly evaluated for the composition and character of the hematopoietic elements, as well as to identify abnormal cellular infiltrates or deposits. To this end, each of the bone

Table 2-4

COMPONENTS OF A COMPLETE BONE MARROW EXAMINATION

Component	Value/Utility
CBC[a] and peripheral blood smear	Assess quantitative blood cell variations, red blood cell indices, leukocyte differential leukocyte differential (absolute count) anomalies, qualitative and maturational abnormalities of each hematolymphoid lineage, presence of atypical circulating cells (e.g., blasts, lymphoma cells), characteristic features suggestive of specific diagnostic processes (e.g., leukoerythroblastic changes) Fresh blood or unstained smears can be used for special studies (see Table 2-5)
Bone marrow aspirate	Quantitative aspects: differential cell count; granulocyte:erythroid ratio; presence of other increased cell types (lymphocytes, plasma cells) Qualitative aspects: maturation changes and/or abnormalities in hematopoietic lineages (e.g., "left-shift," dysplasia); distinct cytologic features of cell types (e.g., blasts, lymphocytes, plasma cells, histiocytes, mast cells); abnormal infiltrates (e.g., nonhematopoietic malignant cells) Fresh bone marrow or unstained slides can be used for special studies (see Table 2-5)
Bone marrow core biopsy	Assess cellularity, general cell distribution (architecture) and composition Critically assess megakaryocyte morphology (determine unusual cellular features [e.g., inclusions, hemophagocytosis]) Evaluate for primary hematologic and lymphoid neoplasms, other infiltrative disorders, or features of infection (e.g., granulomas); especially valuable to identify focal involvement of the bone marrow by disease Determine changes in bone, vascular, or stromal compartments Fresh biopsy can be disaggregated to provide cells for special studies (see Table 2-5)
Bone marrow biopsy touch imprint	Similar utility to bone marrow aspirate, but typically lower quality Useful if aspirate is excessively hemodilute or a dry tap due to fibrosis
Bone marrow aspirate clot section	Similar utility to bone marrow core biopsy, but may be accompanied by abundant aspirated red cell clot; not of use if aspiration was a dry tap Some architectural relationships preserved, but paratrabecular anatomy not present May not be representative of pathologic infiltrates associated with fibrosis in the bone marrow

[a]CBC = complete blood count.

marrow tissue preparations provides valuable information in significantly different ways. The discriminating qualitative and quantitative assessment of bone marrow cell composition is obtained mainly from the aspirate smear, or occasionally, the core biopsy touch preparation. In contrast, the H&E-stained core biopsy section is ideal for determining overall hematopoietic cellularity, distortions in spatial relationships or architecture, the presence and extent of infiltrative lesions, and any changes affecting the supporting stroma, vessels, or trabecular bone. Complete bone marrow examination should ensure that these variables are duly evaluated and that pertinent details concerning any abnormalities are clearly described.

Many hematology laboratories use their own document templates to ensure that the evaluation of a bone marrow sample is adequately comprehensive; guidelines for establishing such checklists have also been put forth by professional organizations (23). By acquiring the breadth of data available, the pathologist can better generate a conclusive diagnosis, or at least guide the selection of appropriate ancillary, specialized investigations to confirm a favored diagnostic impression.

UTILITY OF SPECIAL TECHNIQUES

Ideally, a limited selection of specialized investigations should be based upon a critical evaluation of the clinical and pathologic features of the individual patient presentation in order to optimize diagnostic accuracy and minimize cost. Accordingly, given the range of bone marrow tissue preparations and the choice of a potentially large array of ancillary investigations, the diagnostician must have a thorough knowledge of both technical and interpretive aspects of these tests, as well as the advantages and limitations of each, to ensure the best application of these resources in specific instances.

In practical terms, additional bone marrow tissue is usually obtained at the time of the bone marrow procedure to ensure sufficient material is present for pertinent extra studies and to obviate the undesirable alternative of having to repeat the bone marrow sampling

Table 2-5

UTILITY OF AND SPECIMEN REQUIREMENTS FOR DIAGNOSTIC PROCEDURES IN BONE MARROW EVALUATION

Diagnostic Procedure	Diagnostic Utility	Specimen Requirements
Morphology +/- immuno-histochemistry (IHC)	Quantitative and qualitative cytologic assessment of cell types and maturation (including use of IHC as necessary); identification of some infectious agents (e.g., viruses) by IHC	Air-dried, stained bone marrow aspirate smears and fixed, processed core biopsy
Flow cytometry	Quantitative and qualitative assessment of cell surface and intracellular markers; identification of aberrant or characteristic disease phenotypes	Fresh bone marrow aspirate cells or blood (if sufficient circulating cells of interest)
Special stains:		Bone marrow aspirate smears and core biopsy sections: air-dried,
Iron	Evaluation of storage and erythroid iron	unfixed aspirate smears for iron,
Organism (PAS/GMS/ acid fast)[a]	Identification of bacterial, fungal, or mycobacterial organisms	NSE, MPO, PAS; clot/biopsy core sections for organism stains, and
NSE/MPO/PAS	Lineage characterization of acute leukemias	reticulin (poor for iron)
Reticulin	Assessment of bone marrow fibrosis	
Microbial/viral cultures	Identification and antibiotic sensitivity testing of infectious agents	Fresh sterile bone marrow aspirate cells
Cytogenetics/FISH	Identification of clonal karyotypic abnormalities in malignant hematolymphoid disorders; specialized applications in some congenital bone marrow syndromes (e.g., chromosome breakage studies in Fanconi anemia)	Fresh sterile bone marrow aspirate cells for standard cytogenetics; fresh cells or air-dried unfixed/unstained aspirate or touch preparation slides for FISH
Molecular analysis (PCR)	Complementary to cytogenetics/FISH for evaluation of hematolymphoid tumors; increasing role in revealing specific gene abnormalities associated with constitutional disorders	Fresh or frozen bone marrow aspirate cells; can also extract nucleic acids from air-dried slides and from fixed paraffin tissue

[a]PAS = periodic acid–Schiff; GMS = Gomori methenamine silver; NSE = nonspecific esterase; MPO = myeloperoxidase; FISH = fluorescence in situ hybridization; PCR = polymerase chain reaction.

procedure for these purposes. Many studies beyond routine staining of the bone marrow aspirate can be performed on air-dried aspirate or biopsy touch imprint slides, indicating that an adequate number of additional unstained slides should be made and retained. These air-dried preparations can be utilized for the assessment of iron stores and abnormal inclusions in cells, or for revealing the presence of specific cytosolic enzymes (24). Concerning enzymatic studies (e.g. esterases, acid phosphatase), air-dried slides should be rapidly processed for analysis (within 24 to 48 hours), since many proteins are labile with even short-term storage.

Unstained aspirate smears also provide an excellent source for genomic fluorescence in situ hybridization (FISH) studies, and in some cases, cells can be scraped from the glass slides to isolate DNA (and possibly RNA) for molecular investigations. In contrast, fresh bone marrow aspirate cells are required for flow cytometric cell marker studies, classic cytogenetic studies, many molecular diagnostic assays, and microbial/viral cultures. The fixed, decalcified bone marrow

biopsy (and indeed the aspirate clot section) can be subjected to further investigations by immunohistochemistry or RNA in situ hybridization methods; however, a number of antibody or nucleotide probe reagents may be poorly reactive following decalcification or the use of specific fixatives (e.g., B5), and these limitations must be determined in each laboratory. A summary of the types and uses of ancillary investigations is shown in Table 2-5, and representative examples of several of these specialized studies are illustrated in figures 2-8 to 2-15.

The use of special stains is commonplace in bone marrow evaluation. The presence of storage and erythrocyte iron is an important aspect which can shed light on pathologic bone marrow processes beyond iron deficiency anemia (fig. 2-8). Although classic iron deficiency does not require bone marrow examination for diagnosis, refractory anemias or anemias of uncertain etiology typically require examination of a bone marrow specimen. Of importance, iron staining is not reliable in determining deficiency or sideroblastic pathology when performed on

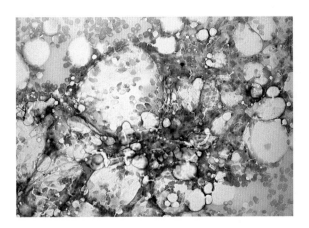
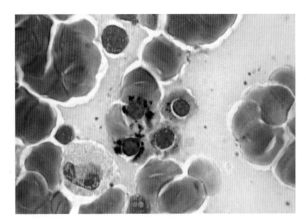

Figure 2-8

IRON STAINS OF BONE MARROW ASPIRATE

Left: A Prussian blue stain of a bone marrow aspirate slide reveals iron deposits within storage macrophages.
Right: There is a pathologic increase in red blood cell precursor or sideroblastic iron, with evidence of ring sideroblasts.

Figure 2-9

ORGANISM STAINS

A,B: Positivity for fungal organisms are demonstrated with periodic acid-Schiff/diastase (PAS/D) (A) and Gomori methenamine silver (GMS) (B) special stains.

C: A Ziehl-Nilsson acid-fast bacillus stain highlights numerous organisms consistent with atypical mycobacteria (e.g., *Mycobacterium avium-intracellulare*).

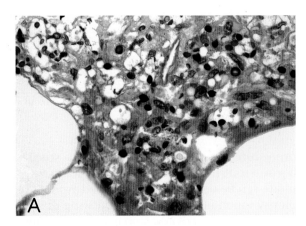

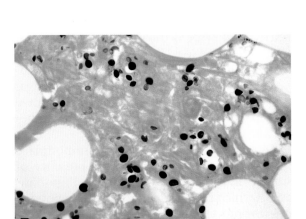
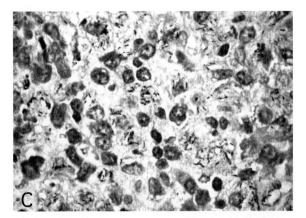

fixed, decalcified tissue sections; a bone marrow aspirate smear preparation represents the optimal specimen type for these purposes. The application of special stains to detect fungal and mycobacterial (acid-fast) organisms can also be invaluable, since some of these infectious agents (notably *Mycobacterium tuberculosis*) may grow poorly or slowly in culture and a rapid diagnosis can be achieved with appropriate stains on core biopsy or clot sections (fig. 2-9). Reticulin

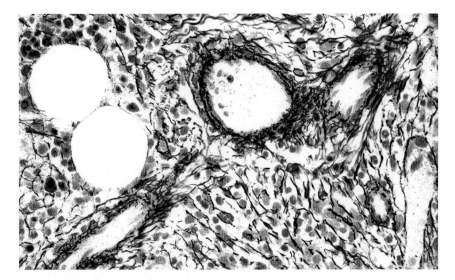

Figure 2-10

RETICULIN STAIN

A reticulin stain of a bone marrow core biopsy shows fibers concentrated around blood vessels and increased in the interstitium.

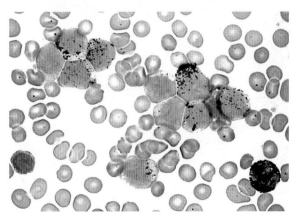
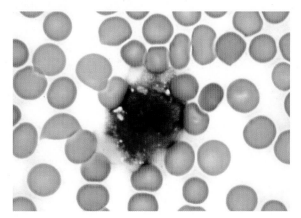

Figure 2-11

CYTOCHEMICAL STAINS IN BONE MARROW

Left: A rapid cytochemical preparation of a bone marrow aspirate slide reveals cytoplasmic myeloperoxidase (MPO) granules in myeloid lineage precursors. Immature myeloid cells and myeloblasts typically show less MPO positivity than more mature forms.

Right: Alpha-naphthyl butyrate esterase (also referred to as nonspecific esterase) cytochemistry on a bone marrow aspirate slide is very useful for demonstrating monocytic differentiation in bone marrow precursor cells.

staining of the core biopsy can be valuable in the setting of a dry-tap aspiration to assess for the presence and degree of bone marrow fibrosis (fig. 2-10).

Although most relevant for neoplastic disorders, air-dried smears or touch preparations can be used for cytochemical stains such as myeloperoxidase and alpha-naphthol butyrate esterase (nonspecific esterase) (Table 2-5; fig. 2-11). Numerous immunohistochemical stains can be performed on bone marrow core biopsy and clot sections. In non-neoplastic biopsy specimens immunohistochemical stains for hematopoietic lineages, blasts, lymphoid cell types, and organisms are most frequently utilized (fig. 2-12). Additional specialized tests, including flow cytometric immunophenotyping, DNA content analysis, in situ hybridization, and polymerase chain reaction techniques, are most often used to evaluate neoplastic disorders, but can be used in selective circumstances in non-neoplastic disorders (figs. 2-13–2-15).

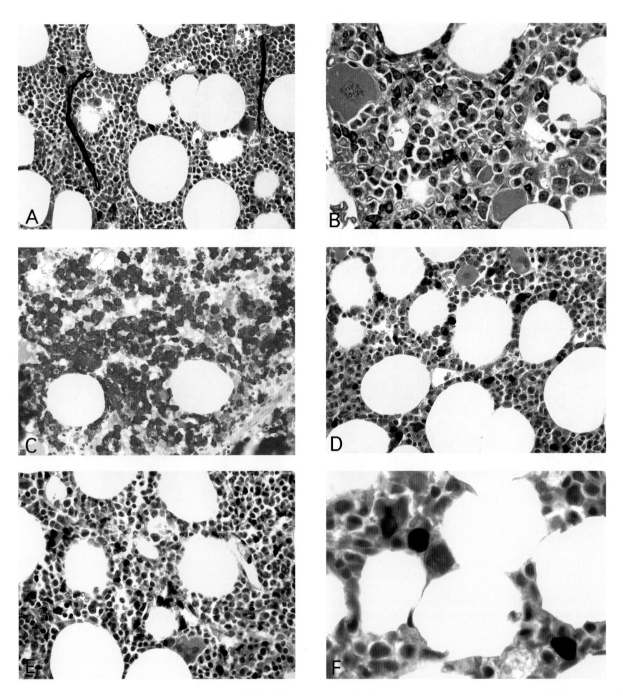

Figure 2-12

IMMUNOHISTOCHEMICAL STAINS OF BONE MARROW

The following images represent commonly applied immunohistochemical reagents used to identify specific cell types.
A: Immunostaining of CD34 antigen-positive blasts and vessels in normal bone marrow.
B: Increased CD34 positivity in a neoplastic bone marrow process (such as myelodysplasia).
C: Numerous erythroid precursors revealed with antihemoglobin A antibody.
D: A scattered population of normal bone marrow B cells demonstrated with anti-CD20 immunostain.
E: Anti-CD3 antibody highlights normal bone marrow T-cell distribution.
F: Immunostaining for parvovirus B19 confirms acute bone marrow infection in a patient with severe erythroid hypoplasia.
(A–F: bone marrow core biopsies.)

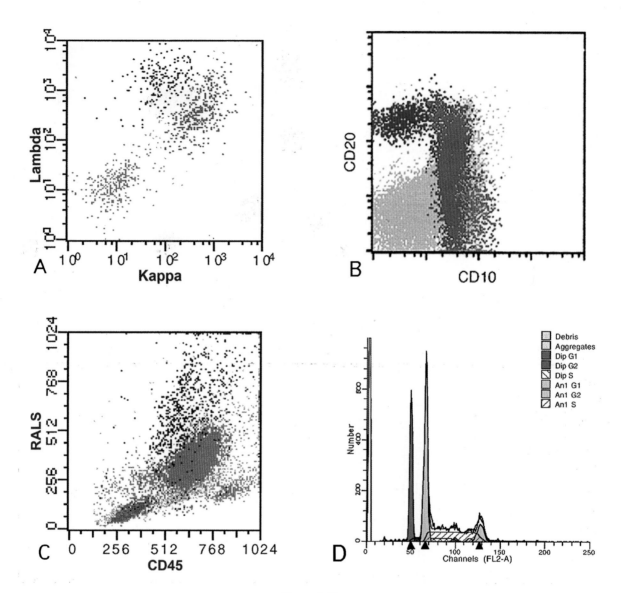

Figure 2-13

FLOW CYTOMETRY IN BONE MARROW EVALUATION

The sensitive and specific characterization of cell populations can be rapidly achieved by flow cytometric techniques using epitope-specific monoclonal antibody reagents.

A: A normal bone marrow study for B-lymphocyte clonality shows both kappa- and lambda-positive B cells (green and blue cell clusters), along with a subpopulation of surface immunoglobulin-negative developing B cells, or hematogones (pink cell cluster).

B: A more detailed analysis of bone marrow hematogones demonstrates a maturational spectrum with CD20 and CD10 B-cell–associated markers.

C: A large abnormal immature blast population (pink cell cluster) is revealed by CD45 (panleukocyte antigen) cell membrane staining and right angle light scatter (or side scatter) profile. This technique allows for improved delineation of normal and abnormal hematolymphoid cell populations in the bone marrow.

D: Another specialized application of flow cytometry, namely, the determination of cellular DNA content. A nuclear preparation of a bone marrow sample is incubated with a DNA intercalating dye (e.g., propidium iodide) and the cell nuclei are evaluated by flow cytometry. A normal distribution of DNA content is reflected by the prominent left red peak profile (G1 phase diploid DNA content), whereas an admixed abnormal aneuploid G1 phase tumor cell DNA content is identified by the left yellow peak. Smaller and broader peaks lying to the right represent G2 phase and mitotic cell populations, which have duplicated (4n) DNA content. The area under the curve between G1 and G2/M regions represents the percentage of cells in synthesis (S-phase) of the cell cycle. These quantitative parameters are determined by dedicated software analysis.

Figure 2-14

IN SITU HYBRIDIZATION TECHNIQUES IN BONE MARROW EVALUATION

In some instances, recognition of a specific cell marker is achieved with high sensitivity by the identification of the transcribed mRNA species. In this image, chromogenic in situ hybridization was employed to detect the presence of Epstein-Barr virus early RNA (EBV-EBER). A similar technical approach is used to detect numerical or structural genetic abnormalities by fluorescence in situ hybridization (FISH), using nuclear preparations of bone marrow cells.

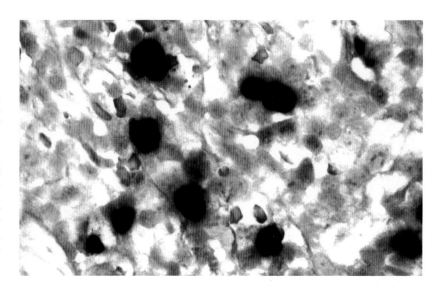

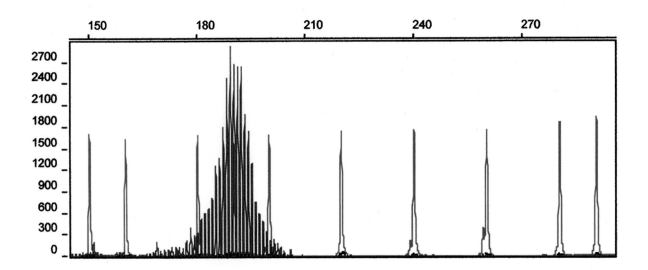

Figure 2-15

MOLECULAR GENETIC TECHNIQUE IN BONE MARROW EVALUATION

The image depicts the results of a DNA polymerase chain reaction (PCR) method to detect antigen receptor gene rearrangements at the T-cell gamma locus. The fluorescently labeled primers amplify a specified region of rearrangement in the T-gamma gene and the PCR products are detected by a post-PCR capillary electrophoresis method. The electropherogram shown indicates a statistically normal distribution of rearranged amplicons, indicative of a polyclonal T-cell process. In contrast, a monoclonal population, consistent with a malignant T-lymphoid disorder, would present as a single (or possibly biallelic) peak profile (not shown). Other commonly employed techniques in clinical molecular diagnostics include reverse-transcription PCR (to detect specific RNA species), DNA ligation-based assays, and genomic Southern blot hybridization.

REFERENCES

Indications for Bone Marrow Evaluation, Procurement, Potential Procedural Complications

1. Bain BJ. Bone marrow aspiration. J Clin Pathol 2001;54:657-63.
2. Bain BJ. Bone marrow biopsy morbidity and mortality. Br J Haematol 2003;121:949-51.
3. Bain BJ. Bone marrow biopsy morbidity and mortality: 2002 data. Clin Lab Haematol 2004; 26:315-8.
4. Bain BJ. Bone marrow trephine biopsy. J Clin Pathol 2001;54:737-42.
5. Bain BJ, Clark DM, Lampert IA, et al. Bone marrow pathology, 3rd ed. Oxford: Blackwell Science Ltd.; 2001.
6. Brynes RK, McKenna RW, Sundberg RD. Bone marrow aspiration and trephine biopsy. An approach to a thorough study. Am J Clin Pathol 1978;70:753-9.
7. Burkle CM, Harrison BA, Koenig LF, Decker PA, Warner DO, Gastineau DA. Morbidity and mortality of deep sedation in outpatient bone marrow biopsy. Am J Hematol 2004;77:250-6.
8. Cotelingam JD. Bone marrow biopsy: interpretive guidelines for the surgical pathologist. Adv Anat Pathol 2003;10:8-26.
9. Devaliaf V, Tudor G. Bone marrow examination in obese patients. Br J Haematol 2004;125:538-9.
10. Foucar K. Hematopoiesis and morphologic review of bone marrow. Bone marrow pathology, 2nd ed. Chicago: ASCP Press; 2001:1-29.
11. Ghosh K. Bone marrow examination in obese patients: CAT or not to CAT! Br J Haematol 2004;127:230-1.
12. Giannoutsos I, Grech H, Maboreke T, et al. Performing bone marrow biopsies with or without sedation: a comparison. Clin Lab Haematol 2004;26:201-4.
13. Marti J, Anton E, Valenti C. Complications of bone marrow biopsy. Br J Haematol 2004;124:557-88.

Sampling, Preparation, Adequacy, Quality Considerations in Bone Marrow Evaluation

14. Barekman CL, Fair KP, Cotelingam JD. Comparative utility of diagnostic bone-marrow components: a 10-year study. Am J Hematol 1997;56:37-41.

15. Bonds LA, Barnes P, Foucar K, Sever CE. Acetic acid-zinc-formalin: a safe alternative to B-5 fixative. Am J Clin Pathol 2005;124:205-11.
16. Novotny JR, Schmucker U, Staats B, Duhrsen U. Failed or inadequate bone marrow aspiration: a fast, simple and cost-effective method to produce a cell suspension from a core biopsy specimen. Clin Lab Haematol 2005;27:33-40.
17. Peterson LC, Brunning RD. Bone marrow specimen processing. In: Knowles DM, ed. Neoplastic hematopathology, 2nd ed. Philadelphia: Lippincott Williams & Wilkins; 2001:1391-406.

Interpretation of the Bone Marrow Aspirate and Biopsy: Qualitative and Quantitative Aspects

18. Bain BJ. Bone marrow aspiration. J Clin Pathol 2001;54:657-63.
19. Bain BJ. Bone marrow trephine biopsy. J Clin Pathol 2001;54:737-42.
20. Barekman CL, Fair KP, Cotelingam JD. Comparative utility of diagnostic bone-marrow components: a 10-year study. Am J Hematol 1997;56:37-41.
21. Cotelingam JD. Bone marrow biopsy: interpretive guidelines for the surgical pathologist. Adv Anat Pathol 2003;10:8-26.
22. Foucar K. Hematopoiesis and morphologic review of bone marrow. In: Bone marrow pathology, 2nd ed. Chicago: ASCP Press; 2001:1-29.
23. Peterson LC, Agosti SJ, Hoyer JD, et al. Protocol for the examination of specimens from patients with hematopoietic neoplasms of the bone marrow: a basis for checklists. Arch Pathol Lab Med 2002;126:1050-6.

Utility of Special Techniques

24. Li CY, Yam LT. Cytochemical, histochemical, and immunohistochemical analysis of the bone marrow. In: Knowles DM, ed. Neoplastic hematopathology, 2nd ed. Philadelphia: Lippincott Williams & Wilkins; 2001:1407-46.

3 LABORATORY EVALUATION OF BLOOD AND BONE MARROW IN NON-NEOPLASTIC DISORDERS

A bone marrow evaluation is incomplete without the concurrent assessment of the peripheral blood. Whenever possible, the peripheral blood smear should be reviewed prior to obtaining the bone marrow sample since it may provide sufficient information to preempt the need for the more invasive procedure. Thrombocytopenia due to ethylene diaminetetraacetic acid (EDTA)-induced platelet clumping is one example of such a situation.

Three primary considerations influence the initial evaluation of the peripheral smear, regardless of whether a bone marrow examination is being contemplated: the age of the patient, whether a quantitative defect involves more than one lineage, and whether associated qualitative changes are present (i.e., change in size, shape, or appearance of cells). This evaluation necessitates correlation with the results of the complete blood count (CBC). The decision to then perform a bone marrow procedure requires integration of the peripheral blood findings with a carefully obtained clinical history, thorough physical examination, and current and historic laboratory data.

PERIPHERAL BLOOD SMEAR EVALUATION

Preparation of high-quality blood smears is crucial to the correct identification of abnormal cell populations, altered cellular distributions (clumping, rouleaux), or cytologic features that can be used to guide further testing. Knowledge of the patient's age and sex, in addition to relevant clinical information, facilitates appropriate and rapid interpretation. The initial review should be systematic and comprehensive. A common practice is to sequentially evaluate the red blood cells, the white blood cells, and then the platelets. Table 3-1 lists the components of a comprehensive peripheral blood smear examination.

Red Blood Cells

Initial evaluation of the red blood cells (RBCs) at low-power microscopy (2X or 4X) and performed within a few fields of the feathered edge of the smear highlights the relationship of the RBCs to one another (figs. 3-1, 3-2). Large gaps between cells suggests anemia whereas minimal spacing between cells reflects possible polycythemia; confirmation with the CBC data is required (figs. 3-3, 3-4). Overlapping of RBCs in this thinner region of the smear, in contrast to thicker areas, is indicative of either true RBC clumping or rouleaux formation (fig. 3-5).

Closer microscopic visualization (10X or 20X) helps identify alterations in RBC color (hypochromic if a central area of pallor is more than one third of the RBC diameter), size, and shape. Any changes in shape should be seen throughout the smear and not isolated to one area to exclude artifacts of smearing or pH change. In anemic patients, a dearth of polychromatophilic cells signals a problem with RBC production, whereas increased polychromatophilic cells implies functional erythropoiesis, which can be further established with a reticulocyte count. Careful evaluation for schistocytes (fragments without central pallor) or spherocytes is particularly indicated in smears with increased polychromasia to assess for hemolysis (fig. 3-6) (see chapter 4). Finally, high power (40X to 100X) examination is best for detecting intracellular inclusions or organisms (*Babesia, Plasmodium*) (see chapters 4 and 10 for illustrations).

White Blood Cells

White blood cells (WBCs) should be similarly assessed at low, intermediate, and high microscopic power for quantitative and qualitative changes. Correlation with CBC data is required, particularly as the quantity of circulating WBCs may be difficult to ascertain if only mildly altered due to a variation in the number of cells trapped at the feathered edge. Scanning the smear to assure accuracy of automated or manual differential counts should be followed by determination of whether the absolute counts for the different leukocyte types are within the appropriate reference ranges. If the

Table 3-1

DOCUMENTATION OF PERIPHERAL BLOOD SMEAR FINDINGS

Cell Type	Quantity[a]	Appearance	Ancillary Tests[b]

Red blood cells (RBCs)	Decreased
	  Hypochromic microcytic
	  Macrocytic
	  Normochromic normocytic
	  Dimorphic
		Anisocytosis: not significant versus mild, moderate, or marked
		Poikilocytosis: not significant versus mild, moderate, or marked; cell types (e.g., schistocytes, spherocytes)
		Polychromasia: not increased versus increased
			Iron; vitamin B_{12} and folate studies; thyroid, renal, and liver function tests; reticulocyte count; hemoglobin electrophoresis; direct antiglobulin test; osmotic fragility; flow cytometry (PNH),[c] RBC enzymes (history of recent treatment or transfusion if dimorphic)

	Normal or increased
	  Normochromic normocytic
	  Hypochromic microcytic
		Document if present: nRBCs, clumping, rouleaux formation, inclusions, organisms	Hemoglobin electrophoresis, arterial oxygen saturation, renal and liver function tests, serum erythropoietin level, carbon monoxide level

White blood cells (WBCs)	Decreased:
	  Neutropenia (adult): mild (1-1.5x10³/µL), moderate (0.5-0.9x10³ /µL), marked (<0.5x10³/µL)
	  Lymphopenia
	  Monocytopenia
	  Normal with normal or abnormal differential count
		Reactive changes: toxic granulation, Döhle bodies, vacuolation, variant or large granular lymphocytes
		Dysplasia–not significant versus present and describe (e.g., pseudo-Pelger-Hüet nuclei, hypogranulation, abnormal nuclear segmentation, immature monocytes)
			Bacterial, fungal, viral cultures/titers; HIV testing; vitamin B_{12} and folate studies; evaluate for autoimmune disorders (serologies, erythrocyte sedimentation rate); immunoglobulin/complement workup

	Increased:
	  Neutrophilia
	  Lymphocytosis
	  Monocytosis
	  Eosinophilia
	  Basophilia
		Document if present: left shift with immature cell type present (e.g., myelocyte), any blasts or atypical cells of unknown type or significance, neutrophil hypersegmentation, WBC clumping	Bacterial, fungal, viral cultures/titers; flow cytometry; tissue biopsy
			Cytogenetic analysis; fluorescence in situ hybridization; molecular studies

Platelets	Decreased: mild (100-149x10³/µL), moderate (50-99x10³/µL), marked (<50x10³/µL)	Size: small, normal, large, giant (larger than a normal RBC) Granularity: normal versus hypogranular[d] Document if present: clumping, satellitism, megakaryocyte nuclei, nuclear fragments	Coagulation studies (including D-dimer) evaluation for autoimmune disorders (serologies, erythrocyte sedimentation rate), renal function tests, mean platelet volume (may help with small platelets, less helpful with large or giant), thyroid tests, HIV testing

	Normal: (150-399x10³/µL)
	Increased:
	  mild (400-699x10³/µL),
	  moderate (700-1,000x10³/µL),
	  marked (>1,000x10³/µL)
			Iron studies, cultures/titers (bacteria, fungus, virus), cytogenetic studies for chronic myeloproliferative disorder

[a]Reference ranges for age and sex (and possibly ethnic group) must be considered.

[b]Please refer to the appropriate chapters in this Fascicle for further discussion of which of the listed ancillary tests are pertinent to perform based on the specific peripheral blood smear findings.

[c]PNH = paroxysmal nocturnal hemoglobinuria; nRBC = nucleated red blood cells; HIV = human immunodeficiency virus.

[d]Platelet hypogranularity may be an artifact of prolonged storage or poor staining.

absolute counts are not provided, they can be easily calculated by multiplying the WBC count times the percent of cell type of interest (i.e., 5 x 10³/µL WBC x 30 percent lymphocytes = 1.5 x 10³/µL absolute lymphocyte count). Absolute cell counts are essential as a lineage may be decreased or increased even in the presence of a normal differential count (percent) or a normal WBC count. This occurs most commonly when one of the less frequent cell types is altered, such as a decrease in monocytes or increase in basophils, or when a decrease in one cell type (such as neutrophils) is offset by an increase in another (lymphocytes). For abnormal WBC counts, determining the cell type or types that are quantitatively changed is essential for establishing an appropriate differential diagnosis.

Further evaluation of leukocyte appearance on the blood film is best performed at intermediate or high power. Neutrophils should be examined

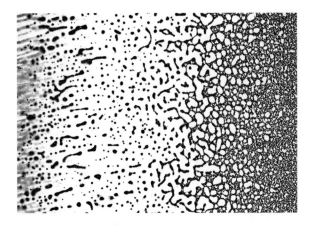

Figure 3-1

FEATHERED EDGE OF PERIPHERAL BLOOD SMEAR

The feathered edge of the peripheral blood smear is an important area to scan for platelet clumps, large cells (cytomegalovirus-infected endothelial cells), and organisms (microfilariae). This is not a good area for visualization of red blood cell (RBC) morphology (Wright stain).

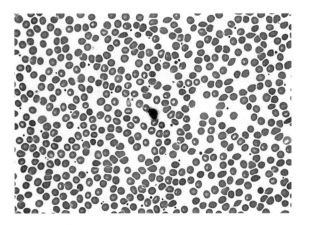

Figure 3-2

NORMAL RED BLOOD CELL DISTRIBUTION

The field immediately adjacent to the cells shown in the previous slide is the optimal area for visualization of RBCs. A thinly spread layer of RBCs allows for estimation of RBC quantity and evaluation of cell distribution (Wright stain).

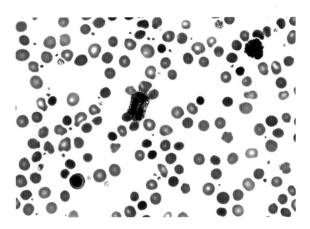

Figure 3-3

ANEMIA

Decreased number of RBCs in a blood film from 84-year-old male with microangiopathic hemolytic anemia (Wright stain).

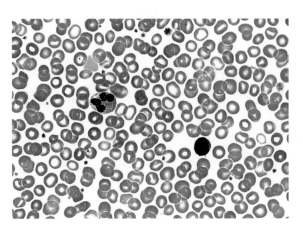

Figure 3-4

INCREASED RED BLOOD CELLS

Increased number of RBCs in a blood film from 52-year-old female receiving phlebotomy for polycythemia vera. The RBCs are hypochromic and microcytic due to iron deficiency (Wright stain).

for features of activation, such as toxic granulation, Döhle bodies, and cytoplasmic vacuolation; features of dysplasia, such as hypogranulation and abnormal nuclear segmentation; features of atypia associated with nutritional deficiencies or metabolic disorders, such as hypersegmentation and cytoplasmic vacuolation; and finally, changes associated with constitutional abnormalities, such as Pelger-Hüet nuclei, increased Döhle bodies (May-Hegglin anomaly), abnormal cytoplasmic granulation (Alder-Reilly

anomaly, Chediak-Higashi inclusions), or neutrophil apoptosis (glycogen storage disease) (see chapter 5 for illustrations) (2,3). Documentation of a left shift is indicated if neutrophilic myeloid precursors prior to the band stage are identified (fig. 3-7).

The assessment of lymphocytes should take into account the increased presence of activated or variant forms (i.e., plasmacytoid, immunoblasts), large granular lymphocytes (if over 15

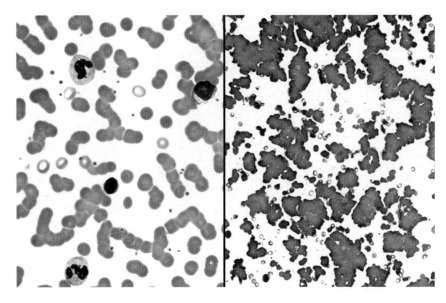

Figure 3-5

ABNORMAL RED BLOOD CELL DISTRIBUTION

RBC distribution abnormalities detected on peripheral blood smears.

Left: Rouleaux formation is identified in a patient with Waldenstrom macroglobulinemia.

Right: RBC clumping is observed in a patient with cold agglutinin, secondary to lymphoma (Wright stain). (Courtesy Dr. C. Sever, Albuquerque, NM.)

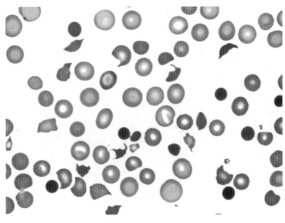

Figure 3-6

RED BLOOD CELL HEMOLYSIS

Increased polychromatophilic cells, schistocytes, and spherocytes are indicative of RBC hemolysis in this patient with thrombotic thrombocytopenic purpura (TTP) (Wright stain).

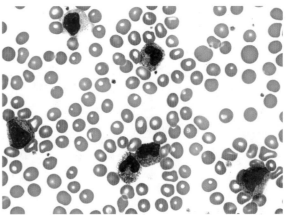

Figure 3-7

NEUTROPHILS WITH LEFT SHIFT

Neutrophilic precursors prior to the band stage are observed in this peripheral blood smear. In addition to the neutrophilic left shift, neutrophils show features of activation, with prominent toxic granulation (Wright stain).

percent of circulating lymphocytes), or unusual granulation or discrete cytoplasmic vacuolation (metabolic or storage disorders) (1,5). Reactive lymphocytes often have a range of morphology within the smear but are larger and have more abundant cytoplasm than normal lymphocytes (see chapter 8 for illustrations).

Monocytes may also show abnormalities in cytoplasmic granulation (Chediak-Higashi syndrome) (4). Monocytic dysplasia is suggested by the finding of nuclear immaturity, a high nuclear to cytoplasmic ratio, and pale cytoplasm.

Plasma cells and basophils are infrequently seen in the peripheral blood and once a plasma cell dyscrasia or myeloproliferative disorder is excluded, these cells are most often associated with chronic infectious or inflammatory conditions. Degranulated basophils may be missed by automated instruments and careful review for the few residual basophilic granules in these cells is required for appropriate cell recognition.

Organisms should always be sought in the cytoplasm of neutrophils and monocytes, as well as circulating extracellularly. Low-power

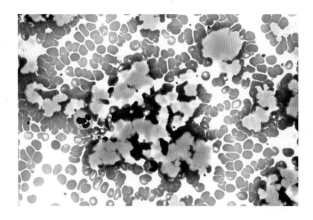

Figure 3-8

CRYOGLOBULIN

The marked cryoglobulin in this peripheral blood smear interferes with the automated cell count (Wright stain).

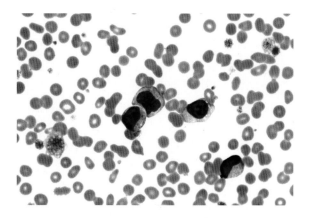

Figure 3-9

PLATELET PLEOMORPHISM

Peripheral blood smear from a patient with a chronic myeloproliferative disorder shows platelet pleomorphism. The platelets vary in size and degree of granulation. Giant platelets, which are larger than RBCs, are present (Wright stain).

review of the lateral margins and feathered edge of the smear is best for detecting circulating microfilaria or large cells with viral inclusions (see chapter 10 for illustrations).

Platelets

Low platelet counts must be confirmed by screening the blood film. Platelet clumps become trapped along the feathered edge of the smear, making this an important area to screen; clumping is more frequent in smears from fingerstick or heelstick blood draws. Platelet clumps must also be distinguished from other extracellular material, such as cryoglobulin (fig. 3-8). Platelets present in clumps or adherent to neutrophils (platelet satellitism) are not counted by the automated hematology instruments and are a common cause for spuriously low platelet counts and, occasionally, pseudoleukocytosis (see chapter 6 for illustrations). This may be a significant problem, as evidenced by Cohen et al. (7), who found 17 percent of their outpatient referrals for evaluation of thrombocytopenia were due to pseudothrombocytopenia.

Platelet clumping and platelet satellitism may be associated with blood collected in EDTA tubes. Renumeration of the platelets using an alternative anticoagulant (such as sodium citrate) usually ameliorates this problem, although citrate, oxalate, and heparin are also infrequently implicated with clumping and satellitism. When the use of an alternative anticoagulant does not resolve the problem, platelet estimation

on a smear from a freshly drawn blood sample without any anticoagulant is necessary.

The pathophysiologic mechanism responsible for platelet clumping and satellitism is hypothesized to be the binding of antibodies of immunoglobulin (Ig)G, IgM, or IgA classes to epitopes on the glycoprotein complex IIb/IIIa that are exposed in the presence of EDTA (or one of the other anticoagulants) (8). Although most cases are not related to specific diseases, reports of pseudothrombocytopenia associated with known infections or during the administration of specific drugs, such as Abciximab for coronary interventions, are well described (9,11). Spuriously low platelet counts may result in unnecessary testing or cancellation of procedures and surgery. Platelet clumps in patients with normal or high platelet counts are of less concern and, although they merit comment, do not have the same clinical impact.

Platelets vary in size and shape, particularly when platelet production is accelerated. Extreme platelet pleomorphism is less commonly seen in reactive than neoplastic conditions (fig. 3-9). A platelet should be considered giant in size only when it is larger than the surrounding RBCs (assuming normal mean corpuscular volume [MCV]). This equates to greater than 7 μm in size as compared to the normal platelet size of 1 to 4 μm. Platelets between these sizes are considered to be large platelets. Small platelets are

Table 3-2

IMPORTANCE OF AGE IN THE INTERPRETATION OF SELECT PERIPHERAL BLOOD FINDINGS

	Finding	Important Considerations Based on Age
Red Blood Cells	Nucleated red blood cells	Newborn: normal
		Others: multifactorial, requires evaluation unless asplenic (e.g., Howell-Jolly bodies)
	Spherocytes	Newborn: maternal antibody mediated
		Infant/child: hereditary spherocytosis
		All ages: warm alloantibody mediated
	Macrocytic anemia, reticulocytopenia	Infant: congenital disorder (Diamond-Blackfan anemia, congenital dyserythro-poietic anemia [+dyserythropoiesis], congenital megaloblastic anemia)
		Children/adults: vitamin B_{12} or folate deficiency, liver disease, postsplenectomy, medication
		Adult: alcoholism, pernicious anemia, myelodysplastic syndrome
	Normochromic normocytic anemia, reticulocytopenia	Infant (<1 year old): Diamond-Blackfan anemia
		Infant/child: often transient (transient erythroblastemia of childhood [usually >1 year old]), parvovirus infection
		All ages: systemic diseases (anemia of chronic disease, endocrine disorders, renal disease), chronic infection (HIV[a]), primary bone marrow disorder (MDS, drug)
	Normochromic normocytic anemia, reticulocytosis	Infant/child: hereditary nonspherocytic hemolytic anemia
		All ages: blood loss
	Sideroblastic anemia	Infant/child: lead poisoning (microcytic), hereditary sideroblastic anemia
		Adults: myelodysplastic syndromes
		All ages: drugs, toxins
	Erythrocytosis	Children: congenital disorder (high oxygen-affinity hemoglobin, methemo-globinemia, increased erythropoietin production)
		Adult: myeloproliferative disorder (polycythemia vera), smoking
		All ages: hypoxia (chronic lung disease), renal or hepatic disease
	Rouleaux formation	Adult: plasma cell dyscrasia
		All ages: increased fibrinogen, protein
White Blood Cells	Immature lymphocytes	Neonate/infant: normal or reactive
		Children/adults: acute lymphoblastic leukemia
	Mature lymphocytosis	Infant/child: pertussis infection
		Adult: lymphoproliferative disorder (e.g., chronic lymphocytic leukemia)
	Reactive lymphocytosis with immunoblasts	Adolescents/young adults (~10-30 yrs): infectious mononucleosis (EBV)
		Adult: (>30 yrs, infectious mononucleosis-like syndrome), hypersensitivity drug reactions (phenytoin), autoimmune disorders
		All ages: viral infections

more difficult to assess but are associated with Wiskott-Aldrich syndrome and an increased incidence of bone marrow–related disease; correlation with the mean platelet volume (MPV) supports the morphologic impression (6,10).

Megakaryocyte nuclei or fragments of nuclei with minimal or no cytoplasm may circulate but are scarce in normal individuals other than newborns. Therefore, identification of nuclear portions of megakaryocytes beyond the neonatal period suggests an alteration in megakaryopoiesis, which may be either reactive or neoplastic in nature.

The assessment of platelet granularity is dependent on the quality and intensity of smear staining. Platelet hypogranularity or reduction in platelet granules can only be confirmed when normally granulated platelets are present on the same slide for comparison. Hypogranular platelets must also be distinguished from small cytoplasmic fragments of other cell types (see chapter 6 for illustrations).

Age-Related Factors

Age is one of the most important factors to consider when reviewing a peripheral smear. Age, ethnicity, and altitude-related reference ranges are critical to the determination of cytopenias and cytoses on which differential diagnoses are based (see Appendix) (12,14). Diagnostic considerations that are dependent on the age of an individual are illustrated in Table 3-2 (13,15). For example, an increase in small lymphocytes with lobated or indented

Table 3-2 (continued)

	Finding	Important Considerations Based on Age
White Blood Cells	Lymphocytopenia	Infant/child: congenital immunodeficiency disorders Adults: autoimmune disorders All ages: iatrogenic (radiation, chemotherapy), renal insufficiency, infection
	Rare blasts	Neonate/infant: severe infections Children/adults: neoplastic disorder, growth factor therapy
	Isolated neutropenia	Neonate: maternal auto- or alloantibody Infant/child: often transient, follow for resolution (viral infections, post immunizations) Adult: multifactorial (if severe and unexplained perform bone marrow)
	Mild chronic neutropenia	Infant/child: congenital disorder (familial neutropenia, leukocyte adhesion defects, Kostman agranulocytosis, Shwachman-Diamond syndrome, Chediak-Higashi syndrome, chronic granulomatous disease) Adult: hypersplenism, autoimmune, chronic myeloproliferative disorder with eosinophilia All ages: drug induced, infection
	Eosinophilia	Infant/child: immunodeficiencies (hyper-IgE syndrome, IgA deficiency, Wiskott-Aldrich syndrome) Adult: collagen vascular disorder, myeloproliferative disorder, mast cell disease All ages: allergic disorders, dermatitis, drug reaction
Platelets	Abrupt onset thrombocytopenia with normal platelet granularity	Neonate: maternal alloimmunization Children: hemolytic uremic syndrome, constitutional disorders Adult: heparin-induced thrombocytopenia (infants—may see after cardiac surgery), autoimmune disorder, pregnancy-induced platelet disorders All ages: idiopathic thrombocytopenic purpura (also large platelets), medication, hypersplenism, infections
	Moderate thrombocytopenia with hypogranular platelets	Infant/children: gray platelet syndrome (alpha storage pool disease) Adult: myelodysplastic syndrome, myeloproliferative disorder
	Thrombocytosis	Neonate: Down syndrome–associated aberrations Adults: myeloproliferative disorders All ages: surgery, tissue injury, blood loss, iron deficiency, postsplenectomy
Multi-lineage	Leukoerythroblastic reaction	Newborn/infant/child: severe infection, hemolytic anemia, cyanotic heart disease, Gaucher disease, fracture Adult: hematopoietic or metastatic malignancy, bone marrow replacement, fibrosis
	Microangiopathic hemolytic anemia and thrombocytopenia	Infant/child: hemolytic uremic syndrome, congenital TTP, Kasabach-Merritt syndrome (kaposiform hemangioendothelioma, tufted angioma) Child/adult: TTP Pregnant women: HELLP, eclampsia All ages: disseminated intravascular coagulation
	Left-shifted neutrophilia with dyspoiesis, eosinophilia or basophilia	Children: juvenile rheumatoid arthritis Adult: myeloproliferative disorder
	Two or three lineages decreased	Children: hereditary disorders (familial aplastic anemia, Fanconi anemia, dyskeratosis, congenital Shwachman-Diamond syndrome) Adults: autoimmune disorders, viral infections (hepatitis C), alcohol All ages: drug effect, viral infections (HIV, parvovirus), aplastic anemia

[a]HIV = human immunodeficiency syndrome; MDS = myelodysplastic syndrome; EBV = Epstein-Barr virus; TTP = thrombotic thrombocytopenic purpura; HELLP= hemolysis, elevated liver enzymes, low platelets.

nuclei in a child suggests pertussis infection, while a similar picture in an older adult more likely represents a lymphoproliferative disorder. Congenital disorders of blood and bone marrow are of greater concern in pediatric patients, while neoplastic processes involving bone marrow increase in incidence as the adult population ages.

Additional Considerations

Cytopenias involving a single lineage, particularly in children, seldom require bone marrow examination unless persistent and nonresolving or severe and unresponsive to treatment. The most common cause of marked thrombocytopenia in the pediatric population

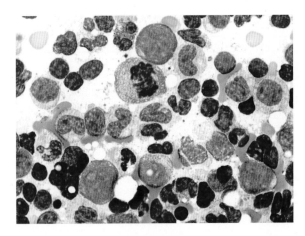

Figure 3-10

TRANSIENT ERYTHROBLASTOPENIA OF CHILDHOOD

The bone marrow aspirate smear from a 15-month-old child with transient erythroblastopenia of childhood shows markedly decreased and left-shifted erythroid precursors (Wright stain).

is immune thrombocytopenic purpura (ITP). Pediatric ITP differs from adult ITP in that platelet counts are often lower, with less likelihood of life-threatening hemorrhage or associated autoimmune disorders, such as systemic lupus erythematosus (21). Spontaneous resolution without treatment usually occurs within 6 months and bone marrow evaluation is only indicated if platelet counts do not return to normal, particularly with therapy. A number of disorders cause reduced platelet counts in adults including, but not limited to, metabolic syndromes, toxin/drug exposure, autoimmune disorders, and acquired problems of bone marrow function (22). Therapy in the adult population, therefore, depends on elucidating the underlying pathophysiology, which often requires bone marrow evaluation.

Severe neutropenia in a child is frequently transitory, whereas in adults it may be a harbinger of a significant bone marrow problem when not linked to recent drug exposure (17). A careful medication history, including both prescribed and over-the-counter medicines, is critical in this scenario. Even mild neutropenia in an adult who presents with splenomegaly and no evidence of cirrhosis, chronic hepatitis, autoimmune disorder, or human immunodeficiency virus (HIV) infection, commonly requires a bone marrow examination to exclude a lymphoproliferative or myeloproliferative disorder.

Anemia is the most common cytopenia for which a bone marrow examination is performed in the adult population. In contrast, Fahri et al. (16) found only 2 percent of bone marrow evaluations were performed for anemia in children less than 12 years of age. The diagnosis in 60 percent of these was transient erythroblastopenia of childhood (fig. 3-10).

Bicytopenias and pancytopenias may be caused by antibody formation or infection (20); however, a more serious bone marrow process, such as a congenital hematopoietic disorder in children, or leukemia, aplastic anemia, or a myelodysplastic syndrome in all age groups, must be considered. A bone marrow evaluation is generally indicated when two or more lineages are abnormal, except in clear diagnoses (thrombotic thrombocytopenic purpura, hemolytic uremic syndrome, drug effect, excess alcohol consumption). The exception is mild multilineage cytopenias in asymptomatic elderly patients whose bone marrow evaluations are seldom contributory to care. Stable cytopenias in these patients are often the result of medications, alcohol consumption, or poorly described autoimmune-mediated mechanisms; therefore, monitoring cell counts usually suffices, with bone marrow evaluation held for deterioration or unexplained alterations in counts (18).

Bone marrow evaluation is rarely revealing for increased cell counts involving a single lineage unless unexplained splenomegaly is present, a chronic myeloproliferative disorder is of concern, or abnormal circulating cells are identified (i.e., blasts, lymphoma cells). The majority of patients with myeloproliferative disorders have at least two increased lineages. An exception is chronic idiopathic myelofibrosis, wherein the finding of leukoerythroblastic features or tear drop-shaped RBCs (dacryocytes) is significant (fig. 3-11). Early chronic myelogenous leukemia may present with thrombocytosis (and basophilia) prior to an increase in WBCs (19). Flow cytometric analysis of peripheral blood may alleviate the need for bone marrow evaluation for particular lymphoproliferative disorders (i.e., chronic lymphocytic leukemia).

The appearance of the cells in the peripheral blood smear provides information regarding the

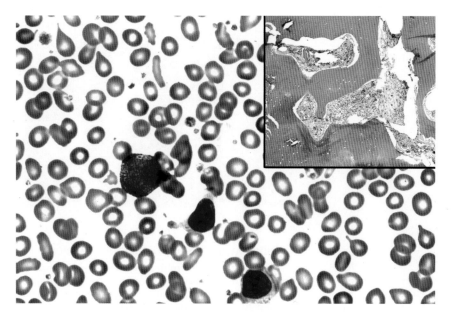

Figure 3-11

CHRONIC IDIOPATHIC MYELOFIBROSIS

Tear drop–shaped RBCs (dacrocytes) and neutrophilic myeloid precursors are present in the peripheral blood smear of this young woman with chronic idiopathic myelofibrosis. The biopsy shows marked osteosclerosis and bone marrow fibrosis (insert) (Wright and hematoxylin and eosin [H&E] stains).

underlying pathologic process, especially for patients with anemia. Determining the size and color (hemoglobinization) of RBCs is imperative for the investigation of RBC production disorders (hypochromic microcytic, normochromic normocytic versus macrocytic) (see chapter 4). The shape of the RBCs helps to elucidate the etiology of a hemolytic anemia (sickle cells, bite cells, spherocytes, schistocytes). In congenital disorders, the appearance of cells may be diagnostic, such as the bilobed or nonsegmented neutrophil nuclei of the Pelger-Hüet anomaly, or the giant cytoplasmic granules seen in leukocytes of Chediak-Higashi syndrome. Less specific features, including increased activated lymphocytes or toxic changes in neutrophils, support an underlying reactive process. Lastly, the observation of cellular alterations in one lineage may serve to explain aberrations in a different lineage. For example, the presence of Howell-Jolly bodies in RBCs of a patient with mild thrombocytosis indicates asplenia as the likely cause for the extra platelets in peripheral circulation (fig. 3-12).

BONE MARROW EVALUATION

Overview

Bone marrow evaluations are indicated when peripheral blood abnormalities are not explainable by the clinical, physical, or laboratory findings (25,28). The importance of the clinical history

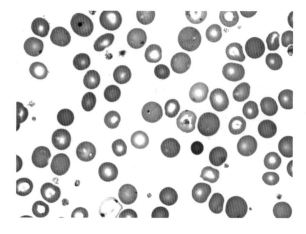

Fig 3-12

ASPLENIA

Mild thrombocytosis in a patient who underwent splenectomy for splenic marginal zone lymphoma. The RBCs contain multiple inclusions including Howell-Jolly bodies and Pappenheimer bodies. Polychromasia and spherocytes are also present (Wright stain).

cannot be overemphasized and should include at the minimum information about past and present illnesses, with additional questions as listed in Table 3-3. If a decision is made not to perform a bone marrow biopsy based on the initial compilation of data, this decision should be reexamined any time the clinical course does not follow the initial presumptive diagnosis (e.g., ITP unresponsive to appropriate therapy). Well-prepared and -stained bone marrow smears

Table 3-3

CLINICAL INFORMATION REQUIRED FOR ADEQUATE BONE MARROW INTERPRETATION

Type and duration of symptomatology including fever, night sweats, weight loss

Distribution of disease

Physical findings including ecchymoses, petechia, jaundice, dysmorphic features, splenomegaly, lymphadenopathy, or other abnormalities

Occupational history and history of exposures to radiation, organic chemicals, heavy metals, current drugs/medications, herbal or cytokine therapy

Recent travel history

Recent exposure to infectious individuals

Personal medical history

Family medical history

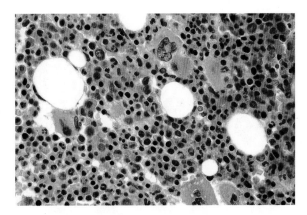

Fig 3-13

IDIOPATHIC THROMBOCYTOPENIC PURPURA

Bone marrow biopsy from a 5-year-old boy with marked thrombocytopenia shows increased megakaryocytes, consistent with the clinical history of immune thrombocytopenic purpura (ITP) (H&E stain).

and biopsy sections are essential for the best interpretation and it is the pathologist's responsibility to optimize the fixation, decalcification, and staining procedures (see chapter 2, Table 2-3). Greater reliance on alternative testing (flow cytometry, immunohistochemistry) is required when bone marrow preparations are of poor quality.

The most common indications for a bone marrow examination are described in chapter 2 (see Table 2-1). Even when a bone marrow biopsy is being performed for the evaluation of a suspected non-neoplastic disorder, neoplastic processes must first be excluded by morphologic evaluation and perhaps ancillary testing (27). The bone marrow analysis then shifts to the assessment of hematopoietic tissue, stroma, and bone, as detailed in chapters 1 and 2. Similar to the peripheral blood examination, a systematic review of aspirate smears and touch imprints for cell composition and cytology, and verification of appropriate maturation is required (23). Evaluation of both storage and erythroid iron incorporation is best made on an iron-stained aspirate smear or imprint preparation. Bone marrow cellularity is then better determined in the clot and core biopsy sections, with confirmation of cell composition, enumeration of megakaryocytes (normally 2 to 4 per 40X high-power fields), and evaluation of stroma, vessels, bone, and abnormal infiltrates (24). When the material is inadequate or of poor technical quality, this should be commented upon

for relevant preparations. Anything considered abnormal or unusual should also be described (e.g., organisms, appearance of histiocytes). Table 3-4 lists key parameters to evaluate for the most common non-neoplastic disorders that prompt a bone marrow examination.

Bone marrow reports must be easy for the clinicians to read and the results described in an orderly manner. The findings pertinent to the clinical question for which the bone marrow examination was performed should be synthesized as part of the diagnosis and final comment. The bone marrow findings should also correlate with the peripheral blood findings or be explainable by the pathologic process present. For instance, megakaryocytic hyperplasia is expected in patients with thrombocytosis, whereas the discordant finding of megakaryocytic hyperplasia and thrombocytopenia may occur secondary to platelet redistribution (splenomegaly) or destruction (ITP) (fig. 3-13). Common causes for discrepancies between peripheral blood and bone marrow findings, or between bone marrow aspirate and biopsy findings, are given in Table 3-5 (26).

Importance of Bone Marrow Cellularity

Special consideration for age-related changes is of utmost importance in the interpretation of bone marrow hematopoietic tissue, as the number and proportion of cells change with age (see Appendix). Overall, hematopoietic tissue and

Table 3-4

FOCUS OF BONE MARROW EXAMINATION FOR SELECTED NON-NEOPLASTIC INDICATIONS

Peripheral Blood Indication for Bone Marrow Examination	Primary Focus of Bone Marrow Examination after Exclusion of Neoplastic Processes

Cytopenia(s) of all types	Evaluate pertinent cell lineage(s)
	  increased, adequate, or decreased
	  appropriate maturation, left shift

Microcytic anemia	Iron studies
	  adequate or decreased storage iron
	  adequate or decreased erythroid iron incorporation (10-15% of normoblasts
	    normally contain 1-2 siderotic granules)

Infection or fever of unknown origin, or immunocompromised individuals	Granulomas, necrosis, lymphohistiocytic aggregates, histiocytic infiltrates, organism stains

Metabolic or autoimmune disorders	Vessels and stroma
	  thrombi (microangiopathic process)
	  vasculitis
	  serous fat atrophy
	  brown fat (diabetes)
	  reticulin fibrosis (autoimmune, postinfarction)
	Lymphoid aggregates, plasmacytosis, granulomas

Congenital hematologic disorders Sickle cell anemia	Necrosis, thrombosis
Lipid/glycogen storage disease	Histiocytic infiltrates[a]
Metabolic bone disease	Trabecular bone osteopenia, normal, osteomalacia Osteoclast and osteoblast number and distribution

[a]Definitive diagnosis of a storage disease requires additional testing for the actual biochemical defect.

Table 3-5

CAUSES OF DISCREPANCIES BETWEEN PERIPHERAL BLOOD AND BONE MARROW FINDINGS

Bone Marrow	Peripheral Blood	Potential Causes
Markedly hypocellular bone marrow	Peripheral blood counts intact or partially intact	Sampling: small biopsy consisting of predominately subcortical marrow in adults Previous radiation therapy to hip (or sternum) Previous biopsy site (bone remodeling, marrow injury with fibrosis) Marked aspiration artifact Focal infarction
Normal bone marrow	Abnormal cells or blasts in circulation	Focal lesions (get step sections of biopsy, sample contralateral iliac crest) Lesion at other tissue site (mediastinum, spleen, lymph node, skin)
Hypercellular bone marrow	Peripheral blood cytopenias	Ineffective hematopoiesis Peripheral cell destruction Splenomegaly
Disparate cell composition in aspirate smear and biopsy preparations		Specimen mislabeling Focal lesions or infiltrates Reticulin fibrosis Nonrepresentative tangentially taken biopsy
"Dry tap" aspiration	Variable peripheral blood counts	Bone marrow fibrosis Hypercellularity (especially due to immature cells)

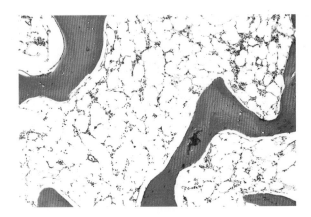

Figure 3-14

TRILINEAGE HYPOPLASIA

Markedly hypocellular bone marrow from 2-year-old female with myeloid, erythroid, and megakaryocytic (trilineage) hypoplasia (H&E stain).

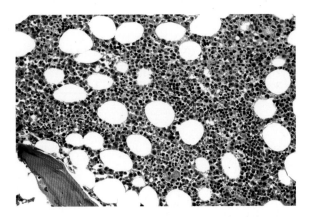

Figure 3-15

EOSINOPHILIC MYELOID HYPERPLASIA

Hypercellular bone marrow from 71-year-old male with eosinophilic myeloid hyperplasia (H&E stain).

Figure 3-16

INCREASED PLASMA CELLS POSITIVE FOR CD138

Normocellular bone marrow clot section from a middle-aged patient with plasma cell myeloma. Myeloid and erythroid hypoplasias are present due to the significant plasma cell infiltrate highlighted by CD138 (insert) (H&E, immunoperoxidase for CD138).

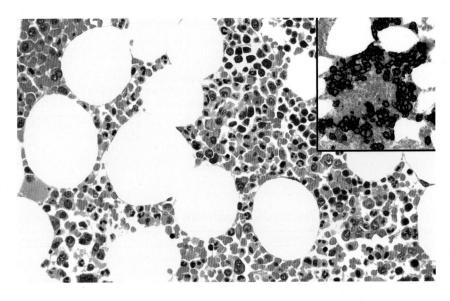

bone mass decrease with age, accompanied by an increase in the number and size of fat cells, which are disproportionately seen in subcortical regions (30). Cellularity is an estimate of the percentage of cells occupying the marrow between bony trabeculae (in contrast to fat, fibrosis, gelatinous transformation, amyloid, or necrosis). Cells are often unevenly distributed in the bone marrow space of adults, and an estimate of average cellularity should exclude the hypocellular subcortical regions normally seen with aging. Cellularity must be compared to age-related norms and documented as being normocellular, hypercellular, or hypocellular (for age), with the corresponding lineage(s) responsible for any alterations described (e.g., myeloid hyperplasia, erythroid hypoplasia) (figs. 3-14, 3-15). A normocellular bone marrow may have lineage-specific hyperplasia and hypoplasia when hypoplasia of one lineage is offset by hyperplasia of another or when an abnormal infiltrate accounts for a significant fraction of the cellularity (fig. 3-16). Knowledge of an absolute increase or decrease in a lineage is of more value than a relative change for deliberation of the underlying etiology.

Once the bone marrow lineage(s) of interest is correctly identified, the appropriate section in this Fascicle can be utilized to further guide the morphologic assessment that differentiates between the diagnostic possibilities. One example is marked erythroid hypoplasia in a child. An underlying parvovirus infection can be recognized by the identification of viral inclusions in erythroblasts and the absence of erythroid maturation (see chapters 4 and 10 for illustrations) (29). However, viral inclusions may not be seen in all cases and appropriate documentation of the marked erythroid hypoplasia with minimal maturation prompts the clinician to pursue additional testing, such as polymerase chain reaction for parvovirus DNA, which may then establish the correct etiology.

Interpretation of Pediatric Bone Marrow Specimens

In the neonatal period, a bone marrow evaluation is primarily used as a tool for assessment of severe and unexplained cytopenias, with the exception of staging for a known neoplasm or for evaluation of a congenital leukemia suspected by a peripheral blood review. Myeloid precursors dominate the bone marrows of normal full-term infants, comprising approximately two thirds of the cellularity at birth but falling to approximately one third of cellularity by 1 month of age (39). Lymphocyte percentages have the opposite trend and account for an average of 15 percent of cellularity at birth and increase up to almost half of bone marrow cellularity by 1 month of age. This expanded lymphocyte population remains stable until approximately 18 months of age, paralleling the peripheral blood findings. Of importance in the evaluation of bone marrows in this age group is the realization that a significant subset of the expanded lymphocyte population is immature B cells (hematogones), which must be differentiated from acute lymphoblastic leukemia (fig. 3-17). These cells are typically not evident in the peripheral blood. Hematogones average 9 percent of the bone marrow cellularity in children less than 2 years of age, dropping to 3.9 percent of cells by 2 to 5 years of age (34). This percentage greatly increases in certain disease states, making it extremely important to distinguish this reactive population from acute leukemia through morphologic review combined with immunophenotypic characteristics and architectural distribution in the bone marrow (see chapter 8) (37).

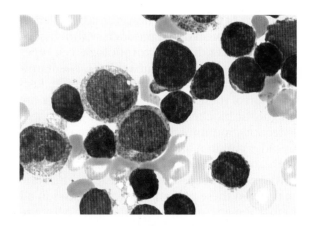

Figure 3-17

HEMATOGONES

This bone marrow aspirate smear shows increased hematogones (Wright stain).

Cytopenias in neonates may be the consequence of maternal factors (medication, infections, hypertension, blood incompatibilities) or obstetric factors (fetal blood loss), in addition to constitutional disorders. These need to be taken into account in the final interpretation of the findings.

Less is known about the bone marrow composition of premature infants. One study suggests that hematogones are the most common lymphoid population in living premature infants, comprising an average of one third of all bone marrow cells, but with a broad range that varies from 10 to 60 percent (38). If hematogones are not recognized as a common component of bone marrow in this age group, these cells may be misinterpreted as a potentially neoplastic infiltrate.

After the neonatal period, T cells predominate in the bone marrow of children (and adults), with hematogone populations primarily seen in association with specific disorders (viral infections, childhood neoplasms, cytopenias) (see chapter 8) (33). Congenital disorders enter more prominently into the differential considerations for hematologic abnormalities during infancy and childhood, and knowledge of the pertinent family history and unusual clinical findings, such as dysmorphic physical features, is important. When assessing for hereditary disorders, careful evaluation of all cell lineages is required (35). For instance, monocytes/histiocytes resembling "storage" cells are seen in a number of conditions; however, accumulation of abnormal breakdown products within histiocytes produces distinct morphologic cell types in the bone marrow (Gaucher cells, Niemann-Pick histiocytes) (fig. 3-18) (see chapter 9). Recognition of these cells allows for the appropriate diagnostic biochemical assays to be performed. Infectious mononucleosis must be considered in older children and adolescents who present with sore throat and fatigue, even when the initial monospot test is negative (32). The bone marrow in these patients shows increases in all hematopoietic elements, sometimes with the presence of granulomas and absence of a significant lymphoid infiltrate (see chapter 10).

Pediatric bone marrows have active bone production and remodeling, with the presence of osteoblasts and occasional osteoclasts. With the exception of patients with renal or endocrine complications, additional or more profound bony alterations in this age group are often congenital. The presence of osteosclerosis is related to osteopetrosis, carbonic anhydrase II deficiency, and pycnodysostosis (31,36). Osteopenia occurs with osteogenesis imperfecta, Marfan syndrome, Ehlers-Danlos syndrome, and homocystinuria (see chapters 9 and 11 for illustrations) (40).

Interpretation of Adult Bone Marrow Specimens

With advancing age, the bone marrow cellularity decreases in association with a reduction in trabecular bone volume and the number of associated endosteal cells and osteocytes (see Appendix). A study of 4,902 bone marrow evaluations in adults referred to a tertiary center found that 75 percent of the patients were referred for staging of carcinoma or lymphoma; evaluation for acute leukemia; or for cytopenias (17 percent), particularly anemia (44 percent of cytopenias) (42). This highlights the greater emphasis on evaluation for neoplastic processes as people age (45).

Infiltrating lymphocytes in adult bone marrow reflect the proportions seen in peripheral blood, with T cells accounting for 65 to 75 percent and B cells for 10 to 15 percent of bone marrow lymphocytes (47). Lymphoid aggregates increase in frequency after 50 years of age, and reach an incidence of 20 to 40 percent in elderly

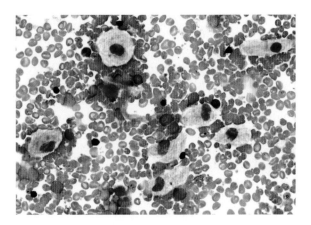

Figure 3-18

GAUCHER DISEASE

Large histiocytes with striated tubular-shaped inclusion bodies, consistent with Gaucher cells, are present in the bone marrow aspirate smear of a patient with Gaucher disease (Wright stain). (Courtesy of P. Izadi, Los Angeles, CA.)

patients (46). The incidence is also increased in association with immune or hematologic disorders, systemic infections, and drug therapy (see chapter 8) (50). A random rather than paratrabecular distribution, well-delineated outlines, close association with small blood vessels, and polymorphous composition with varying numbers of associated histiocytes, mast cells, eosinophils, and plasma cells help to distinguish reactive lymphoid aggregates from lymphoma (fig. 3-19) (51). Germinal centers are rare and more common in females than males (ratio, 5 to 1), and in association with follicular lymphoma (41,44). Reticulin fibers are intertwined with lymphocytes in aggregates, making the associated lymphocytes more difficult to aspirate than the normal bone marrow elements. Lipogranulomas are also a common finding in the elderly (see chapters 8 and 9 for illustrations) (49).

Increased monocyte/histiocyte populations in noninfected adults are most often seen in conditions with high cell turnover and ineffective hematopoiesis. Increased storage iron in untreated patients is commonly pathogenic (anemia of chronic disease or myelodysplasia) or may be seen in hemochromatosis.

Bone mass peaks between 20 to 30 years of age, and loss may begin as early as the 3rd decade depending on the patient's genetic background, sex, weight, lifestyle, medications, and other

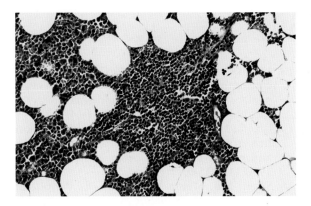

Figure 3-19

BENIGN LYMPHOID AGGREGATE

A benign lymphoid aggregate in the bone marrow clot section is relatively well-circumscribed, associated with small blood vessels, and composed of a polymorphous population of lymphocytes (H&E stain).

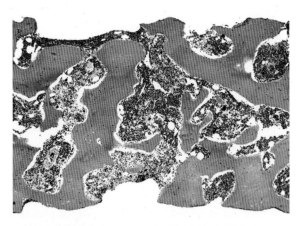

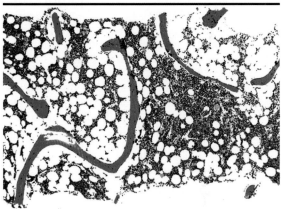

Figure 3-20

BONE ALTERATIONS

Bone marrow core biopsies from patients with chronic myeloproliferative disorders show alterations in bone thickness including osteosclerosis (top) and osteopenia (bottom) (H&E stain).

factors. The presence of osteoclasts and osteoblasts is unusual in older individuals. These are seen in disorders with unbalanced bony remodeling, such as Paget disease (thickened bone), renal osteodystrophy, primary hyperparathyroidism, and metastatic bone disease (48). Osteosclerosis is found in adults with endocrine disorders, primary hematopoietic disorders, and those taking certain medications, while osteopenia is common in postmenstrual women, immobilized individuals, and those with metabolic, nutritional, and gastrointestinal disorders (fig. 3-20) (see chapters 9 and 11 for illustrations) (43).

DOCUMENTATION

Information gleaned from astute observation of all parts of the peripheral blood and bone marrow examination must be documented, as even subtle findings may hold the clue to the underlying pathology (e.g., circulating vacuolated lymphocytes in rare storage diseases). Bone marrow is one of the few specimens for which a specific diagnosis may be difficult to ascertain, particularly in nonneoplastic conditions, and learning to recognize the normal and describe the abnormal is often the best approach. Providing differential considerations in a comment is preferable to forcing a diagnosis when findings are not specific. Based on the bone marrow results, additional directed

testing may then provide the answer that leads to a final diagnosis. Therefore, incomplete documentation of even normal findings limits the data for others to review and compile. Poor specimen quality also leads to significant data limitations so every attempt must be made to optimize handling, processing, and staining of peripheral blood and bone marrow specimens. Overinterpretation of difficult to read or inadequate specimens is worse than no interpretation and examination of additional material should be requested when clinically indicated.

REFERENCES

White Blood Cells

1. Anderson G, Smith VV, Malone M, Sebire NJ. Blood film examination for vacuolated lymphocytes in the diagnosis of metabolic disorders; retrospective experience of more than 2,500 cases from a single centre. J Clin Pathol 2005;58:1305-10.
2. Chetty-Raju N, Cook R, Erber WN. Vacuolated neutrophils in ethanol toxicity. Br J Haematol 2004;127:478.
3. Kuijpers TW, Maianski NA, Tool AT, et al. Apoptotic neutrophils in the circulation of patients with glycogen storage disease type 1b (GSD1b). Blood 2003;101:5021-4.
4. Shiflett SL, Kaplan J, Ward DM. Chediak-Higashi syndrome: a rare disorder of lysosomes and lysosome related organelles. Pigment Cell Res 2002;15:251-7.
5. von Bassewitz DB, Bremer HJ, Bourgeois M, Grobe H, Stoermer J. Vacuolated lymphocytes in type II glycogenosis—a diagnostic approach? Eur J Pediatr 1977;127:1-7.

Platelets

6. Bowles KM, Cooke LJ, Richards EM, Baglin TP. Platelet size has diagnostic predictive value in patients with thrombocytopenia. Clin Lab Haematol 2005;27:370-3.
7. Cohen AM, Cycowitz Z, Mittelman M, Lewinski UH, Gardyn J. The incidence of pseudothrombocytopenia in automatic blood analyzers. Haematologia (Budap) 2000;30:117-21.
8. Fiorin F, Steffan A, Pradella P, Bizzaro N, Potenza R, DeAngelis V. IgG platelet antibodies in EDTA-dependent pseudothrombocytopenia bind to platelet membrane glycoprotein IIb. Am J Clin Pathol 1998;110:178-83.
9. Hsieh AT, Chao TY, Chen YC. Pseudothrombocytopenia associated with infectious mononucleosis. Arch Pathol Lab Med 2003;127:e17-8.
10. Orange JS, Stone KD, Turvey SE, Krzewski K. The Wiskott-Aldrich syndrome. Cell Mol Life Sci 2004;61:2361-85.
11. Wool RL, Coleman TA, Hamill RL. Abciximab-associated pseudothrombocytopenia. Am J Med 2002;113:697-8.

Age-Related Factors

12. Cheng CK, Chan J, Cembrowski GS, van Assendelft OW. Complete blood count reference interval diagrams derived from NHANES III: stratification by age, sex, and race. Lab Hematol 2004;10:42-53.

13. Latvala J, Parkkila S, Niemela O. Excess alcohol consumption is common in patients with cytopenia: studies in blood and bone marrow cells. Alcohol Clin Exp Res 2004;28:619-24.
14. Saxena S, Wong ET. Heterogeneity of common hematologic parameters among racial, ethnic, and gender subgroups. Arch Pathol Lab Med 1990;114:715-9.
15. Streiff MB, Mehta S, Thomas DL. Peripheral blood count abnormalities among patients with hepatitis C in the United States. Hepatology 2002;35:947-52.

Additional Considerations

16. Farhi DC, Luebbers EL, Rosenthal NS. Bone marrow biopsy findings in childhood anemia: prevalence of transient erythroblastopenia of childhood. Arch Pathol Lab Med 1998;122:638-41.
17. Foucar K, Duncan MH, Smith KJ. Practical approach to the investigation of neutropenia. Clin Lab Med 1993;13:879-94.
18. Izaks GJ, Remarque EJ, Becker SV, Westendorp RG. Lymphocyte count and mortality risk in older persons. The Leiden 85-Plus Study. J Am Geriatr Soc 2003;51:1461-5.
19. Kamada N, Uchino H. Chronologic sequence in appearance of clinical and laboratory findings characteristic of chronic myelocytic leukemia. Blood 1978;51:843-50.
20. Malyangu E, Abayomi EA, Adewuyi J, Coutts AM. AIDS is now the commonest clinical condition associated with multilineage blood cytopenia in a central referral hospital in Zimbabwe. Cent Afr J Med 2000;46:59-61.
21. Tarantino MD, Buchanan GR. The pros and cons of drug therapy for immune thrombocytopenic purpura in children. Hematol Oncol Clin North Am 2004;18:1301-14, viii.
22. van den Bemt PM, Meyboom RH, Egberts AC. Drug-induced immune thrombocytopenia. Drug Saf 2004;27:1243-52.

Bone Marrow Evaluation—Overview

23. Aboul-Nasr R, Estey EH, Kantarjian HM, et al. Comparison of touch imprints with aspirate smears for evaluating bone marrow specimens. Am J Clin Pathol 1999;111:753-8.
24. Brynes RK, McKenna RW, Sundberg RD. Bone marrow aspiration and trephine biopsy. An approach to a thorough study. Am J Clin Pathol 1978;70:753-9.

25. Foucar K. Bone marrow examination: indications and techniques. Bone marrow pathology, 2nd ed. Chicago: ASCP Press; 2001:30-48.

26. Navone R, Colombano MT. Histopathological trephine biopsy findings in cases of 'dry tap' bone marrow aspirations. Appl Pathol 1984;2: 264-71.

27. Ozkalemkas F, Ali R, Ozkocaman V, et al. The bone marrow aspirate and biopsy in the diagnosis of unsuspected nonhematologic malignancy: a clinical study of 19 cases. BMC Cancer 2005; 5:144.

28. Sills RH. Indications for bone marrow examination. Pediatr Rev 1995;16:226-8.

Importance of Bone Marrow Cellularity

29. Garewal G, Ahluwalia J, Das R, Marwaha RK. Parvovirus B19-associated transient red cell aplasia in children: the role of bone marrow examination in unusual presentations. Pediatr Hematol Oncol 2004;21:505-11.

30. Rozman C, Reverter JC, Feliu E, Berga L, Rozman M, Climent C. Variations of fat tissue fraction in abnormal human bone marrow depend both on size and number of adipocytes: a stereologic study. Blood 1990;76:892-5.

Interpretation of Pediatric Bone Marrows

31. Bruder E, Stallmach T, Peier K, Superti-Furga A, Vezzoni P. Osteoclast morphology in autosomal recessive malignant osteopetrosis due to a TCIRG1 gene mutation. Pediatr Pathol Mol Med 2003;22:3-9.

32. Ebell MH. Epstein-Barr virus infectious mononucleosis. Am Fam Physician 2004;70:1279-87.

33. McKenna RW, Asplund SL, Kroft SH. Immunophenotypic analysis of hematogones (B-lymphocyte precursors) and neoplastic lymphoblasts by 4-color flow cytometry. Leuk Lymphoma 2004;45:277-85.

34. McKenna RW, Washington LT, Aquino DB, Picker LJ, Kroft SH. Immunophenotypic analysis of hematogones (B-lymphocyte precursors) in 662 consecutive bone marrow specimens by 4-color flow cytometry. Blood 2001;98:2498-507.

35. Nurden AT. Qualitative disorders of platelets and megakaryocytes. J Thromb Haemost 2005; 3:1773-82.

36. Quarello P, Forni M, Barberis L, et al. Severe malignant osteopetrosis caused by a GL gene mutation. J Bone Miner Res 2004;19:1194-9.

37. Rimsza L, Larson R, Winter S, et al. Benign hematogone-rich lymphoid proliferations can be distinguished from B-lineage acute lymphoblastic leukemia by integration of morphology, immunophenotype, adhesion molecule expression, and architectural features. Am J Clin Pathol 2000;114:66-75.

38. Rimsza LM, Douglas VK, Tighe P, et al. Benign B-cell precursors (hematogones) are the predominant lymphoid population in the bone marrow of preterm infants. Biol Neonate 2004;86:247-53.

39. Rosse C, Kraemer MJ, Dillon TL, McFarland R, Smith NJ. Bone marrow cell populations of normal infants; the predominance of lymphocytes. J Lab Clin Med 1977;89:1225-40.

40. Vignery A. Bone cell defects in osteogenesis imperfecta. Connect Tissue Res 1995;31:275-8.

Interpretation of Adult Bone Marrows

41. Arber DA, George TI. Bone marrow biopsy involvement by non-Hodgkin's lymphoma: frequency of lymphoma types, patterns, blood involvement, and discordance with other sites in 450 specimens. Am J Surg Pathol 2005;29:1549-57.

42. Barekman CL, Fair KP, Cotelingam JD. Comparative utility of diagnostic bone-marrow components: a 10-year study. Am J Hematol 1997;56:37-41.

43. Chakkalakal DA. Alcohol-induced bone loss and deficient bone repair. Alcohol Clin Exp Res 2005;29:2077-90.

44. Farhi DC. Germinal centers in the bone marrow. Hematol Pathol 1989;3:133-6.

45. Imbert M, Scoazec JY, Mary JY, Jouzult H, Rochant H, Sultan C. Adult patients presenting with pancytopenia: a reappraisal of underlying pathology and diagnostic procedures in 213 cases. Hematol Pathol 1989;3:159-67.

46. Navone R, Valpreda M, Pich A. Lymphoid nodules and nodular lymphoid hyperplasia in bone marrow biopsies. Acta Haematol 1985;74:19-22.

47. O'Donnell LR, Alder SL, Balis UJ, Perkins SL, Kjeldsberg CR. Immunohistochemical reference ranges for B lymphocytes in bone marrow biopsy paraffin sections. Am J Clin Pathol 1995;104:517-23.

48. Reddy SV. Etiologic factors in Paget's disease of bone. Cell Mol Life Sci 2006;63:391-8.

49. Rywlin AM, Ortega R. Lipid granulomas of the bone marrow. Am J Clin Pathol 1972;57:457-62.

50. Thiele J, Kvasnicka HM, Schmitt-Graeff A, et al. Bone marrow changes in chronic myelogenous leukaemia after long-term treatment with the tyrosine kinase inhibitor STI571: an immunohistochemical study on 75 patients. Histopathology 2005;46:540-50.

51. Thiele J, Zirbes TK, Kvasnicka HM, Fischer R. Focal lymphoid aggregates (nodules) in bone marrow biopsies: differentiation between benign hyperplasia and malignant lymphoma—a practical guideline. J Clin Pathol 1999;52:294-300.

4 NON-NEOPLASTIC ERYTHROID LINEAGE DISORDERS

ERYTHROPOIESIS

As detailed in chapter 1, the production of erythrocytes is a highly regulated process, and normal red blood cell (RBC) count and hemoglobin/hematocrit levels are maintained by the appropriate balance between erythrocyte production and erythrocyte destruction (4). The commitment of progenitor cells to the erythroid lineage and their subsequent maturation are under the control of cytokines, growth factors, and bone marrow microenvironment signaling, which direct nuclear transcription factors which, in turn, direct gene expression. *GATA1* encodes a major nuclear transcription factor directing erythropoiesis (3,4,6). Erythropoietin, required for the survival, proliferation, and differentiation of erythroid progenitor cells, is an obligate growth factor for erythropoiesis (1). This growth factor is produced by specialized cells within the kidney in response to hypoxia. The binding of erythropoietin to its transmembrane protein receptor initiates intracellular events that simultaneously inhibit apoptosis while stimulating the proliferation of erythroid progenitor cells (5).

The earliest morphologically recognizable erythroid precursor cell, the erythroblast (pronormoblast), is characterized by large overall size, moderate amounts of deeply basophilic cytoplasm, and a large round nucleus with dispersed chromatin and generally inconspicuous nucleoli (fig. 4-1). Subsequent maturation of the nucleus is characterized by progressive nuclear shrinkage and pyknosis with ultimate nuclear extrusion, while cytoplasmic maturation is characterized by progressive reduction in basophilia as hemoglobin is synthesized, ultimately producing the uniformly red, hemoglobin-rich cytoplasm of a mature anuclear erythrocyte (figs. 4-2, 4-3). Immature erythrocytes, termed reticulocytes, are the initial anucleate RBC. Reticulocyte maturation into mature biconcave erythrocytes is characterized by the final synthesis of hemoglobin and other proteins, reduction in size to biconcave discoid cells, and degradation of cytoplasmic organelles (fig. 4-4) (2).

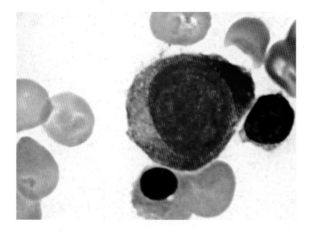

Figure 4-1

ERYTHROBLAST

High magnification shows an erythroblast with deeply basophilic cytoplasm and round nuclear contours in a bone marrow aspirate smear (Wright stain).

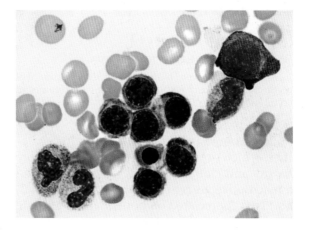

Figure 4-2

STAGES OF ERYTHROID MATURATION

Multiple stages of erythroid maturation are evident including erythroblast, basophilic normoblasts, and orthochromic normoblasts (Wright stain).

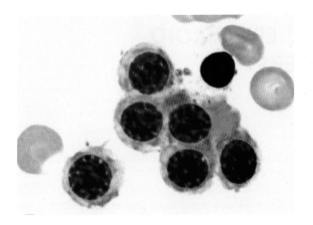

Figure 4-3

EXTRUDED ORTHOCHROME NUCLEUS

An extruded orthochrome nucleus is adjacent to polychromatophilic normoblasts (Wright stain).

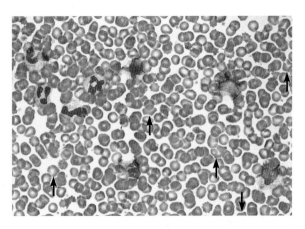

Figure 4-4

POLYCHROMASIA IN NORMAL TERM INFANT

A peripheral blood smear from a normal term infant shows prominent polychromasia indicative of abundant reticulocytes (arrows) (Wright stain).

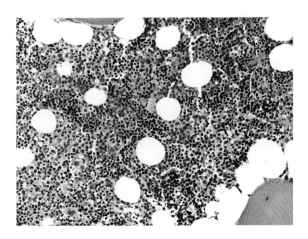

Figure 4-5

ERYTHROID HYPERPLASIA

A bone marrow core biopsy section shows prominent erythroid hyperplasia with distinct dark blue colonies of erythroid precursors (hematoxylin and eosin [H&E] stain).

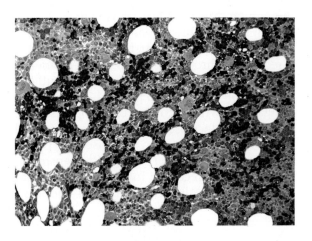

Figure 4-6

ERYTHROID HYPERPLASIA

Hemoglobin A immunoperoxidase stain highlights erythroid colony formation in a bone marrow core biopsy section.

Erythropoiesis occurs within distinct colonies, which are evident on bone marrow core biopsy and clot sections (figs. 4-5, 4-6). Often a macrophage is central within these colonies, and best appreciated on bone marrow aspirate smears (fig. 4-7). The stages of erythroid maturation have been designated as erythroblast, basophilic normoblast, orthochromic normoblast, polychromatophilic RBC (reticulocyte), and mature RBC based on the nuclear features and amount of hemoglobin present.

NUMERICAL AND MORPHOLOGIC ABNORMALITIES OF ERYTHROID ELEMENTS

Blood

Table 4-1 highlights the systematic assessment of the erythron (the total body RBC production capacity) based on both peripheral blood and bone marrow findings (see chapter 3 for a comprehensive discussion of blood smear review and chapters 1 and 2 for bone marrow evaluation). A complete blood count (CBC) is

Table 4-1

ASSESSMENT OF THE ERYTHRON[a]

Blood (Instrument-Generated Data, Morphologic Review, and Additional Tests)

Numerical assessment of RBC, Hgb, Hct[b]
  RBC size: MCV (mean corpuscular volume)
  RBC hemoglobin concentration: MCHC (mean corpuscular hemoglobin concentration)
  Uniformity of RBCs: RDW (red cell distribution width)
  New RBC production: reticulocyte count

Age-related and altitude-related normal ranges in RBC, Hgb, Hct, MCV, and reticulocyte count
Smear review for RBC morphology and unique shape abnormalities (spherocytes, fragmented RBCs, elliptocytes, sickle cells)
Smear review for RBC inclusions (malaria, babesiosis, Howell-Jolly bodies, Cabot rings)
Additional laboratory testing for iron, folate, vitamin B_{12}, and other parameters on a case-by-case basis
Bone Marrow (Morphologic Review and Additional Tests)
Overall cellularity
Proportion of erythroid elements
Maturation pyramid of erythroid lineage
Storage and erythroid iron assessment
Morphologic features of erythroid elements: left shift, megaloblastic change, dyserythropoiesis
Numerical and morphologic features of other hematopoietic lineages
Additional testing including cytogenetics and flow cytometry on a case-by-case basis

[a]Complete assessment of blood and bone marrow involves the evaluation of all cell types and all lineages. (See chapter 3 for a discussion of all lineages in blood and chapters 1 and 2 for hematopoiesis in bone marrow.)
[b]RBC = red blood cell; Hgb = hemoglobin; Hct = hematocrit.

the initial step in assessing erythropoiesis; by automated instrumentation numerous RBC parameters related to number, size, amount of hemoglobin, cell uniformity, and new erythrocyte production, are delineated. This instrument-generated data can be used to determine whether the patient has anemia or, less commonly, erythrocytosis, in addition to providing evidence to suggest nutritional deficiencies and to assess bone marrow erythrocyte production capability. Because of age-, sex-, and altitude-related variations in normal range, it is essential to correlate CBC findings with patient age and locally established normal ranges. Morphologic review of blood smears is critical for detecting distinctive shape abnormalities (spherocytes, fragmented RBCs, sickle cells, and elliptocytes) as well as finding erythrocyte inclusions such as Howell-Jolly bodies, Pappenheimer bodies, Cabot rings, or even microbial agents such as *Plasmodium* and *Babesia* organisms (figs. 4-8–4-12).

The production of new erythrocytes can be estimated by the degree of polychromasia (young erythrocytes with incomplete hemoglobiniza-

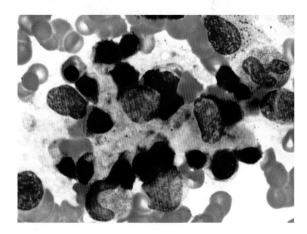

Figure 4-7

ERYTHROID CELLS SURROUNDING MACROPHAGE

Erythroid cells surround macrophages on a bone marrow aspirate smear (Wright stain).

tion), although a quantitative reticulocyte count is the best measure of effective RBC production (fig. 4-13). Since an erythrocyte abnormality may be one part of a multilineage disorder,

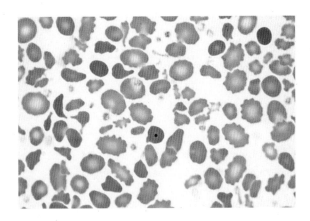

Figure 4-8

MARKED ERYTHROCYTE FRAGMENTATION

A peripheral blood smear shows marked erythrocyte fragmentation with microspherocytes in a patient with hereditary pyropoikilocytosis (Wright stain).

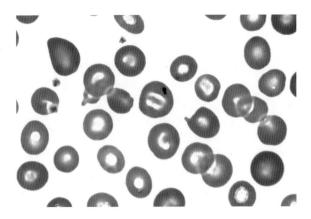

Figure 4-9

HOWELL-JOLLY BODY IN ERYTHROCYTE

A Howell-Jolly body is evident in a central reticulocyte postsplenectomy (Wright stain).

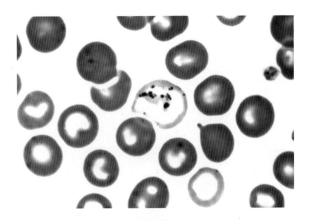

Figure 4-10

PAPPENHEIMER BODIES IN ERYTHROCYTE

Pappenheimer bodies are evident in erythrocytes in a patient with sideroblastic anemia (Wright stain).

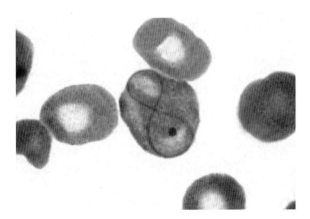

Figure 4-11

CABOT RING IN ERYTHROCYTE

An erythrocyte-containing Cabot ring is seen in a patient with high-grade myelodysplasia (Wright stain).

it is essential to evaluate all other peripheral blood elements, using both quantitative and morphologic parameters.

Bone Marrow

Bone marrow examination is not necessary for most patients with erythrocyte disorders so long as the cause of the abnormality can be adequately explained by clinical, hematologic, and other laboratory parameters. If a bone marrow examination is required, a systematic assessment of a bone marrow aspirate and core biopsy is optimal in conjunction with an evaluation of erythroid and storage iron (Table 4-1).

Evaluation of erythropoiesis integrates overall cellularity as well as the features of other lineages. The stages of maturation as well as the nuclear and cytoplasmic features of all lineages need to be reviewed. A wide spectrum of morphologic erythroid abnormalities may be evident, and these stimulate various differential diagnostic considerations. These changes include erythroid hypoplasia with scattered erythroblasts, which typifies red cell aplasias; dispersed sieve-like chromatin, which characterizes megaloblastic anemias; reduced storage and erythroid iron of iron deficiency anemia; and a host of primarily nuclear shape abnormalities such as karyorrhexis,

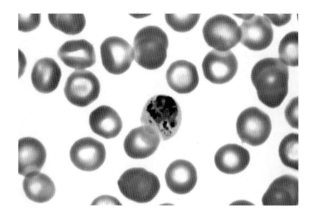

Figure 4-12

MALARIA IN ERYTHROCYTE

Plasmodium vivax organisms are present in the peripheral blood of a patient with malaria (Wright stain).

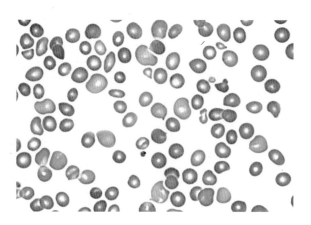

Figure 4-13

POLYCHROMASIA

Prominent polychromasia, reflecting new RBC production, is evident in this peripheral blood smear from a patient recovering from induction chemotherapy (Wright stain).

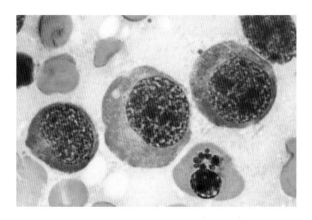

Figure 4-14

DYSERYTHROPOIESIS IN MEGALOBLASTIC ANEMIA

The sieve-like dispersed nuclear chromatin of megaloblastic erythroid precursors is evident in this bone marrow aspirate smear from a patient with megaloblastic anemia (Wright stain).

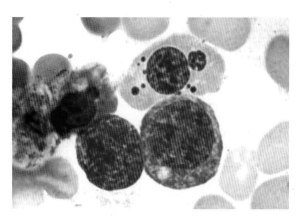

Figure 4-15

DYSERYTHROPOIESIS IN MEGALOBLASTIC ANEMIA

Karyorrhexis and nuclear lobulation of erythroid precursors are evident in this bone marrow aspirate smear from a patient with megaloblastic anemia (Wright stain).

lobulation, multinucleation, and nuclear budding, which constitute the broad designation of dyserythropoieses (figs. 4-14, 4-15) (7). These numerical and morphologic features of the erythroid lineage provide essential information for diagnostic decision making and further laboratory testing strategies in patients with non-neoplastic erythroid disorders.

OVERVIEW OF ANEMIAS

Anemia is defined as RBC count, and hemoglobin and hematocrit levels below age-related normal values. Anemias are categorized as mild, moderate, or severe based on comparison to predicted or locally established age-, sex-, and race-based normal ranges (8). A comprehensive discussion of all types of non-neoplastic anemias is beyond the scope of this Fascicle; instead, an overview of anemia classification, emphasizing strategies to approach anemia, is provided. Greater detail is given for those anemias for which bone marrow examination is typically required (8–10).

Normal hemoglobin and hematocrit values are achieved by adequate erythrocyte proliferation

Table 4-2

MECHANISTIC CLASSIFICATION OF ANEMIA

Type of Abnormality	Exemplary Types	Comments
Production defect	Red cell aplasia Aplastic anemia Bone marrow suppression from therapy, other causes	Inadequate erythroid elements in bone marrow to maintain sufficient erythrocyte production Increased erythropoietin levels, except in renal disorders associated with impaired erythropoietin production Normocytic/normochromic anemia with inadequate reticulocyte production
Cytoplasmic maturation defect	Iron deficiency anemia Sideroblastic anemia Thalassemias	Erythroid hyperplasia in bone marrow, but hemoglobin production impaired due to deficiency of iron, defective production of globin chains, or porphyrin ring defects Increased erythropoietin levels Microcytic/hypochromic anemia with inadequate reticulocyte production
Nuclear maturation defect	Megaloblastic anemia secondary to vitamin B_{12} or folate deficiency	Panhyperplasia in bone marrow. Due to deficiency of either folate or vitamin B_{12}, mitoses can't be completed, intramedullary cell death involving all lineages Florid megaloblastic changes in erythroid and myeloid lineages Erythroid lineage changes can be masked by concurrent iron deficiency Increased erythropoietin levels Macrocytic/normochromic anemia with oval macrocytes, fragmented erythrocytes and hypersegmented neutrophils
Survival defect due to intrinsic erythrocyte abnormality	Sickle cell anemia Hereditary spherocytosis/elliptocytosis Pyruvate kinase deficiency	Erythroid hyperplasia in bone marrow Increased erythropoietin levels Brisk polychromasia (reticulocytosis) in blood Erythrocyte abnormalities vary by type of disorder
Survival defect due to external (extracorpuscular) abnormality	Immune-mediated hemolytic anemia Hemolytic uremic syndrome Thrombotic thrombocytopenic purpura Other angiopathies	Erythroid hyperplasia in bone marrow Increased erythropoietin levels Brisk polychromasia (reticulocytosis) in blood Spherocytes in all subtypes with fragmentation common in angiopathies

in bone marrow, successful production of hemoglobin, and normal duration of erythrocyte survival. A mechanistic approach to diagnosing anemia segregates cases into the broad categories of erythrocyte production defects, cytoplasmic or nuclear maturation defects, or survival defects (Table 4-2). The delineation of a specific mechanism can often be determined by the integration of hematologic (erythrocyte size and hemoglobin content) features, specific erythrocyte shape abnormalities, reticulocyte count, and other laboratory/clinical parameters (direct antiglobulin test positivity, nutrient levels, splenomegaly, recent therapy, and others).

Cytoplasmic maturation defects affect only erythrocytes, while nuclear maturation defects affect all proliferating cell lineages. Production defects may be attributed to either iso-lated erythrocyte lineage abnormalities or to multilineage hematopoietic failure disorders. Erythropoietin levels are increased in virtually all types of anemia, except those that are the consequence of the failure of the kidney to produce adequate amounts of erythropoietin as in chronic renal failure.

Erythrocyte survival defects are caused by either an intrinsic RBC defect that results in decreased survival time or an extrinsic disorder such as an abnormality of blood flow caused by vascular malformations, cardiac defects, microangiopathies, or alloantibodies/autoantibodies and infectious agents. In the latter circumstance, the erythrocytes produced in the bone marrow are normal and would survive normally if transfused into another host. The decreased erythrocyte survival time is the consequence of erythrocyte disruption from these underlying disorders/conditions.

Table 4-3

CAUSAL CLASSIFICATION OF ACQUIRED ANEMIAS

Cause	Comments
Chronic infection/inflammatory disorder	Anemia of chronic disease[a] results from sustained inflammatory molecule production including interleukin 1 and hepcidin Anemia linked to interrelated proliferation, maturation, and survival defects
Nutritional deficiency	Iron deficiency results in microcytic/hypochromic anemia due to impaired hemoglobin production Folate/vitamin B_{12} deficiency results in macrocytic/normochromic anemia due to impaired mitotic activity; all proliferating lineages affected
Autoantibody production	Immune-mediated hemolytic anemia linked to collagen vascular (rheumatologic) disorders, medications, lymphoid neoplasms, and other disorders Spherocytosis and polychromasia (reticulocytosis) prominent
Turbulent blood flow	Vascular anomalies, thermal injury, and small vessel microthrombi linked to erythrocyte fragmentation, microspherocytosis, and polychromasia (reticulocytosis)
Parvovirus infection	Pure red cell aplasia results from incorporation of parvovirus into erythroid lineage nuclei resulting in cell death Anemia results if viral infection sustained as occurs in immunocompromised patients
Toxic or immune assault on bone marrow	Loss of hematopoietic elements following toxic- or immune-mediated progenitor cell destruction results in panhypoplasia with inadequate production of all hematopoietic lineages Pancytopenia with an inadequate reticulocyte response
Acute hemorrhage	Abrupt blood loss in short time period results in normocytic/normochromic anemia

[a]See chapter 11 for more details on anemia of chronic disease.

It is also helpful to classify anemias based on cause (Table 4-3). This causal classification strategy is most applicable to acquired anemias rather than genetic/constitutional anemias, which are discussed next. Anemia is a frequent development in patients with sustained infections or other chronic inflammatory conditions; anemia of chronic disease results from complex, interrelated pathophysiologic mechanisms (see next section and chapter 11). Nutritional deficiency–related anemias are commonly encountered in clinical practice, especially iron deficiency anemia. Megaloblastic anemias secondary to either folate or vitamin B_{12} (cobalamin) deficiency are important to recognize and exhibit very distinctive blood and bone marrow features (see next section). Other causes of anemia include parvovirus-induced RBC aplasia, immune-mediated or turbulent blood flow–mediated hemolytic anemia, and idiopathic or toxin-induced aplastic anemia (Table 4-3).

In addition to these pathophysiologic classification schemes, it is essential to determine whether an anemia is acquired or the result of a constitutional disorder. Patients with constitutional anemias characteristically demonstrate a common profile of features including onset at birth or early infancy, positive family history, other phenotypic abnormalities (especially common in constitutional bone marrow failure syndromes), and underlying genetic defects. Broad categories of constitutional anemias including hemoglobinopathies, erythrocyte enzyme defects, single or multilineage bone marrow failure disorders, erythrocyte membrane defect disorders, as well as miscellaneous types of constitutional anemia are listed in Table 4-4. Red cell aplasias, aplastic anemias, megaloblastic anemias, and sideroblastic anemias may be either constitutional or acquired; typically, acquired types predominate.

A pathophysiologic classification of anemia incorporating both constitutional and acquired types is presented in Table 4-5. Although this type of classification is useful, some anemias (e.g., anemia of chronic disease) have a multifactorial etiology, while in disorders such as paroxysmal nocturnal hemoglobinuria, the primary mechanism of the anemia may vary over time.

ACQUIRED ANEMIAS

Anemia of Chronic Disease

Definition. Patients with sustained infections and other immunostimulatory disorders

Table 4-4

CONSTITUTIONAL ANEMIAS

Category	Examples/Comments
Hemoglobinopathies	Thalassemias (multiple types of globin chain production defects) Sickle cell anemia Numerous other infrequent types of hemoglobinopathy
Enzyme deficiency disorders	Pyruvate kinase deficiency Glucose-6-phosphate dehydrogenase deficiency Other infrequent enzyme defect disorders
Erythrocyte membrane disorders	Hereditary spherocytosis Hereditary elliptocytosis Hereditary pyropoikilocytosis
Single or multilineage bone marrow failure disorders[a]	Diamond-Blackfan anemia (red cell aplasia) Fanconi anemia (eventual aplasia) Shwachman-Diamond syndrome (frequent aplasia) Dyskeratosis congenita (frequent aplasia) High incidence of multiorgan system anomalies
Miscellaneous types of constitutional anemias	Congenital megaloblastic anemia (multiple genetic types) Congenital sideroblastic anemia Congenital dyserythropoietic anemia (multiple types) Erythropoietic protoporphyria Orotic aciduria Other rare types

[a]See chapter 7 for detailed discussion.

commonly develop anemia about 2 to 4 months after disease onset; the designation *anemia of chronic disease* has been applied to anemias developing in this clinical situation (see also chapter 11) (12,15). Anemia of chronic disease is very common and may be the most frequently encountered type of anemia in some clinical practices.

Pathologic Findings. The hematologic profile of anemia of chronic disease has been well recognized for decades. This anemia is typically mild to moderate in severity, and the erythrocytes are generally normocytic and normochromic; the severity of the anemia tends to parallel the activity of the associated disease (14). The reticulocyte count is not appropriately elevated for the degree of anemia. Bone marrow examination demonstrates a unique disparity between storage and erythroid iron, in that storage iron is typically substantially increased, while erythroid iron is significantly reduced (fig. 4-16).

Pathogenesis. Only recently has the pathogenesis of anemia of chronic disease been elucidated. Four major pathologic processes are involved, including a mild decrease in erythrocyte survival time, a blunted erythropoietin response, impaired erythropoiesis, and pathologic

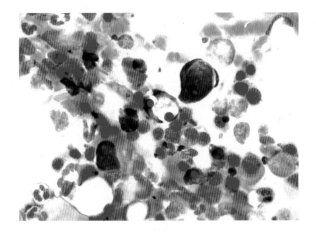

Figure 4-16

ANEMIA OF CHRONIC DISEASE: IRON STAINING PATTERN

An iron stain of a bone marrow aspirate smear shows markedly increased storage iron yet reduced erythroid iron, characteristic of anemia of chronic disease. Abundant Prussian blue–positive macrophage fragments are present. (Courtesy of Dr. C. Sever, Albuquerque, NM.)

iron homeostasis (12,14,15). Multiple cytokines and regulatory factor defects are linked to these complex interrelated pathologic processes. Major roles in producing anemia of chronic disease are postulated for the proinflammatory

Table 4-5

PATHOPHYSIOLOGIC CLASSIFICATION OF CONGENITAL AND ACQUIRED ANEMIAS[a]

Mechanism	Congenital	Acquired
Proliferation defect	Fanconi anemia Diamond-Blackfan anemia Dyskeratosis congenita Shwachman-Diamond syndrome	Aplastic anemia Red cell aplasia (some secondary to viral infection or underlying T-cell large granular lymphocytic leukemia) Anemia of chronic disease[b] Transient erythroblastopenia of childhood Bone marrow replacement by neoplasm or fibrosis Bone marrow suppression from chemotherapy, radiation, infection, or alcohol Renal failure, endocrine deficiency Paroxysmal nocturnal hemoglobinuria[c]
Maturation defect (nuclear or cytoplasmic)	Thalassemia (cytoplasmic) Congenital dyserythropoietic anemia (nuclear) Congenital sideroblastic anemia (cytoplasmic) Erythropoietic protoporphyria (cytoplasmic) Transcobalamin II deficiency (nuclear) Congenital megaloblastic anemia (nuclear) Orotic aciduria (nuclear)	Nutritional deficiency Iron (cytoplasmic) Vitamin B_{12} (nuclear) Folate (nuclear) Acquired sideroblastic anemia (cytoplasmic) Alcohol-induced (cytoplasmic)
Survival defect	Intrinsic red blood cell defects Membrane, e.g., hereditary spherocytes Enzyme, e.g., glucose-6-phosphate dehydrogenase deficiency Hemoglobin, e.g., sickle cell anemia	Intrinsic red blood cell (RBC) defect Paroxysmal nocturnal hemoglobinuria[c] Extrinsic (environmental) defects Immune-mediated hemolytic anemia: autoimmune, secondary immune, drug-related RBC fragmentation disorders: microangiopathies, thermal injury, clostridial sepsis, heart valve dysfunction, vascular malformation

[a]Data from references 8–10.
[b]Complex, multifactorial etiology includes production, maturation, and survival defects (see chapter 11).
[c]Highly variable bone marrow picture ranging from aplasia (production defect predominates) to erythroid hyperplasia (survival defect predominates).

cytokine/regulatory factors such as interleukin (IL)1, IL6, and IL10; tumor necrosis factor-alpha; transforming growth factor-beta; several interferons; and hepcidin, an iron-regulatory protein (11,13–15).

Iron Deficiency Anemia

Definition. Insufficient iron for hemoglobin production can be the consequence of inadequate intake for host requirements, accelerated iron loss, or a combination of both. Only rarely is either inadequate absorption of dietary iron or defective iron transport the primary cause of iron deficiency, although iron absorption is clearly an issue in patients with inflammatory bowel disease or malabsorption disorders associated with rapid transit time (21,25). *Iron deficiency anemia* is very common in clinical practice and may be the most common type of anemia worldwide (17,23,25,28). Key factors linked to iron deficiency anemia include inadequate iron intake, rapid growth conditions (prematurity, adolescence), pregnancy, heavy menses, and other chronic blood loss, especially from the gastrointestinal tract (18,23).

Pathologic Findings. The blood features of iron deficiency anemia include microcytic/hypochromic erythrocyte indices in conjunction with ovalocytes (fig. 4-17). The reticulocyte count is not appropriately elevated for the degree of anemia. The RBC distribution width (RDW) is typically elevated, reflecting the range in erythrocyte size that characterizes the dynamic variations in iron availability as iron deficiency evolves (19,23). Mild thrombocytosis is common in patients with iron deficiency anemia; the etiology for this association is unclear (fig. 4-18) (22).

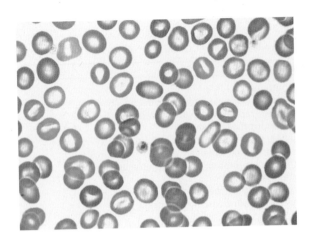

Figure 4-17

IRON DEFICIENCY ANEMIA

A peripheral blood smear from a 73-year-old woman with gastrointestinal bleeding and iron deficiency anemia shows hypochromic erythrocytes and admixed hypochromic elliptocytes (Wright stain).

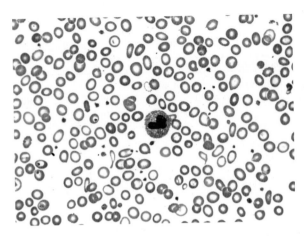

Figure 4-18

IRON DEFICIENCY ANEMIA

Thrombocytosis accompanies severe iron deficiency anemia. Microcytic hypochromic erythrocytes are present (Wright stain).

A combination of erythrocyte parameters and laboratory tests can be used to distinguish iron deficiency anemia from thalassemias and anemia of chronic disease (16,17,19,23,26). In recent years, soluble transferrin receptor levels have been used to distinguish iron deficiency anemia (increased soluble transferrin receptor levels) from other anemias, notably anemia of chronic disease (normal soluble transferrin receptor levels). Problems with this methodology, however, have been identified, and the measurement of sequential soluble transferrin receptor levels may be necessary (16,17,24). The ratio of soluble transferrin receptor levels to log ferritin may be more useful in distinguishing iron deficiency anemia (ratio over 2) from anemia of chronic disease (ratio under 1) (26).

Although bone marrow examination is not generally required in patients with straightforward iron deficiency anemia, expected findings include an abundance of maturing erythroid elements with absent storage and erythroid iron; storage and erythroid iron assessment is best performed on Prussian blue stains of bone marrow aspirate smears that contain sufficient particles. The evaluation of core biopsy specimens for iron is complicated by the possible leaching out of iron during decalcification and processing. Recently, functional iron deficiency has been noted in patients with stainable bone marrow storage iron, despite elevated soluble plasma transferrin receptor levels (20).

Differential Diagnosis. The differential diagnosis of iron deficiency anemia includes other microcytic erythrocyte disorders such as thalassemia and other hemoglobinopathies such as hemoglobin E, lead poisoning, and anemia of chronic disease (23,25). Rare disorders such as congenital sideroblastic anemia, copper deficiency–associated anemia, and congenital atransferrinemia are also characterized by microcytic anemia (23,27). The integration of clinical findings, family history, and comprehensive laboratory results can generally distinguish these microcytic anemias.

Megaloblastic Anemia

Definition. *Megaloblastic anemia* occurs when the coenzyme forms of either folate or vitamin B_{12} (cobalamin) are deficient. The resultant defective DNA synthesis impairs the ability of all proliferating cells to synthesize enough DNA per unit of time to allow for mitosis; as a consequence, ineffective hematopoiesis results in high rates of intramedullary cell death in a setting of bone marrow hypercellularity (33,37).

Although impaired production of hematopoietic elements is the major clinical manifestation of vitamin B_{12} and folate deficiency, other disorders, especially neuropsychiatric,

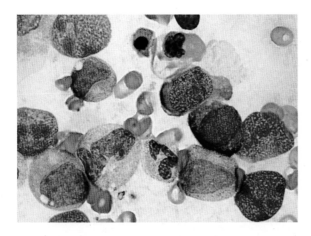

Figure 4-19

INFANTILE MEGALOBLASTIC ANEMIA

This bone marrow aspirate smear is from a 7-month-old infant exclusively breastfed by a vegan mother who developed vitamin B_{12} deficiency–associated megaloblastic anemia (Wright stain). (Courtesy of Dr. C. Kjeldsberg, Salt Lake City, UT.)

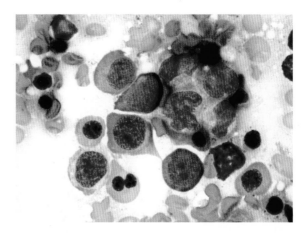

Figure 4-20

MEGALOBLASTIC ANEMIA

Prominent megaloblastic changes are evident in the granulocytic and erythroid cells in this bone marrow aspirate smear from a patient with megaloblastic anemia (Wright stain).

also can develop and even precede or occur in the absence of hematologic manifestations (33). Megaloblastic anemias may be either constitutional or acquired; acquired cases are much more commonly encountered in clinical practice. Even cases of megaloblastic anemia manifesting in infancy and early childhood are more likely to be the consequence of dietary factors (maternal or infant feeding practices) rather than constitutional factors (see below).

Except in infants, total body stores of vitamin B_{12} are abundant and are sufficient to adequately supply the host for 2 to 5 years. Likewise, except in infants, total body stores of folate are moderate and are sufficient to maintain normal cellular proliferation for approximately 3 to 5 months. In addition to lower baseline stores, folate is heat labile and is destroyed readily in the cooking process. Consequently, the incidence of folate deficiency secondary to inadequate intake is substantially greater than that of vitamin B_{12} deficiency. Because of lower baseline stores, a deficiency of either vitamin B_{12} or folate develops more rapidly in children, especially infants. Consequently, there is a clearcut association between maternal vitamin B_{12} intake and status during pregnancy and fetal storage of this vitamin during gestation; maternal dietary factors are often the cause of infantile megaloblastic anemia (33,40,43).

The diagnosis of infantile megaloblastic anemia is problematic because failure to thrive is often the only clinical abnormality (figs. 4-19–4-21). Older infants with severe vitamin B_{12} deficiency may manifest with severe pancytopenia and neurologic deficits with regression of motor functions (40). At the other age extreme, an increased incidence of megaloblastic anemia has been noted in elderly patients; cryptic neurologic/neuropsychiatric symptoms may predominate in these patients, rendering a clinical diagnosis challenging (31,32).

Pathogenesis. There are five basic mechanisms leading to vitamin B_{12} deficiency: inadequate intake, increased requirement, defective absorption, defective transport, and disorders of vitamin B_{12} metabolism. By far, the most common mechanism is defective absorption (33). Requirements for vitamin B_{12} absorption are complex and include an adequate amount of intrinsic factor, R-binders, and pancreatic enzymes, and an intact intestinal mucosa. Although abnormalities in any of these components can result in defective absorption, the one most commonly encountered in clinical practice is decreased intrinsic factor in patients with pernicious anemia, an autoimmune disorder associated with chronic atrophic gastritis and autoantibody production (33). Although vitamin B_{12} deficiency may occur secondary to insufficient dietary intake, a

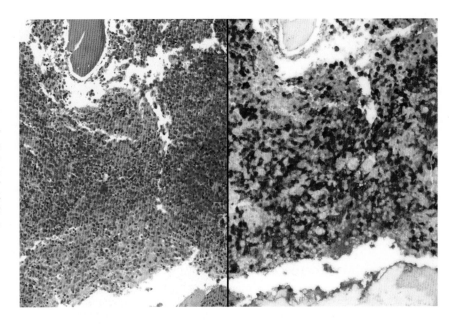

Figure 4-21

INFANTILE MEGALOBLASTIC ANEMIA, HEMOGLOBIN A

This composite of a core biopsy (left) and immunoperoxidase stain for hemoglobin A (right) is from a 7-month-old with megaloblastic anemia secondary to vitamin B_{12} deficiency (H&E and immunoperoxidase stain for HgbA). (Courtesy of Dr. X. Yao, Sacramento, CA.)

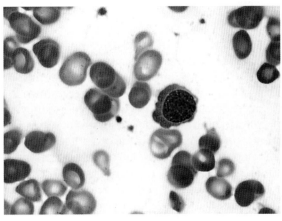

Figure 4-22

MEGALOBLASTIC ANEMIA

A peripheral blood smear shows circulating erythroid precursors with sieve-like chromatin and moderate anisopoikilocytosis (Wright stain).

stringent diet deficient in all meat, egg, and milk products must be followed for a sustained period for this to occur. Infants born to mothers following restrictive diets or to mothers with pernicious anemia have deficient vitamin B_{12} stores and may manifest severe megaloblastic anemia if fed breast milk exclusively (40).

The major causes of folate deficiency include dietary deficiency and increased requirement, although defective absorption and disorders of metabolism are occasionally responsible for folate deficiency. A dietary deficiency of folate is com-

mon in chronic alcoholics, drug addicts, and patients in low socioeconomic conditions who consume inadequate diets. Excessive cooking destroys folate. Increased folate is required by infants, pregnant and lactating women, and patients with either malignancies or chronic hemolytic anemias. Premature infants have very low folate stores and are highly susceptible to folate deficiency. Infants of mothers on restricted diets are also highly susceptible to folate deficiency, which typically manifests as failure to thrive (33).

Pathologic Findings. The prototypic peripheral blood features of megaloblastic anemia include macrocytic/normochromic anemia with oval macrocytes and disrupted erythrocytes in conjunction with pancytopenia and hypersegmented neutrophils (figs. 4-22–4-24) (29,30,33,34). Due to the combination of macrocytosis and disrupted erythrocytes, the RDW is markedly elevated in megaloblastic anemia.

Differential Diagnosis. Other causes of macrocytosis that should be considered in the differential diagnosis include drug treatments, reticulocytosis, alcohol abuse, liver disease, myelodysplasia, and rare constitutional disorders (Table 4-6) (34,38,39). With the exception of antiretroviral therapy in patients with human immunodeficiency virus (HIV)-1, a mean corpuscular value (MCV) exceeding 120 μm^3 is more characteristic of megaloblastic anemia than other macrocytic disorders (33). The florid erythroid lineage abnormalities in the blood

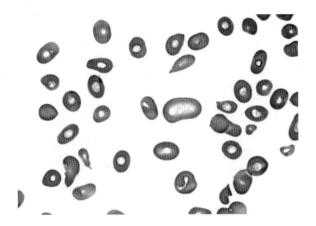

Figure 4-23

MEGALOBLASTIC ANEMIA

Profound anemia with oval macrocytes and erythrocyte fragmentation in a patient with megaloblastic anemia (Wright stain).

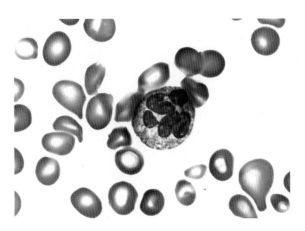

Figure 4-24

MEGALOBLASTIC ANEMIA

Hypersegmentation of neutrophils in a patient with megaloblastic anemia (Wright stain).

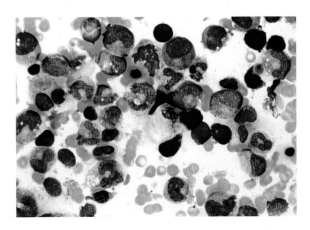

Figure 4-25

CONCURRENT IRON DEFICIENCY AND MEGALOBLASTIC ANEMIA

A hypercellular bone marrow aspirate smear from a patient with concurrent iron deficiency and folate deficiency shows striking granulocytic megaloblastic changes and less conspicuous erythroid megaloblastic changes (Wright stain).

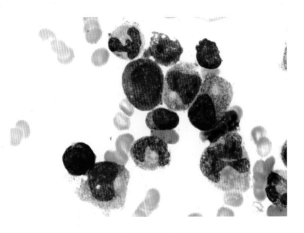

Figure 4-26

CONCURRENT IRON DEFICIENCY AND MEGALOBLASTIC ANEMIA

The bone marrow aspirate smear shows granulocytic megaloblastic changes with less conspicuous erythroid abnormalities (Wright stain).

and bone marrow of patients with megaloblastic anemia may be masked by concurrent iron deficiency (figs. 4-25, 4-26) (34).

The bone marrow in patients with florid megaloblastic anemia is characteristically markedly hypercellular, with erythroid and granulocytic hyperplasia (figs. 4-27, 4-28). Mitotic activity is abundant, but there is significant intramedullary cell death secondary to the nuclear maturation defect. The proliferating erythroid and myeloid cell lines show megaloblastic changes. In the erythroid elements, the major morphologic manifestation is nuclear-cytoplasmic asynchrony, in which the nuclei are large with finely dispersed chromatin, whereas the cytoplasm is more mature with effective hemoglobinization (fig. 4-29) (33,44). The dominant myeloid abnormalities are giantism of bands and metamyelocytes, and nuclear hypersegmentation

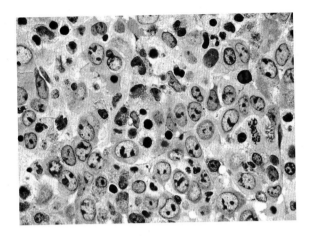

Figure 4-27

MEGALOBLASTIC ANEMIA

This hypercellular bone marrow core biopsy section is from an adult with megaloblastic anemia. Striking hyperplasia of erythroid precursor cells, dispersed nuclear chromatin, and oblong nucleoli are seen (H&E stain).

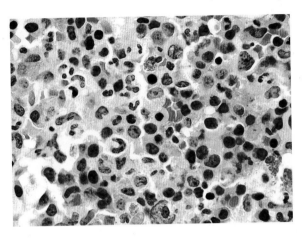

Figure 4-28

MEGALOBLASTIC ANEMIA

This hypercellular bone marrow biopsy section is from an adult with megaloblastic anemia. The erythroid and granulocytic elements are increased and giant bands are present (H&E stain).

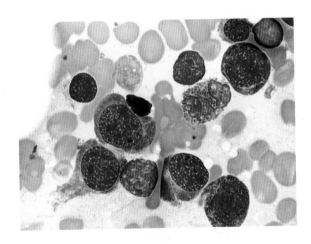

Figure 4-29

MEGALOBLASTIC ANEMIA

Finely dispersed, sieve-like nuclear chromatin characterizes the proliferating erythroid progenitor cells in a patient with megaloblastic anemia (Wright stain).

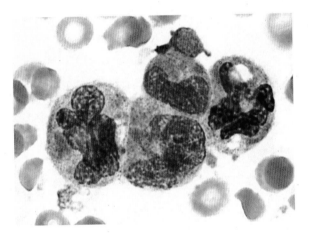

Figure 4-30

MEGALOBLASTIC ANEMIA

Marked enlargement of the band and neutrophil nuclei, along with hypersegmentation and giant bands, in a patient with megaloblastic anemia (Wright stain).

of mature granulocytes (fig. 4-30). Large megakaryocytes also have been described.

Erythroid megaloblastosis can be masked because of concomitant iron deficiency or other confounding causes of anemia, although the megaloblastic changes in the granulocytic cell line persist (see figs. 4-25, 4-26). Other causes of bone marrow megaloblastosis include both constitutional and acquired disorders (Table 4-6).

The primary laboratory tests used in the diagnosis of megaloblastic anemia are measurements of serum vitamin B_{12}, fasting serum folate, RBC folate, serum methylmalonic acid, and serum homocysteine levels (Table 4-7). Recent studies, however, suggest a lack of concordance between laboratory evidence of vitamin deficiency and response to therapy (35,41). A variety of supplementary tests provide additional sensitivity and specificity in the diagnosis of either vitamin B_{12} or folate deficiency, as well as in determining the likely cause of the vitamin B_{12} deficiency, such as pernicious anemia. These tests measure intrinsic factor antibodies, antiparietal cell antibodies, and levels of gastrin, serum lactic dehydrogenase, and homocysteine (33,36,42).

Hemolytic Anemias

Acquired hemolytic anemias are the consequence of either intrinsically defective erythrocytes or altered environmental factors. Unlike constitutional hemolytic anemias, however, acquired hemolytic anemias due to intrinsic erythrocyte defects are very uncommon. In fact, the only type of acquired hemolytic anemia due to an intrinsic erythrocyte abnormality is *paroxysmal nocturnal hemoglobinuria* (PNH), an acquired, clonal hematopoietic stem cell disorder caused by a somatic mutation of phosphatidylinositol glycan-class A (*PIG-A*) on the X chromosome (63,66). As a consequence of this mutation, glycosylphosphatidylinositol (GPI) synthesis is blocked; GPI is a critical cell membrane–anchoring constituent responsible for binding proteins to the cell membrane of hematopoietic elements. In PNH, hematopoietic cells fail to express GPI-anchored proteins, notably CD55 and CD59, which protect cells against complement-mediated destruction (54,55,63,66). Flow cytometric immunophenotyping is the method of choice to assess erythrocytes, neutrophils, monocytes, and even B lymphocytes for cell surface membrane expression of various GPI-anchored proteins (fig. 4-31) (49,63,67). The reduced expression of various anchoring proteins such as CD55 and CD59 reflects failed synthesis of GPI. In some patients with PNH,

complement-mediated nocturnal hemolysis is the main disease manifestation (figs. 4-32, 4-33) (55,65); other PNH disease manifestations include thrombosis and bone marrow failure with eventual aplasia (figs. 4-34–4-36) (47,55).

The association of PNH type cellular defects with aplastic anemia and myelodysplasia is well-recognized, although precise pathogenic mechanisms are not clearcut and likely vary by type of disease association. Autoantibody production in PNH-associated aplastic anemia

---

Table 4-6

CAUSES OF BONE MARROW MEGALOBLASTOSIS[a]

Acquired Megaloblastic Disorders

Megaloblastic anemia (vitamin B_{12} or folate deficiency)

Myelodysplastic syndromes

Acute myelogenous leukemia, especially erythroid leukemias

Chemotherapeutic agents that primarily interfere with purine or pyrimidine synthesis

Antiretroviral agents

Drugs associated with impaired absorption or other causes of decreased availability of vitamin B_{12} or folate (anticonvulsants, antibiotics, antimalarial agents, oral contraceptives, alcohol)

Toxins (benzene, arsenic)[b]

Rare Constitutional Genetic Disorders

Congenital megaloblastic anemia

Orotic aciduria

Transcobalamin II deficiency

Congenital dyserythropoietic anemia

Congenital sideroblastic anemia

Homocysteinosis

[a]Data from references 29, 33, 42, and 44.
[b]Marked karyorrhexis is also present.

Table 4-7

TESTS USEFUL IN THE DIAGNOSIS AND DISTINCTION OF VITAMIN B_{12} AND FOLATE DEFICIENCY[a]

Disorder	Serum Cobalamin	Serum Folate	RBC[b] Folate	Methylmalonic Acid (Serum)	Homocysteine (Serum)
Vitamin B_{12} deficiency	↓	NR, ↑	↓, NR	↑	↑
Folate deficiency	NR	↓	↓	NR	↑
Combined vitamin B_{12}/folate deficiency	↓	↓	↓	↑	↑

[a]Data from references 29, 33, 35, and 41. Recent studies suggest a lack of concordance between laboratory assessment of cobalamin adequacy and response to pharmacologic vitamin B_{12} therapy in that a significant number of anemic patients with laboratory values within normal range respond to vitamin B_{12} therapy (41).
[b]RBC = red blood cell; NR = normal.

Granulocyte Gate

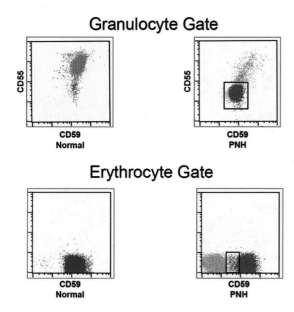

Erythrocyte Gate

Figure 4-31

FLOW CYTOMETRY FOR PAROXYSMAL NOCTURNAL HEMOGLOBINURIA (PNH)

Flow cytometric histograms compare normal populations to those with PNH. Reduced expression of surface membrane antigens is seen in the patient with PNH. (Boxes highlight abnormal populations.) (Multicolor flow cytometry for CD55 and CD59 expression.)

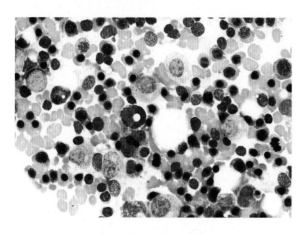

Figure 4-33

PAROXYSMAL NOCTURNAL HEMOGLOBINURIA

Marked erythroid hyperplasia in a bone marrow aspirate smear from a patient with PNH (Wright stain).

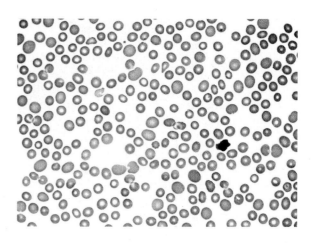

Figure 4-32

PAROXYSMAL NOCTURNAL HEMOGLOBINURIA

Peripheral blood smear shows anemia with polychromasia in patient with PNH (Wright stain).

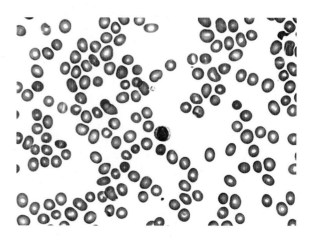

Figure 4-34

PAROXYSMAL NOCTURNAL HEMOGLOBINURIA: HYPOCELLULAR PHASE

Peripheral blood smear of the hypocellular phase shows profound anemia without significant polychromasia (Wright stain).

may result in the immune-mediated destruction of bone marrow stem cells (52).

The bone marrow in cases of PNH with dominant complement-mediated intravascular hemoly-sis exhibits hypercellularity with marked erythroid hyperplasia, without dysplastic features. Polychromasia, a peripheral blood feature, is validated by a marked increase in the reticulocyte count (see figs. 4-32, 4-33) (47,51).

Acquired hemolytic anemias secondary to extrinsic (environmental) defects are much more commonly encountered in clinical practice than intrinsic anemias. Extrinsic factor–related hemolytic anemia occurs in patients of all ages, including fetuses and neonates.

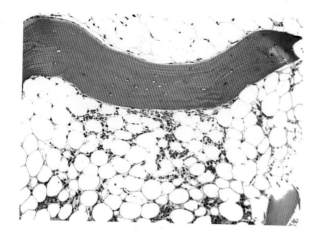

Figure 4-35

PAROXYSMAL NOCTURNAL HEMOGLOBINURIA: HYPOCELLULAR PHASE

Bone marrow core biopsy from a patient with hypoplastic PNH shows decreased overall cellularity (H&E stain).

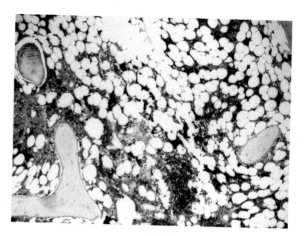

Figure 4-36

PAROXYSMAL NOCTURNAL HEMOGLOBINURIA: HYPOCELLULAR PHASE, HEMOGLOBIN A STAIN

Immunoperoxidase stain for hemoglobin A on hypocellular PNH specimen shows small islands of residual erythroid elements.

The transplacental passage of maternal immunoglobulin (Ig)G antibody directed against paternally derived fetal erythrocyte antigens produces *hemolytic disease of the newborn*, a disease that can be averted by preventing maternal sensitization to these paternally derived fetal antigens. The most common scenario is the development of anti-D antibodies in an Rh-negative mother (58,70). The mother is exposed to fetal erythrocytes from minor fetal-maternal hemorrhages that typically occur late in pregnancy or during delivery. Once sensitization occurs, there is significant risk of the immune-mediated hemolysis of fetal erythrocytes in subsequent pregnancies. Affected neonates may be severely anemic, with striking polychromasia, normoblastosis, and spherocytosis (fig. 4-37). Significant central nervous system (CNS) complications from hyperbilirubinemia occur if exchange transfusion (whether in utero or after delivery) is not promptly undertaken. The incidence of this dramatic immune-mediated hemolytic anemia has decreased markedly with the institution of Rh immune globulin therapy to prevent maternal sensitization. Recombinant anti-RhD antibody is also available for clinical use, obviating transfusion-related risks (58).

Many other types of *immune-mediated hemolytic anemia* have been described. In some cases the disorder is idiopathic; other specific associations include collagen vascular diseases, lymphoproliferative disorders, viral or myco-

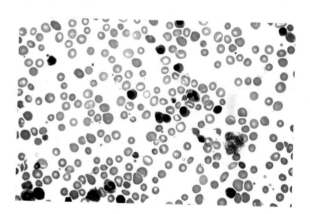

Figure 4-37

HEMOLYTIC DISEASE OF THE NEWBORN

The peripheral blood smear shows striking polychromasia, spherocytes, numerous nucleated red blood cells, and severe anemia (Wright stain).

plasma infections, immunizations, or certain medications (48,53,56,69,70). Rare cases of *autoimmune hemolytic anemia* following stem cell transplantation have been described (62). Depending upon antibody characteristics, autoimmune hemolytic anemias can be classified as warm antibody, cold agglutinin, biphasic antibody, or drug-induced subtypes (56). Successful treatment of refractory immune-mediated hemolytic anemia with rituximab, an antibody directed against CD20-positive B cells, has been documented in children and adults (68,71).

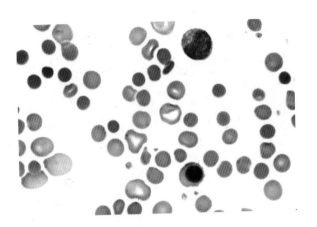

Figure 4-38

DIRECT ANTIGLOBULIN–POSITIVE HEMOLYTIC ANEMIA

Marked anemia, spherocytosis, polychromasia, and circulating erythroid precursors are seen (Wright stain).

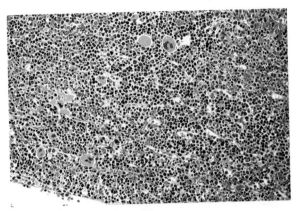

Figure 4-40

CHRONIC HEMOLYSIS

This low magnification photomicrograph of a bone marrow core biopsy showing markedly increased erythroid cells is from a patient with chronic hemolysis (H&E stain).

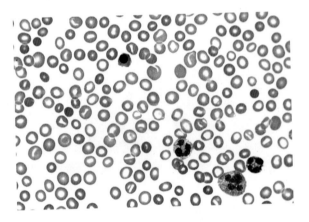

Figure 4-39

HEMOLYTIC ANEMIA AND THROMBOCYTOPENIA IN EVAN SYNDROME

Marked thrombocytopenia, prominent polychromasia, spherocytes, and occasional nucleated red blood cells are evident in this peripheral blood smear from a patient with systemic lupus erythematosus and Evan syndrome, status postsplenectomy (Wright stain).

In immune-mediated hemolytic anemias, the peripheral blood smear shows a distinctive combination of findings. The anemia may be macrocytic due to marked reticulocytosis, marked polychromasia, and spherocytosis; significant erythrocyte fragmentation is absent (fig. 4-38). Immune-mediated destruction of both erythrocytes and platelets may occur (fig. 4-39). In rare cases, a reticulocytosis is not evident, presumably due to autoantibody-mediated destruction of developing erythroid elements;

hyperuricemia may be evident in these cases (56). An autoantibody is usually documented by the direct antiglobulin test, although more elaborate testing may be necessary to diagnose drug-induced or complement-induced hemolytic anemia (50,53,69). Bone marrow examination is generally not required for the diagnosis of straightforward immune-mediated hemolytic anemia; erythroid hyperplasia is, however, a predicted morphologic feature of these disorders (figs. 4-40, 4-41).

Paroxysmal cold hemoglobinuria (PCH) is the rarest form of autoimmune hemolytic anemia, and distinctive peripheral blood findings characterize this disorder (59,70). In addition to erythrocyte agglutination, erythrocyte fragmentation, and spherocytosis, florid erythrophagocytosis by neutrophils and monocytes may be evident (figs. 4-42, 4-43). This disorder results from a cold-reacting IgG antibody (Donath-Landsteiner antibody). Paroxysmal cold hemoglobinuria usually manifests as an abrupt onset, transient hemolytic anemia in young children who have a history of antecedent infection caused by viruses, mycoplasma, or bacteria (53,59,70). Exposure to cold may trigger hemolysis in these patients; hemoglobinuria is typical, producing dark urine. Both intravascular and extravascular hemolytic mechanisms are operative in patients with PCH. The direct antiglobulin test is typically negative unless complement binding to erythrocytes is assessed.

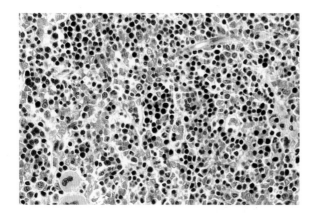

Figure 4-41

CHRONIC HEMOLYSIS

Prominent and confluent islands of erythroid precursors are evident on high magnification of this bone marrow core biopsy section from a patient with chronic hemolysis (H&E stain).

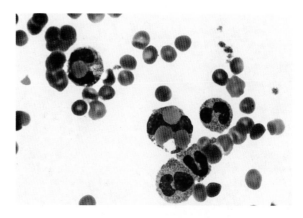

Figure 4-42

PAROXYSMAL COLD HEMOGLOBINURIA

The peripheral blood smear shows profound anemia with ingestion of erythrocytes by white blood cells, including neutrophils and monocytes (Wright stain). (Courtesy of Dr. A. Blenc, Royal Oak, MI.)

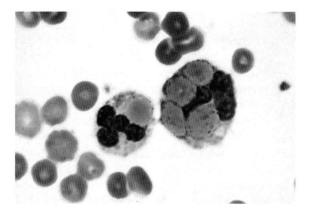

Figure 4-43

PAROXYSMAL COLD HEMOGLOBINURIA

This peripheral blood smear is from a 2-year-old child with paroxysmal cold hemoglobinuria who developed severe anemia. There is prominent ingestion of erythrocytes by monocytes and neutrophils (Wright stain). (Courtesy of Dr. A. Blenc, Royal Oak, MI.)

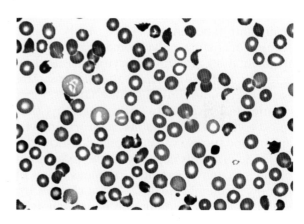

Figure 4-44

THROMBOTIC THROMBOCYTOPENIC PURPURA

The peripheral blood smear shows marked polychromasia, anemia, microspherocytes, and fragmented forms in an adult male with thrombotic thrombocytopenic purpura (Wright stain).

Premature erythrocyte destruction can also be the consequence of turbulent blood flow and microangiopathies. *Macroangiopathic* and *microangiopathic hemolytic anemias* consist of erythrocyte fragmentation, spherocytes, and polychromasia, the consequence of these vascular anomalies (fig. 4-44). Microangiopathic hemolytic anemia may be evident at birth in neonates with hemangioendotheliomas or other vascular anomalies (60). Associated coagulopathy with platelet trapping in these vascular lesions results in thrombocytopenia, elevated D-dimer levels, and reduced fibrinogen, producing the so-called Kasabach-Merritt syndrome (60). Similarly, macroangiopathic/microangiopathic hemolytic anemia with associated thrombocytopenia and coagulopathy may occur in patients with acquired disorders such as thrombotic thrombocytopenic purpura, hemolytic uremic syndrome, obstetrical vasculopathies, heart valve damage, and

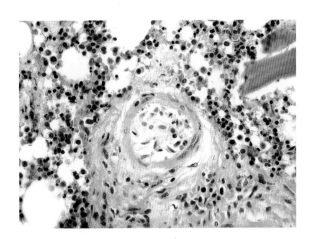

Figure 4-45

THROMBOTIC THROMBOCYTOPENIC PURPURA

The bone marrow core biopsy specimen shows a thrombosed vessel with an organizing thrombus in a fatal case of thrombotic thrombocytopenic purpura (H&E stain).

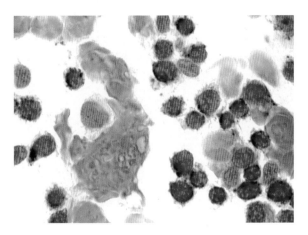

Figure 4-46

SIDEROBLASTIC ANEMIA

Erythroid hyperplasia with a predominance of ringed sideroblasts is seen in a bone marrow aspirate smear from a patient with sideroblastic anemia (Prussian blue stain).

malignant hypertension (45,46,61,64). Similar features of anemia, polychromasia, erythrocyte fragmentation, and thrombocytopenia are characteristic in these patients, and diagnoses are based on unique clinical manifestations.

Infection, especially with organisms that infect erythrocytes, is another cause of hemolytic anemia and shows a variable worldwide incidence (57). The diagnosis depends on the recognition of the infectious organisms. Infectious causes of hemolytic anemia are discussed in chapter 10.

Bone marrow examination is not generally required for diagnosis, but would show erythroid hyperplasia. In rare cases of thrombotic thrombocytopenic purpura, fibrin thrombi may be noted in the lumens of bone marrow vessels (fig. 4-45) (61).

Sideroblastic Anemia

Definition. The detection of iron granules encircling normoblast nuclei on Prussian blue–stained bone marrow aspirate smears is a unique finding that is encountered in both acquired and constitutional disorders (fig. 4-46). If a substantial proportion (usually over 20 percent) of erythroid precursors are ringed sideroblasts, a diagnosis of *sideroblastic anemia* is likely.

Pathogenesis. Electron microscopy has confirmed that the unique perinuclear ring of iron granules results from iron deposition within perinuclear mitochondria (fig. 4-47). Indeed, mi-

tochondria play a unique role in iron metabolism in that the final step of heme biosynthesis occurs in the mitochondrial matrix (72). Hemoglobin is comprised of three constituents (iron, protoporphyrin IX, and globin) which are produced in proportional amounts within developing erythroid elements. Imbalances in the availability of any of these three constituents typically results in a hypochromic, microcytic erythrocyte (fig. 4-48). As noted earlier, acquired iron deficiency anemias are commonly encountered in clinical practice, while thalassemias (globin chain production defects) and sideroblastic anemias (porphyrin ring defects) are much less commonly seen, except in geographic areas of high prevalence of hemoglobinopathies including thalassemia (see later section of this chapter).

Differential Diagnosis. Ringed sideroblasts are a fairly common component of primary myeloid neoplasms such as myelodysplasia, hybrid myelodysplastic/myeloproliferative disorders, and overt acute myeloid leukemia, often in conjunction with other dysplastic features such as periodic acid–Schiff (PAS) positivity of erythroid cells (fig. 4-49). Ringed sideroblasts are especially likely to be encountered in therapy-related myeloid neoplasms. In addition, a variety of toxic exposures or medications have been associated with abundant ringed sideroblasts in bone marrow. These toxins include alcohol, benzene, lead, arsenic, and high doses of zinc. The

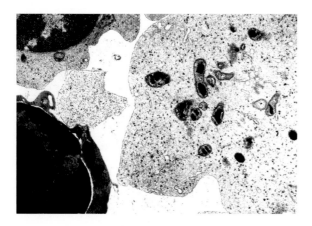

Figure 4-47

SIDEROBLASTIC ANEMIA

The electron micrograph shows iron within the perinuclear mitochondria.

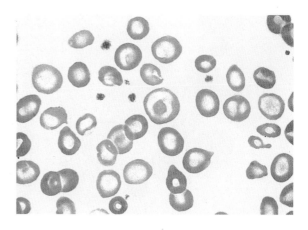

Figure 4-48

SIDEROBLASTIC ANEMIA

The peripheral blood smear shows prominent hypochromia with variably sized erythrocytes and mild anisopoikilocytosis (Wright stain).

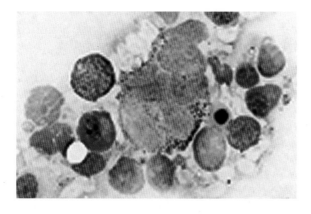

Figure 4-49

THERAPY-RELATED ACUTE MYELOGENOUS LEUKEMIA

Abnormal erythroid elements that are PAS positive is one component of the multilineage dysplasia in a bone marrow aspirate smear from patient with therapy-related acute myelogenous leukemia.

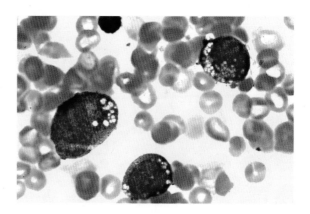

Figure 4-50

COPPER DEFICIENCY

Prominent vacuolization of erythroblasts and myeloblasts is evident in this bone marrow aspirate smear from a child on total parenteral nutrition who developed marked copper deficiency. Occasional ringed sideroblasts were also present (not illustrated) (Wright stain).

latter produces zinc therapy–induced copper deficiency, which results in sideroblastic anemia often with associated neutropenia, cytoplasmic vacuolization of myeloid and erythroid precursors, and neuropathy (figs. 4-50, 4-51) (74–76). Numerous other causes of copper deficiency have been described ranging from dietary deficiency to constitutional disorders (76). Other medications linked to the development of significant ringed sideroblasts in the bone marrow include isoniazid, pyrazinamide, azathioprine, chloramphenicol, and cycloserine (73,75).

Red Cell Aplasia and Other Hypoplastic Disorders

Red Cell Aplasia. *Red cell aplasia* is a dramatic event characterized by a marked reduction in erythroid precursors within the bone marrow. Often only scattered erythroblasts (pronormoblasts) are evident, while all other successive maturation stages of the erythroid lineage are conspicuously absent (figs. 4-52, 4-53). Depending upon the duration of the red cell aplasia

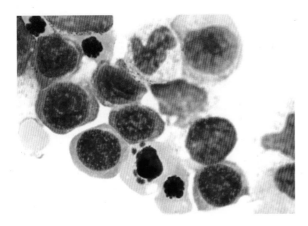

Figure 4-51

**DYSERYTHROPOIESIS SECONDARY
TO ARSENIC TOXICITY**

Erythroid hyperplasia and karyorrhexis are seen in the bone marrow aspirate (Wright stain). (Courtesy of Dr. R. Brynes, Los Angeles, CA.)

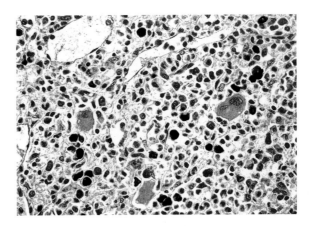

Figure 4-53

ACQUIRED RED CELL APLASIA

Only rare isolated erythroblasts are highlighted in an adult with acquired red cell aplasia (immunoperoxidase stain for HgbA).

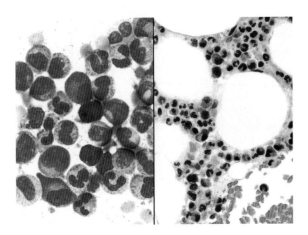

Figure 4-52

ACQUIRED RED BLOOD CELL APLASIA

A composite of the bone marrow aspirate and core biopsy in a renal transplant patient with acquired red cell aplasia secondary to antierythropoietin antibody production (Wright and H&E stains). (Courtesy of Dr. Q.Y. Zhang, Albuquerque, NM.)

and the patient's baseline erythrocyte survival time, a progressively severe reticulocytopenic normocytic/normochromic anemia results (fig. 4-54). The majority of cases of red cell aplasia encountered in clinical practice are acquired; constitutional red cell aplasias are rare and are discussed in a later section of this chapter.

Clinical factors such as patient age, underlying disorders, and medication history weigh heavily in the diagnostic approach to acquired red cell aplasia.

Transient Erythroblastopenia of Childhood. In young, previously healthy children, a self-limited, temporary red cell aplasia may develop that characteristically follows a febrile illness (fig. 4-55). The term *transient erythroblastopenia of childhood* (TEC) has been applied to this disorder, which has been described in children under 6 months of age, although most children are between 1 and 4 years of age (96,99,102). Spontaneous recovery in 1 to 2 months is typical, and therapy is not generally required. While a viral etiology for TEC is suspected, recent studies have failed to identify a common viral agent in successive children with this disorder (102). Some case reports confirm parvovirus B19 infection in spontaneously remitting TEC (100). Neutropenia is a common associated finding, again suggesting an underlying viral illness (82,86).

As expected, red cell aplasia with only scattered erythroblasts is a predicted bone marrow feature in children with TEC, although bone marrow examination is not generally necessary. Some authors report large numbers of hematogones in these pediatric specimens, again a predicted finding in this patient age group (see fig. 4-55) (86).

Parvovirus Infection. Parvovirus infection, a common cause of acquired red cell aplasia, also demonstrates some predictable clinical profiles

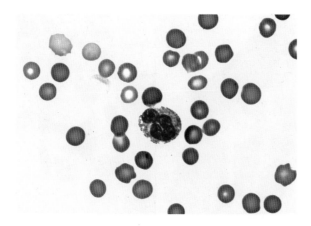

Figure 4-54

**HEREDITARY SPHEROCYTOSIS WITH
SECONDARY PARVOVIRUS INFECTION**

The peripheral blood smear shows profound spherocytic anemia with the absence of polychromasia (Wright stain).

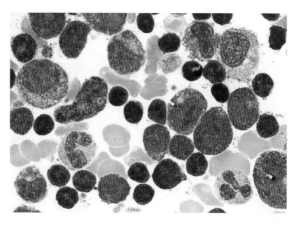

Figure 4-55

TRANSIENT ERYTHROBLASTOPENIA OF CHILDHOOD

A bone marrow aspirate smear in a 16-month-old female shows only rare erythroid precursor cells and numerous hematogones (Wright stain).

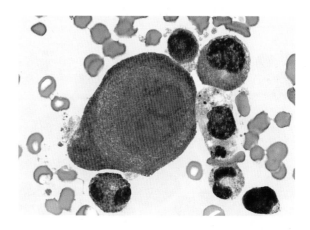

Figure 4-56

PARVOVIRUS INFECTION–INDUCED RED CELL APLASIA

A bone marrow aspirate smear from an immunosuppressed patient developing secondary parvovirus infection shows a giant erythroblast with an intranuclear inclusion (Wright stain).

(87,104). In some patients, acute parvovirus infection complicates chronic hemolytic disorders. Because of the reduced erythrocyte survival time from the primary disorder, a severe reticulocytopenic anemia can develop precipitously (see fig. 4-54). Patients with an underlying immunodeficiency also have an increased incidence of parvovirus-induced red cell aplasia (93). Due to underlying immunocompromise, an appropriate immune response against this virus cannot be mounted, and the infection becomes chronic, with sustained red cell aplasia. Viral inclusions within enlarged erythroblasts may be evident on either bone marrow aspirate smears or core biopsy sections; immunohistochemical techniques highlight these rare, virally infected erythroblasts (figs. 4-56–4-58) (92,94). A wave of regenerating erythroblasts characterizes early recovery in patients who are successful at mounting an immune response to the parvoviral infection (figs. 4-59, 4-60).

In rare immunosuppressed patients, erythroid elements are numerous and show abundant intranuclear inclusions (83). Case reports describe parvovirus-induced red cell aplasia developing as either a late consequence of bone marrow transplantation or following rituximab therapy. Rare cases of acute parvovirus infection mimic congenital dyserythropoietic anemia (80,91,101). See chapter 10 for a detailed discussion of bone marrow in patients with systemic infectious disorders.

Other Red Cell Aplasias. Isolated, acquired red cell aplasia has also been associated with T-cell large granular lymphocytic leukemia, thymoma, antierythropoietin antibody formation in patients receiving recombinant erythropoietin, other autoimmune disorders, other (nonparvoviral) viral infections, and a variety of medications (phenytoin, chloramphenicol, azathioprine, procainamide, sulfonamide, sodium valproate, mycophenolate mofetil) (fig. 4-61) (77–79,81,84,85,87,89,95,99). The association of T-cell large granular lymphocytic leukemia

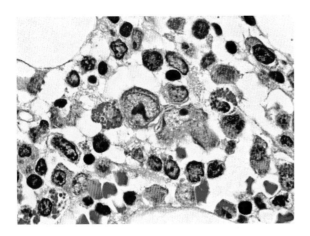

Figure 4-57

PARVOVIRUS INFECTION

The bone marrow core biopsy shows several giant erythroblasts in a patient with underlying immunodeficiency who developed parvovirus infection. Note the dissolution of the right erythroblast (H&E stain).

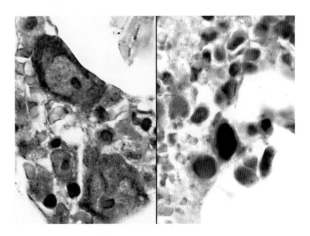

Figure 4-58

PARVOVIRUS INFECTION

Immunoperoxidase stains for hemoglobin A (left) and parvovirus (right) in an immunodeficient patient who developed secondary parvovirus infection–induced red cell aplasia.

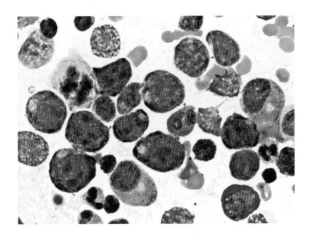

Figure 4-59

ERYTHROBLAST RECOVERY

A wave of erythroblast recovery in patient with acute parvovirus infection (Wright stain).

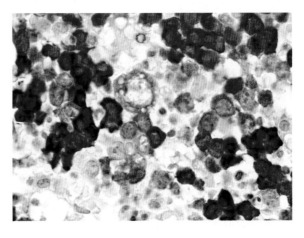

Figure 4-60

ERYTHROID RECOVERY

The immunoperoxidase stain for hemoglobin A highlights the wave of erythroid recovery in a patient with acute parvovirus infection. There is a persistent cytopathic effect with giant erythroblasts.

with acquired red cell aplasia is sufficiently common to warrant routine immunophenotypic assessment of blood or bone marrow for increased cytotoxic suppressor T cells (fig. 4-61).

Finally, red cell aplasia may be a component of a multilineage hypoplastic or aplastic process. Acquired multilineage hypoplasias or aplasias can occur as an idiopathic, presumed autoimmune, disorder or following infections, drug treatments, or toxin exposure. In addition, progressive multilineage hypoplasia may occur in patients with paroxysmal nocturnal hemoglobinuria (fig. 4-62) (88,97,98,103). Constitutional and single/multilineage disorders are discussed briefly later in this chapter and comprehensively in chapter 7.

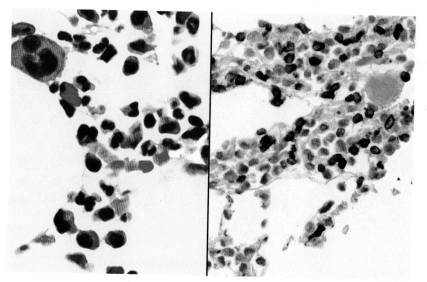

Figure 4-61

RED CELL APLASIA SECONDARY TO T-CELL LARGE GRANULAR LYMPHOCYTIC LEUKEMIA

This composite illustrates the morphology (left) and increase in T cells (right) in a patient with acquired red cell aplasia–associated T-cell large granular lymphocytic leukemia (H&E and immunoperoxidase stain for CD3).

CONSTITUTIONAL ANEMIAS

Hemoglobinopathies/Erythrocyte Enzyme Deficiency Disorders

Adult hemoglobin is a tetramer comprised of two alpha- and two beta-globin chains which are bound to heme (111). In normal adults, hemoglobin A ($\alpha_2\beta_2$) constitutes 95 percent of hemoglobin; the remainder consists of hemoglobin A_2 ($\alpha_2\delta_2$) (less than 3.5 percent) and hemoglobin F ($\alpha_2\gamma_2$) (1 percent) (111). The alpha-globin chain is encoded by four genes, while the gamma, delta, and beta chains are encoded by two genes (115). *Hemoglobinopathies* result from either reduced synthesis of one or more globin chains or from the production of a genetically acquired defective globin chain (111). Coinheritance of various types of hemoglobinopathy is common. Most hemoglobinopathies can be detected by polymerase chain reaction (PCR)-based techniques (111,121). Increased resistance to malarial infections in patients with mild disease is the likely explanation for the high prevalence of these disorders in various populations and ethnic groups (106,112).

Thalassemia. The various *thalassemia disorders* result from reduced globin chain synthesis (either alpha or beta). The resulting microcytic, hypochromic RBCs are due to the inadequate availability of either alpha- or beta-globin chains for hemoglobin production. Thalassemias exhibit an autosomal recessive inheritance pattern and generally affect populations residing in the ma-

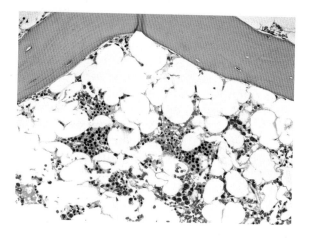

Figure 4-62

HYPOCELLULAR PAROXYSMAL NOCTURNAL HEMOGLOBINURIA

Bone marrow core biopsy shows overall hypocellularity with reduced granulocytic elements and small residual erythroid islands (H&E stain).

laria belt (115,125). Numerous genetic variants of thalassemia have been described; thalassemia is among the most common genetic disorders worldwide (125). A detailed discussion of these disorders is beyond the scope of this Fascicle. This chapter focuses on blood and bone marrow features in patients with thalassemia.

For patients with mild thalassemic disorders (so-called *thalassemia minor*), the RBC count is typically elevated, and the microcytic, hypochromic erythrocytes are characteristically uniform in size (figs. 4-63, 4-64). Consequently,

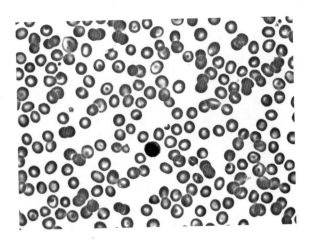

Figure 4-63

BETA-THALASSEMIA MINOR

Mild anemia is seen on the peripheral blood smear as well as relative uniformity of erythrocyte size and moderate targeting (Wright stain).

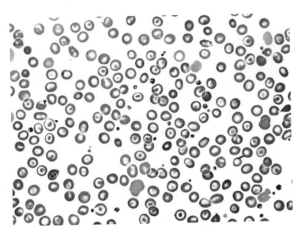

Figure 4-64

BETA-THALASSEMIA MINOR

Mild to moderate anemia is seen on the peripheral blood smear, with prominent targeting and apparent microcytosis, which is best determined by automated instrument techniques (Wright stain).

the RDW is normal or near normal. In patients with milder thalassemias, the differential diagnosis often focuses on iron deficiency anemia versus thalassemia minor. In this situation, the RBC count, RDW, and serum iron assessment are all useful methods to distinguish these two causes of microcytic/hypochromic anemia (119). Hemoglobin electrophoresis is also useful in this situation in that elevations in hemoglobin A$_2$ are characteristic of *beta (β)-thalassemias* (122). Definitive diagnosis, however, relies on PCR techniques (111,122). Bone marrow examination is not generally necessary in patients with thalassemia minor (124,127).

In more severe genetic forms of thalassemia, the blood picture is much more atypical, with severe anemia, nucleated RBCs, and marked hypochromia (fig. 4-65). Bone marrow examination may be necessary to assess for chronic transfusion-related iron overload or other possible disorders. Erythropoietin-driven erythroid hyperplasia is a predicted bone marrow finding in patients with thalassemia; other findings vary depending upon transfusion requirements and secondary infections (127). Recently, gene therapy techniques have been proposed for the correction of the β-thalassemia major phenotype; other treatment strategies include fetal-hemoglobin enhancing agents (117,124,125).

Sickle Cell Anemia. *Sickle cell anemia* is a constitutional hemolytic anemia resulting

from a single amino acid mutation in the beta-globin gene, producing hemoglobin S, which abnormally polymerizes under conditions of decreased pH or oxygen tension (111,126). Coinheritance of the sickle cell and β-thalassemia genes is common (128). Although patients with heterozygous disease (sickle cell trait) experience few, if any, symptoms while benefitting from increased resistance to malarial infections, patients with homozygous (SS) disease have severe, debilitating complications of lifelong painful sickle crises, recurrent infections, and severe pulmonary, CNS, and renal complications adversely impacting survival time (106,107,126).

Vasoocclusive crises result from irreversible sickling of erythrocytes under conditions of deoxygenation, which cause polymerization of hemoglobin S. Numerous therapeutic strategies to reduce hemoglobin polymerization and associated erythrocyte dehydration have been developed, including agents that induce increased levels of protective hemoglobin F, agents that prevent erythrocyte dehydration, and agents that allosterically shift oxygen equilibrium curves (105,107–109,118,126).

In the acute crisis stage of sickle cell anemia, the peripheral blood smear is dramatic (figs. 4-66, 4-67). In addition to features of acute stress such as neutrophilia with a mild left shift and

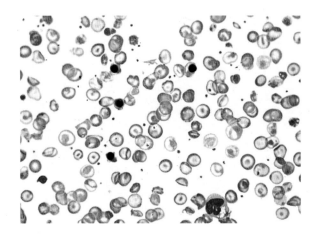

Figure 4-65

SEVERE THALASSEMIA

Severe thalassemia is manifested by striking erythrocyte changes and nucleated red blood cells on a peripheral blood smear (Wright stain).

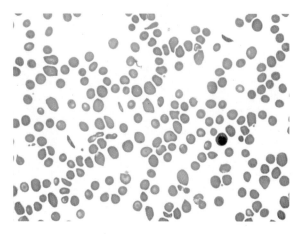

Figure 4-66

SICKLE CELL ANEMIA

Marked polychromasia and moderate numbers of sickle cells are evident on a peripheral blood smear (Wright stain).

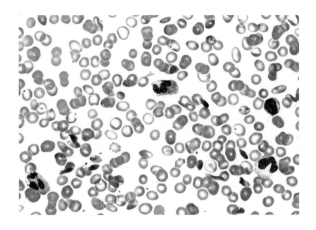

Figure 4-67

SICKLE CELL ANEMIA IN CRISIS

Striking red blood cell changes are seen in conjunction with neutrophilia (Wright stain).

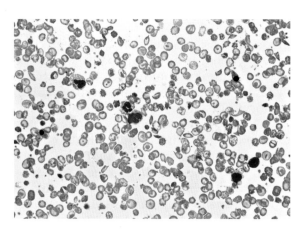

Figure 4-68

SICKLE CELL ANEMIA/THALASSEMIA

Sickle cells, prominent targeting, nucleated red blood cells, and polychromasia are present on the peripheral blood smear (Wright stain).

thrombocytosis, striking erythrocyte pathology is evident. Numerous sickle cells are present in association with marked polychromasia and significant anemia. Variable erythrocyte targeting may be evident depending upon concurrent thalassemia or underlying organ pathology such as liver disease (fig. 4-68). Profound reticulocytopenic anemia can result if the patient develops concurrent parvovirus-induced red cell aplasia.

A bone marrow examination is not required to establish a diagnosis of sickle cell anemia, but may be necessary to assess for secondary complications, such as the bone marrow necrosis with systemic embolization that produces the acute chest syndrome, an acute respiratory disorder caused by pulmonary emboli (fig. 4-69) (107,110,113,116). Predicted bone marrow findings in patients with sickle cell anemia include marked erythroid hyperplasia and abnormal medullary blood vessels (120).

Other Hemoglobinopathies. Other hemoglobinopathies include *hemoglobin C* and *hemoglobin E diseases*. Hemoglobin E disease predominates

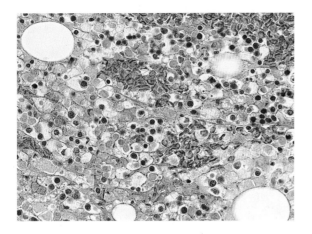

Figure 4-69

BONE MARROW NECROSIS, ACUTE CHEST SYNDROME

The bone marrow biopsy shows necrosis of the normal hematopoietic elements in a patient with sickle cell anemia/thalassemia who developed fatal acute chest syndrome (H&E stain).

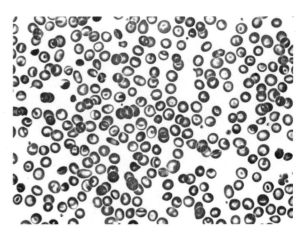

Figure 4-70

HOMOZYGOUS HEMOGLOBIN E

Peripheral blood smear from a Southeast Asian patient with homozygous hemoglobin E shows mild anemia with monotonous, targeted, small erythrocytes (Wright stain).

in Southeast Asian populations and is the second most prevalent hemoglobinopathy worldwide (115). Features of homozygous hemoglobin E disease include mild anemia, erythrocytosis, microcytosis, and erythrocyte targeting (fig. 4-70). These patients are typically asymptomatic. Coinheritance of other hemoglobin disorders is common in this population. Similarly, hemoglobin C disease, when homozygous, is associated with mild clinical manifestations, mild to moderate anemia, microcytosis, and targeting. Coinheritance with other hemoglobin mutations, especially hemoglobin S, is common. Acute chest syndrome, secondary to bone marrow necrosis with systemic embolization, is relatively common in patients with hemoglobin S/C disease (fig. 4-69).

Erythrocyte Enzyme Deficiencies. The two most common constitutional erythrocyte enzyme deficiencies that produce hemolytic anemia are *glucose-6-phosphate dehydrogenase* (G6PD) and *pyruvate kinase deficiencies* (114,123,129). In patients with G6PD deficiency, an X-linked oxidative enzyme deficiency affecting over 400 million patients worldwide, the hemolytic episodes may be intermittent since they are precipitated by oxidant exposures (123). In these patients, an erythrocyte fragmentation syndrome with "bite cells," resulting from splenic removal of Heinz bodies, may be evident on blood smear review

(fig. 4-71). In patients with pyruvate kinase deficiency, an autosomal dominant glycolytic enzyme deficiency affecting only a small proportion of the population, a sustained reticulocytosis secondary to chronic nonspherocytic hemolysis is the typical blood picture (123,129). In both disorders, erythropoietin-induced erythroid hyperplasia is a predicted bone marrow finding, although bone marrow examination is not required for the diagnosis of these disorders unless complications develop.

Hereditary Spherocytosis and Other Erythrocyte Membrane Disorders

Hereditary Spherocytosis. *Hereditary spherocytosis* is the most common constitutional hemolytic anemia in Caucasian populations, especially those of northern European heritage (131,132,134). Hereditary spherocytosis results from a deficiency or dysfunction of one of the constituents of the RBC cytoskeleton. Many different genetic variants have been described affecting ankyrin, AE1 transmembrane transport protein, or various spectrin proteins, and all of these mutations result in the decreased stability of the RBC membrane cytoskeleton (131,132,134). The inheritance patterns for all of these diverse mutations are typically autosomal dominant (134).

The clinical picture is variable, with mild, moderate, and severe forms characterized by

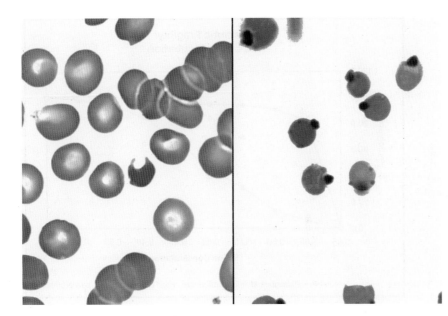

Figure 4-71

G6PD DEFICIENCY WITH HEINZ BODY PREP

The red blood cell pathology includes "bite cells" (left), while Heinz bodies are noted after oxidant stress (right) (Wright and Heinz body preparation.)

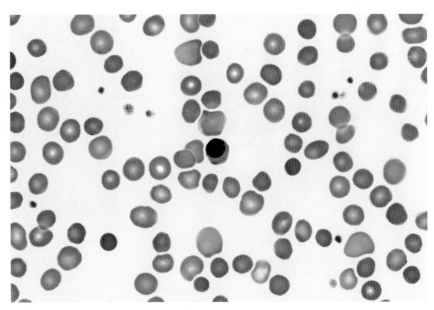

Figure 4-72

HEREDITARY SPHEROCYTOSIS

Profound spherocytic anemia with polychromasia and circulating nucleated red blood cells in a patient with hereditary spherocytosis (Wright stain). (Courtesy of Dr. S. Kroft, Milwaukee, WI.)

variably severe anemia, reticulocytosis, and abundant dense spherocytes in the absence of significant erythrocyte fragmentation (fig. 4-72) (135). Spherocytes are characterized by decreased MCV and increased mean corpuscular hemoglobin concentration (MCHC) levels (134). The osmotic fragililty test provides diagnostic specificity for the presence of spherocytes beyond the morphologic assessment by documenting the increased osmotic fragility of these RBCs compared to normal erythrocytes (fig. 4-73) (132). Incubation prior to the performance of the

osmotic fragility test results in improved detection of spherocytes. Direct hyperbilirubinemia is typical, and cholelithiasis is a frequent clinical manifestation of the chronic hemolysis (134). Splenectomy, usually delayed until the patient is at least 3 years old, alleviates hemolysis in patients with clinically significant disease (132).

A bone marrow examination is not generally required in patients with hereditary spherocytosis, unless necessary to assess for a complication such as parvovirus-induced red cell aplasia. Erythroid hyperplasia is a predicted bone marrow

Figure 4-73

OSMOTIC FRAGILITY CURVE

The osmotic fragility curve shows the increased hemolysis characteristic of spherocytes in a patient with hereditary spherocytosis compared to normal erythrocytes.

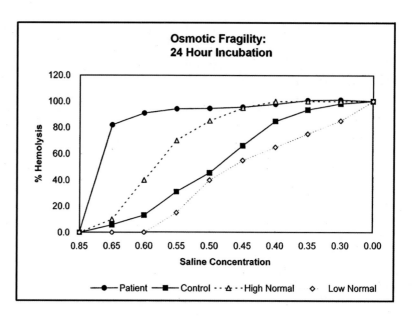

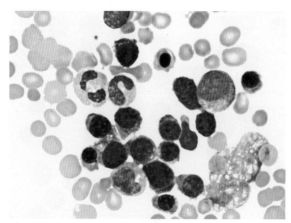

Figure 4-74

ERYTHROID HYPERPLASIA IN HEREDITARY SPHEROCYTOSIS

A bone marrow aspirate smear shows marked erythroid hyperplasia (Wright stain). (Courtesy of Dr. S. Kroft, Milwaukee, WI.)

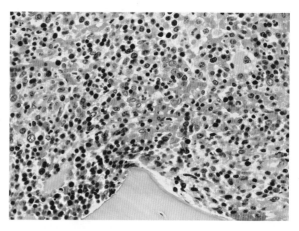

Figure 4-75

ERYTHROID HYPERPLASIA IN HEREDITARY SPHEROCYTOSIS

The bone marrow core biopsy shows markedly hypercellular bone marrow with marked erythroid hyperplasia (H&E stain). (Courtesy of Dr. S. Kroft, Milwaukee, WI.)

finding in patients with hereditary spherocytosis (figs. 4-74, 4-75).

Hereditary elliptocytosis is usually an autosomal dominant shape disorder resulting from mutations in RBC cytoskeletal proteins; oblong elliptocytes predominate on the blood smear (133,134). A spectrum of clinical and genetic disorders produces this common erythrocyte shape abnormality which concurs resistance to malarial infection and is thus more common in individuals of African and Mediterranean an-

cestry, although hereditary elliptocytosis occurs in all ethnic populations (133,134). Multiple genetic loci have been identified including mutations in *alpha-spectrin, beta-spectrin, protein 4.1,* and *glycophorin C* genes (133,134). Hemolytic anemia, of varying severity, results from either mechanical weakness or increased fragility of the elliptocytes; the clinical spectrum ranges from asymptomatic carriers (the majority of cases) to patients with severe transfusion-dependent hemolytic anemia (133,134).

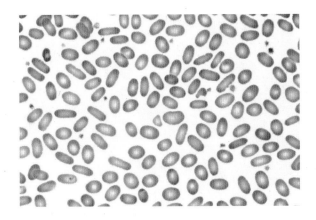

Figure 4-76

HEREDITARY ELLIPTOCYTOSIS

A peripheral blood smear shows abundant, monotonous elliptocytes (Wright stain).

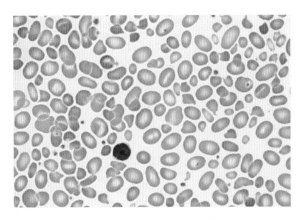

Figure 4-77

HEREDITARY PYROPOIKILOCYTOSIS

A peripheral blood smear shows profound erythrocyte fragmentation (Wright stain).

There is marked elliptocytosis, variable reticulocytosis, and variable anemia in the peripheral blood smear (fig. 4-76). Bone marrow examination is not generally required but would show erythroid hyperplasia proportional to the reduction in erythrocyte survival time.

One variant of hereditary elliptocytosis, *hereditary pyropoikilocytosis*, produces a dramatic blood picture in neonates and infants. In these patients, erythrocytes are highly mechanically unstable due to instability of the RBC cytoskeleton, resulting in extreme erythrocyte fragmentation, a microspherocytic hemolytic picture similar to that seen in association with thermal injury (figs. 4-77, 4-78) (131,133,134).

Elliptocytes may be evident on blood smears in many other conditions, generally in association with other erythrocyte abnormalities. In addition to hereditary elliptocytosis, elliptocytes may be prominent in iron deficiency anemia, megaloblastic anemia, myelodysplasia, myelophthistic anemias, and other constitutional erythrocyte disorders such as pyruvate kinase deficiency, sickle cell anemia, and thalassemias (fig. 4-79) (133).

Congenital Dyserythropoietic Anemia

The *congenital dyserythropoietic anemias* (CDAs) are a rare heterogeneous group of disorders characterized by ineffective erythropoiesis, marked dyserythropoiesis of circulating erythrocytes, and marked dyspoiesis of bone marrow erythroid elements (fig. 4-80) (142,149,150).

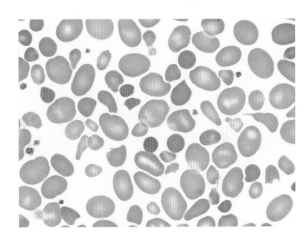

Figure 4-78

HEREDITARY PYROPOIKILOCYTOSIS

Striking red blood cell fragmentation and microspherocytes are seen in the peripheral blood smear (Wright stain).

Three variants, CDA I, II, and III, were initially described, although other variants have been described subsequently (139,143,149,150). All types of congenital dyserythropoietic anemia are uncommon in clinical practice.

A combination of blood, bone marrow, ultrastructural, and electrophoretic features is used to classify these disorders. Bone marrow examination is generally required for their subclassification (Table 4-8). The inheritance pattern, typical morphologic features, and genetic defects in the three established subtypes have been delineated (Table 4-8) (136,138,140,143,145,149,

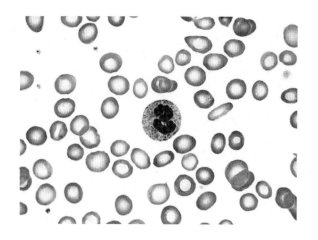

Figure 4-79

IRON DEFICIENCY ANEMIA WITH ELLIPTOCYTES

The peripheral blood smear from a patient with iron deficiency anemia shows elliptocytes (Wright stain).

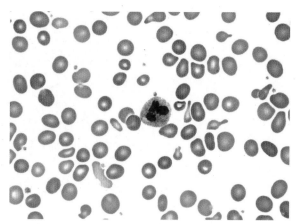

Figure 4-80

CONGENITAL DYSERYTHROPOIETIC ANEMIA

A peripheral blood smear shows prominent dyserythropoiesis (Wright stain). (Courtesy of P. Izadi, Los Angeles, CA.)

Table 4-8

PERIPHERAL BLOOD AND BONE MARROW FINDINGS IN PATIENTS WITH CONGENITAL DYSERTHROPOIETIC ANEMIAS[a]

	CDA I	CDA II[b]	CDA III
Blood			
RBC[c] size	Macrocytic	Normocytic	Usually macrocytic
RBC morphology	Anisopoikilocytosis	Anisopoikilocytosis	Anisopoikilocytosis
Anemia	Mild to severe	Mild to severe	Mild to moderate
Bone Marrow			
Erythroid hyperplasia	Prominent	Prominent	Prominent
Erythroid morphology	Megaloblastic	Normoblastic	Megaloblastic "giganto-blasts" (up to 12 nuclei)
	Internuclear chromatin bridging	Bi/multinucleated normoblasts	
	Nuclear budding	Nuclear karyorrhexis	Nuclear karyorrhexis
	Occasional binucleate forms		
Ultrastructure of erythroid cells	"Swiss cheese" nuclear changes	Peripheral cisternae derived from endoplasmic reticulum	Not characterized
Other lineages	Usually normal	Usually normal	Usually normal
Inheritance	Autosomal recessive	Autosomal recessive	Autosomal dominant, sporadic form
Genetic localization	15q15.1-15.3, codanin-1 mutations	20q11.2	15q21-25

[a]Data from references 136, 138–147, 149, and 150.
[b]The designation HEMPAS (hereditary erythroblastic multinuclearity with positive acidified serum [test]) is sometimes applied to patients with CDA II.
[c]RBC = red blood cell.

150). Electron microscopy reveals unique "Swiss cheese"-like heterochromatin in CDA I, as well as peripheral cisternae (double membranes) that appear to be derived from endoplasmic reticulum (fig. 4-81) (143,149). In CDA II, hemolysis of erythrocytes by ABO-compatible sera at an acid pH is caused by a naturally occurring IgM antibody that recognizes CDA II RBCs (142,149).

CDA III is characterized by marked multinucleation with erythroblast gigantism in both familial and sporadic cases (148,150).

Neonatal and even in utero complications have been noted in patients with CDA I. The other types of congenital dyserythropoietic anemia tend to manifest later in childhood (143,147,149). A mutation in the *CDAN-1* (Codanin-1) gene was

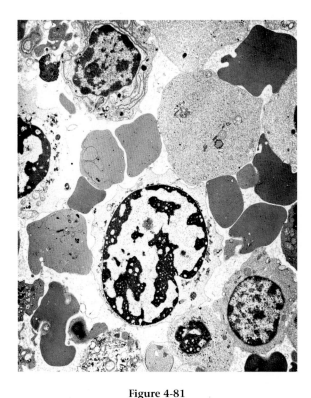

Figure 4-81

CONGENITAL DYSERYTHROPOIETIC ANEMIA

An electron micrograph of the bone marrow from a patient with congenital dyserythropoietic anemia shows "Swiss cheese"-like heterochromatin.

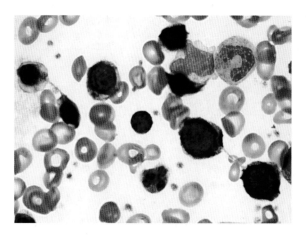

Figure 4-82

CONGENITAL DYSERYTHROPOIETIC ANEMIA

Erythroid hyperplasia with intercellular bridging is seen in the bone marrow (Wright stain). (Courtesy of P. Izadi, Los Angeles, CA.)

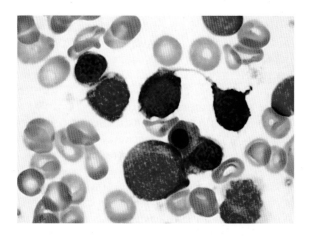

Figure 4-83

CONGENITAL DYSERYTHROPOIETIC ANEMIA

Prominent intercellular bridging is present in the bone marrow (Wright stain). (Courtesy of P. Izadi, Los Angles, CA.)

identified in all CDA I patients of Bedouin ethnicity in one recent study (138,143,147). CDA II is the most common of these rare disorders. Registries of CDA II patients document long-term complications such as cholelithiasis and secondary hemochromatosis (142).

Morphologic features of erythroid lineage in the bone marrow are crucial for the diagnosis of congenital dyserythropoietic anemia; consequently, bone marrow examination is routinely performed on these patients (150). The predominant bone marrow findings in CDA I are intercellular bridging and bi/multinucleation; karyorrhexis typifies CDA II; gigantoblastic erythroid precursors with up to 12 nuclei are found in CDA III (figs. 4-82–4-84).

Congenital dyserythropoietic anemia is a diagnosis of exclusion, unless documented within well-established kindreds. Because macrocytosis is a common finding, other causes of macrocytic anemia with dyserythropoiesis must be excluded (fig. 4-85). Rare reports of acute parvovirus infection mimicking congenital dyserythropoietic anemia have been published, and marked dyserythropoiesis is noted occasionally in patients with myelodysplasia (137).

Congenital (Hereditary) Megaloblastic Anemia

Congential megaloblastic anemias are rare disorders resulting from various constitutional defects in absorption, transportation, or utilization of either vitamin B_{12} or folate (Table 4-9) (151–157). These autosomal recessive disorders often manifest in infancy or early childhood,

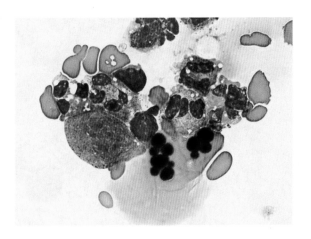

Figure 4-84

**MULTINUCLEATION IN CONGENITAL
DYSERYTHROPOIETIC ANEMIA**

A bone marrow aspirate smear shows multinucleation
(Wright stain). (Courtesy of Dr. R. Larson, Albuquerque, NM.)

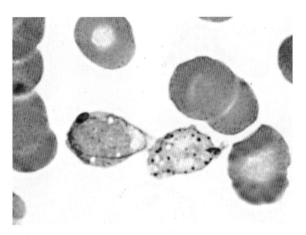

Figure 4-85

HIGH-GRADE MYELODYSPLASIA

Marked dyserythropoiesis is highlighted by these two
dysplastic macrocytic erythrocytes in the peripheral blood of
a patient with high-grade myelodysplasia (Wright stain).

although a spectrum of disease manifestations
and age of onset characterizes some of these
hereditary disorders. As predicted, the dominant
features tend to be hematologic and neurologic,
but nonspecific symptoms such as failure to
thrive are common in infants.

Distinguishing these constitutional disorders
from vitamin B_{12}/folate deficiency resulting from
maternal factors such as maternal dietary restrictions or maternal pernicious anemia is essential.
Infants born with reduced vitamin B_{12}/folate
because of these maternal factors can manifest
symptomatology similar to infants with various
constitutional defects. Treatment with vitamin
B_{12} or folate results in complete resolution of
hematologic abnormalities in children with
acquired deficiency, although neurologic abnormalities may persist. Treatment for the rare,
diverse constitutional disorders listed on Table
4-9 is much more problematic, if available at all.
If bone marrow examination is performed, florid
megaloblastosis is a predicted finding.

Congenital Sideroblastic Anemia. Sideroblastic anemias are characterized by the presence
of ringed sideroblasts, i.e., perinuclear localization
of iron granules, on Prussian blue staining of bone
marrow aspirate smears. By electron microscopy,
this perinuclear iron is localized within mitochondria (159,162). The three components of hemoglobin—iron, protophoryrin IX, and globin—are
physiologically coordinated to insure that ap-

propriate amounts are available for hemoglobin
production without excess or deficiency of any
one constituent. The terminal step in heme biosynthesis, the incorporation of iron into protophoryrin IX by the enzyme ferrochetalase, occurs
within the mitochondria (159). The inefficient
utilization of mitochondrial iron results in the
accumulation of excess iron within mitochondria,
producing ringed sideroblasts (159).

Although most cases of sideroblastic anemia are acquired, multiple genetic types of
congenital sideroblastic anemia have been described, and these predominate in the pediatric
population. All are rare in clinical practice, and
numerous mutations have been identified in
these patients (159). For example, over 20 dis-
ease-causing mutations in 5-aminolevulinic acid
synthase have been described in kindreds with
X-linked sideroblastic anemia (159–162). Similar
to acquired sideroblastic anemia, the characteristic hematologic manifestations of X-linked
sideroblastic anemia include hypochromic
anemia with a dimorphic erythrocyte picture,
Pappenheimer bodies, and erythroid hyperplasia with ringed sideroblasts within bone marrow
(figs. 4-86–4-89) (162). Overall bone marrow
hypercellularity with erythroid hyperplasia and
significant anemia characterize the ineffective
erythropoiesis in these patients. In addition to
increased erythroid iron with numerous ringed
sideroblasts, storage iron is also markedly increased

Table 4-9

CONGENITAL (HEREDITARY) MEGALOBLASTIC ANEMIAS[a]

Defect	Mutation	Inheritance Pattern	Clinical/Epidemiologic Features
Intrinsic factor (IF) deficiency (defective cobalamin absorption)	Human *IF* on chromosome 11	Autosomal recessive	Megaloblastic anemia by age 2, developmental delay, myelopathy
Defect in intestinal absorption of IF-cobalamin complex (Imerslund-Grasbeck syndrome)	Two mutations noted: *Cubilin* gene at chromosome 10p12.1 *AMN* (amnionless) gene at 14q32	Autosomal recessive	Megaloblastic anemia due to cobalamin malabsorption, proteinuria, neurologic manifestations Scandinavian and Middle Eastern kindreds described
Decreased synthesis of transcobalamins (defective cobalamin transport)	Several genetic variants of transcobalamin I and transcobalamin II deficiency	Autosomal recessive	Manifest in early infancy, failure to thrive, weakness, diarrhea, eventual neurologic manifestations Other variants have different manifestations
Functional defect in mitochondrial methylmalonyl coenzyme A (CoA) mutase (defective cobalamin utilization)	Multiple mutations described	Autosomal recessive	Severe metabolic acidosis with accumulation of methylmalonic acid in blood, urine, spinal fluid Prenatal diagnosis possible Treatment with protein restricted diet
Deficiency of adenosylcobalamin (defective cobalamin utilization)	Multiple mutations described	Autosomal recessive	Severe manifestations in early infancy; some subtypes respond to cyanocobalamin therapy
Hereditary folate malabsorption	Not characterized	Probable autosomal recessive	Megaloblastic anemia, failure to thrive, diarrhea, mouth ulcers, progressive neurological deterioration Linked to consanguinity
Methylenetetrahydrofolate reductase deficiency (defective folate utilization)	Multiple mutations described, usually missense	Probable autosomal recessive	Wide spectrum of disease manifestations and age of onset; usually develops in first year of life
Glutamate formiminotransferase deficiency (defective folate utilization)	Not characterized	Probable autosomal recessive	Wide spectrum of disease manifestations and age of onset; mild and severe phenotypes

[a]Data from references 151–157.

(162). Response to pyridoxine therapy is well described in this patient population (159).

Other rare types of congenital sideroblastic anemia include *X-linked sideroblastic anemia with ataxia, thiamine-responsive megaloblastic anemia* (with ringed sideroblasts), and *Pearson marrow-pancreas syndrome* (158,159,162). Pearson marrow-pancreas syndrome is a unique type of congenital sideroblastic anemia thought to be maternally derived and due to mutations in mitochondrial DNA that result in defective cellular energy production (159,162). These patients have pancytopenia with severe macrocytic anemia in conjunction with exocrine pancreatic dysfunction and variable hepatic and renal impairment (159,161,162). In addition to ringed sideroblasts, both myeloid and erythroid precursors have distinct cytoplasmic vacuoles (fig. 4-90). Although most of these disorders manifest in infancy, milder cases may not manifest until adulthood (160,162).

Constitutional Single and Multilineage Bone Marrow Failure Disorders with Anemia

Diamond-Blackfan Anemia. *Diamond-Blackfan anemia* is the prototypic constitutional red cell aplasia for which the hematologic, inheritance, and genetic features are reasonably well characterized (Table 4-10). This rare disorder typically manifests at birth as severe, usually macrocytic anemia in conjunction with profound reticulocytopenia, although clinically silent cases have been identified in kindred studies (fig. 4-91) (166,169,170). Early in the disease course, the dominant bone marrow pathology is isolated profound erythroid hypoplasia with only scattered, morphologically

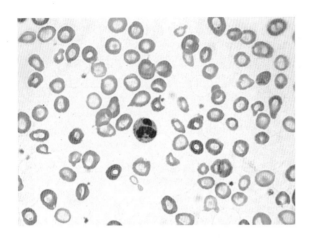

Figure 4-86

CONGENITAL SIDEROBLASTIC ANEMIA

A peripheral blood smear from a child with congenital sideroblastic anemia shows variable erythrocyte size and hemoglobin concentration (Wright stain). (Courtesy of P. Izadi, Los Angeles, CA.)

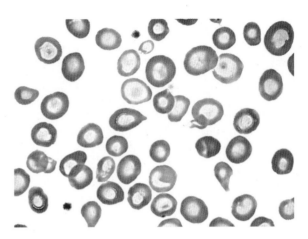

Figure 4-87

CONGENITAL SIDEROBLASTIC ANEMIA

The peripheral blood smear shows dimorphic erythrocytes (Wright stain). (Courtesy of P. Izadi, Los Angeles, CA.)

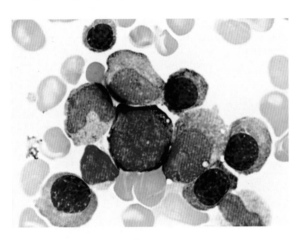

Figure 4-88

ERYTHROID HYPERPLASIA IN CONGENITAL SIDEROBLASTIC ANEMIA

The bone marrow aspirate smear shows erythroid hyperplasia in a child with congenital sideroblastic anemia (Wright stain). (Courtesy of P. Izadi, Los Angeles, CA.)

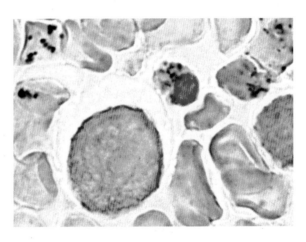

Figure 4-89

RINGED SIDEROBLAST IN CONGENITAL SIDEROBLASTIC ANEMIA

Numerous ringed sideroblasts with dysplastic erythroid iron, even in mature erythrocytes, are evident in this bone marrow aspirate smear from a child with congenital sideroblastic anemia (Prussian blue stain). (Courtesy of P. Izadi, Los Angeles, CA.)

unremarkable erythroblasts (fig. 4-92). Increased benign lymphoid precursor cells, hematogones, are a frequent nonspecific feature in bone marrow specimens from infants (see chapter 8). In studies of long-term survivors of Diamond-Blackfan anemia, the majority of patients develop moderate to severe multilineage hypoplasia with associated neutropenia and thrombocytopenia

(166). Other features of Diamond-Blackfan anemia are highlighted on Table 4-10.

Multilineage Constitutional Abnormalities. Anemia is a common manifestation in patients with various constitutional multilineage bone marrow failure disorders such as *Fanconi anemia, Shwachman-Diamond syndrome*, and *dyskeratosis congenita*. The salient hematologic, clinical, and

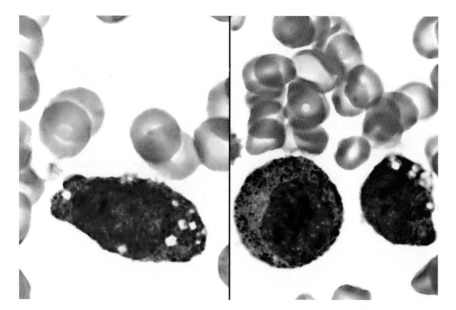

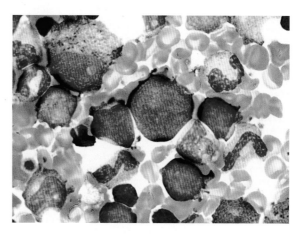

Figure 4-90

PEARSON SYNDROME

Vacuolated myeloid and erythroid precursors are seen in an infant with Pearson syndrome (Wright stain). (Courtesy of Dr. L. Contis, Pittsburgh, PA.)

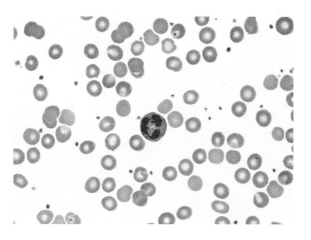

Figure 4-91

DIAMOND-BLACKFAN ANEMIA

The peripheral blood smear from an infant with Diamond-Blackfan anemia shows profound normocytic and normochromic anemia without significant polychromasia (Wright stain). (Courtesy of P. Izadi, Los Angeles, CA.)

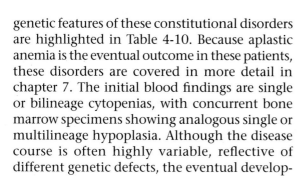

Figure 4-92

RED CELL APLASIA IN DIAMOND-BLACKFAN ANEMIA

The bone marrow aspirate smear shows only occasional erythroblasts in a child with Diamond-Blackfan anemia (Wright stain). (Courtesy of P. Izadi, Los Angeles, CA.)

genetic features of these constitutional disorders are highlighted in Table 4-10. Because aplastic anemia is the eventual outcome in these patients, these disorders are covered in more detail in chapter 7. The initial blood findings are single or bilineage cytopenias, with concurrent bone marrow specimens showing analogous single or multilineage hypoplasia. Although the disease course is often highly variable, reflective of different genetic defects, the eventual develop-ment of profound multilineage hypoplasia is characteristic.

OVERVIEW OF ERYTHROCYTOSIS

Classification of Erythrocytosis

Erythrocytosis is defined by hemoglobin, hema-tocrit, and RBC counts that exceed age-related and altitude-related normal ranges. In some cases, the increase in erythrocytes is the physiologically

Table 4-10

CONSTITUTIONAL SINGLE AND MULTILINEAGE BONE MARROW FAILURE DISORDERS WITH ANEMIA[a]

Hematolgic Features	Bone Marrow	Other Findings	Inheritance Pattern	Genetic Features
Diamond-Blackfan Anemia				
Severe, usually macrocytic anemia w/ reduced reticulocytes Normal to mildly ↓ WBCs[b], platelets Multilineage hematologic failure may develop in long-term survivors	Profound erythroid lineage hypoplasia w/only rare erythroblasts May progress to multilineage hypoplasia	Onset at birth or early infancy Skeletal abnormalities and growth retardation in 30% Increased HgbF[b], RBC[b] adenosine, and EPO[b] levels Clinically silent phenotype noted in some family kindreds (broad spectrum)	Minority familial (both autosomal dominant and recessive types described); remainder sporadic Autosomal dominant more common than autosomal recessive for familial cases	Mutations in small ribosomal protein S19 (19q13) in 25%; other gene mutations likely Genetic defect results in intrinsic defect in erythroid differentiation
Franconi Anemia (see chapter 7)				
Single lineage defect w/gradual progression to pancytopenia	Single lineage failure (hypoplasia) with gradual progression to multilineage hematopoietic failure Variable time course in development of aplastic picture linked to genetic subtypes	Range in clinical disease spectrum likely linked to specific genetic subtype Short stature, thumb abnormalities, skin lesions Cancer susceptibility with ↑ of leukemias and carcinomas in adolescence and adulthood (cancer type and age at onset linked to genetic subtypes)	Autosomal recessive	Inherited chromosomal instability with spontaneous chromosomal breakage DNA repair defect w/ specific genetic defects described in 11 complementation types
Shwachman-Diamond Syndrome (see chaper 7)				
Neutropenia, often dominant cytopenia early in disease course; progression to pancytopenia common	May be initially normal; early pathologic features; myeloid hypoplasia w/paucity of mature neutrophils Eventual progression to aplastic anemia common	Pancreatic dysfunction, metaphyseal dysplasia, small thoracic cage, and recurrent infections 1/3 of patients develop myelodysplasia or AML[b]	Autosomal recessive	90% of patients have mutations in *SBDS* gene on 7q11
Dyskeratosis Congenita (see chapter 7)				
Initial blood abnormalities: anemia and thrombocytopenia Eventual development of severe neutropenia	Initial normocellular w/megaloblastic features Eventual aplasia common	Skin, nail, and mucosal abnormalities, mental retardation Subsequent AML and carcinomas, esp. squamous cell carcinoma	X-linked, autosomal dominant/ autosomal recessive types	At least 3 genetic subtypes Gene products involved in telomere maintenance

[a]Data from references 163–170.
[b]WBC = white blood cell; HgbF = hemoglobin F; RBC = red blood cell; EPO = erythropoietin; AML = acute myeloid leukemia.

predicted response to increased erythropoietin levels (secondary erythrocytosis), while other cases of erythrocytosis result from autonomous erythrocyte overproduction (primary erythrocytosis). Both constitutional and acquired types of erythrocytosis have been described; acquired, primary erythrocytotic disorders are frequently clonal neoplastic processes (Table 4-11). Some-times, elevated levels of RBC parameters do not reflect an actual increase in erythrocyte mass, but are instead the consequence of disorders linked to decreased plasma volume, so-called relative or apparent erythrocytosis. By convention, erythrocytosis and polycythemia are often used interchangeably, but for clarity, the term erythrocytosis is used to describe isolated RBC

Table 4-11

CLASSIFICATION OF ERYTHROCYTOTIC DISORDERS[a]

Category	Pathophysiologic Mechanism(s)	RBC[b] Mass	EPO Level[c]	Other Features
Congenital, primary erythrocytosis	Familial erythrocytotic disorders linked to mutations of EPO receptor, or defects in EPO signal transduction pathway downstream of receptor Usually autosomal dominant inheritance, but variable	Increased	Varies by specific genetic disorder, usually normal to decreased	Other hematopoietic lineages unremarkable Phlebotomies may be required to control symptoms
Acquired, primary erythrocytosis	Acquired autonomous overproduction of erythrocytes is dominant component in polycythemia vera, a clonal hematopoietic disorder Intrinsic defect in hematopoiesis, especially erythroid progenitor cells in polycythemia vera	Increased	Decreased	Multilineage abnormalities common, especially megakaryocyte/platelet aberrations
Congenital, secondary erythrocytosis	High oxygen affinity hemoglobinopathy results in physiologic hypoxia Congenital disorder of oxygen sensing (Chuvash polycythemia) linked to homozygous mutation in von Hippel-Lindau gene, a negative regulator of hypoxia sensing	Increased	Increased	Specialized tests required to detect hemoglobin/other mutations
Acquired secondary erythrocytosis	Both physiologically appropriate and physiologically inappropriate types; caused by factors extrinsic to erythroid progenitor cells			
	Physiologically appropriate secondary erythrocytotic disorders are linked to chronic hypoxia; include many cardiopulmonary disorders, sleep apnea, and residence at high altitude	Increased	Increased	Other clinicopathologic disease manifestations may dominate clinical picture
	Physiologically inappropriate secondary erythrocytotic disorders are not clearly hypoxia-mediated and consist of various neoplasms: leiomyomas, cerebellar hemangioblastoma, hepatoma, various endocrine neoplasms (pheochromocytoma, aldosterone-producing adenoma); other renal, endocrine, hepatic, and renal lesions (such as renal cysts, renal vascular lesions, transplantation)	Increased	Increased	Other manifestations of neoplasms may dominate clinical picture
Relative erythrocytosis	Diverse causes of decreased plasma volume include fluid loss (emesis, diarrhea), other causes of dehydration, chronic diuretic therapy Gaisbock syndrome encompasses patients with relative erythrocytosis, hypertension, obesity, stress, and current smoking	Normal	Normal	Other lineages generally unremarkable

[a]Data from references 171–178.
[b]RBC = red blood cell; EPO = erythropoietin.
[c]The utility of EPO levels in classification of erythrocytotic disorders has been challenged (6).

abnormalities, while the term polycythemia is used to describe disorders characterized by multilineage elevations (cytoses).

Congenital erythrocytosis is the consequence of mutations in the erythropoietin receptor, in erythropoietin signal transduction pathways, in hemoglobin or hemoglobin-associated enzymes, or in genes regulating oxygen sensing (Table 4-11) (171,173,178). Congenital erythrocytosis is associated with increased erythrocyte parameters and elevated RBC mass, but erythropoietin levels vary by the type of defect. Erythropoietin is decreased in familial erythrocytoses mediated by mutations in the erythropoietin receptor genes, while serum levels are increased in patients with congenital disorders of hypoxia sensing (Chuvash polycythemia). Although bone marrow examination is not required for diagnosis, erythroid hyperplasia is a predicted finding in these patients.

Acquired erythrocytosis may be primary or secondary. The primary disorders result from clonal

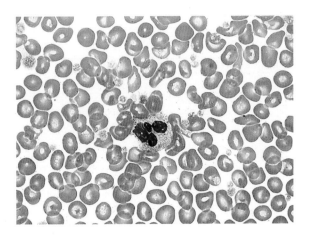

Figure 4-93

POLYCYTHEMIA VERA

The peripheral blood smear from patient with polycythemia vera shows erythrocytosis in conjunction with other lineage abnormalities (Wright stain).

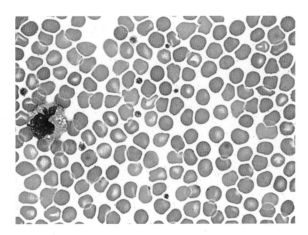

Figure 4-95

SECONDARY ERYTHROCYTOSIS FROM CHRONIC HYPOXIA

A peripheral blood smear in a patient with secondary erythrocytosis from chronic hypoxia shows polychromasia (Wright stain).

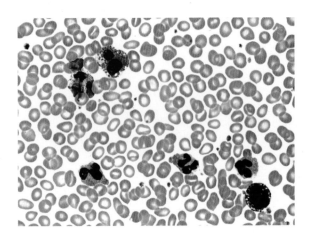

Figure 4-94

IRON DEFICIENT POLYCYTHEMIA VERA

The iron deficient polycythemia vera is secondary to chronic phlebotomy. The white blood cells have myeloproliferative features, including basophilia (Wright stain).

defects in hematopoietic progenitor cells, with *polycythemia vera* being the prototypic acquired primary erythrocytotic disorder. Polycythemia vera is characterized by multilineage proliferation in bone marrow, while erythrocytosis with left shift, thrombocytosis, and variable leukocytosis with left shift comprise the hematologic profile (figs. 4-93, 4-94).

The acquired secondary erythrocytoses encompass a broad spectrum of physiologically appropriate and physiologically inappropriate erythropoietin overproduction (fig. 4-95). Erythroid elements within bone marrow respond to increased erythropoietin with excess production of erythrocytes. The overproduction of erythropoietin may be hypoxia mediated (i.e., physiologically appropriate) or linked to erythropoietin production by various neoplasms or renal lesions (i.e., physiologically inappropriate) (Table 4-11). Although bone marrow examination is not generally required for diagnosis, erythroid hyperplasia with intact maturation is a predicted finding in these patients. Other hematopoietic lineages are typically unremarkable.

Decreased plasma volume is the primary pathophysiologic mechanism linked to *relative erythrocytosis* (Table 4-11). Although the cause of the decreased plasma volume is generally readily apparent clinically, in some patients the etiology is less clearcut, and these patients may undergo assessment for possible chronic myeloproliferative disorders. A cohort of patients with erythrocytosis and common clinical findings, including obesity, history of smoking, hypertension, and stress (Gaisbock syndrome) has been described (fig. 4-96) (175,177). Bone marrow examination with cytogenetic assessment may be performed in patients with relative erythrocytosis if clinical and hematologic findings mimic chronic myeloproliferative disorders. In these patients, the overall cellularity,

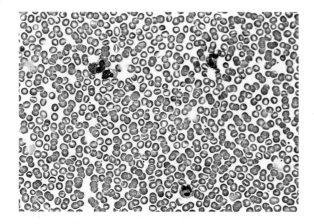

Figure 4-96

ERYTHROCYTOSIS IN GAISBOCK SYNDROME

The peripheral blood smear shows erythrocytosis without significant abnormalities in white blood cells and platelets (Wright stain).

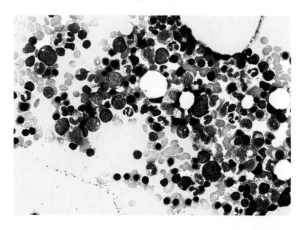

Figure 4-97

ERYTHROID HYPERPLASIA IN GAISBOCK SYNDROME

The bone marrow aspirate shows normal overall cellularity and normal hematopoietic elements with mild erythroid hyperplasia (Wright stain).

megakaryocyte morphology and distribution, and relative proportion of erythroid elements are normal, unlike typical chronic myeloproliferative disorders (figs. 4-97, 4-98).

Isolated Erythrocytosis Versus Multilineage Abnormalities

The detection of multilineage hematologic abnormalities in a patient with erythrocytosis raises the clinical suspicion for a clonal chronic myeloproliferative disorder, unless these hematologic aberrations can be explained by the clinical circumstances in a given patient. Although thrombocytosis and absolute neutrophilia are common sequelae in patients with a wide spectrum of conditions, the detection of a myeloid left shift, circulating myeloblasts, circulating erythroid precursors, and absolute basophilia suggest a chronic myeloproliferative disorder (fig. 4-99). Appropriate studies (genetics, bone marrow examination, and other laboratory tests) must be undertaken to assess for a clonal hematopoietic disorder such as polycythemia vera. In patients with chronic myeloproliferative disorders, the bone marrow is typically initially hypercellular, with increased, clustered, and morphologically abnormal megakaryocytes in conjunction with multilineage abnormalities and variable bony changes and fibrosis (fig. 4-100). If a chronic myeloproliferative disorder is a viable clinical suspicion, genetic testing is indicated, including evaluation for *BCR/ABL*-

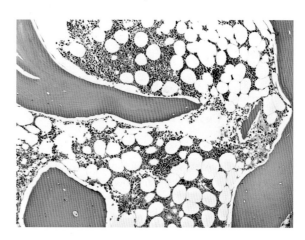

Figure 4-98

NORMOCELLULAR BONE MARROW IN GAISBOCK SYNDROME

The bone marrow core biopsy shows overall normal cellularity without myeloproliferative features (H&E stain).

related disease (chronic myelogenous leukemia) and *JAK2* mutations (other chronic myeloproliferative disorders) (172).

ERYTHROID MANIFESTATIONS OF SYSTEMIC DISORDERS

Anemia is the most common erythroid lineage abnormality in patients with either chronic infections or noninfectious systemic disorders. Anemia of chronic disease is very common and is discussed in detail in chapter 11 and earlier

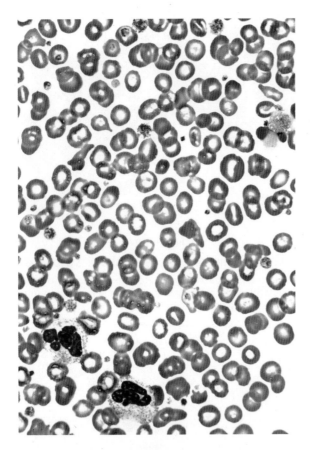

Figure 4-99

CHRONIC MYELOPROLIFERATIVE DISORDER

The peripheral blood smear shows erythrocytosis and other features of a chronic myeloproliferative disorder compatible with polycythemia vera (Wright stain).

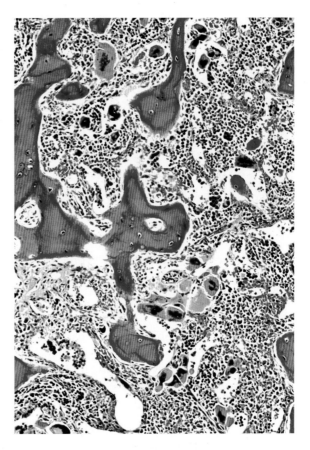

Figure 4-100

**BONE MARROW FIBROSIS IN
LONGSTANDING POLYCYTHEMIA VERA**

Bone marrow core biopsy from 53-year-old woman with longstanding polycythemia vera who developed post-polycythemic myelofibrosis with osteosclerosis, dilated sinuses, and clustered pleomorphic megakaryocytes (H&E stain).

in this chapter. Other unique erythroid manifestations in infectious diseases are reviewed in detail in chapter 10 and include intraerythrocyte parasitic diseases such as malaria and babesiosis, as well as the distinctive parvoviral inclusions in bone marrow erythroid precursors in patients who develop sustained parvovirus-induced red cell aplasia.

In addition to anemia of chronic disease, another erythroid lineage abnormality in patients with noninfectious systemic illnesses is immune-mediated hemolytic anemia with spherocytes and polychromasia on blood smears and erythroid hyperplasia in bone marrow. The physiologically appropriate and inappropriate causes of sustained secondary erythrocytosis in patients with diverse cardiac, pulmonary, endocrine, hepatic, and renal disorders were reviewed in a previous section of this chapter.

TREATMENT-RELATED
ERYTHROID LINEAGE EFFECTS

The development of an erythroid lineage abnormality in patients undergoing therapy for underlying conditions should always prompt consideration of a pathogenic link between the therapeutic agent and the new onset erythroid abnormality. Erythroid cells in bone marrow are highly susceptible to toxic chemotherapeutic agents, and may result in dyspoietic features such as nuclear budding and megaloblastic changes (see chapter 11) (fig. 4-101). In addition, noncytotoxic medications have been linked to acquired red cell aplasia, sideroblastic anemia, hemolytic anemia, and, rarely, erythrocytosis, while marked macrocytosis has been linked to

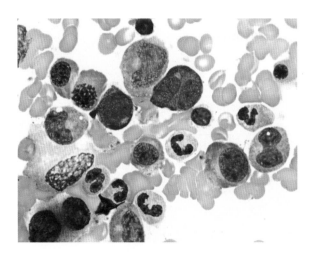

Figure 4-101

METHOTREXATE THERAPY

The bone marrow aspirate smear shows mild megaloblastic changes secondary to methotrexate therapy (Wright stain). (Courtesy of Dr. C. Sever, Albuquerque, NM.)

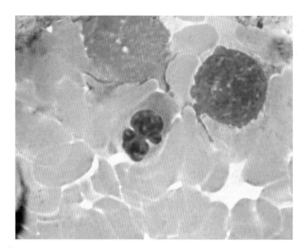

Figure 4-102

ABNORMAL ERYTHROID CELL IN ACQUIRED IMMUNODEFICIENCY SYNDROME (AIDS)

Bone marrow aspirate smear shows abnormal erythrocyte lobulation (Wright stain).

antiretroviral therapy. Bone marrow changes in patients with acquired immunodeficiency syndrome (AIDS) include megaloblastic changes and variable dyserythropoiesis (figs. 4-102, 4-103).

DIFFERENTIAL DIAGNOSIS OF ERYTHROID DISORDERS

The approach to the differential diagnosis for patients with erythroid disorders must be directed toward defining the pathophysiologic mechanism of the disorder in conjunction with determining whether a given disorder is constitutional or acquired. Anemias may be the consequence of a defect in production, maturation, or survival of erythrocytes; they may result from constitutional/genetic aberrations or they may be acquired. The diagnostic algorithm used in the assessment of anemia varies by subtype and follows a logical sequence based on MCV, RDW, reticulocyte count, and clinical parameters based on age of onset and family history. A similar algorithmic approach is utilized in the differential diagnostic approach to erythrocytoses and encompasses congenital versus acquired and primary versus secondary types of erythrocytosis (fig. 4-104). Bone marrow examination may or may not be required for the diagnosis, depending upon the specific disorder and the evidence that can be gleaned from clinical and laboratory assessments.

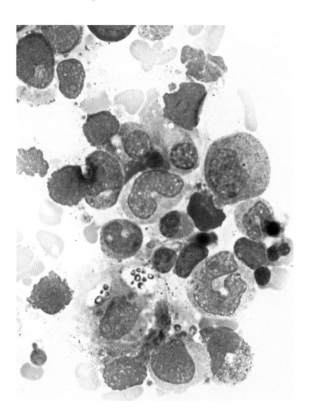

Figure 4-103

AIDS-ASSOCIATED DYSPLASIA

The bone marrow aspirate smear from a patient with AIDS shows erythroid abnormalities including nuclear lobulation as well as giant metamyelocytes. Fungal organisms are present (Wright stain).

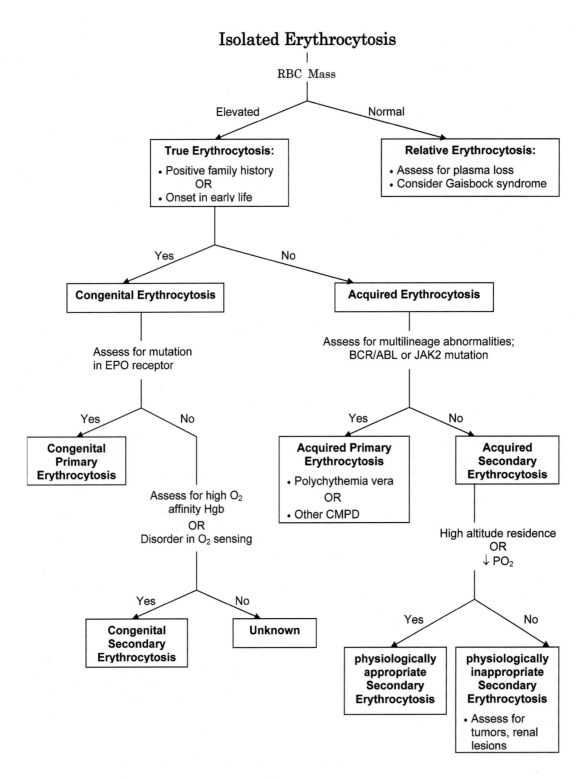

Figure 4-104

ERYTHROCYTOSIS ALGORITHM

The algorithm highlights the decision-making process in erythrocytosis. RBC = red blood cell; EPO = erythropoietin; Hgb = hemoglobin.

REFERENCES

Erythropoiesis

1. Beleslin-Cokic BB, Cokic VP, Yu X, Weksler BB, Schechter AN, Noguchi CT. Erythropoietin and hypoxia stimulate erythropoietin receptor and nitric oxide production by endothelial cells. Blood 2004;104:2073-80.
2. Koury MJ, Koury ST, Kopsombut P, Bondurant MC. In vitro maturation of nascent reticulocytes to erythrocytes. Blood 2005;105:2168-74.
3. Suzuki N, Suwabe N, Ohneda O, et al. Identification and characterization of 2 types of erythroid progenitors that express GATA-1 at distinct levels. Blood 2003;102:3575-83.
4. Testa U. Apoptotic mechanisms in the control of erythropoiesis. Leukemia 2004;18:1176-99.
5. Walrafen P, Verdier F, Kadri Z, Chretien S, Lacombe C, Mayeux P. Both proteasomes and lysosomes degrade the activated erythropoietin receptor. Blood 2005;105:600-8.
6. Welch JJ, Watts JA, Vakoc CR, et al. Global regulation of erythroid gene expression by transcription factor GATA-1. Blood 2004;104:3136-47.

Numerical and Morphologic Abnormalities of Erythroid Elements

7. Foucar K. Anemias. In: Bone marrow pathology, 2nd ed. Chicago: ASCP Press; 2001:88-108.

Overview of Anemias

8. Beutler E, Waalen J. The definition of anemia: what is the lower limit of normal of the blood hemoglobin concentration? Blood 2006;107:1747-50.
9. Foucar K. Anemias. In: Bone marrow pathology, 2nd ed. Chicago: ASCP Press; 2001:88-108.
10. Perkins SL. Pediatric red cell disorders and pure red cell aplasia. Am J Clin Pathol 2004;122 (Suppl):S70-86.

Anemia of Chronic Disease

11. Dallalio G, Fleury T, Means RT. Serum hepcidin in clinical specimens. Br J Haematol 2003;122:996-1000.
12. Dallalio G, Law E, Means RT Jr. Hepcidin inhibits in vitro erythroid colony formation at reduced erythropoietin concentrations. Blood 2006;107:2702-4.
13. Ganz T. Hepcidin, a key regulator of iron metabolism and mediator of anemia of inflammation. Blood 2003;102:783-8.
14. Means RT Jr. Hepcidin and anaemia. Blood Rev 2004;18:219-25.
15. Weiss G, Goodnough LT. Anemia of chronic disease. N Engl J Med 2005;352:1011-23.

Iron Deficiency Anemia

16. Baillie FJ, Morrison AE, Fergus I. Soluble transferrin receptor: a discriminating assay for iron deficiency. Clin Lab Haematol 2003;25:353-7.
17. Cook JD, Flowers CH, Skikne BS. The quantitative assessment of body iron. Blood 2003;101:3359-64.
18. Donovan A, Andrews NC. The molecular regulation of iron metabolism. Hematol J 2004;5:373-80.
19. Eldibany MM, Totonchi KF, Joseph NJ, Rhone D. Usefulness of certain red blood cell indices in diagnosing and differentiating thalassemia trait from iron-deficiency anemia. Am J Clin Pathol 1999;111:676-82.
20. Ervasti M, Kotisaari S, Romppanen J, Punnonen K. In patients who have stainable iron in the bone marrow an elevated plasma transferrin receptor value may reflect functional iron deficiency. Clin Lab Haematol 2004;26:205-9.
21. Iolascon A, d'Apolito M, Servedio V, Cimmino F, Piga A, Comaschella C. Microcytic anemia and hepatic iron overload in a child with compound heterozygous mutations in DMT1 (SCL11A2). Blood 2006;107:349-54.
22. Racke FK. EPO and TPO sequences do not explain thrombocytosis in iron deficiency anemia. J Pediatr Hematol Oncol 2003;25:919-20.
23. Sandoval C, Jayabose S, Eden AN. Trends in diagnosis and management of iron deficiency during infancy and early childhood. Hematol Oncol Clin North Am 2004;18:1423-38.
24. Siebert S, Williams BD, Henley R, Ellis R, Cavill I, Worwood M. Single value of serum transferrin receptor is not diagnostic for the absence of iron stores in anaemic patients with rheumatoid arthritis. Clin Lab Haematol 2003;25:155-60.
25. Umbreit J. Iron deficiency: a concise review. Am J Hematol 2005;78:225-31.
26. Weiss G, Goodnough LT. Anemia of chronic disease. N Engl J Med 2005;352:1011-23.
27. Willis M, Monaghan S, Miller M, et al. Zinc-induced copper deficiency: a report of three cases initially recognized on bone marrow examination. Am J Clin Pathol 2005;123:125-31.
28. Yurdakok K, Temiz F, Yalcin SS, Gumruk F. Efficacy of daily and weekly iron supplementation on iron status in exclusively breast-fed infants. J Pediatr Hematol Oncol 2004;26:284-8.

Megaloblastic Anemia

29. Carmel R. Megaloblastic anemias: disorders of impaired DNA synthesis. In: Greer JP, Foerster J, Lukens J, et al., eds. Wintrobe's clinical hematology, 11th ed. Philadelphia: Lippincott Williams & Wilkins; 2004:1367-95.

30. Carmel R, Green R, Jacobsen DW, Qian GD. Neutrophil nuclear segmentation in mild cobalamin deficiency: relation to metabolic tests of cobalamin status and observations on ethnic differences in neutrophil segmentation. Am J Clin Pathol 1996;106:57-63.

31. Dharmarajan TS, Adiga GU, Norkus EP. Vitamin B12 deficiency. Recognizing subtle symptoms in older adults. Geriatrics 2003;58:30-4, 37-8.

32. Figlin E, Chetrit A, Shahar A, et al. High prevalences of vitamin B12 and folic acid deficiency in elderly subjects in Israel. Br J Haematol 2003;123:696-701.

33. Foucar K. Megaloblastic anemia. In: Kjeldsberg C, ed. Practical diagnosis of hematologic disorders, 4th ed. Chicago: ASCP Press; 2006:61-78.

34. Frenkel EP, Yardley DA. Clinical and laboratory features and sequelae of deficiency of folic acid (folate) and vitamin B12 (cobalamin) in pregnancy and gynecology. Hematol Oncol Clin North Am 2000;14:1079-100.

35. Green R. Unreliability of current assays to detect cobalamin deficiency: "nothing gold can stay". Blood 2005;105:910.

36. Klee GG. Cobalamin and folate evaluation: measurement of methylmalonic acid and homocysteine vs vitamin B(12) and folate. Clin Chem 2000;46(Pt 2):1277-83.

37. Koury MJ, Price JO, Hicks GG. Apoptosis in megaloblastic anemia occurs during DNA synthesis by a p53-independent, nucleoside-reversible mechanism. Blood 2000;96:3249-55.

38. Latvala J, Parkkila S, Niemela O. Excess alcohol consumption is common in patients with cytopenia: studies in blood and bone marrow cells. Alcohol Clin Exp Res 2004;28:619-24.

39. Savage DG, Ogundipe A, Allen RH, Stabler SP, Lindenbaum J. Etiology and diagnostic evaluation of macrocytosis. Am J Med Sci 2000;319:343-52.

40. Simsek OP, Gonc N, Gumruk F, Cetin M. A child with vitamin B12 deficiency presenting with pancytopenia and hyperpigmentation. J Pediatr Hematol Oncol 2004;26:834-6.

41. Solomon LR. Cobalamin-responsive disorders in the ambulatory care setting: unreliability of cobalamin, methylmalonic acid, and homocysteine testing. Blood 2005;105:978-85.

42. Ward PC. Modern approaches to the investigation of vitamin B12 deficiency. Clin Lab Med 2002;22:435-45.

43. Weiss R, Fogelman Y, Bennett M. Severe vitamin B12 deficiency in an infant associated with a maternal deficiency and a strict vegetarian diet. J Pediatr Hematol Oncol 2004;26:270-1.

44. Wickramasinghe SN. Diagnosis of megaloblastic anaemias. Blood Rev 2006;20:299-318.

Hemolytic Anemia

45. Allford SL, Hunt BJ, Rose P, et al. Guidelines on the diagnosis and management of the thrombotic microangiopathic haemolytic anaemias. Br J Haematol 2003;120:556-73.

46. Bick RL. Syndromes of disseminated intravascular coagulation in obstetrics, pregnancy, and gynecology. Objective criteria for diagnosis and management. Hematol Oncol Clin North Am 2000;14:999-1044.

47. Boschetti C, Fermo E, Bianchi P, Vercellati C, Barraco F, Zanella A. Clinical and molecular aspects of 23 patients affected by paroxysmal nocturnal hemoglobinuria. Am J Hematol 2004;77:36-44.

48. Coppo P, Clauvel JP, Bengoufa D, et al. Autoimmune cytopenias associated with autoantibodies to nuclear envelope polypeptides. Am J Hematol 2004;77:241-9.

49. Cui W, Fan Y, Yang M, Zhang Z. Expression of CD59 on lymphocyte and the subsets and its potential clinical application for paroxysmal nocturnal hemoglobinuria diagnosis. Clin Lab Haematol 2004;26:95-100.

50. Domen RE. Warm red blood cell autoantibodies and the direct antiglobulin test revisited. Am J Clin Pathol 2004;122:673-4.

51. Elebute MO, Rizzo S, Tooze JA, et al. Evaluation of the haemopoietic reservoir in de novo haemolytic paroxysmal nocturnal haemoglobinuria. Br J Haematol 2003;123:552-60.

52. Feng X, Chuhjo T, Sugimori C, et al. Diazepam-binding inhibitor-related protein 1: a candidate autoantigen in acquired aplastic anemia patients harboring a minor population of paroxysmal nocturnal hemoglobinuria-type cells. Blood 2004;104:2425-31.

53. Gehrs BC, Friedberg RC. Autoimmune hemolytic anemia. Am J Hematol 2002;69:258-71.

54. Hill A, Ridley SH, Esser D, et al. Protection of erythrocytes from human complement-mediated lysis by membrane-targeted recombinant soluble CD59: a new approach to PNH therapy. Blood 2006;107:2131-7.

55. Hillmen P, Hall C, Marsh JC, et al. Effect of eculizumab on hemolysis and transfusion requirements in patients with paroxysmal nocturnal hemoglobinuria. N Engl J Med 2004;350:552-9.

56. Jastaniah WA, Pritchard SL, Wu JK, Wadsworth LD. Hyperuricemia and reticulocytopenia in association with autoimmune hemolytic anemia in two children. Am J Clin Pathol 2004;122:849-54.

57. Layez C, Nogueira P, Combes V, et al. Plasmodium falciparum rhoptry protein RSP2 triggers destruction of the erythroid lineage. Blood 2005;106:3632-8.

58. Miescher S, Spycher MO, Amstutz H, et al. A single recombinant anti-RhD IgG prevents RhD immunization: association of RhD-positive red blood cell clearance rate with polymorphisms in the FcgammaRIIA and FcgammaIIIA genes. Blood 2004;103:4028-35.

59. Mukhopadhyay S, Keating L, Souid AK. Erythrophagocytosis in paroxysmal cold hemoglobinuria. Am J Hematol 2003;74:196-7.

60. Mulliken JB, Anupindi S, Ezekowitz RA, Mihm MC. Case records of the Massachusetts General Hospital. Weekly clinicopathological exercises. Case 13-2004. A newborn girl with a large cutaneous lesion, thrombocytopenia, and anemia. N Engl J Med 2004;350:1764-75.

61. Nabhan C, Kwaan HC. Current concepts in the diagnosis and management of thrombotic thrombocytopenic purpura. Hematol Oncol Clin North Am 2003;17:177-99.

62. O'Brien TA, Eastlund T, Peters C, et al. Autoimmune haemolytic anaemia complicating haematopoietic cell transplantation in paediatric patients: high incidence and significant mortality in unrelated donor transplants for non-malignant diseases. Br J Haematol 2004;127:67-75.

63. Parker C, Omine M, Richards S, et al. Diagnosis and management of paroxysmal nocturnal hemoglobinuria. Blood 2005;106:3699-709.

64. Safdar N, Said A, Gangnon RE, Maki DG. Risk of hemolytic uremic syndrome after antibiotic treatment of Escherichia coli O157:H7 enteritis: a meta-analysis. JAMA 2002;288:996-1001.

65. Schwartz RS. Black mornings, yellow sunsets—a day with paroxysmal nocturnal hemoglobinuria. N Engl J Med 2004;350:537-8.

66. Takahashi Y, McCoy JP Jr, Carvallo C, et al. In vitro and in vivo evidence of PNH cell sensitivity to immune attack after nonmyeloablative allogeneic hematopoietic cell transplantation. Blood 2004;103:1383-90.

67. Thomason RW, Papiez J, Lee RV, Szczarkowski W. Identification of unsuspected PNH-type cells in flow cytometric immunophenotypic analysis of peripheral blood and bone marrow. Am J Clin Pathol 2004;122:128-34.

68. Webster D, Ritchie B, Mant MJ. Prompt response to rituximab of severe hemolytic anemia with both cold and warm autoantibodies. Am J Hematol 2004;75:258-9.

69. Wheeler CA, Calhoun L, Blackall DP. Warm reactive autoantibodies: clinical and serologic correlations. Am J Clin Pathol 2004;122:680-5.

70. Winkelstein A, Kiss JE. Immunohematologic disorders. JAMA 1997;278:1982-92.

71. Zecca M, Nobili B, Ramenghi U, et al. Rituximab for the treatment of refractory autoimmune hemolytic anemia in children. Blood 2003;101:3857-61.

Sideroblastic Anemia

72. Fleming MD. The genetics of inherited sideroblastic anemias. Semin Hematol 2002;39:270-81.

73. Foucar K. Anemias. In: Bone marrow pathology, 2nd ed. Chicago: ASCP Press; 2001:88-108.

74. Mullally AM, Vogelsang GB, Moliterno AR. Wasted sheep and premature infants: the role of trace metals in hematopoiesis. Blood Rev 2004;18:227-34.

75. Perkins SL. Pediatric red cell disorders and pure red cell aplasia. Am J Clin Pathol 2004;122(Suppl): S70-86.

76. Willis M, Monaghan S, Miller M, et al. Zinc-induced copper deficiency: a report of three cases initially recognized on bone marrow examination. Am J Clin Pathol 2005;123:125-31.

Red Cell Aplasia and Other Hypoplastic Disorders

77. Arbeiter K, Greenbaum L, Balzar E, et al. Reproducible erythroid aplasia caused by mycophenolate mofetil. Pediatr Nephrol 2000;14:195-7.

78. Bennett CL, Cournoyer D, Carson KR, et al. Long-term outcome of individuals with pure red cell aplasia and antierythropoietin antibodies in patients treated with recombinant epoetin: a follow-up report from the Research on Adverse Drug Events and Reports (RADAR) Project. Blood 2005;106:3343-7.

79. Bennett CL, Luminari S, Nissenson AR, et al. Pure red-cell aplasia and epoetin therapy. N Engl J Med 2004;351:1403-8.

80. Carpenter SL, Zimmerman SA, Ware RE. Acute parvovirus B19 infection mimicking congenital dyserythropoietic anemia. J Pediatr Hematol Oncol 2004;26:133-5.

81. Casadevall N, Nataf J, Viron B, et al. Pure red-cell aplasia and antierythropoietin antibodies in patients treated with recombinant erythropoietin. N Engl J Med 2002;346:469-75.

82. Cherrick I, Karayalcin G, Lanzkowsky P. Transient erythroblastopenia of childhood. Prospective study of fifty patients. Am J Pediatr Hematol Oncol 1994;16:320-4.

83. Crook T, Barton Rogers B, McFarland R, et al. Unusual bone marrow manifestations of parvovirus B19 infection in immunocompromised patients. Hum Pathol 2000;31:161-8.

84. Elimelakh M, Dayton V, Park KS, et al. Acquired pure red cell aplasia associated with alemtuzumab, mycophenolate, and daclizumab immunosuppression after pancreas transplant. Blood 2005;106:308a.

85. Erslev AJ, Soltan A. Pure red-cell aplasia: a review. Blood Rev 1996;10:20-8.

86. Farhi DC, Luebbers EL, Rosenthal NS. Bone marrow biopsy findings in childhood anemia: prevalence of transient erythroblastopenia of childhood. Arch Pathol Lab Med 1998;122:638-41.

87. Fisch P, Handgretinger R, Schaefer HE. Pure red cell aplasia. Br J Haematol 2000;111:1010-22.

88. Foucar K. Aplastic and hypoplastic anemias and miscellaneous types of anemia. In: Kjeldsberg C, ed. Practical diagnosis of hematologic disorders, 4th ed. Chicago: ASCP Press; 2006:43-60.

89. Go RS, Li CY, Tefferi A, Phyliky RL. Acquired pure red cell aplasia associated with lymphoproliferative disease of granular T lymphocytes. Blood 2001;98:483-5.

90. Gustavsson P, Klar J, Matsson H, et al. Familial transient erythroblastopenia of childhood is associated with the chromosome 19q13.2 region but not caused by mutations in coding sequences of the ribosomal protein S19 (RPS19) gene. Br J Haematol 2002;119:261-4.

91. Hayes-Lattin B, Seipel TJ, Gatter K, Heinrich MC, Maziarz RT. Pure red cell aplasia associated with parvovirus B19 infection occurring late after allogeneic bone marrow transplantation. Am J Hematol 2004;75:142-5.

92. Koduri PR. Novel cytomorphology of the giant proerythroblasts of parvovirus B19 infection. Am J Hematol 1998;58:95-9.

93. Koduri PR, Kumapley R, Valladares J, Teter C. Chronic pure red cell aplasia caused by parvovirus B19 in AIDS: use of intravenous immunoglobulin—a report of eight patients. Am J Hematol 1999;61:16-20.

94. Liu W, Ittmann M, Liu J, et al. Human parvovirus B19 in bone marrows from adults with acquired immunodeficiency syndrome: a comparative study using in situ hybridization and immunohistochemistry. Hum Pathol 1997;28:760-6.

95. Masuda M, Arai Y, Okamura T, Mizoguchi H. Pure red cell aplasia with thymoma: evidence of T-cell clonal disorder. Am J Hematol 1997;54:324-8.

96. Miller R, Berman B. Transient erythroblastopenia of childhood in infants < 6 months of age. Am J Pediatr Hematol Oncol 1994;16:246-8.

97. Mortazavi Y, Merk B, McIntosh J, et al. The spectrum of PIG-A gene mutations in aplastic anemia/paroxysmal nocturnal hemoglobinuria (AA/PNH): a high incidence of multiple mutations and evidence of a mutational hot spot. Blood 2003;101:2833-41.

98. Packman CH. Pathogenesis and management of paroxysmal nocturnal haemoglobinuria. Blood Rev 1998;12:1-11.

99. Perkins SL. Pediatric red cell disorders and pure red cell aplasia. Am J Clin Pathol 2004;122(Suppl):S70-86.

100. Prassouli A, Papadakis V, Tsakris A, et al. Classic transient erythroblastopenia of childhood with human parvovirus B19 genome detection in the blood and bone marrow. J Pediatr Hematol Oncol 2005;27:333-6.

101. Sharma VR, Fleming DR, Slone SP. Pure red cell aplasia due to parvovirus B19 in a patient treated with rituximab. Blood 2000;96:1184-6.

102. Skeppner G, Kreuger A, Elinder G. Transient erythroblastopenia of childhood: prospective study of 10 patients with special reference to viral infections. J Pediatr Hematol Oncol 2002;24:294-8.

103. Young NS. Hematopoietic cell destruction by immune mechanisms in acquired aplastic anemia. Semin Hematol 2000;37:3-14.

104. Young NS, Brown KE. Parvovirus B19. N Engl J Med 2004;350:586-97.

Hemoglobinopathies, Thalassemias, and Erythrocyte Enzyme Deficiency Disorders

105. Abdulmalik O, Safo MK, Chen Q, et al. 5-hydroxymethyl-2-furfural modifies intracellular sickle haemoglobin and inhibits sickling of red blood cells. Br J Haematol 2005;128:552-61.

106. Ayi K, Turrini F, Piga A, Arese P. Enhanced phagocytosis of ring-parasitized mutant erythrocytes: a common mechanism that may explain protection against falciparum malaria in sickle trait and beta-thalassemia trait. Blood 2004;104:3364-71.

107. Bakanay SM, Dainer E, Clair B, et al. Mortality in sickle cell patients on hydroxyurea therapy. Blood 2005;105:545-7.

108. Bonds DR. Three decades of innovation in the management of sickle cell disease: the road to understanding the sickle cell disease clinical phenotype. Blood Rev 2005;19:99-110.

109. Brugnara C. Sickle cell disease: from membrane pathophysiology to novel therapies for prevention of erythrocyte dehydration. J Pediatr Hematol Oncol 2003;25:927-33.

110. Castro O, Brambilla DJ, Thorington B, et al. The acute chest syndrome in sickle cell disease: incidence and risk factors. The Cooperative Study of Sickle Cell Disease. Blood 1994;84:643-9.

111. Clark BE, Thein SL. Molecular diagnosis of haemoglobin disorders. Clin Lab Haematol 2004;26:159-76.

112. Cooke BM, Mohandas N, Coppel RL. Malaria and the red blood cell membrane. Semin Hematol 2004;41:173-88.

113. Dang NC, Johnson C, Eslami-Farsani M, Haywood LJ. Bone marrow embolism in sickle cell disease: a review. Am J Hematol 2005;79:61-7.

114. Janssen WJ, Dhaliwal G, Collard HR, Saint S. Clinical problem-solving. Why "why" matters. N Engl J Med 2004;351:2429-34.

115. Jeng MR, Vichinsky E. Hematologic problems in immigrants from Southeast Asia. Hematol Oncol Clin North Am 2004;18:1405-22, x.

116. Kaur N, Motwani B, Sivasubramaniam D, et al. Potential role of the ventilation and perfusion (V/Q) lung scan in the diagnosis of acute chest syndrome in adults with sickle cell disease. Am J Hematol 2004;77:407-9.

117. Lal A, Vichinsky E. The role of fetal hemoglobin-enhancing agents in thalassemia. Semin Hematol 2004;41:17-22.

118. Lavelle DE. The molecular mechanism of fetal hemoglobin reactivation. Semin Hematol 2004;41:3-10.

119. Liu TC, Seong PS, Lin TK. The erythrocyte cell hemoglobin distribution width segregates thalassemia traits from other nonthalassemic conditions with microcytosis. Am J Clin Pathol 1997;107:601-7.

120. Manci EA, Culberson DE, Gardner JM, et al. Perivascular fibrosis in the bone marrow in sickle cell disease. Arch Pathol Lab Med 2004;128:634-9.

121. Naja RP, Kaspar H, Shbaklo H, Chakar N, Makhoul NJ, Zalloua PA. Accurate and rapid prenatal diagnosis of the most frequent East Mediterranean beta-thalassemia mutations. Am J Hematol 2004;75:220-4.

122. Old JM. Screening and genetic diagnosis of haemoglobin disorders. Blood Rev 2003;17:43-53.

123. Perkins SL. Pediatric red cell disorders and pure red cell aplasia. Am J Clin Pathol 2004;122(Suppl): S70-86.

124. Puthenveetil G, Scholes J, Carbonell D, et al. Successful correction of the human beta-thalassemia major phenotype using a lentiviral vector. Blood 2004;104:3445-53.

125. Rund D, Rachmilewitz E. Beta-thalassemia. N Engl J Med 2005;353:1135-46.

126. Saunthararajah Y, DeSimone J. Clinical studies with hemoglobin-enhancing agents in sickle cell disease. Semin Hematol 2004;41:11-6.

127. Thein SL. Genetic insights into the clinical diversity of beta thalassaemia. Br J Haematol 2004;124:264-74.

128. Tyagi S, Choudhry VP, Saxena R. Subclassification of HbS syndrome: is it necessary? Clin Lab Haematol 2003;25:377-81.

129. Zanella A, Fermo E, Bianchi P, Chiarelli LR, Valentini G. Pyruvate kinase deficiency: the genotype-phenotype association. Blood Rev 2007;21:217-31.

Hereditary Spherocytosis and Other Erythrocyte Membrane Disorders

130. Costa DB, Lozovatsky L, Gallagher PG, Forget BG. A novel splicing mutation of the alpha-spectrin gene in the original hereditary pyropoikilocytosis kindred. Blood 2005;106:4367-9.

131. Delaunay J. The molecular basis of hereditary red cell membrane disorders. Blood Rev 2007;21:1-20.

132. Eber S, Lux SE. Hereditary spherocytosis—defects in proteins that connect the membrane skeleton to the lipid bilayer. Semin Hematol 2004;41:118-41.

133. Gallagher PG. Hereditary elliptocytosis: spectrin and protein 4.1R. Semin Hematol 2004;41:142-64.

134. Perkins SL. Pediatric red cell disorders and pure red cell aplasia. Am J Clin Pathol 2004;122(Suppl): S70-86.

135. Rocha S, Costa E, Catarino C, et al. Erythropoietin levels in the different clinical forms of hereditary spherocytosis. Br J Haematol 2005;131:534-42.

Congenital Dyserythropoietic Anemia

136. Alloisio N, Texier P, Denoroy L, et al. The cisternae decorating the red blood cell membrane in congenital dyserythropoietic anemia (type II) originate from the endoplasmic reticulum. Blood 1996;87:4433-9.

137. Carpenter SL, Zimmerman SA, Ware RE. Acute parvovirus B19 infection mimicking congenital dyserythropoietic anemia. J Pediatr Hematol Oncol 2004;26:133-5.

138. Dgany O, Avidan N, Delaunay J, et al. Congenital dyserythropoietic anemia type I is caused by mutations in codanin-1. Am J Hum Genet 2002;71:1467-74.

139. Foucar K. Anemias. In: Bone marrow pathology, 2nd ed. Chicago: ASCP Press; 2001:88-108.

140. Gasparini P, Miraglia del Giudice E, Delaunay J, et al. Localization of the congenital dyserythropoietic anemia II locus to chromosome 20q11.2 by genomewide search. Am J Hum Genet 1997;61:1112-6.

141. Geller J, Kronn D, Jayabose S, Sandoval C. Hereditary folate malabsorption: family report and review of the literature. Medicine (Baltimore) 2002;81:51-68.

142. Heimpel H, Anselstetter V, Chrobak L, et al. Congenital dyserythropoietic anemia type II: epidemiology, clinical appearance, and prognosis based on long-term observation. Blood 2003;102:4576-81.

143. Heimpel H, Schwarz K, Ebnother M, et al. Congenital dyserythropoietic anemia type I (CDA I): molecular genetics, clinical appearance, and prognosis based on long-term observation. Blood 2006;107:334-40.

144. Kostaridou S, Polychronopoulou S, Premetis E, Papassotiriou I, Stamoulakatou A, Haidas S. Ineffective erythropoiesis underlies the clinical heterogeneity of congenital dyserythropoietic anemia type II (CDA II). Pediatr Int 2004;46:274-9.

145. Lind L, Sandstrom H, Wahlin A, et al. Localization of the gene for congenital dyserythropoietic anemia type III, CDAN3, to chromosome 15q21-q25. Hum Mol Genet 1995;4:109-12.

146. Perkins SL. Pediatric red cell disorders and pure red cell aplasia. Am J Clin Pathol 2004;122(Suppl): S70-86.

147. Shalev H, Kapelushnik J, Moser A, Dgany O, Krasnov T, Tamary H. A comprehensive study of the neonatal manifestations of congenital dyserythropoietic anemia type I. J Pediatr Hematol Oncol 2004;26:746-8.

148. Sigler E, Shaft D, Shtalrid M, Shvidel L, Berrebi A, Resnitzky P. New sporadic case of congenital dyserythropoietic anemia type III in an aged woman: detailed description of ultrastructural findings. Am J Hematol 2002;70:72-6.

149. Wickramasinghe SN. Congenital dyserythropoietic anemias. Curr Opin Hematol 2000;7:71-8.

150. Wickramasinghe SN, Wood WG. Advances in the understanding of the congenital dyserythropoietic anaemias. Br J Haematol 2005;131:431-46.

Congenital (Hereditary) Megaloblastic Anemia

151. Aminoff M, Carter JE, Chadwick RB, et al. Mutations in CUBN, encoding the intrinsic factor-vitamin B12 receptor, cubilin, cause hereditary megaloblastic anaemia 1. Nat Genet 1999;21:309-13.

152. Fyfe J, Madsen M, Hojrup P, et al. The functional cobalamin (vitamin B12)–intrinsic factor receptor is a novel complex of cubilin and amnionless. Blood 2004;103:1573-1579.

153. Geller J, Kronn D, Jayabose S, Sandoval C. Hereditary folate malabsorption: family report and review of the literature. Medicine (Baltimore) 2002;81:51-68.

154. Kozyraki R, Kristiansen M, Silahtaroglu A, et al. The human intrinsic factor-vitamin B12 receptor, cubilin: molecular characterization and chromosomal mapping of the gene to 10p within the autosomal recessive megaloblastic anemia (MGA1) region. Blood 1998;91:3593-600.

155. Kristiansen M, Aminoff M, Jacobsen C, et al. Cubilin P1297L mutation associated with hereditary megaloblastic anemia 1 causes impaired recognition of intrinsic factor-vitamin B(12) by cubilin. Blood 2000;96:405-9.

156. Rosenblatt DS, Whitehead VM. Cobalamin and folate deficiency: acquired and hereditary disorders in children. Semin Hematol 1999;36:19-34.

157. Solans A, Estivill X, de la Luna S. Cloning and characterization of human FTCD on 21q22.3, a candidate gene for glutamate formiminotransferase deficiency. Cytogenet Cell Genet 2000; 88:43-9.

Congenital Sideroblastic Anemia

158. Fleming JC, Tartaglini E, Steinkamp MP, Schorderet DF, Cohen N, Neufeld EJ. The gene mutated in thiamine-responsive anaemia with diabetes and deafness (TRMA) encodes a functional thiamine transporter. Nat Genet 1999;22:305-8.

159. Fleming MD. The genetics of inherited sideroblastic anemias. Semin Hematol 2002;39:270-81.

160. Furuyama K, Harigae H, Kinoshita C, et al. Late-onset X-linked sideroblastic anemia following hemodialysis. Blood 2003;101:4623-4.

161. Odoardi F, Rana M, Broccolini A, et al. Pathogenic role of mtDNA duplications in mitochondrial diseases associated with mtDNA deletions. Am J Med Genet A 2003;118:247-54.

162. Perkins SL. Pediatric red cell disorders and pure red cell aplasia. Am J Clin Pathol 2004;122(Suppl): S70-86.

Constitutional Single and Multilineage Bone Marrow Failure Disorders with Anemia

163. Draptchinskaia N, Gustavsson P, Andersson B, et al. The gene encoding ribosomal protein S19 is mutated in Diamond-Blackfan anaemia. Nat Genet 1999;21:169-75.

164. Dror Y, Sung L. Update on childhood neutropenia: molecular and clinical advances. Hematol Oncol Clin North Am 2004;18:1439-58.

165. Gazda HT, Zhong R, Long L, et al. RNA and protein evidence for haplo-insufficiency in Diamond-Blackfan anaemia patients with RPS19 mutations. Br J Haematol 2004;127:105-13.

166. Giri N, Kang E, Tisdale J, et al. Clinical and laboratory evidence for a trilineage haematopoietic defect in patients with refractory Diamond-Blackfan anaemia. Br J Haematol 2000;108:167-75.

167. Levitus M, Rooimans MA, Steltenpool J, et al. Heterogeneity in Fanconi anemia: evidence for 2 new genetic subtypes. Blood 2004;103:2498-503.

168. Ohene-Abuakwa Y, Orfali KA, Marius C, Ball SE. Two-phase culture in Diamond Blackfan anemia: localization of erythroid defect. Blood 2005;105:838-46.

169. Orfali KA, Ohene-Abuakwa Y, Ball SE. Diamond Blackfan anaemia in the UK: clinical and genetic heterogeneity. Br J Haematol 2004;125:243-52.

170. Perkins SL. Pediatric red cell disorders and pure red cell aplasia. Am J Clin Pathol 2004;122(Suppl): S70-86.

Erythrocytosis

171. Gordeuk VR, Sergueeva AI, Miasnikova GY, et al. Congenital disorder of oxygen sensing: association of the homozygous Chuvash polycythemia VHL mutation with thrombosis and vascular abnormalities but not tumors. Blood 2004;103:3924-32.

172. Kralovics R, Passamonti F, Buser AS, et al. A gain-of-function mutation of JAK2 in myeloproliferative disorders. N Engl J Med 2005;352:1779-90.

173. Kralovics R, Skoda RC. Molecular pathogenesis of Philadelphia chromosome negative myeloproliferative disorders. Blood Rev 2005;19:1-13.

174. McMullin MF, Percy MJ. Erythropoietin receptor and hematological disease. Am J Hematol 1999;60:55-60.

175. Means RT. Erythrocytosis. In: Greer J, Foerster J, Lukens J, et al, eds. Wintrobe's clinical hematology, 11th ed. Philadelphia: Lippincott Williams & Wilkins; 2004:1495-508.

176. Messinezy M, Westwood NB, El-Hemaidi I, Marsden JT, Sherwood RS, Pearson TC. Serum erythropoietin values in erythrocytoses and in primary thrombocythaemia. Br J Haematol 2002;117:47-53.

177. Pearson TC. Apparent polycythaemia. Blood Rev 1991;5:205-13.

178. Van Maerken T, Hunninck K, Callewaert L, Benoit Y, Laureys G, Verlooy J. Familial and congenital polycythemias: a diagnostic approach. J Pediatr Hematol Oncol 2004;26:407-16.

5

NON-NEOPLASTIC GRANULOCYTIC AND MONOCYTIC DISORDERS

GENERAL CONCEPTS

Abnormalities of the myeloid lineage are often first detected during peripheral blood evaluation. When quantitative or qualitative abnormalities of the leukocytes are present, concurrent evaluation of red blood cells (RBCs) and platelets provides clues to the possible etiology. Similar to many of the other non-neoplastic entities described in this Fascicle, non-neoplastic disorders affecting the neutrophils, eosinophils, basophils, and monocytes usually do not require bone marrow evaluation for diagnosis (see chapter 3), although there are exceptions.

Normal cell counts vary depending on age, sex, ethnic background, smoking status, and altitude of residence (1,3,5–7). An absolute neutrophilia with a left shift is normal at birth (fig. 5-1), but at 1 week of age and extending throughout early childhood, a predominance of lymphocytes is normal (2,4). Neutrophils again dominate in older children, teenagers, and adults. Absolute cell counts generally considered normal are listed in the Appendix. More refined reference ranges must be established in each laboratory based on the patient population (ethnic background) and instrumentation.

A bone marrow examination becomes imperative in the evaluation of sustained leukocytosis after correlation with clinical, laboratory, or radiographic findings is unrevealing. Bone marrow evaluation is important for the cytogenetic and molecular studies that help diagnose a primary hematopoietic malignancy or a nonhematopoietic neoplasm that secondarily stimulates myelopoiesis. A second significant role for a bone marrow examination in the workup of leukocytosis is to uncover an infectious process, especially in a patient with fever of unknown origin who has negative blood cultures and serologies, and white blood cell (WBC) findings suggestive of infection. Obtaining both a bone marrow aspirate specimen for cultures and a biopsy for the morphologic evaluation of

granulomas or organisms provides useful information, as further described in chapter 10.

The primary cause of leukopenia, except during infancy and young childhood, is a decrease in the neutrophils that normally dominate the WBC differential. The clinical consequences of neutropenia are more profound than for other types of leukopenia, thus bringing patients more quickly to medical attention and subsequent bone marrow evaluation. Neutropenia may be classified as either constitutional or acquired based on the bone marrow and clinical findings.

Qualitative abnormalities of leukocytes are seen in both hereditary and acquired disorders. Rare hereditary conditions that are not diagnosed by a combination of peripheral blood smear morphology, family history, and clinical examination, are usually discovered during bone marrow evaluation for an unrelated concern. These patients are often asymptomatic and may not have altered peripheral blood cell counts. In contrast, abnormally appearing leukocytes associated with acquired disorders

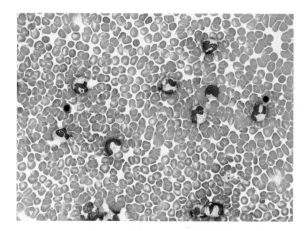

Figure 5-1

NEWBORN PERIPHERAL BLOOD SMEAR

A normal peripheral blood smear from a newborn shows the characteristic high neutrophil count with left shift and circulating nucleated red blood cells (Wright stain).

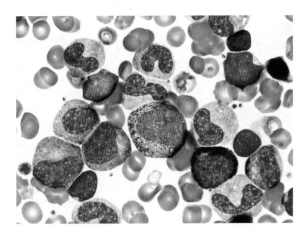

Figure 5-2

NORMAL NEUTROPHILIC MYELOID MATURATION

Spectrum of normally developing neutrophilic myeloid cells with intact maturation in a well-prepared and -stained bone marrow aspirate smear (Wright stain).

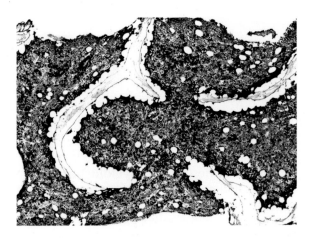

Figure 5-3

MYELOPEROXIDASE STAIN FOR GRANULOCYTIC LINEAGE

A myeloperoxidase immunostain (brown) highlights the normal peritrabecular and perivascular localization of immature neutrophilic myeloid precursors in a trephine biopsy section.

elicit more concern, as qualitative abnormalities are frequently associated with neoplastic disorders, particularly myelodysplastic syndromes or chronic myeloproliferative disorders. A bone marrow evaluation helps to exclude these processes and may suggest an alternative underlying etiology (viral infection, alcohol toxicity, copper deficiency).

Abnormalities in granulocytic maturation are best evaluated in well-prepared bone marrow aspirate smears (fig. 5-2). The Appendix lists the relative proportions of myeloid cells seen in normal bone marrow. Differential counts must be related to the total bone marrow cellularity, as best determined in biopsy specimens, for the determination of absolute counts (see chapter 3). The localization of the cells in the bone marrow biopsy sections provides additional information in the assessment of maturational abnormalities (see chapter 1) (fig. 5-3).

MYELOPOIESIS

The term myeloid is derived from the Greek word for marrow, reflecting the predominance of myeloid (nonlymphoid) cells in the bone marrow of neonates, adolescents, and adults (see chapter 3). The myeloid lineage arises from the extremely small population of pluripotent hematopoietic stem cells that have the ability to differentiate into multiple cell types (see chapter 1). More than a dozen transcription factors play crucial roles in regulating the pluripotent hematopoietic stem cell to undergo divisions that yield committed myeloid progenitor cells (a common myeloid progenitor with differentiation into a granulocyte-monocyte progenitor or eosinophil-basophil progenitor) (see fig. 1-1) (11,12). Transcription factors interact with transcriptional coactivators and repressor molecules to regulate myeloid genes. These interactions remodel the nuclear chromatin of the cells, which acts to limit gene accessibility to transcription factors and other regulatory proteins as cells develop (10,14).

Committed myeloid progenitor cells have the capacity to proliferate to meet the peripheral requirements of their mature circulating progeny through activation of intracellular signal transduction pathways (12a). Terminal differentiation into neutrophils, monocytes, eosinophils, and basophils occurs in response to specific colony-stimulating factors (CSFs) (8,9). The key CSF for neutrophil production is the cytokine granulocyte (G)-CSF. In contrast, the cytokine granulocyte-monocyte (GM)-CSF acts at an earlier level to effect multilineage stimulation.

Two of the most important transcriptional regulators for neutrophil production are PU.1 and C/EBPα (13). They are specifically required

Table 5-1

CAUSES OF ACQUIRED NON-NEOPLASTIC NEUTROPHILIA
WITH ASSOCIATED PERIPHERAL BLOOD AND BONE MARROW FINDINGS[a]

Condition	Mechanism	Peripheral Blood Findings	Bone Marrow Neutrophilic Myelopoiesis
Exercise Acute emotional stress Acute trauma Physical stress Epinephrine, adrenaline, or cortisol Hypoxia	Demargination	Mildly increased, segmented neutrophils without toxic features	Normal
Pregnancy and labor Asplenia Corticosteroids	Decreased apoptosis Decreased egress from circulation	Mildly increased segmented neutrophils and bands Possible features of activation	Normal to slightly increased
Acute infection—primarily bacterial	Initial shift from bone marrow storage pool (hours)	Mild increase in neutrophils	Normal to slightly decreased Left shifted with fewer cells
Inflammation—colitis, dermatitis, gout, nephritis Tissue necrosis—burns, wounds surgery, trauma, infarction Autoimmune disorders, collagen vascular disorders Infection	Increased bone marrow production (days) Possible decreased apoptosis	Mild to marked increase in neutrophilic cells Features of activation Usually left shift (to promyelocyte stage except for neonates may see blasts)	Increased Possible left shift and toxic changes depending on duration and etiology
Drugs—lithium, beta agonists Exogenous CSF[b] therapy Metabolic disorders—uremia, ketoacidosis, eclampsia	↓	↓	↓
Chronic smoking Tumors—carcinomas, rarely Hodgkin lymphoma, plasma cell myeloma	Endogenous CSF production	↓	↓

[a]Data from references 16, 17, 30, 36, and 41.
[b]CSF = colony-stimulating factor.

for myeloid lineage development through the regulation of numerous myeloid genes. Abnormal expression or mutations of these two transcriptional regulators contribute to the development of some acute myeloid leukemias (12b). A final key determinate to normal granulopoiesis is the bone marrow microenvironment; the bone marrow stroma is essential for appropriate development of hematopoietic cells (see chapter 9).

NEUTROPHILIA

The major causes of non-neoplastic *neutrophilia* are listed in Table 5-1. The time course and the magnitude of the neutrophilic response help in the differential diagnosis. Mild transient neutrophilia is frequently caused by exercise, emotional stress, or other conditions that increase the production of epinephrine, norepinephrine, or cortisol (29). This induces downregulation of adhesion molecules on neutrophils normally attached to blood vessel walls (17,34). Detachment or demargination of these cells quickly acts to increase the number of nonreactive-appearing segmented neutrophils in the circulation (36). This "marginated pool" of neutrophils accounts for approximately half of the neutrophils normally present in blood vessels.

Neutrophilia is the most common finding in patients presenting with bacterial, some viral, and rare fungal infections. This includes recently identified infections such as severe acute respiratory syndrome (SARS) (43) and hantavirus cardiopulmonary syndrome (see chapter 10) (fig. 5-4).

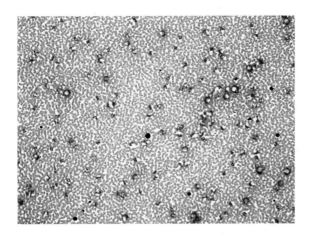

Figure 5-4

NEUTROPHILIA IN HANTAVIRUS INFECTION

Neutrophilia with a left shift in the peripheral blood smear from a middle-aged man with hantavirus pulmonary syndrome (Wright stain).

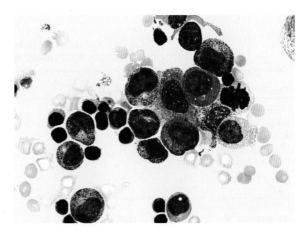

Figure 5-6

LEFT-SHIFTED NEUTROPHILIC MYELOID MATURATION

A bone marrow aspirate smear shows increased immature neutrophilic myeloid elements due to the release of mature forms in response to tissue injury (Wright stain).

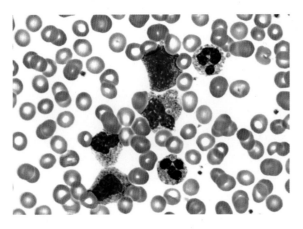

Figure 5-5

LEFT-SHIFTED NEUTROPHILIA IN BACTERIAL SEPSIS

A peripheral blood smear from a woman with bacterial sepsis shows a left shift in neutrophilic cells to the promyelocyte stage (Wright stain).

In patients with acute infectious or inflammatory conditions, a more robust neutrophil response is required than that provided by demargination. Factors elicited by the inciting process, such as glucocorticoids, endotoxins, tumor necrosis factors, or interleukin (IL)1, stimulate the release from bone marrow of predominately bands and segmented neutrophils, with occasional neutrophilic metamyelocytes, myelocytes, and rare promyelocytes (fig. 5-5) (20,35). This response occurs within hours of stimulation. Because neutrophils normally circulate for only 6 hours

before tissue migration, the bone marrow has a large reservoir of more mature neutrophilic progenitors. Neutrophilic myeloid hyperplasia ensues in the bone marrow, in which more mature neutrophilic cells may be decreased due to their rapid release into the peripheral blood (fig. 5-6). Any cause of tissue injury can evoke this response, whether related to infection, burn, thromboemboli, malignancy, surgery, or exercise-induced injury, for example, among marathon runners (25,34).

Beyond the neonatal period, a neutrophilic left shift in the blood is best identified by observing metamyelocytes or myelocytes in the circulation (fig. 5-7). Separating bands from segmented neutrophils in differential counts is not justifiable due to poor reproducibility in distinguishing between these two cell types (19,39). The percentage of band neutrophils is still used by neonatologists to evaluate for stress and infection in the neonatal period (fig. 5-8), although the few studies performed in this age group suggest this is inappropriate given the documented problems with this analysis (37). Different morphologic features have been described to distinguish between bands and segmented forms, despite the limited reproducibility in surveys using these criteria. One feature is the identification of a thin filament separating at least two nuclear lobes in a segmented neutrophil (fig. 5-9). If the filament is hidden due to extensive nuclear folding or the manner in which

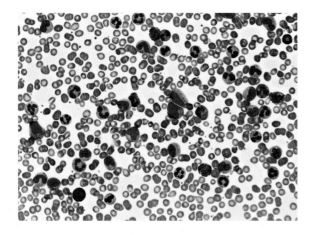

Figure 5-7

CIRCULATING NEUTROPHILIC MYELOID PRECURSORS

A granulocytic left shift in a peripheral blood smear shows numerous neutrophilic metamyelocytes, occasional neutrophilic myelocytes, and promyelocytes (Wright stain).

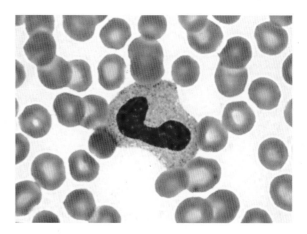

Figure 5-8

BAND NEUTROPHIL

A band neutrophil contains a nucleus without filaments, lobation, or constrictions (Wright stain).

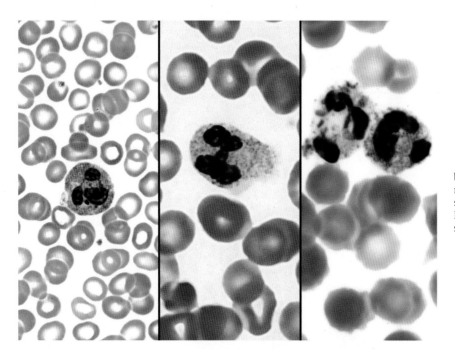

Figure 5-9

SEGMENTED NEUTROPHILS

The nuclear lobes are connected by thin filaments (left). The nuclear folding hides the thin separating filaments (middle). Lobes are separated (right) (Wright stain).

the nucleus is laying, segmentation is considered present if constriction between two lobes is observed or the margins of two adjacent lobes are completely separated (33).

Stimulated neutrophils are hyperfunctional, have shortened transit times, and have morphologic features of activation, such as toxic granulation and Döhle bodies (Table 5-2; fig. 5-10) (28). Toxic granules are larger and stain more darkly than the normal neutrophilic secondary granules. When specimens are fresh and not altered by neutrophil degeneration in ethylenediaminetetraacetic acid (EDTA) anticoagulant, the presence of prominent neutrophil cytoplasmic vacuoles with sharp borders that sometimes coalesce is associated with sepsis (fig. 5-11) (15,31). Circulating fragments of neutrophil cytoplasm may additionally be seen in septic shock (fig. 5-12) (26). Less specific features of sepsis are toxic granulation, seen in up to 75

Table 5-2	
MORPHOLOGIC FEATURES OF NEUTROPHIL ACTIVATION[a]	
Toxic granulation	Controversial, either retained primary granules or altered uptake of stain by secondary granules
Döhle bodies[b]	Gray-blue fusiform inclusions formed from lamellar aggregates of rough endoplasmic reticulum or denatured ribosomes; retained from more immature state of maturation
Cytoplasmic vacuoles	Degenerative feature associated with sepsis in fresh specimens

[a]Data from references 23, 31, 32, 38, and 44.
[b]Döhle bodies in hypogranular cells are suggestive of myelodysplastic syndromes.

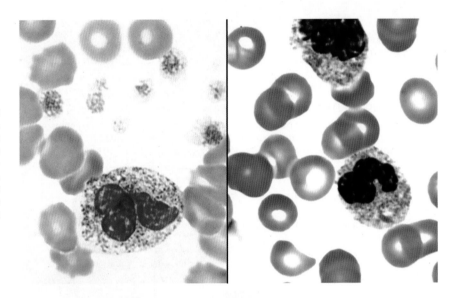

Figure 5-10

ACTIVATED NEUTROPHILS

Neutrophils with toxic granulation in a patient with a bacterial infection. Coarse azurophilic cytoplasmic granules are larger and darker than normal secondary granules. A Döhle body (blue rectangular inclusion) is prominent in the neutrophil in the right image (Wright stain).

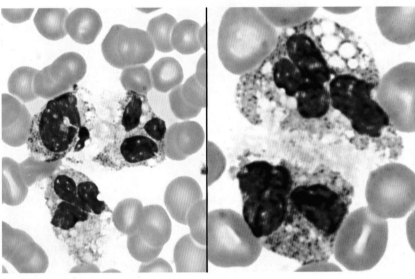

Figure 5-11

SEPSIS

A peripheral smear from a patient with an acute urinary tract infection shows many neutrophils with prominent cytoplasmic vacuoles, indicative of sepsis (Wright stain).

percent of patients, and Döhle bodies, found in only one third (27).

For a sustained increased in neutrophils, augmented bone marrow production is required. This process is predominately regulated and stimulated by the binding of G-CSF to receptors on the granulocytic stem cells (see chapter 1). This type of bone marrow response is frequently seen in cigarette smokers with mild chronic neutrophilia (40,41). If an individual presents with unexplained

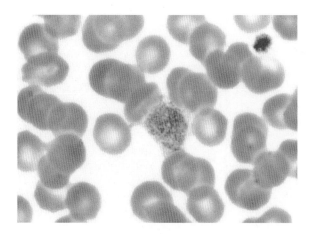

Figure 5-12

CYTOPLASMIC FRAGMENTS IN SEPTIC SHOCK

Fragments of cell cytoplasm are observed in the peripheral blood smear from an adult with fatal septic shock (Wright stain).

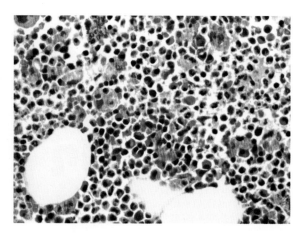

Figure 5-13

**NEUTROPHILIA ASSOCIATED
WITH PLASMA CELL MYELOMA**

Hypercellular bone marrow clot section from a patient with plasma cell myeloma, neutrophilic myeloid hyperplasia, and associated neutrophilia (hematoxylin and eosin [H&E] stain).

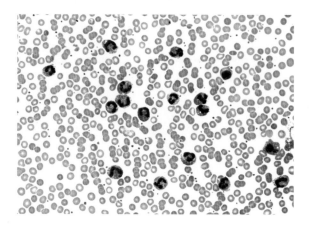

Figure 5-14

NEUTROPHILIA ASSOCIATED WITH CARCINOMA

Marked toxic neutrophilia is secondary to cytokine production in a 68-year-old woman with adrenocortical carcinoma (Wright stain). (Courtesy of Dr. C. Sever, Albuquerque, NM.)

persistent mature neutrophilia, such that a chronic myeloproliferative disorder is considered, a bone marrow evaluation with serum and urine electrophoresis may help to exclude additionally an underlying multiple myeloma (18). The bone marrow will be markedly hypercellular, with prominent neutrophilic myeloid hyperplasia and increased plasma cells (fig. 5-13) (21). Other tumors, such as those that invade the genitourinary tract, liver, gastrointestinal tract, or bone marrow, may be associated with mild to marked chronic neutrophilia and bone marrow hyperplasia, especially if necrotic from overgrowth of the blood supply (figs. 5-14, 5-15) (22,24,42).

Growth Factor Effect in Bone Marrow

The binding of G-CSF to receptors on granulocytic progenitor cells stimulates and regulates neutrophil production. G-CSF is produced primarily by monocytes/macrophages, fibroblasts, and endothelial cells (50). Therapeutic doses of G-CSF or GM-CSF act similarly on the granulocytic lineage, with an initial marked left-shifted neutrophilic myeloid hyperplasia in the bone marrow, accelerated neutrophil release to the blood, a possible leukoerythroblastic blood picture with blasts (usually less than 3 percent unless there is marked neutropenia), and an antiapoptotic effect on mature neutrophils (54,55,57,60,65). In neutropenic patients, G-CSF also helps to upregulate phagocyte function (50). G-CSF is a

significantly more potent stimulator of neutrophilic myelopoiesis than GM-CSF.

GM-CSF stimulates multipotent progenitor cells, depending on the concentration: the lowest doses stimulate monocyte precursors while increasing concentrations stimulate granulocytic, erythroid, eosinophilic, megakaryocytic, and multipotent progenitors (66). Associated eosinophilia and monocytosis are therefore

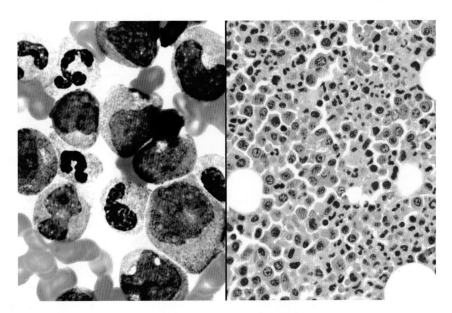

Figure 5-15

CARCINOMA-RELATED NEUTROPHILIC MYELOID HYPERPLASIA

The bone marrow aspirate smear (left) and biopsy (right) from a woman with adrenocortical carcinoma show marked myeloid hyperplasia with all stages of neutrophilic myeloid maturation (Wright, H&E stains). (Courtesy of Dr. C. Sever, Albuquerque, NM.)

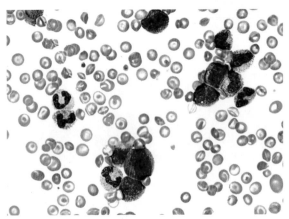

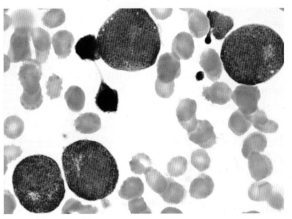

Figure 5-16

GRANULOCYTE–COLONY-STIMULATING FACTOR (G-CSF) THERAPY

A 40-year-old female recently received G-CSF after chemotherapy for pancreatic cancer. In the peripheral blood, the neutrophilic cells are shifted to the left and show features of activation (Wright stain).

Figure 5-17

G-CSF THERAPY

A bone marrow aspirate smear shows early neutrophilic myeloid regeneration with a predominance of promyelocytes and blasts in a patient treated with G-CSF for therapy-related bone marrow aplasia (Wright stain). (Courtesy of Dr. A. M. Blenc, Royal Oak, MI.)

more often seen with GM-CSF therapy, while G-CSF causes monocytosis at higher doses.

Early in the course of CSF therapy, the percentage of promyelocytes and myelocytes in the bone marrow and peripheral blood may be substantial (figs. 5-16, 5-17). Regenerating promyelocytes are best distinguished from acute promyelocytic leukemia by the lack of nuclear lobulation, absence of Auer rods, and presence of distinct perinuclear hofs (fig. 5-18) (49,51). Additional morphologic findings associated with

cytokine-induced activation of neutrophil production are listed in Table 5-3. Later in therapy, a greater proportion of more mature myeloid precursors are present, which may suggest a chronic myeloproliferative disorder, although concurrent basophilia is not observed (figs. 5-19, 5-20). Correlation with the clinical history is imperative in such cases.

One feature that helps in the identification of a G-CSF or GM-CSF effect is intense azurophilic granulation, along with Döhle bodies

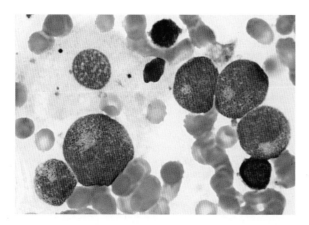

Figure 5-18

MYELOID REGENERATION AFTER G-CSF THERAPY

Increased promyelocytes in a bone marrow aspirate after G-CSF therapy. The promyelocytes have benign features, with minimal nuclear irregularity, distinct perinuclear hofs, and no Auer rods (Wright stain). (Courtesy of Dr. A. M. Blenc, Royal Oak, MI.)

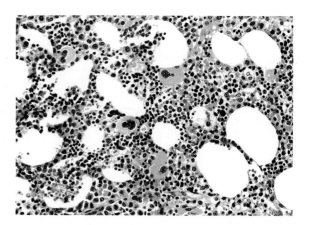

Figure 5-19

CHRONIC G-CSF THERAPY

The bone marrow biopsy is from a 58 year-old male with advanced human immunodeficiency virus (HIV) infection who is receiving chronic G-CSF therapy. The bone marrow is slightly hypercellular and shows mild trilineage hyperplasia with maturation of neutrophilic myeloid cells (H&E stain).

and vacuolation in the more mature neutrophilic cells (fig. 5-21). As recombinant G-CSF is the mainstay of treatment for patients with prolonged neutropenia due to chemotherapy, stem cell transplantation, infections such as with human immunodeficiency virus (HIV), autoimmune disorders, myelodysplastic syndromes, and constitutional neutropenic disorders (47,48,58,62), the peripheral blood and bone marrow may also show quantitative and qualitative changes associated with the underlying condition. Significant myeloblast and immature monocytic proliferations have been reported in rare patients treated with G-CSF or GM-CSF for myelodysplastic syndromes or acute myeloid leukemia (56,59). For patients with a myelodysplastic syndrome, discontinuation of therapy with bone marrow reevaluation may prevent a misdiagnosis of refractory anemia with excess blasts or acute myeloid leukemia. Similarly, acute myeloid leukemic blasts may be difficult to distinguish from regenerating cells.

When additional studies such as flow cytometric or fluorescence in situ hybridization (FISH)/cytogenetic analysis fail to differentiate between these processes, bone marrow reevaluation, after allowing time for granulocytic maturation, is indicated (usually 1 to 2 weeks). The bone marrow myeloid to erythroid ratio may

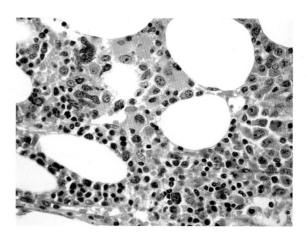

Figure 5-20

IMMUNOHISTOCHEMICAL STAIN FOR CD34

The bone marrow from an HIV-positive male receiving G-CSF therapy shows a mildly increased number of CD34-positive blasts, reminiscent of a chronic myeloproliferative or myelodysplastic syndrome.

not return to normal until 4 to 8 weeks after CSF therapy. Of consideration is the increased risk for the development of myelodysplastic syndrome or acute myeloid leukemia in rare patients receiving G-CSF for congenital neutropenia (see below) or after intensive anti-acute lymphoblastic leukemia therapy that includes etoposide and G-CSF (61).

Table 5-3

PERIPHERAL BLOOD AND BONE MARROW FINDINGS IN PATIENTS RECEIVING RECOMBINANT COLONY-STIMULATING FACTOR THERAPY (rhG-CSF AND rhGM-CSF)[a,b]

	Peripheral Blood	Bone Marrow
Cellularity and neutrophilic myeloid lineage	Increased neutrophils with left shift Usually <2% myeloblasts but transient increase up to 40% possible (rare)[c]	Hypo- to hypercellular bone marrow Increased neutrophilic myelopoiesis after CSF administration (↑ M:E ratio)[d] with initial increase in promyelocytes and myelocytes (18-52%). Later M:E ratio normalizes and more maturation seen (increased bands) Myeloblasts usually <3% but transient increase up to 40% possible (rare)[c]. Immature monocytes may also be increased
Neutrophil and neutrophilic precursor morphology	Intense azurophilic granulation, Döhle bodies (+/- multiple per cell, may coalesce) +/– cytoplasmic vacuolation +/– abnormal nuclear segmentation with hyposegmented, hypersegmented, and ringed forms[e] +/– giant tetraploid neutrophils (macropolycytes) +/– circulating cytoplasmic fragments from neutrophilic precursors (G-CSF)	No Auer rods in myeloblasts +/– enlarged promyelocytes, myelocytes, possible binucleation (G-CSF) Intense azurophilic granulation, Döhle bodies +/– nuclear to cytoplasmic asynchronous maturation, cytoplasmic basophilia
Other lineages	+/– monocytosis, eosinophilia, lymphocytosis, basophilia (GM-CSF) Enlarged platelets +/– transient decrease in platelets +/– subsequent thrombocytosis (GM-CSF)	+/– increased erythropoiesis, megakaryopoiesis, monocytes, eosinophils, lymphocytes, basophils (GM-CSF) +/– histiocytic proliferation (rare) No significant dysplastic features unless underlying MDS
Miscellaneous	+/– leukoerythroblastic picture	Increased neutrophilic myelopoiesis adjacent to bony trabeculae (also interstitium in hypocellular bone marrows) Bone marrow necrosis (rare)

[a]Data from references 46, 52–55, 59, 63, 65, and 69.

[b]Similar morphologic features may be seen with either rhG-CSF or rhGM-CSF unless indicated in parentheses. Morphologic findings are dependent on CSF dose, recent treatment, and underlying condition. Interleukin (IL)3 therapy has similar but milder effects than GM-CSF.

[c]Case reports in patients with underlying hematopoietic disorders.

[d]M:E = myeloid to erythroid ratio; MDS = myelodysplastic syndrome.

[e]Greater nuclear abnormalities are seen after high-dose chemotherapy.

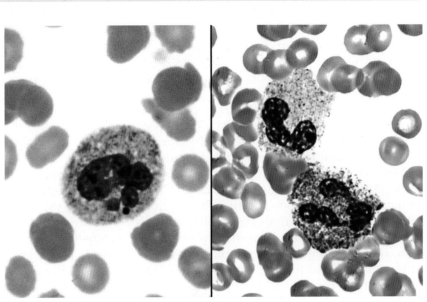

Figure 5-21

G-CSF THERAPY

Neutrophils show intense azurophilic granulation, with Döhle bodies (left) and mild vacuolization (right) in a patient given G-CSF (Wright stain).

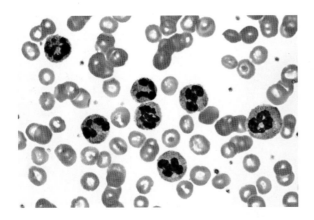

Figure 5-22

NEUTROPHILIA ASSOCIATED WITH CARCINOMA

A peripheral blood smear from an adult male with recently diagnosed transitional cell carcinoma of the bladder shows a striking cytokine-induced neutrophilia, with hypersegmented neutrophils (white blood cells [WBC] 69,800/μL) (Wright stain).

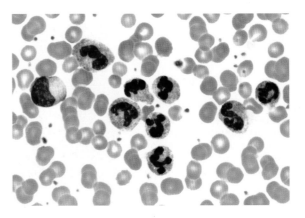

Figure 5-23

LEUKEMOID REACTION

A leukemoid reaction is seen in a patient with a surgical wound infection. The peripheral blood smear has increased neutrophils with only a few neutrophilic metamyelocytes (one shown) and myelocytes (Wright stain).

If CSF-like peripheral blood features are observed in the absence of CSF therapy, and an infection is excluded, evaluation for a growth factor–producing tumor is indicated. In particular, transitional cell carcinoma of the bladder produces G-CSF and must be considered in the differential diagnosis for older men (fig. 5-22) (67,68). G-CSF–producing carcinomas make a variety of additional growth factors and chemokines that also stimulate granulopoiesis (45,64).

Leukemoid Reaction versus Chronic Myelogenous Leukemia

During severe tissue injury, a marked elevation in the WBC count may occur, resembling leukemia. The WBC count usually does not exceed 50,000/μL and is composed predominantly of segmented neutrophils with toxic changes, and fewer numbers of circulating neutrophilic myeloid precursors (fig. 5-23). This *leukemoid reaction* is caused by the numerous cytokines released during tissue injury and is not specific to any particular insult (70,72). It may also be seen rarely in association with severe hemorrhage or acute hemolysis (75a).

The primary differential diagnosis is a chronic myeloproliferative disorder (CMPD), most commonly chronic myelogenous leukemia (CML). Because CMPDs are clonal stem cell disorders, quantitative abnormalities of multiple cell

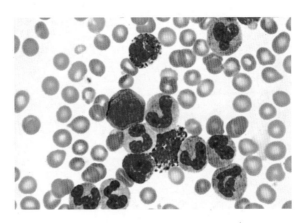

Figure 5-24

CHRONIC MYELOGENOUS LEUKEMIA

Peripheral blood smear from a 2-year-old boy who presented with hepatosplenomegaly and a high WBC count. The blood shows a left-shifted neutrophilia with occasional blasts, increased basophils, and eosinophils. Cytogenetic analysis was positive for the Philadelphia chromosome, confirming the diagnosis of chronic myelogenous leukemia (Wright stain).

lineages occur. The WBC count in CML often exceeds 50,000/μL and a greater proportion of neutrophilic myeloid precursors and blasts are present than typical for a leukemoid reaction (77). Basophilia, eosinophilia with possible eosinophilic myelocytes, and absence of significant toxic features in the neutrophilic cells help to distinguish CML from a leukemoid reaction (fig. 5-24). If the cause of sustained reactive neutrophilia is

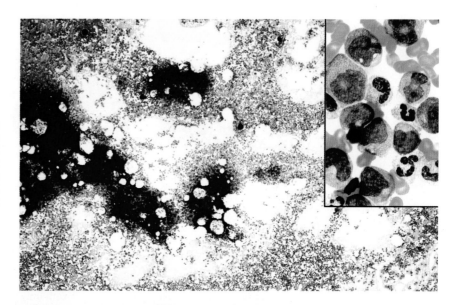

Figure 5-25

LEUKEMOID REACTION

A slightly hypercellular bone marrow aspirate smear from a patient with a leukemoid reaction. Neutrophilic myeloid and megakaryocytic hyperplasias are present without increased basophils or eosinophils (insert) (Wright stain).

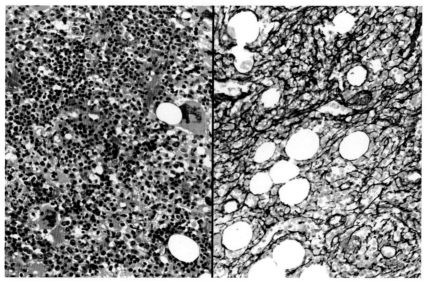

Figure 5-26

AUTOIMMUNE MYELOFIBROSIS

A hypercellular bone marrow core biopsy with neutrophilic myeloid hyperplasia (left) and reticulin fibrosis (autoimmune myelofibrosis) (right) from a patient with systemic lupus erythematosus (Wright reticulin stain).

not identified, especially after evaluation for an underlying malignant disease, bone marrow examination with cytogenetic/molecular analysis is indicated (74).

The bone marrow in a leukemoid reaction is most often mildly hypercellular due to neutrophilic myeloid hyperplasia and sometimes megakaryocytic hyperplasia (fig. 5-25). Megakaryocytes are normal in appearance, unlike the predominately small cells seen in CML, and basophilia is not observed. Additional findings such as lymphoid aggregates, increased polyclonal plasma cells, and granulomas suggest an inflammatory disorder, especially viral, and autoimmune disorders, or an alternative infec-

tious process (described in chapters 10 and 11). Reticulin fibrosis may be a feature of one of these reactive processes (e.g., autoimmune myelofibrosis) or a CMPD, and is therefore not a helpful finding (fig. 5-26).

A consideration of *chronic neutrophilic leukemia* in a patient with prolonged neutrophilia and splenomegaly is one of exclusion (figs. 5-27, 5-28) (73,75). This entity is extremely rare and for this diagnosis, the clonality of the neutrophils or the presence of a *JAK2 V617F* mutation should be demonstrated whenever possible (76). As only 10 percent of patients have cytogenetic abnormalities, this study is often normal. Evaluation of blood neutrophils

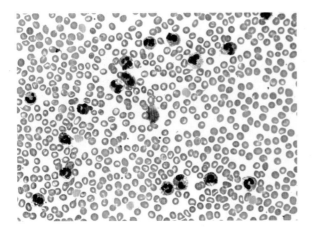

Figure 5-27

CHRONIC NEUTROPHILIC LEUKEMIA

A peripheral blood smear from a middle-aged male with splenomegaly and a 1-year history of marked neutrophilia. The neutrophils have mild toxic changes with a minimal left shift. Extensive evaluations for autoimmune, infectious, and neoplastic disorders were negative, suggesting probable chronic neutrophilic leukemia (with normal cytogenetic studies) (Wright stain).

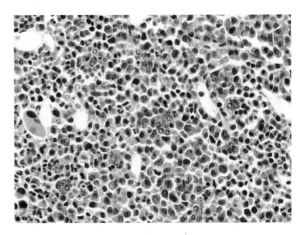

Figure 5-28

CHRONIC NEUTROPHILIC LEUKEMIA

Marked neutrophilic myeloid hyperplasia with dilated sinuses in the hypercellular bone marrow biopsy from the male with probable chronic neutrophilic leukemia (see fig. 5-27). Macrophages are ingesting neutrophils and cellular debris (H&E stain).

using human androgen-receptor gene (HU-MARA) assays may establish clonality among female patients (71).

Neutrophilic Disorders that Imitate Neoplastic Processes in Children

A *transient myeloproliferative disorder* occurs in 10 percent of neonates and infants with Down syndrome and infrequently in phenotypically normal mosaic infants with trisomy 21 identified in the blast cells (see chapters 6 and 11) (80,81). The patients are usually under 6 months of age and are clinically healthy except for the frequent presence of hepatosplenomegaly. Affected infants present with WBC counts that may exceed 50,000/μL and can include up to 50 percent blasts in a background of increased neutrophils and neutrophilic myeloid precursors (fig. 5-29). The blasts have a heterogeneous appearance and immunophenotype, often consisting of megakaryoblasts or erythroblasts in conjunction with myeloblasts (82). RBC and platelet counts are usually not significantly depressed. The bone marrows from these infants may have lower blast counts than the peripheral blood and evidence of appropriate neutrophilic myeloid maturation without dysplasia or Auer rods (79).

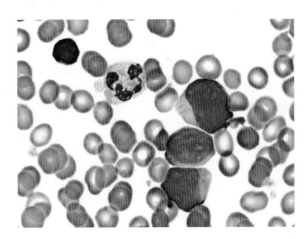

Figure 5-29

TRANSIENT MYELOPROLIFERATIVE DISORDER

A peripheral blood smear from a newborn with transient myeloproliferative disorder associated with trisomy 21 mosaicism and *GATA1* mutation. An initial WBC count was over 50,000 cells/μL with 41 percent blasts. The blasts have variable myeloid, erythroid, and megakaryocytic features (Wright stain).

Approximately 20 to 30 percent of infants with transient myeloproliferative disorder subsequently develop acute myeloid leukemia (usually of acute megakaryoblastic type) between 6 months and 3 years of age. The blasts in this disorder frequently have *GATA1* mutations; these mutations, coupled with the overexpression of genes on

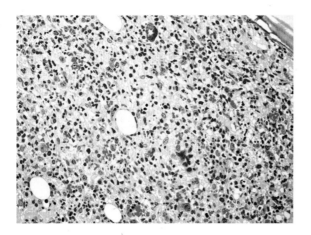

Figure 5-30

CYTOMEGALOVIRUS (CMV) INFECTION

Bone marrow biopsy from a patient with CMV infection mimics a chronic myeloproliferative disorder, with left-shifted neutrophilic myeloid hyperplasia, increased monocytes, and lymphocytes (H&E stain).

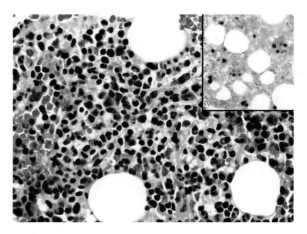

Figure 5-31

EPSTEIN-BARR VIRUS (EBV) INFECTION WITH POSITIVE IN SITU HYBRIDIZATION

Hypercellular bone marrow clot section from an older woman with reactivated EBV infection. The bone marrow shows neutrophilic myeloid and monocytic hyperplasias with lymphocytosis and EBV-encoded RNA (EBER)-positive cells (insert) (Wright stain).

chromosome 21, likely lead to the differentiation arrest and later shift towards megakaryocytic lineage (78,80).

Chronic viral infection, most commonly Epstein-Barr virus (EBV) or cytomegalovirus (CMV), and rarely, juvenile rheumatoid arthritis, can cause left-shifted neutrophilia and monocytosis that may mimic a neoplastic process (83,84). These findings are often associated with hepatosplenomegaly and lymphadenopathy. The bone marrow shows neutrophilic myeloid and monocytic hyperplasia, often with increased immature cells and lymphocytosis (figs. 5-30, 5-31).

Congenital Neutrophilia

Neutrophilia caused by a constitutional disorder is extremely rare, and usually presents in infancy or early childhood secondary to a defect in neutrophil adhesion. Abnormal neutrophil adherence to the endothelium prevents egress of circulating neutrophils into the tissue, with secondary accumulation of neutrophils in the blood. Patients with leucocyte adhesion deficiency (LAD) type 1 present with severe recurrent bacterial and fungal infections and poor wound healing (87a,88). Case reports of LAD type II describe associated severe growth and mental retardation, Bombay blood group type, and a defect in fucose metabolism, in addition to recurrent infections (85). Neutrophils may

show features of activation in peripheral blood smears. Bone marrow findings are unremarkable and show an intact neutrophilic myeloid lineage with appropriate maturation.

Additional rare causes of neutrophilia include hereditary neutrophilia, described in a few individuals with hepatosplenomegaly and increased alkaline phosphatase (87), and neutrophilia induced by cold exposure in individuals with familial cold urticaria, concurrent fever, and urticarial rashes (86).

NEUTROPENIA

The definition of *neutropenia* varies by patient age, sex, and ethnic background and appropriate reference ranges must be considered in this determination (see Appendix). Before 1 week of age to after approximately 5 years of life, neutrophils are the most prevalent leukocyte in circulation, and are thus the most common cause of a decreased WBC count. Among Caucasians, neutropenia is present if absolute neutrophil counts are less than 7,000/μL in neonates, less than 2,500/μL in infants, and less than 1,500/μL in children and adults. Latinos have slightly higher and blacks slightly lower neutrophil counts (89,94,95). Approximately one fourth of asymptomatic children and adults of African descent have neutrophil counts considered to be mildly decreased (1,000

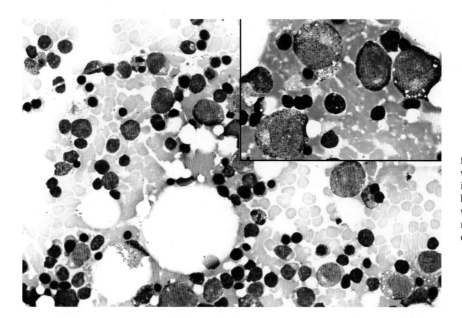

Figure 5-32

LEFT-SHIFTED NEUTROPHILIC MYELOPOIESIS

A bone marrow aspirate smear from an 84-year-old female who developed metoclopramide-induced agranulocytosis. The bone marrow shows regeneration with left-shifted neutrophilic myelopoiesis after discontinuation of the drug (Wright stain).

to 1,500/µL) based on Caucasian reference ranges. Myelopoiesis appears to be less productive in those of African heritage in contrast to the previous consideration that increased neutrophil margination accounts for race variations (90,99). Therefore, race must be strongly considered, particularly when an otherwise healthy individual is considered for bone marrow evaluation for an isolated mild neutropenia. In patients of African descent, mild neutrophilic myeloid hypoplasia, in the absence of dysplastic features, is likely inconsequential. This is also true for a patient of any race with a documented family history of mild neutropenia in multiple family members without clinical sequelae.

Acquired causes of neutropenia are more common than constitutional disorders, even among neonates and infants, as listed in Table 5-4 (91). They are most often transient or chronic and self-resolving, as many are infectious or immunologic in nature.

Acquired Neutropenia in Adults

Neutropenia in adults is produced by a number of mechanisms with a diversity of causes (Table 5-4). Broad categories of neutropenia are drug-induced neutropenia, primary and secondary immune neutropenia, and nonimmune chronic idiopathic neutropenia (104). Neutropenia in a given individual may be multifactorial, as observed in HIV-infected patients on drug therapy (see chapter 10).

Drugs are the most common cause of neutropenia in adults (110,114,123). In an outpatient setting, an idiosyncratic drug reaction is the primary reason for unexpected isolated neutropenia. The onset of *drug-induced neutropenia* is unpredictable, but most frequently occurs 1 to 2 weeks after initial drug exposure or immediately after drug reexposure. Patients have an increased rate of infectious complications and a high mortality rate of 10 percent (109). The most common offending drugs are antithyroid medications and sulfonamides (107,122); however, several additional types of drug have been implicated including sedatives and antimicrobial, cardiovascular, anticonvulsant, and antiinflammatory agents. If drug-related neutropenia is suspected, research of all drugs and over-the-counter medications taken by the patient is important. Discontinuation of all nonessential drugs and substitution of essential medications are required if the potential offending drug is not identified. The idiosyncratic drug reaction may be due to increased myeloid precursor sensitivity to a normal drug concentration in susceptible individuals (110). Alternatively, toxic levels of a drug or its metabolites may accumulate in the bone marrow of individuals with intrinsic abnormalities in drug metabolism or breakdown. Metabolites of certain drugs, such as clozapine, cause neutrophilic myeloid apoptosis in this subset of patients (120,124). The bone marrow then shows neutrophilic myeloid hypoplasia

Table 5-4

DISORDERS AND MECHANISMS CAUSING ACQUIRED NEUTROPENIA[a]

Disorder[b]	Mechanisms	Morphology

Drug induced:
Antibiotics, antipyretics, chemo-therapeutics, anticonvulsants, sedatives, antidepressants, antithyroid, antimalarials, cardio-vascular
	Inadequate production
	  interference with protein synthesis or cell replication
	  toxic effect by free radicals or drug metabolites (apoptosis)
	  immune-mediated destruction
	Survival defect
	  immune-mediated destruction
		Hypocellular bone marrow
		  >1 lineage decreased or
		  isolated neutrophilic myeloid aplasia
		  possibly only blasts and promyelocytes
		  +/– peripheral blood monocytosis
		
		Neutrophilic myeloid hyperplasia with decreased mature cells

Infection:
Viral—HIV[c,] RSV, EBV, CMV, parvovirus, influenza, measles, mumps, rubella
Bacterial- rickettsia, bartonella, typhoid, brucellosis, tularemia, typhus, military TB, gram negative (neonates)
Protozoa—malaria, kala-azar, trypanosomes
Fungus—histoplasmosis
	Inadequate production[d]
	  infects progenitor cells or endo-thelial cells
	  insufficient proliferation (neonates)
	Survival defect
	  antineutrophil antibodies
	Distribution
	  increased neutrophil adherence to altered endothelium
	  secondary splenomegaly
	  increased utilization at infection site
		Pancytopenia with >1 lineage decreased
		Adequate or increased neutrophilic myelopoiesis with relatively decreased mature cells
		Decreased myelopoiesis (neonates)

Nutritional deficiency:
  Vitamin B$_{12}$ (cobalamin)
  Folic acid
  Copper
	Ineffective production
	  maturational defect
	  production defect (copper)
		Hypercellular bone marrow (B vitamins)
		  erythroid and often myeloid hyperplasia
		  megaloblastic features in multiple lineages
		  (giant serpentine bands)
		  hypersegmented neutrophils
		  anemia and possible thrombocytopenia
		Hypocellular bone marrow (copper)
		  megaloblastic erythropoiesis
		  vacuolation in precursors
		  sideroblastic anemia

Autoimmune:
Primary—AIN
Secondary—rheumatoid arthritis, polyarteritis nodosa, primary biliary cirrhosis, scleroderma, Castleman disease, Sjögren syndrome
	Inadequate production (rare)
	  increased apoptosis (SLE)
	Survival defect
	  antineutrophil antibodies
	  antigen-antibody complexes
	  complement activation
		Neutrophilic myeloid hypoplasia (rare)
		Normocellular or hypercellular
		Neutrophilic myeloid hyperplasia
		  relative decrease in mature cells
		  possible neutrophil ingestion by macrophages

Alloimmune: Neonatal alloimmune neutropenia	Survival defect maternal antineutrophil antibodies	Normal or increased neutrophilic myelopoiesis with decreased mature cells
Chronic idiopathic neutropenia	Possible inadequate production increased apoptosis (cytokine mediated)	Hypocellular, normocellular, or hypercellular Possible neutrophilic myeloid hypoplasia with left shift
Endocrine/metabolic disorders: Addison disease, hyperthyroidism, hypopituitarism, Hyperglycemia, acidemias, tyrosinemia, glycogen storage disease type 1B	Inadequate production toxic effect of metabolites?	Decreased neutrophilic myelopoiesis
Splenomegaly: Portal hypertension, hyperplasia, secondary disease (TB, malaria kala-azar, sarcoid, Gaucher disease)	Distribution alteration	Normocellular or hypercellular bone marrow often anemia and thrombocytopenia

Table 5-4 (Continued)

Disorder[b]	Mechanisms	Morphology

Bone marrow infiltration:
Neoplasm—carcinoma, leukemia, lymphoma, myeloma
Granulomatous diseases
Fibrotic processes
	Inadequate production
	  marrow replacement
	  cytokine-mediated suppression
		Normocellular or hypercellular
		  >1 lineage often decreased
		  possible anemia, thrombocytopenia

Hematologic malignancies:
Aplastic anemia
Paroxysmal nocturnal hemoglobinuria (PNH)
T-large granular lymphocytic leukemia (T-LGL)
	Inadequate production
	  cytokine-mediated suppression
	  mutation of hematopoietic stem cell
	Survival defect
	  antibody-mediated destruction
	  complement-mediated destruction
		Hypocellular bone marrow
		  trilineage hypoplasia (aplastic)
		Possible erythroid hyperplasia (PNH)
		Hypercellular bone marrow (T-LGL)
		Left-shifted neutrophilic myelopoiesis
		Decreased M:E ratio[e]

Miscellaneous:
Radiation
Toxins, alcohol
Burns
Hemodialysis
Maternal hypertension (newborn)
Twin to twin transfusion
	Variable
	Inadequate production
	  toxic damage
	Survival defect
	Distribution alteration
		Neutrophilic myeloid hypoplasia
		  >1 lineage often decreased anemia,
		  thrombocytopenia, or lymphopenia
		Normocellular or hypercellular bone marrow
		Possible neutrophilic myeloid hyperplasia
		  with left shift

[a]Data from references 91–93, 96, 97, 100, 101, and 113.
[b]The disorders listed are not inclusive and represent examples of each major type of disorder.
[c]HIV = human immunodeficiency virus; RSV = respiratory syncytial virus; EBV = Epstein-Barr virus; CMV = cytomegalovirus; TB = tuberculosis; AIN = autoimmune idiopathic neutropenia; SLE = systemic lupus erythematosus.
[d]Acute and chronic infections cause neutropenia through multiple mechanisms.
[e]M:E ratio = myeloid to erythroid ratio.

with a left shift in myelopoiesis (fig. 5-32). Drugs may induce antineutrophil antibodies or immune complexes that attach to neutrophils and ultimately lead to their destruction (102,104). Bone marrows from such individuals are normal or hypercellular, with neutrophilic myeloid hyperplasia.

Primary autoimmune neutropenia (AIN) is most commonly seen in children and is therefore discussed in the next section. Adults more frequently have *secondary forms of AIN* that can be evaluated with tests for antineutrophil antibodies, and often relate to underlying rheumatologic syndromes (121). A bone marrow evaluation is rarely necessary unless the underlying mechanism for the neutropenia is unclear and therapy is required. For example, patients with systemic lupus erythematosus have a high incidence of neutropenia that may be antibody mediated (immune complex and neutrophil antigen specific), but also may be due to increased neutrophil apoptosis and decreased bone marrow production (104,108). The bone marrow may, therefore, show neutrophilic myeloid hypoplasia or autoimmune myelofibrosis (decreased production)

in contrast to the expected neutrophilic myeloid hyperplasia seen with antibody-mediated peripheral destruction (119).

Felty syndrome and *T-cell large granular lymphocytic leukemia* likely represent a spectrum of the same disorder and are commonly associated with rheumatoid arthritis (103,105). In these disorders, the neutropenia occurs through the decreased production (diminished granulocyte colony growth), antibody-mediated destruction, and distribution alterations (sequestration in spleen) of neutrophils (104,111). Nevertheless, the bone marrow in affected individuals often shows mild neutrophilic myeloid hypoplasia with a left shift in maturation and increased numbers of T cells that express CD2, CD3, CD8, CD57, T-cell restricted intercellular antigen (TIA)-1, granzyme B, and to a variable degree, CD16, CD56, CD11b, and CD11c (fig. 5-33) (106,107a,112,113).

Nonimmune chronic idiopathic neutropenia is the chronic neutropenia associated with a relatively benign clinical course and no evidence of neutrophil antibodies, infections, underlying autoimmune diseases, nutritional disorders, or neoplastic processes (normal bone marrow

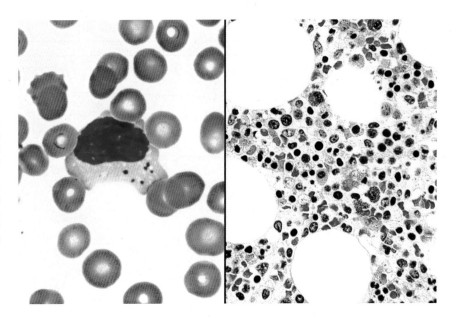

Figure 5-33

T-CELL LARGE GRANULAR LYMPHOCYTIC LEUKEMIA

Left: A large granular lymphocyte in the peripheral blood smear from a markedly neutropenic male with T-cell large granular lymphocytic leukemia.

Right: The bone marrow contains maturing neutrophilic myeloid cells and an inconspicuous increase in interstitial large granular lymphocytes (Wright and H&E stains).

karyotypes). It is seen more frequently in females than males; rare spontaneous remissions occur. The bone marrow may be unremarkable or may show either neutrophilic myeloid hyperplasia or neutrophilic myeloid hypoplasia. The etiology is unclear but is likely multifactorial (116–118). Among individuals with neutrophilic myeloid hypoplasia, an underlying inflammatory process, with the increased production of cytokines that destroy neutrophilic myeloid progenitors, has been postulated (115). G-CSF is the preferred treatment when necessary.

Acquired Neutropenia in Infancy and Childhood

Neonatal alloimmune neutropenia is caused by maternal sensitization to paternal antigens on fetal neutrophils. The resulting immunoglobin (Ig)G antibodies produced by the mother cross the placenta to the fetus and cause transient neutropenia, lasting from 2 to 4 months (average, 11 weeks). The neutropenia varies from relatively mild to severe; thus, the affected neonate may be either asymptomatic or extremely neutropenic, requiring G-CSF administration at birth (130). Granulocyte agglutination (GAT) or immunofluorescent (GIFT) tests are usually sufficient to make the diagnosis. Antibodies are most often directed against human neutrophil antigen (HNA)-1 antigens (128). The number of postpartum women having granulocyte-specific antigens (1 to 2 percent) is greater than the incidence of neonatal neutropenia, suggesting that many of the antibodies are clinically irrelevant. A bone marrow examination is usually not required to make this diagnosis, but if performed, shows normal to increased cellularity with a decrease in mature neutrophils.

Primary autoimmune neutropenia (AIN), also called *autoimmune neutropenia of childhood*, is a rare disorder; however, it is the most common cause of chronic neutropenia in infants and children. It generally affects infants and children from 3 to 38 months of age and remits spontaneously in 95 percent of patients within 7 to 24 months (125,127). The neutropenia is moderate to marked, and the associated infections are usually mild or less severe than expected for the degree of neutropenia. Evaluation of sera for autoantibodies by GAT, or if negative, by GIFT, is diagnostic. Repeat testing may be required for autoantibody detection. The majority of patients develop IgG antibodies directed against HNA-1 or, less commonly, HNA-2 (126). Bone marrow evaluation is indicated if additional abnormalities are identified on the blood film or if a child is older than typical for this disorder. The bone marrow is normocellular to hypercellular, often with left-shifted neutrophilic myelopoiesis and a decrease in mature neutrophils (127,131).

Additional causes of neutropenia in infancy and childhood are often infectious or drug related (described above, see also chapter 10). An acute episode of neutropenia may develop

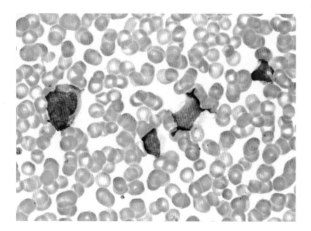

Figure 5-34

EPSTEIN-BARR VIRUS INFECTION AND NEUTROPENIA

Activated lymphocytes in EBV infection with associated neutropenia (Wright stain).

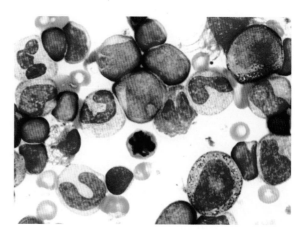

Figure 5-35

CYCLIC NEUTROPENIA

Bone marrow regeneration is observed in the aspirate smear from a patient with known cyclic neutropenia and an *ELA2* mutation. The neutrophilic myeloid lineage is increased and left shifted but shows maturation prior to the next cycle of neutropenia (Wright stain).

within 48 hours of a viral infection and persist up to 6 days. Neutrophils are primarily lost from the circulation by extensive infiltration into infected tissues. Splenic sequestration or antineutrophil antibody formation (such as EBV-infection related) may accelerate neutrophil destruction. The peripheral blood smear shows activated lymphocytes in addition to the neutropenia (fig. 5-34). Monitoring peripheral blood cell counts for evidence of recovery is usually sufficient. A bone marrow examination shows normal or increased left-shifted neutrophilic myelopoiesis. Transient neutropenia of unknown mechanism may be seen in neonates of hypertensive women (129).

Congenital Neutropenias

The term *congenital neutropenia* is generally used to describe neutropenia secondary to inherited genetic mutations and not simply neutropenia present at birth (see chapter 7). The pathophysiologic mechanism responsible for many hereditary neutropenias is the accelerated apoptosis of neutrophil precursors in the bone marrow, which causes ineffective neutrophil production and often recurrent infections (143). Several of the genetic defects have been identified (Table 5-5). Two of the most frequent congenital neutropenias, cyclic neutropenia and severe congenital neutropenia (SCN), are associated with inherited or spontaneously appearing mutations in the *ELA2* gene encoding for neutrophil elastase (138,147a). *ELA2* mutations are

implicated in a majority of cyclic neutropenias and 35 to 84 percent of SCNs (136,137).

Cyclic neutropenia, also called benign *familial neutropenia*, is characterized by cyclic episodes of severe neutropenia recurring at 21-day intervals (intervals vary from 14 to 36 days). Neutrophil counts at the nadir of the cycle approach zero and at the peak are normal. Severe infections accompany the 3- to 4-day neutropenic nadir, unless the individual is treated with G-CSF, which shortens the cycle and raises the neutrophil count throughout the cycle. The identification of bone marrow neutrophilic myeloid hypoplasia with a marked left shift in maturation prior to the period of severe peripheral neutropenia supports the diagnosis (fig. 5-35). The diagnosis is more easily established, however, by monitoring serial neutrophil counts over a 6- to 8-week period. A procedure to detect the most common *ELA2* mutations is also available. Symptoms often improve in patients with cyclic neutropenia as they grow older (141). Accelerated apoptosis of the bone marrow progenitor cells is found in all stages of the cycle, with insufficient neutrophilic myeloid output (134,155).

Severe congenital neutropenia, also termed *Kostmann syndrome*, was first described by Kostmann in 1956 (151a). He described the autosomal recessive form of this disease, which presents

Table 5-5

PERIPHERAL BLOOD AND BONE MARROW FINDINGS IN SELECT CONSTITUTIONAL NEUTROPENIAS[a]

Disorder	Inheritance	Peripheral Blood Findings	Bone Marrow Findings	Genetics
Cyclic neutro-penia	Autosomal dominant Sporadic cases (new mutations)	Marked neutropenia and monocytosis in in 21-day cycle Possible eosinophilia, reticulocytosis, thrombocytosis	Cyclic neutrophilic myeloid aplasia or arrest at neutrophilic myelocyte stage during periods of neutropenia	*ELA2* mutations on chromosome 19p13.3 encoding neutrophil elastase △V161-F170 most common
Severe congenital neutropenia (Kostmann syndrome)	Heterogenous	Isolated static neutropenia Rare cases with circulating myeloid progenitors and lymphopenia (GFI1) Possible monocytosis	Decreased granulopoiesis with few cells past the myelocyte stage Possible enlarged multinucleated myeloid precursors Increased monocytes, eosinophils, macrophages, plasma cells	*ELA2* mutations (35-84%) G185R associated with poor prognosis Rare—*GFI1, WASP* mutations
Chediak-Higashi syndrome	Autosomal recessive	Chronic neutropenia Large cytoplasmic inclusion bodies in granulocytes	Cytoplasmic granules/inclusion bodies in granulated cells that are myeloperoxidase and CD63 positive	*CHS1/LYST* gene on chromosome 1q42 encodes large protein with un-known function
Myelokathexis	Unknown	Chronic severe neutro-penia Hypersegmented neutro-phils with cytoplasmic vacuoles and degenera-tive changes	Neutrophilic myeloid hyperplasia with hypersegmented myeloid precursors and fine interlobar bridging Apoptotic nuclear features Cytoplasmic vacuolation	Molecular defect unknown ↓ bcl-x in myeloid precursors
Shwachman-Diamond syndrome	Autosomal recessive	Cyclic, often moderate neutropenia (<1000/μl) but variable Possible anemia, throm-bocytopenia	Variable neutrophilic myeloid hypoplasia with possible left shift in maturation May develop multilineage failure	*SBDS* mutations on chromosome 7q11

[a]See chapter 7 for a more complete discussion of bone marrow failure disorders.

as severe persistent neutropenia in infancy, associated with a few cells that mature beyond the promyelocyte stage in the bone marrow due to increased apoptosis (figs. 5-36, 5-37) (139,153). SCN is more genetically diverse than this initial description, with many cases arising sporadically and others arising in an autosomal dominant, or rarely, sex-linked manner of inheritance (132). Infants may develop severe infections in the first month of life and often die by 3 years of age unless they undergo bone marrow transplantation or receive chronic G-CSF treatment (164). A higher dose of G-CSF is required for SCN than cyclic neutropenia to achieve a similar response. Improvements in survival by G-CSF therapy are offset by the development of a myelodysplastic syndrome or acute myeloid leukemia (158a). The incidence of adverse events increases significantly with cumulative time or therapy, particularly among patients less responsive to G-CSF (144a,158a).

SCN patients with *ELA2* mutations generally have worse disease, with lower neutrophil counts and a higher incidence of secondary malignancy, than those without these mutations. Alternative mutations (*GFI1, WASP*) in rare cases of SCN also affect the processing and transporting of a neutrophil elastase (137). A smaller group of patients has mutations in the G-CSF receptor. These individuals are refractory to G-CSF treatment and have a high risk of leukemic transformation (144,146).

Chediak-Higashi syndrome (CHS) is a rare autosomal recessive disorder characterized by severe immunologic defects that lead to frequent and severe pyogenic infections (149). CHS is caused by a mutation in the *CHS1/LYST* gene on chromosome 1 (163). Patients with this syndrome exhibit partial oculocutaneous albinism, peripheral neuropathies, and easy bruisability due to a deficiency of platelet dense bodies. The classic diagnostic feature of CHS is the presence

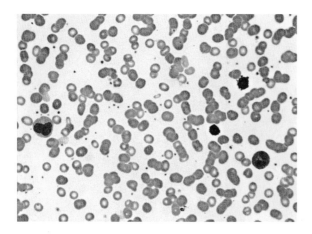

Figure 5-36

SEVERE CONGENITAL NEUTROPENIA

There is profound neutropenia with predominantly monocytes and lymphocytes present in the peripheral blood smear (Wright stain). (Courtesy of P. Izadi, Los Angeles, CA.)

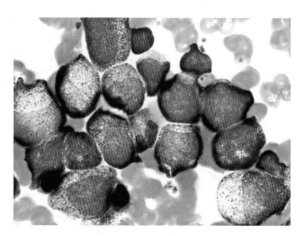

Figure 5-37

SEVERE CONGENITAL NEUTROPENIA

Bone marrow aspirate smear shows a cellular bone marrow with little neutrophilic myeloid maturation beyond the myelocyte stage (Wright stain). (Courtesy of P. Izadi, Los Angeles, CA.)

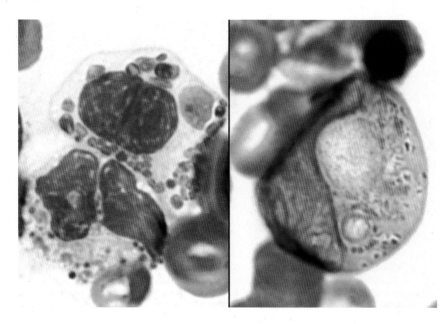

Figure 5-38

CHEDIAK-HIGASHI SYNDROME

Abnormally enlarged granules/inclusion bodies are present in myeloid precursors and blasts in a bone marrow aspirate smear from a patient with Chediak-Higashi syndrome (Wright stain). (Courtesy of Dr. R. Brynes, Los Angeles, CA.)

of huge cytoplasmic azurophilic granules within granulocytes and other granule-producing cells, including large granular lymphocytes in peripheral blood and bone marrow (figs. 5-38, 5-39) (150). The abnormal granules lead to poor mobilization and chemotaxis deficits among the neutrophils (148). Natural killer cells and T-cell large granular lymphocytes also function poorly. Without bone marrow transplantation, the disease is usually fatal in the first decade of life (147). Patients die from either frequent

bacterial infections or accelerated disease associated with a multiorgan lymphohistiocytic infiltrate. The lymphoproliferation resembles lymphoma or is associated with a hemophagocytic syndrome.

A disturbed balance between proapoptotic and antiapoptotic intracellular proteins, such as downregulation of bcl-2 family members or upregulation of the Fas death receptor, has been implicated in neutropenias associated with myelokathexis, Shwachman-Diamond syndrome,

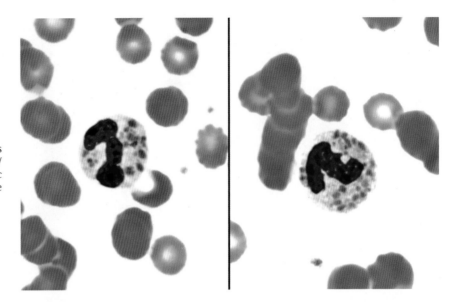

Figure 5-39

CHEDIAK-HIGASHI SYNDROME

Circulating neutrophils with abnormally large granules/inclusion bodies are characteristic of the Chediak-Higashi syndrome (Wright stain).

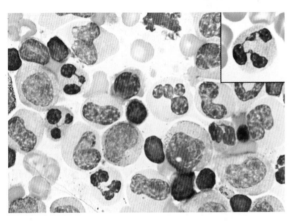

Figure 5-40

MYELOKATHEXIS

Peripheral blood (insert) and bone marrow aspirate smears from a 19-year-old Hispanic female with profound chronic neutropenia (absolute neutrophil count [ANC] 154/µL) and myelokathexis. Neutrophilic myelopoiesis is increased, with some elongate filamentous strands in the neutrophil nuclei (Wright stain). (Courtesy of Dr. S. Kroft, Milwaukee, WI.)

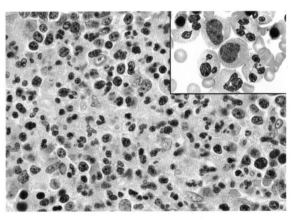

Figure 5-41

MYELOKATHEXIS

The bone marrow approximately 4 years later from the patient in figure 5-40 shows a markedly hypercellular bone marrow with neutrophilic myeloid hyperplasia and karyorrhexis. The neutrophilic myeloid lineage now shows greater atypia with hypersegmentation, fine interlobar bridging, and occasional cytoplasmic vacuolation (Wright, H&E stains). (Courtesy of Dr. S. Kroft, Milwaukee, WI.)

and acquired chronic idiopathic neutropenia of adults (156). *Myelokathexis* is attributed to the downregulation of the bcl-x protein, but the genetic basis is not yet known (133). Distinctive and specific changes are observed in the bone marrow myeloid series in these patients, secondary to the accelerated apoptosis (see Table 5-7; figs. 5-40, 5-41) (133,160). Hypogammaglobulinemia is seen in some cases, particularly in association with the WHIM (warts, hypogamma-

globulinemia, infections, and myelokathexis) syndrome. Patients often have severe recurrent upper respiratory tract infections with frequent mutations of the *CXCR4* gene (142).

Shwachman-Diamond syndrome (SDS) is a rare autosomal recessive, multisystem disorder presenting in infancy with intermittent (often cyclic) neutropenia, pancreatic insufficiency, and skeletal abnormalities (metaphyseal dysostosis) (see also chapter 7). Affected infants invariably

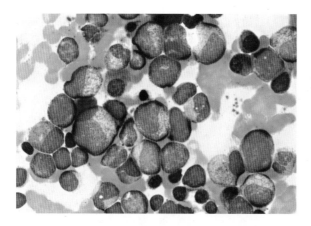

Figure 5-42

SHWACHMAN-DIAMOND SYNDROME

Despite profound peripheral neutropenia, the bone marrow aspirate from this patient with Shwachman-Diamond syndrome has abundant neutrophilic myeloid precursors. Maturation is left shifted, suggesting faulty maturation and possibly cyclical features (Wright stain). (Courtesy of P. Izadi, Los Angeles, CA.)

have failure to thrive with growth retardation and increased infections. Infections occur independent of the presence of neutropenia due to a functional neutrophil chemotaxis defect. T-cell and B-cell abnormalities and bone marrow stromal defects are also common. Hemoglobin F levels are increased. Mutations of the *SBDS* gene locus are responsible for SDS in a majority of patients (157,162). While the function of this gene has not been elucidated, an RNA metabolism deficiency essential for the development of the exocrine pancreas, hematopoiesis, and chondrogenesis is speculated (135). The bone marrow of affected children shows abnormally increased apoptosis mediated through the Fas pathway, and possibly faulty proliferative activity with abnormal granulocyte-monocyte colony formation (fig. 5-42) (145,152). An increased propensity to develop a myelodysplastic syndrome or acute myeloid leukemia has been observed, with G-CSF therapy likely accelerating this progression, similar to SCN. Approximately 25 percent of patients develop aplastic anemia.

Dyskeratosis congenita is a multisystem disorder that affects proliferating tissues with high turnover rates, such as skin, mucus membranes, and blood. Although neutropenia is often the presenting hematologic manifestation, approximately 80 to 90 percent of patients de-

velop bone marrow failure (159a). Therefore, this disorder is more fully described with the bone marrow failure syndromes in chapter 7. Additionally, patients with Fanconi anemia; inherited immunodeficiency disorders, such as reticular dysgenesis and cartilage-hair hypoplasia (140,158); metabolic disorders, such as Barth syndrome, glycogen storage disease type 1B, Hermansky-Pudlak syndrome type 2, and Cohen syndrome; and triple A syndrome (Allgrove syndrome) (151,154,159,161) may present with neutropenia.

ABNORMAL NEUTROPHIL MORPHOLOGY

Morphologic changes may be seen in the neutrophilic myeloid lineage in conditions that do not necessarily alter the total neutrophil count. These primarily include abnormalities in nuclear segmentation or in cytoplasmic granulation.

Nuclear Segmentation

A distinctive abnormality of neutrophil segmentation is the *Pelger-Hüet anomaly* (PHA). This anomaly may be inherited or acquired and must be distinguished from potential misinterpretation on blood films as a neutrophilic left shift. In the autosomal dominant inherited form, segmentation abnormalities are seen in the bone marrow from the myelocyte stage onward (fig. 5-43) (167). The appearance of circulating neutrophils depends upon whether the patient has the heterozygous or the relatively rare homozygous form of PHA. Neutrophils in the heterozygous form have nuclei with a spectacle-like "pince-nez," dumbbell shape, or bilobed shape; coarse condensed nuclear chromatin; and unremarkable cytoplasmic features (fig. 5-44). Neutrophils in the rare homozygous PHA are similar but contain only rounded or slightly indented nuclei without segmentation. The frequency of PHA varies throughout the world and has been linked to laminin B receptor mutations on chromosome 1q41-43 (166,171,176). It is considered to be a benign condition without effect on individual longevity.

Acquired PHA differs from inherited PHA in that only a subset of neutrophils has the appearance of heterozygous type Pelger-Hüet cells (167). These pseudo-Pelger-Hüet cells may be seen in association with a number of conditions, as well as with the use of a variety of medications

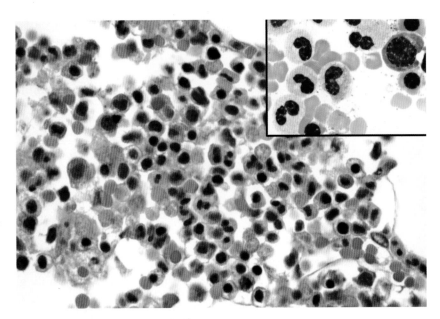

Figure 5-43

PELGER-HÜET ANOMALY

Bone marrow aspirate (insert) and clot section from a patient with familial Pelger-Hüet anomaly originally misdiagnosed as a myelodysplastic syndrome (normal karyotype, 46XX). Abnormal nuclear hyposegmentation is observed in the myeloid lineage after the myelocyte stage of maturation (Wright, H&E stains). (Courtesy of Dr. S. Kroft, Milwaukee, WI.)

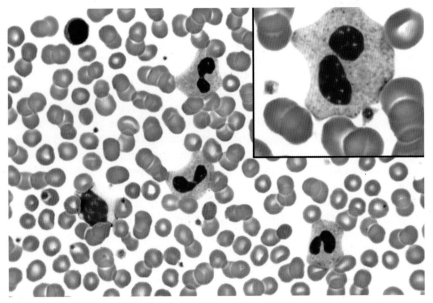

Figure 5-44

PELGER-HÜET ANOMALY

An individual with the heterozygous form of familial Pelger-Hüet anomaly has neutrophils with predominately dumbbell-shaped or bilobed nuclei circulating in the peripheral blood (Wright stain). (Courtesy of Dr. S. Kroft, Milwaukee, WI.)

and chemicals, such as ibuprofen, sulfonamide, ganciclovir, mycophenolate mofetil, valproic acid, and tacrolimus (165,168,170,173,193). Pseudo-Pelger-Hüet cells may also be seen in conjunction with infections (HIV infection, tuberculosis, influenza, mycoplasma pneumonia) (fig. 5-45) (188) and nonhematologic disorders (systemic lupus erythematosus, muscular dystrophy). In acquired PHA, benign causes must be separated from neoplastic processes since pseudo-Pelger-Hüet cells are one of the most common dysplastic markers for myelodysplastic syndromes (190). The presence of additional cy-topenias, cytoses, and other lineage abnormalities in the peripheral blood and bone marrow become important for excluding an associated myelodysplastic syndrome, CMPD, leukemia, or lymphoma (180).

The finding of neutrophil hypersegmentation is most characteristic of *megaloblastic anemia* due to either vitamin B_{12} or folic acid deficiency (see chapter 4) (194). The bone marrow myeloid lineage shows megaloblastoid nuclear features with the formation of giant metamyelocytes and band neutrophils (figs. 5-46, 5-47) (181). Circulating hypersegmented neutrophils are

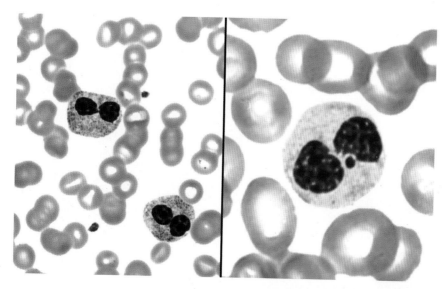

Figure 5-45

ACQUIRED PELGER-HÜET ANOMALY

Pseudo-Pelger-Hüet cells in the peripheral blood smear from an HIV-infected patient with an unknown medication history (left), and from a patient with a myelodysplastic syndrome, which also shows cytoplasmic hypogranulation (right). (Wright stain). (Courtesy of Dr. S. Kroft, Milwaukee, WI.)

Figure 5-46

MEGALOBLASTIC ANEMIA

A hypersegmented neutrophil with at least six nuclear lobes (left) and megaloblastic granulopoiesis with giant neutrophilic metamyelocytes and bands (right), from a patient with florid megaloblastic anemia (Wright stain).

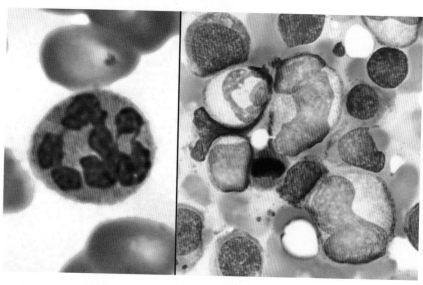

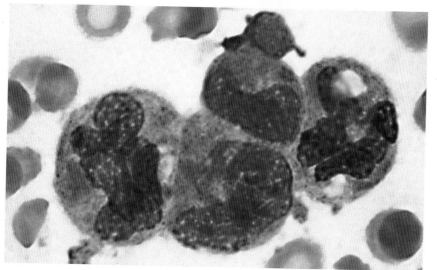

Figure 5-47

MEGALOBLASTIC ANEMIA

Bone marrow aspirate smear from a 7-month-old infant with vitamin B_{12} deficiency. Megaloblastic changes and abnormal nuclear segmentation are evident in the neutrophilic myeloid lineage (Wright stain).

149

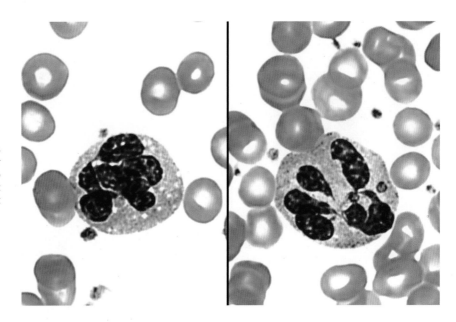

Figure 5-48

METHOTREXATE THERAPY

Hypersegmented neutrophils in a peripheral blood smear from a child with sarcoma who received chemotherapy that included methotrexate (Wright stain).

increased in size and have at least six nuclear lobes. Similar bone marrow and peripheral blood findings may be seen whenever reduced DNA synthesis but adequate RNA synthesis occurs during myelopoiesis. This may happen with infections (particularly HIV), with iron deficiency, and with corticosteroid therapy or certain chemotherapeutic agents, especially methotrexate or hydroxyurea (fig. 5-48) (169,191). Detached nuclear fragments resembling Howell-Jolly bodies may be seen in HIV-infected individuals and after chemotherapy (see chapter 10) (172,178,192). Ring-shaped nuclei are occasionally found in smears from severe alcoholics (179).

Cytoplasmic Granulation and Vacuolization

Constitutional disorders with abnormal neutrophil cytoplasmic granulation include myosin heavy chain (MYH) 9-related diseases and the Alder-Reilly anomaly. The *MYH9-related diseases* are caused by mutations in the *MYH9* gene on chromosome 22q11.2 that encodes for nonmuscle myosin heavy chain IIA (188). MYH9-related diseases are autosomal dominant disorders, among which the *May-Hegglin anomaly* has the most distinctive peripheral blood and bone marrow morphologic features. Neutrophils in May-Hegglin anomaly, as well as some eosinophils, basophils, and monocytes, contain basophilic bodies made of aggregated nonmuscle myosin heavy chain IIa, and resemble Döhle bodies (fig. 5-49) (182,185). These

differ in appearance from true Döhle bodies by their larger size, better-defined borders, and more intense blue staining. Peripheral blood findings include variable thrombocytopenia with giant, poorly granulated platelets. *Sebastian syndrome* and *Fechtner syndrome* are related MYH9 diseases that may also have granulocytic inclusions that are less prominent and lighter in color (185).

Alder-Reilly anomaly, also termed *Alder granulation anomaly*, is a granulation abnormality in all blood leukocytes, originally described by Alder in 1939 (174) and Reilly in 1941 (187). The four patients originally described by Alder had "gargoylism," which in retrospect likely represented an associated mucopolysaccharide disorder. Abnormal neutrophil granules are seen most frequently as uniform and dense, dark lilac or azurophilic granules in a background of pink cytoplasm, without Döhle bodies (fig. 5-50) (181). Similar granulation is found, to a lesser extent, in monocytes and lymphocytes, including small lymphocytes with minimal cytoplasm. Eosinophils have the most unique appearance as they contain unusually large and coarse red-violet granules resembling the color of basophilic granules (termed "pseudobasophils" by Alder) (fig. 5-51). These cells are distinguishable from basophils by myeloperoxidase positivity (basophils are normally myeloperoxidase negative). Basophils in this disorder have a reduced number of granules that may be either small or large in size. Bone marrow precursors of all lineages

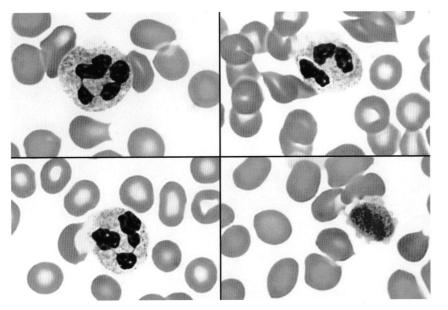

Figure 5-49

MAY-HEGGLIN ANOMALY

The neutrophils contain bright blue spindled cytoplasmic inclusions resembling Döhle bodies. No associated toxic granulation is observed. A large platelet is present (lower right) (Wright stain).

Figure 5-50

ALDER-REILLY ANOMALY

Intense granulation of neutrophils in a patient with the Alder-Reilly anomaly in association with Maroteaux-Lamy syndrome (mucopolysaccharidosis VI). Lymphocytes contain fewer granules, which may appear as distinct inclusions with halos (insert) (Wright stain). (Courtesy of Dr. C. Hanson, Rochester, MN.)

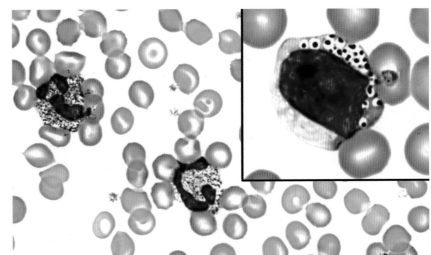

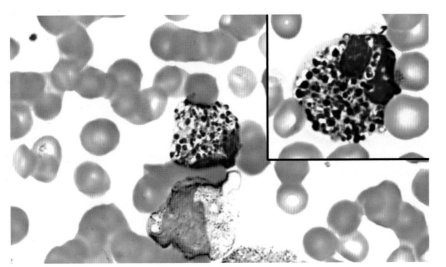

Figure 5-51

ALDER-REILLY ANOMALY

Distinctive eosinophils contain coarse basophilic granules that resemble "pseudobasophils" (Wright stain). (Courtesy of Dr. C. Hanson, Rochester, MN.)

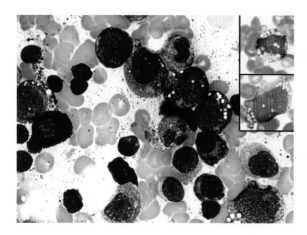

Figure 5-52

COPPER DEFICIENCY

Vacuolated neutrophilic myeloid and erythroid precursors in bone marrow aspirates from a 52-year-old alcoholic woman with low ceruloplasmin level, and a 1-year-old boy on total parenteral nutrition for microvillous inclusion disease (inserts). The findings are consistent with copper deficiency (Wright stain).

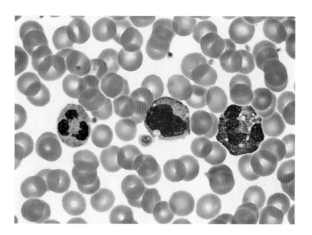

Figure 5-53

EOSINOPHIL

An eosinophil (right) is distinguishable from other hematopoietic cells by the prominent coarse, orange-red cytoplasmic granules. The granules of a neutrophil (left) are smaller, less refractile, and have a lilac-beige coloration (Wright stain).

show similar distinct granulation alterations that may be striking (183). The Alder-Reilly anomaly is frequently associated with the acid mucopolysaccharidoses, which are autosomal recessive inherited disorders caused by deficiencies of the lysosomal enzymes needed to degrade mucopolysaccharides (183,184). Patients with mucopolysaccharidoses generally have additional unique findings in the blood and bone marrow, such as inclusions in marrow plasma cells (Buhot cells) and metachromatic granules in mononuclear cells (174).

Vacuolation of myeloid precursors in bone marrow aspirate smears is most commonly seen with acute alcohol ingestion. Additional reactive causes include severe infections and drug-induced marrow damage. Evaluation for *copper deficiency* should be performed when both erythroid and neutrophilic myeloid precursor vacuolization is observed in bone marrow specimens, possibly mimicking a myelodysplastic syndrome, albeit neutrophilic myeloid precursor vacuolization is not a typical feature of myelodysplasia (fig. 5-52) (195). Copper deficiency is a rare complication of total parenteral nutrition or excess zinc ingestion; the development of cytopenias usually prompts the bone marrow evaluation (175,177,195). A few congenital disorders may also show myeloid

vacuolization, such as *Jordan anomaly (familial vacuolation of leukocytes)* (186).

EOSINOPHILIA

Eosinophils are distinguishable from neutrophils and neutrophilic myeloid precursors in the peripheral blood and bone marrow by their uniform, coarse, orange-red refractile granules (fig. 5-53). Eosinophils are postulated to derive from a hybrid eosinophil/basophil precursor cell with nuclear maturation capitulating that seen in the neutrophilic myeloid lineage (fig. 5-54) (204). Type 1 and 2 T-helper cells (Th1 and Th2) promote early eosinophil development through IL3 and GM-CSF production, while IL5 plays an important subsequent role (225).

The first recognizable bone marrow precursor of the eosinophil is the eosinophilic myelocyte. This may contain a few primary, azurophilic granules in addition to the characteristic orange-red granules. Nuclear maturation ends with nuclear segmentation; approximately 80 percent of mature eosinophils have two equally sized nuclear lobes (fig. 5-55). The remaining eosinophils contain predominately three lobes but up to five lobes may be seen. Eosinophils and precursors are often unevenly distributed in bone marrow biopsy sections, with a greater concentration adjacent to granulomas and

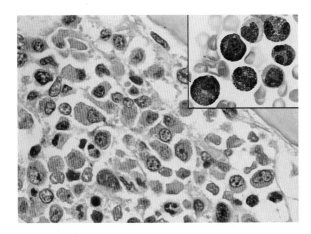

Figure 5-54

EOSINOPHILIC MATURATION

Bone marrow aspirate (insert) and biopsy section show different stages of eosinophil differentiation. The large cells with rounded nuclear contours are eosinophilic myelocytes (Wright, H&E stains).

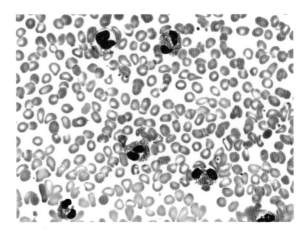

Figure 5-55

EOSINOPHILS

Circulating eosinophils most commonly have bilobed nuclei (Wright stain).

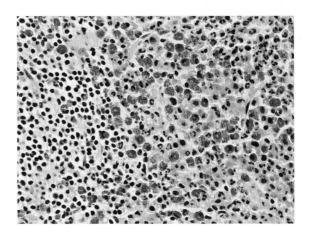

Figure 5-56

BONE MARROW EOSINOPHILS

Eosinophils and precursors are unevenly distributed and concentrated adjacent to lymphoid aggregates in this bone marrow biopsy section (H&E stain).

lymphoid or neoplastic infiltrates (fig. 5-56). In bone marrow aspirate smears, eosinophils concentrated within more cellular parts of spicules will be missed during the counting of peripheral areas. Charcot-Leyden crystals infrequently form in hypercellular bone marrow with marked eosinophilia.

An absolute eosinophil count of greater than 500/µL is defined as eosinophilia for all age groups. Arbitrarily assigned absolute eosinophilia counts based on the degree of eosinophilia include: mild (500 to 1,500/µL), moderate (1,500 to 5,000/µL), and severe (over 5,000/µL) (199). Eosinophilia may be secondary (reactive) or primary (clonal or idiopathic) in etiology (225).

Reactive eosinophilia in the blood and bone marrow is cytokine mediated and caused by a number of inciting factors, as listed in Table 5-6. The most common causes are allergic disorders in industrialized countries, parasitic organisms that invade tissue in other countries, and drug reactions among hospitalized patients (224,229). In patients with allergic disorders, particularly asthma, allergen exposure activates Th2 cells to orchestrate the secretion of growth factors, particularly IL5 and IL3, and chemokines, such as eotaxin (221). IL5 stimulation of bone marrow creates a robust increase in circulating eosinophils. Some of the highest levels of bone

marrow eosinophils are seen with complications of asthma, such as in patients with Churg-Strauss syndrome (primary systemic vasculitis) or secondary *Aspergillus* infection (210,217). Inappropriate release of eosinophilic granules in tissues, especially major basic protein, causes tissue damage, fibrosis, peripheral neuropathy, and endothelial cell damage with thromboembolism formation. In contrast to the many detrimental effects seen with tissue infiltration by eosinophils in allergic disorders, eosinophils play a more beneficial

Table 5-6

CAUSES OF REACTIVE EOSINOPHILIA[a,b]

Disorders	Examples
Drug hyper-sensitivity	Numerous drugs (antibiotics, anticonvulsants, aspirin, sulfonamides, allopurinol, chemotherapeutics) Interleukin-2 and recombinant cytokine therapy Eosinophilia/myalgia syndrome—caused by contaminated L-tryptophan
Allergic	Asthma Hayfever Allergic rhinitis and sinusitis
Infection	Helminths (*Filaria*, hookworm, *Ascaris*, schistosomes, *Trichinella*, *Strongyloides*; often increased serum IgE level) Protozoa (*Isospora belli*, *Dientamoeba fragilis*) Bacteria (*Borrelia burgdorferi*) Fungal (*Cryptococcus*, *Aspergillus*)
Immune	Polyarteritis nodosa Churg-Strauss syndrome Sarcoidosis Scleroderma Systemic lupus erythematosus Kimura disease Eosinophilic fasciitis Other collagen vascular diseases
Skin	Atopic dermatitis Urticaria Bullous pemphigoid Pemphigus Angiolymphoid hyperplasia
Gastrointestinal	Celiac disease Inflammatory bowel disease Chronic pancreatitis
Pulmonary	Loeffler syndrome Hypersensitivity pneumonitis Bronchiectasis Chronic idiopathic eosinophilia
Neoplastic	Classical Hodgkin lymphoma T-cell lymphoma T-cell clonal disorder (T-cell dyscrasia in bone marrow) Langerhans cell histiocytosis Acute lymphoblastic leukemia (when associated with t(5;14); eosinophils probably reactive but appear dysplastic) Solid tumors (lung, stomach)

[a]Data from references 202, 203, 208, 209, 211, 214, 217, 220, 221, 223, and 224–228.
[b]With the exception of eosinophilia secondary to a neoplastic or autoimmune disorder, the bone marrow cellularity is generally near normal with unremarkable findings in other lineages, absence of bony changes, and absence of megakaryocytic clustering or atypia.

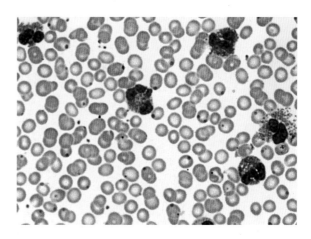

Figure 5-57

EOSINOPHILIA WITH CYTOKINE THERAPY

Peripheral blood eosinophilia in a patient receiving interleukin (IL)2 and IL4 therapy (Wright stain).

role in host defense against tissue invasion by helminthic parasites (201,205).

When an obvious cause of eosinophilia cannot be identified, evaluation of recent drug, herbal, or other treatments is essential. As bone marrow examinations are rarely performed for either parasitic or allergic disorders in the United States, a drug effect or neoplasm is the most common cause of increased bone marrow eosinophils in clinical practice (fig. 5-57). Numerous drugs are associated with eosinophilia, due in part to certain drugs acting as haptens that trigger a Th2 response. Rashes, pulmonary infiltrates, and interstitial nephritis are some of the related findings. Patients with the DRESS syndrome, characterized by drug rash, eosinophilia (with possible atypical lymphocytosis), and systemic symptoms, often present with delayed onset (2 to 6 weeks) after receiving the offending drugs. Systemic symptoms consist of fever, pneumonia, edema, lymphadenopathy, hepatitis, renal failure, and arthritis. Multiple drugs cause DRESS syndrome, including cephalosporins, vancomycin, and phenytoin (196,225,230).

A variety of hematopoietic and solid tumors secrete cytokines, including IL5, that cause reactive eosinophilia. Circulating eosinophils may show cytologic atypia indistinguishable from a primary neoplastic process, with both nuclear and cytoplasmic abnormalities. After the exclusion of known reactive causes for eosinophilia, a bone marrow evaluation is indicated for any

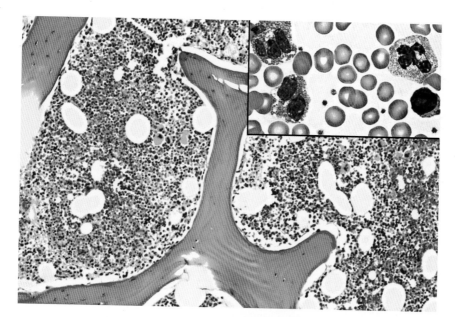

Figure 5-58

HYPEREOSINOPHILIA

A T-cell clone was detected in the bone marrow of this 26-year-old female with marked hypereosinophilia. The peripheral blood (insert) and bone marrow show no evidence of T-cell lymphoma or leukemia (Wright, H&E stains). (Courtesy of Dr. C. Sever, Albuquerque, NM.)

Figure 5-59

HYPEREOSINOPHILIA

Peripheral blood smear from a 67-year-old male with hypereosinophilia of greater than 1 year duration. Prominent eosinophilic atypia including nuclear hyposegmentation and cytoplasmic hypogranulation. Studies for T-cell clonality, karyotypic abnormalities, and a *FIP1L1-PDGFRA* fusion gene were negative. Other lineages were morphologically unremarkable (Wright stain).

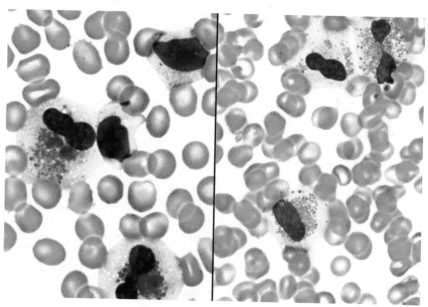

patient with organomegaly, lymphadenopathy, elevated tryptase levels, or additional abnormal peripheral blood findings. A clonal T-cell process (T-cell dyscrasia) may be found by gene rearrangement studies in the absence of an overt T-cell malignancy (fig. 5-58). These patients need to be carefully followed for the development of a T-cell neoplasm and treated for any adverse effects of the hypereosinophilia (200,227a).

Unexplained eosinophilia of over 1,500/μL that persists for more than 6 months is termed *hypereosinophilia* and may be primary (clonal or idiopathic) rather than secondary in origin

(206,222). As previously discussed, it may be difficult to make this distinction based on the appearance of the eosinophils (fig. 5-59). The identification of primary eosinophilia requires the detection of a cytogenetic/molecular abnormality (Table 5-7) or bone marrow histologic evidence of a hematologic malignancy upon which eosinophils are likely part of the neoplastic clone (CMPD, myelodysplastic syndrome, or acute myeloid leukemia) (198,218). Immunohistochemical staining with tryptase and/or CD117 (c-kit) helps to identify neoplastic mast cell infiltrates (fig. 5-60) (219). The features that

Table 5-7

MOLECULARLY DEFINED CAUSES OF NEOPLASTIC/CLONAL EOSINOPHILIA[a,b]

Disorders	Examples
BCR-ABL[c]	Chronic myelogenous leukemia
FIP1L1-PDGFRA mutations[d]	Hypereosinophilic syndrome Chronic eosinophilic leukemia Eosinophilia-associated systemic mastocytosis
PDGFRA—rearranged eosinophilic disorders	Chronic myeloproliferative disorders with t(4:22)(q12;q11) Atypical chronic myelogenous leukemia
PDGFRB—rearranged eosinophilic disorders	Atypical chronic myelogenous leukemia with translocations involving 5q33 Hybrid myeloproliferative/myelodysplastic disorder (CMML, JMML), frequently with eosinophilia Chronic eosinophilic leukemia
FGFR1—rearranged eosinophilic disorder	Chronic myeloproliferative disorders with 8p11, frequently with eosinophilia and T-cell lymphoblastic lymphoma
Kit mutations	Systemic mastocytosis

[a]Data from references 198, 206, 212, 215, 216, 218, 219, 225, and 226.
[b]The examples listed are the most common diagnoses described for each molecular abnormality. Morphologic overlap exists between the molecular entities and some cases of secondary eosinophilia.
[c]*BCR-ABL* = breakpoint cluster region Abelson; *FIP1L1-PDGFR* = Fip1-like-1 platelet-derived growth factor receptor; *FGFR1* = fibroblast growth factor receptor 1; CMML = chronic myelomonocytic leukemia; JMML = juvenile myelomonocytic leukemia.
[d]Mutation is cytogenetically occult and requires reverse transcription-polymerase chain reaction (RT-PCR) or fluorescence in situ hybridization (FISH) for identification.

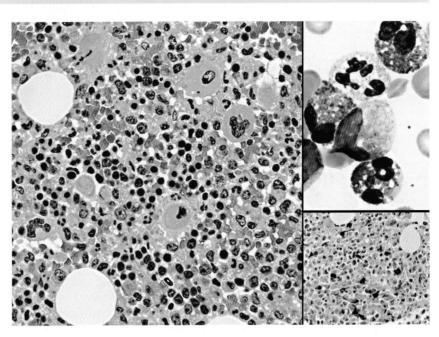

Figure 5-60

CHRONIC EOSINOPHILIC LEUKEMIA WITH TRYPTASE-POSITIVE MAST CELLS

Hypercellular bone marrow with markedly increased megakaryocytes from a patient with chronic eosinophilic leukemia. A tryptase stain (lower right) highlights an increase in mast cells without evidence of systemic mast cell disease (Wright, H&E, and immunoperoxidase stains for tryptase). (Courtesy of Dr. C. Sever, Albuquerque, NM.)

favor a hematologic malignancy are cytologic atypia involving multiple lineages; peripheral blood with basophilia, monocytosis, thrombocytosis, neutrophilia, increased blasts, or neutrophilic myeloid precursors; hypercellular bone marrow; bony changes; and eosinophils beyond the myelocyte stage containing prominent basophilic granulation or showing positive cytochemical staining with periodic acid-Schiff (PAS) or naphthyl-ASD chloroacetate esterase (negative in reactive eosinophils) (fig. 5-61).

In many cases, it may still be difficult to distinguish neoplastic from secondary causes of hypereosinophilia. Cases with similar clonal

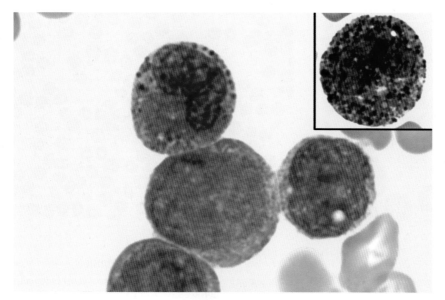

Figure 5-61

BASOPHILIC GRANULES IN EOSINOPHILIC PRECURSORS

The eosinophilic precursors contain basophilic granules in a patient with acute mye-lomonocytic leukemia with increased eosinophils (Wright stain).

Figure 5-62

SYSTEMIC MAST CELL DISEASE WITH EOSINOPHILIA

Bone marrow biopsy from a patient with systemic mast cell disease and striking eosinophilia who subsequently responded to imatinab (Gleevec) therapy (H&E stain). (Courtesy Dr. C. Sever, Albuquerque, NM.)

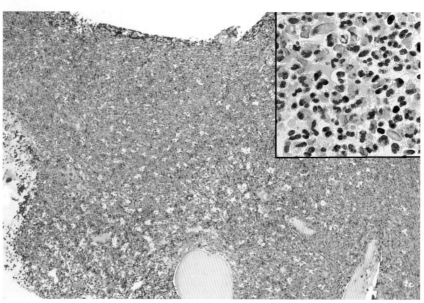

aberrations have overlapping morphologic features (particularly systemic mast cell disease and CMPD), indicating that a molecular/cytogenetic classification is required for therapeutic decisions (225). Patients with *FIP1L1-PDGFRA* mutations, *FLT3* (non-*FLT3*^{D816V}) mutations, and rearrangements of *PDGFRA/B* are imatinib (Gleevec) responsive (fig. 5-62) (197,206,207,226).

The term *hypereosinophilic syndrome* continues to be used when a definitive cause for persistent eosinophilia cannot be determined and there is no molecular or cytogenetic evidence of clonality. Bone marrows are without mastocytosis, mono-

cytosis, increased blasts, or significant dysplasia (226). Some patients have a relatively asymptomatic clinical course that lasts for decades, while others quickly develop severe organ damage.

Familial eosinophilia is a rare autosomal dominant disorder caused by a gene mapped to a cytokine gene cluster region on chromosome 5q31-33. This region is also a major genetic susceptibility locus for genes encoding Th2–secreting growth factors in patients with asthma. Patients with this rare disorder have a reasonably benign clinical course that may be related to a lack of significant eosinophil activation (213).

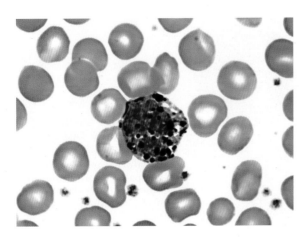

Figure 5-63

BASOPHIL

The circulating basophil has a segmented nucleus with cytoplasmic granules that vary in size and show a range in color from red-purple to blue-black (Wright stain).

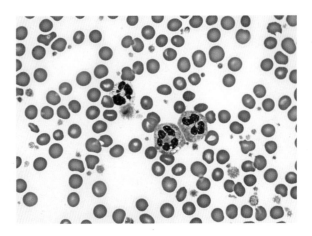

Figure 5-64

DEGRANULATED BASOPHIL

A degranulated basophil is adjacent to a giant platelet in this peripheral blood smear from a woman with a chronic myeloproliferative disorder. The basophil is distinguishable from the neutrophils by the absence of neutrophilic secondary granulation and the presence of a few remaining small basophilic granules (Wright stain).

BASOPHILIA

Basophils are linked to eosinophils through their common derivation from CD34-positive eosinophil/basophil progenitor cells. IL3 is the primary stimulus for basophil growth and differentiation (233,245). Basophilic myelocytes are the first recognizable stage in the bone marrow. Basophils and precursors contain dense purple granules that vary in size and shape, and may obscure the nucleus (fig. 5-63) (248). Basophil granules are metachromatic with the toluidine blue and Alcian blue stains. They are myeloperoxidase negative, rarely chloroacetate esterase positive, and monoclonal antibody 97A6 positive, similar to mast cells (235,236). Basophils have similar adhesion proteins and chemotactic factors as eosinophils, and secrete cytokines, such as IL4 and IL13, to promote the Th2 response and IgE synthesis (243,244). Basophil membranes have high affinity IgE Fc receptors that trigger anaphylactic degranulation when cross-linked by bound IgE antibodies (234,243a).

Basophils account for less than 2 percent of circulating WBCs and are the least common of both blood and bone marrow leukocytes. Despite variations with age, gender, season, and time of day (increased in afternoon/evening), the absolute basophil number in blood remains low (239). Therefore, peripheral blood reference ranges are standard among groups: basophilia

is defined as an absolute basophil count greater than 100/μL. Peripheral blood basophilia is usually associated with bone marrow basophilia, and is typically only modestly increased in reactive disorders (232). Basophil degranulation may be present in the blood films of patients with IgE-mediated reactive disorders or neoplastic disorders (such as CMPD), in addition to being an artifact induced by specimen handling. Inexperienced morphologists may not recognize degranulated basophils; these are best appreciated by the presence of a few remaining basophilic granules and the absence of neutrophilic secondary granulation (fig. 5-64).

Reactive basophilia is most frequently associated with hypersensitivity and inflammatory reactions (Table 5-8) (237,242). Additional findings are dependent upon the underlying disorder (232). For example, concurrent eosinophilia is common with food and drug allergies while hypochromic microcytic RBCs are indicative of iron deficiency (241). The clinical history and the presence of target cells help to identify the frequent finding of basophilia among patients with chronic renal failure. In the majority of disorders with basophilia, a bone marrow evaluation is not indicated unless a relatively high absolute basophil count, abnormalities in other cell lineages suggestive of an underlying neoplastic hematopoietic process, or splenomegaly is identified (fig. 5-65) (240). While circulating and bone marrow basophils commonly appear similar in reactive and malignant conditions, the finding of circulating immature basophils or numerous basophilic precursors in bone marrow suggests a neoplastic process and warrants bone marrow evaluation. After exclusion of a CMPD, bone marrow basophils are most frequently seen in erythrocytic disorders, such as iron deficiency

anemia and aplastic anemia (232). Basophils are distinguishable from mast cells in bone marrow by their slightly smaller size (10 to 15 μm versus 15 to 30 μm), less abundant and more unevenly distributed metachromatic granules, and greater nuclear irregularity with nuclear segmentation in mature cells (fig. 5-66).

MONOCYTES

Monocytes comprise between 2 and 9 percent of circulating WBCs, with an absolute count of 200 to 800/μL. They are the key mediators of immunity and inflammatory responses. They are derived from a committed granulocyte-monocyte progenitor in bone marrow (265). Pluripotent hematopoietic stem cells divide to form common myeloid progenitors from which the committed granulocyte-monocyte progenitor is produced (see fig. 1-1). Differentiation into monocytes is strongly influenced by cytokines, particularly monocyte-CSF (M-CSF) and GM-CSF (256).

The first identifiable stage of monocyte differentiation in bone marrow is the monoblast, followed by promonocytes and mature monocytes (see chapter 1). Mature monocytes are the predominant form present in both normal peripheral blood and bone marrow. These cells are slightly larger than neutrophils, with a diameter of approximately 12 to 15 μm, and have gray to pale blue cytoplasm with possible pseudopod-like extensions and vacuolation (fig. 5-67). Increased fine azurophilic granules may impart

Table 5-8

CAUSES OF REACTIVE PERIPHERAL BLOOD AND BONE MARROW BASOPHILIA[a]

Hypersensitivity reactions	Drug and food hypersensitivity Allergic rhinitis Erythroderma Solid organ transplant rejection
Inflammation	Chronic renal disease Ulcerative colitis Rheumatoid arthritis Collagen vascular disease
Infection	Influenza Chickenpox Tuberculosis *Helicobacter pylori* Smallpox
Endocrinopathy	Diabetes mellitus Estrogen administration Hypothyroidism (myxedema) Iron deficiency anemia
Secondary to carcinoma (rare)	Lung cancer

[a]Data from references 231, 232, 238, 246, and 247.

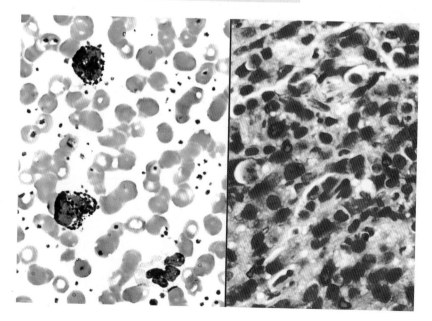

Figure 5-65

BASOPHILIA IN BLAST PHASE OF CHRONIC MYELOGENOUS LEUKEMIA

Striking basophilia and thrombocytosis are observed in this peripheral blood smear (left) from a teenage boy who had blast phase of chronic myelogenous leukemia on bone marrow evaluation (right) (Wright and H&E stains).

Figure 5-66

BASOPHIL VERSUS MAST CELL

Comparison of basophils (left) and mast cells (right) in bone marrow. Basophils are smaller and have nuclei that vary from round to segmented. Mast cells have only round to oval nuclei with purple cytoplasmic granules, which may obscure the nucleus and cytoplasmic borders. Mast cell cytoplasmic granules are more numerous and evenly distributed than those seen in basophils. Mast cells are rarely observed in the peripheral blood of patients with chronic myeloproliferative disorders (Wright stain).

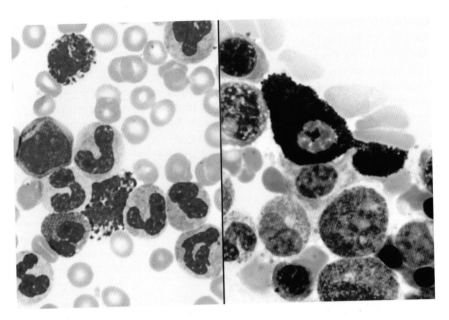

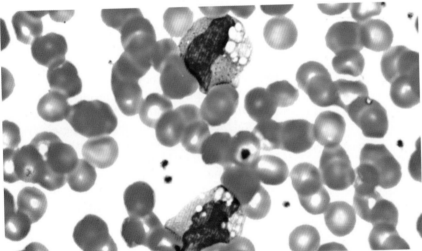

Figure 5-67

MONOCYTES

Normal monocytes in the peripheral blood have abundant pale blue cytoplasm with vacuoles and fine azurophilic granules. The nuclei are reniform, with fine chromatin strands bridging areas of chromatin clumping (Wright stain).

Figure 5-68

NONSPECIFIC ESTERASE STAIN

The nonspecific esterase stain shows diffuse positivity of normal monocytes and patchy weak positivity of occasional neutrophils.

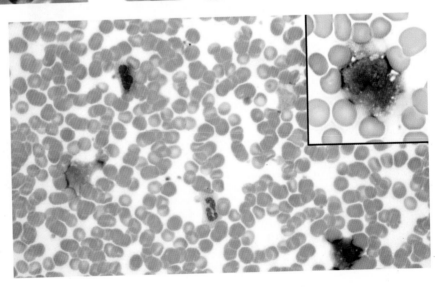

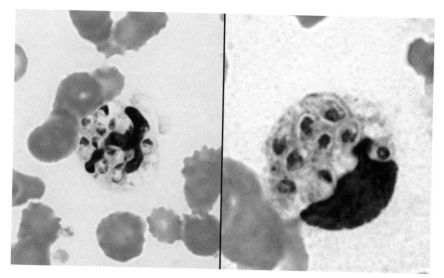

Figure 5-69

HISTOPLASMOSIS IN MONOCYTES

Phagocytosis of yeast by monocytes in an immunosuppressed patient with disseminated histoplasmosis (Wright stain). (Courtesy of Dr. D. O'Malley, Irvine, CA.)

a pink coloration to the cytoplasm. Cytoplasmic granules contain enzymes, such as acid-phosphatase, collagenase, and elastase, which play a role in antimicrobial function. The granule contents contribute to the lysozyme, weakly periodic acid-Schiff (PAS), and nonspecific esterase positivity seen with specialized staining (fig. 5-68) (261). The monocyte nucleus occupies approximately half the area of the cell and is customarily eccentrically placed and indented or reniform in shape.

Circulating monocytes have a propensity to adhere to surfaces and marginate along vessel walls. Monocytes are effective phagocytes that are involved in the ingestion of a variety of organisms (fig. 5-69). They respond to chemotactic and other stimuli by diapedesis across vessel walls into tissues or bone marrow where they mature into a variety of cell types. These include members of the monocyte/histiocyte/immune accessory cell system, which functions in both cellular and humoral immunity. These cells have greater phagocytic capacity than monocytes and secrete numerous chemical mediators and regulators of immune function and hematopoiesis, including interferons, interleukins, tumor necrosis factors, prostaglandins, complement, and CSFs.

Monocytosis

Monocytosis is an absolute monocyte count of over 800/μL in adults and over 3,500/μL in neonates. Reactive monocytosis is most commonly seen in response to chronic infection due to bacterial, viral, fungal, or parasitic organisms.

Table 5-9

CAUSES OF REACTIVE PERIPHERAL BLOOD AND BONE MARROW MONOCYTOSIS[a]

Collagen vascular disease	Systemic lupus erythematosus Rheumatoid arthritis Polyarteritis nodosa Temporal arteritis Myositis
Gastrointestinal disorder	Regional enteritis Ulcerative colitis Alcoholic liver disease Sprue
Infection[b]	Viral (CMV[c], EBV, varicella, parvovirus) Subacute bacterial endocarditis Tuberculosis, malaria Brucellosis, visceral leishmaniasis Syphilis Rare protozoa (visceral leishmaniasis) Rare rickettsia (Rocky mountain spotted fever)
Hematologic disorders	Chronic or drug-related neutropenia Hemolytic anemia Idiopathic thrombocytopenia purpura Lymphoma (Hodgkin and non-Hodgkin) Sarcoidosis Plasma cell myeloma MDS (possible monocytic nodules)
Miscellaneous	Postsplenectomy M-CSF secreting tumors Thermal injury Acute myocardial infarction Marathon running CSF therapy

[a]Data from references 249–254, 258, 262–264, and 267.
[b]Most commonly associated with chronic infections.
[c]CMV = cytomegalovirus; EBV = Epstein-Barr virus; MDS = myelodysplastic syndrome; M-CSF = monocyte–colony-stimulating factor.

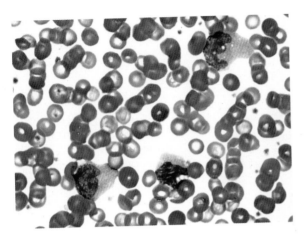

Figure 5-70

MONOCYTOSIS IN CYCLIC NEUTROPENIA

Compensatory peripheral blood monocytosis during a period of marked neutropenia in a patient with cyclic neutropenia (Wright stain).

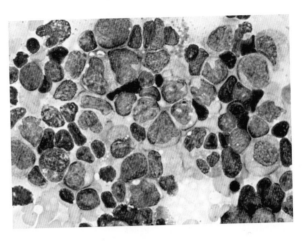

Figure 5-71

LEFT-SHIFTED MONOCYTOSIS WITH G-CSF THERAPY

Increased bone marrow monocytes with immature forms are seen during G-CSF therapy in a young girl with severe congenital neutropenia (Wright stain). (Courtesy of Dr. J. Choi, Philadelphia, PA.)

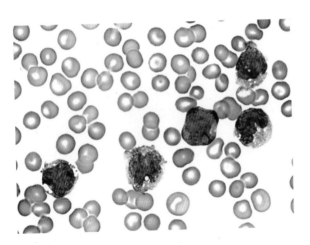

Figure 5-72

ACUTE MYELOMONOCYTIC LEUKEMIA

Monoblasts and promonocytes in the peripheral blood of an older woman with neutropenia, anemia, and acute myelomonocytic leukemia (Wright stain).

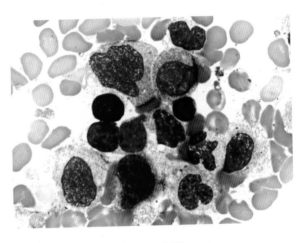

Figure 5-73

PARVOVIRUS B19 INFECTION

Bone marrow aspirate smear from a young child with parvovirus B19 infection shows increased monocytes and lymphocytes, granulocytic atypia, and absence of erythroid precursors (Wright stain).

Additional causes of reactive monocytosis are listed in Table 5-9. Monocytoses may be observed secondary to lymphoma, immune-mediated disorders such as collagen vascular diseases, gastrointestinal disorders, and thermal injury. Patients with marked neutropenia respond with transient monocytosis until recovery from their agranulocytosis (fig. 5-70). Monocyte production as well as granulocyte production is stimulated by CSF therapy with either G-CSF or GM-CSF (fig. 5-71).

The resulting increase in circulating monocytes may include a subset of immature forms that have finer nuclear chromatin and prominent nucleoli. Monocytosis is also commonly associated with hematologic malignancies and these must be excluded based on peripheral blood and possibly bone marrow evaluations.

A bone marrow examination is indicated when monocyte immaturity or atypia is present without

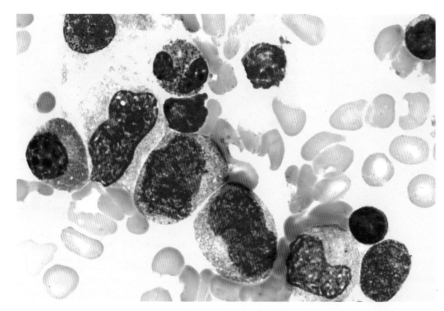

Figure 5-74

MONOCYTIC MATURATION

Different stages of monocyte maturation are easy to identify in this well-stained bone marrow aspirate smear (Wright stain).

Figure 5-75

MONOCYTOSIS AFTER AGRANULOCYTOSIS

Bone marrow aspirate (insert) and biopsy show increased monocytes and early neutrophilic myeloid regeneration after an episode of agranulocytosis (Wright, H&E stains).

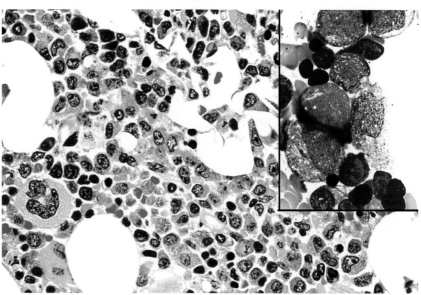

explanation, and when quantitative or morphologic abnormalities are observed in the other lineages (fig. 5-72). One exception is parvovirus B19 infection in which trilineage atypia of the peripheral blood and bone marrow may be seen in conjunction with monocytosis and anemia; evaluation for parvovirus B19 should be performed in such a scenario (fig. 5-73) (see chapter 10) (270).

An increase in bone marrow monocytes accompanies peripheral blood monocytoses. Monocytes are best appreciated in bone marrow aspirate smears or touch preparations (fig. 5-74). Monoblasts and promonocytes are typically

insignificant in number unless coupled with bone marrow regeneration after an episode of aplasia (fig. 5-75). In animal models of thermal injury, augmented expression of M-CSF receptor drives increased growth of monocyte progenitors to the detriment of neutrophilic myeloid progenitor formation. Similar findings are likely in human thermal injury and burn sepsis (266). The presence of monocyte atypia along with abnormalities of the other hematopoietic lineages necessitates the exclusion of chronic myelomonocytic leukemia, juvenile myelomonocytic leukemia, acute myeloid leukemia

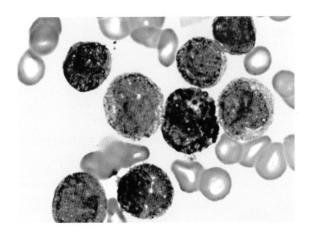

Figure 5-76

**ACUTE MYELOMONOCYTIC
LEUKEMIA WITH EOSINOPHILIA**

Immature monocytic cells and eosinophil precursors containing basophilic granules are seen in the bone marrow of a patient with acute myelomonocytic leukemia with eosinophilia (Wright stains).

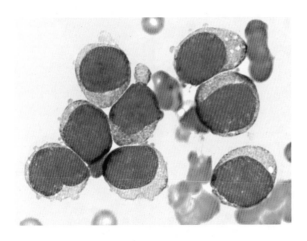

Figure 5-77

ACUTE MONOBLASTIC LEUKEMIA

The peripheral blood from a young man with acute monoblastic leukemia shows immature monocytes with a high nuclear to cytoplasmic ratio, immature chromatin configuration, and variably prominent nucleoli (Wright stain).

with a monocytic component, or a CMPD (fig. 5-76). Atypical or immature monocytes have a higher nuclear to cytoplasmic ratio, variably prominent nucleoli, and a looser chromatin configuration than normal (fig. 5-77).

Bone marrow monocytes express CD4, CD13, CD15, CD33, CD36, and CD38, and variably express CD11b and CD14 (269). Reactive monocytes

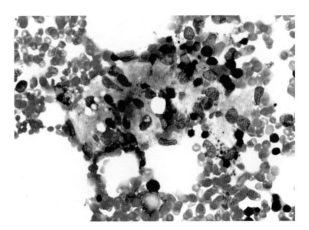

Figure 5-78

GRANULOMA

Small granuloma in a bone marrow aspirate smear from a child on therapy for acute lymphoblastic leukemia (Wright stain).

may have aberrant antigen expression usually isolated to one antigen, such as coexpression of CD56 and CD2, or underexpression of human leukocyte antigen (HLA)-DR or CD13. In contrast, aberrations in antigen expression are typical of neoplastic monocytes and frequently involve multiple antigens (252,257,269).

An increase in bone marrow macrophages (histiocytes) occurs with a variety of hematologic and nonhematologic conditions as outlined in chapter 9. These include infectious and rheumatologic/collagen vascular disorders that may be associated with granuloma formation (fig. 5-78). Stimulation of macrophage production also occurs with GM-CSF therapy or in connection with a cytokine-producing neoplasm. Macrophages vary in appearance from immature cells showing little phagocytic activity to large mature cells with the appearance of tingible body type macrophages or foam cells. The presence of tingible body-like macrophages denotes increased bone marrow turnover, most often occurring with hematopoietic cell destruction or ineffective hematopoiesis (fig. 5-79). The distinctive finding of macrophage hyperplasia with increased phagocytosis of RBCs, granulocytes, platelets, and other hematopoietic cells is termed the *hemophagocytic syndrome* (see chapters 9 and 10) (fig. 5-80). The alternative presence of abnormal breakdown products within the macrophage cytoplasm leads to

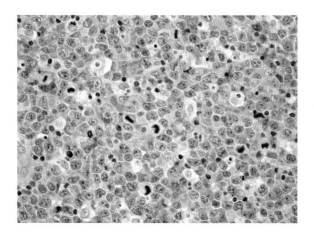

Figure 5-79

TINGIBLE BODY TYPE MACROPHAGES

Tingible body type macrophages ingest cellular debris in a bone marrow replaced by leukemia (H&E stain).

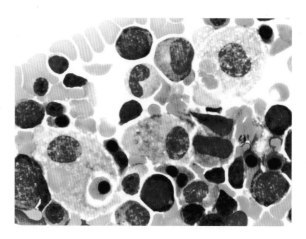

Figure 5-80

HEMOPHAGOCYTIC SYNDROME

Macrophages are ingesting erythroid cells in a patient with hemophagocytic syndrome (Wright stain).

unique morphologic features among marrow histiocytes that help in the identification of storage diseases (see chapter 9).

Monocytopenia

Significant *monocytopenia*, defined as an absolute monocyte count under 200/µL for children and adults, does not occur in isolation. It is a feature of bone marrow failure or replacement, especially infiltration by hairy cell leukemia. The monocytopenia characteristic of hairy cell leukemia results from insufficient production of CSF (255). Glucocorticoid therapy also causes monocytopenia and decreased monocyte migration into tissue sites of inflammation (259).

As monocytes have antibacterial, antiviral, antifungal, and antiparasitic capabilities, their absence predisposes an individual to serious infection. Patients with monocytopenia are particularly susceptible to infections associated with granuloma formation such as with mycobacteria, *Listeria*, and *Brucella* (260). Neutrophils, T cells, endothelial cells, and other cell types attempt to substitute for some monocyte functions in their absence (268).

REFERENCES

General Concepts

1. Abel GA, Hays JT, Decker PA, Croghan GA, Kuter DJ, Rigotti NA. Effects of biochemically confirmed smoking cessation on white blood cell count. Mayo Clin Proc 2005;80:1022-8.
2. Brugnara C. Reference values in infancy and childhood. In: Nathan DG, Orkin SH, Ginsburg D, et al, eds. Nathan and Oski's hematology of infancy and childhood, 6th ed, Vol 2. Philadelphia: Saunders; 2003;1848-51.
3. Cheng CK, Chan J, Cembrowski GS, van Assendelft OW. Complete blood count reference interval diagrams derived from NHANES III: stratification by age, sex, and race. Lab Hematol 2004;10:42-53.
4. Foucar K. Neonatal hematopathology: special considerations. In: Collins R, Swerdlow S, eds. Pediatric hematopathology. New York: Churchill Livingstone; 2001:173-84.
5. Rezvani K, Flanagan AM, Sarma U, Constantinovici N, Bain BJ. Investigation of ethnic neutropenia by assessment of bone marrow colony-forming cells. Acta Haematol 2001;105:32-7.

6. Saxena S, Wong ET. Heterogeneity of common hematologic parameters among racial, ethnic, and gender subgroups. Arch Pathol Lab Med 1990;114:715-9.

7. Thake CD, Mian T, Garnham AW, Mian R. Leukocyte counts and neutrophil activity during 4 h of hypocapnic hypoxia equivalent to 4000 m. Aviat Space Environ Med 2004;75:811-7.

Myelopoiesis

8. Barreda DR, Hanington PC, Belosevic M. Regulation of myeloid development and function by colony stimulating factors. Dev Comp Immunol 2004;28:509-54.

9. Bjerregaard MD, Jurlander J, Klausen P, Borregaard N, Cowland JB. The in vivo profile of transcription factors during neutrophil differentiation in human bone marrow. Blood 2003;101:4322-32.

10. Cerny J, Quesenberry PJ. Chromatin remodeling and stem cell theory of relativity. J Cell Physiol 2004;201:1-16.

11. Friedman AD. Transcriptional regulation of myelopoiesis. Int J Hematol 2002;75:466-72.

12. Kawamoto H, Minato N. Myeloid cells. Int J Biochem Cell Biol 2004;36:1374-9.

12a. Miranda MB, Johnson DE. Signal transduction pathways that contribute to myeloid differentiation. Leukemia 2007;21:1366-77.

12b. Mueller BU, Pabst T. C/ERBPalpha and the pathophysiology of acute myeloid leukemia. Curr Opin Hematol 2006;13:7-14.

13. Rosmarin AG, Yang Z, Resendes KK. Transcriptional regulation in myelopoiesis: hematopoietic fate choice, myeloid differentiation, and leukemogenesis. Exp Hematol 2005;33:131-43.

14. Tagoh H, Melnik S, Lefevre P, Chong S, Riggs AD, Bonifer C. Dynamic reorganization of chromatin structure and selective DNA demethylation prior to stable enhancer complex formation during differentiation of primary hematopoietic cells in vitro. Blood 2004;103:2950-5.

Neutrophilia

15. Amato M, Howald H, von Muralt G. Qualitative changes of white blood cells and perinatal diagnosis of infection in high-risk preterm infants. Pediatr Pathol 1988;23:129-34.

16. Boggs DR, Joyce RA. The hematopoietic effects of lithium. Semin Hematol 1983;20:129-38.

17. Brenner I, Shek PN, Zamecnik J, Shephard RJ. Stress hormones and the immunological responses to heat and exercise. Int J Sports Med 1998;19:130-43.

18. Cehreli C, Undar B, Akkoc N, Onvural B, Altungoz O. Coexistence of chronic neutrophilic leukemia with light chain myeloma. Acta Haematol 1994;91:32-4.

19. Cornbleet PJ. Clinical utility of the band count. Clin Lab Med 2002;22:101-36.

20. Dinarello CA. The IL-1 family and inflammatory diseases. Clin Exp Rheumatol 2002;20:S1-13.

21. Dincol G, Nalcaci M, Dogan O, et al. Coexistence of chronic neutrophilic leukemia with multiple myeloma. Leuk Lymphoma 2002;43:649-51.

22. Ito T, Shimamura K, Shoji K, et al. Urinary bladder carcinoma producing granulocyte colony stimulating factor (G-CSF): a case report with immunohistochemistry. Virchows Arch A Pathol Anat Histopathol 1993;422:487-90.

23. Itoga T, Laszlo J. Dohle bodies and other granulocytic alterations during chemotherapy with cyclophosphamide. Blood 1962;20:668-74.

24. Kitamura H, Kodama F, Odagiri S, Nagahara N, Inoue T, Kanisawa M. Granulocytosis associated with malignant neoplasms: a clinicopathologic study and demonstration of colony-stimulating activity in tumor extracts. Hum Pathol 1989;20:878-85.

25. Kratz A, Lewandrowski KB, Siegel AJ, et al. Effect of marathon running on hematologic and biochemical laboratory parameters, including cardiac markers. Am J Clin Pathol 2002;118:856-63.

26. Krauss JS, Dover RK, Khankhanian NK, Tom GD. Granulocytic fragments in sepsis. Mod Pathol 1989;2:301-5.

27. Kroft SH. Infectious diseases manifested in the peripheral blood. Clin Lab Med 2002;22:253-77.

28. Lee KY, Suh BG, Kim JW, et al. Varying expression levels of colony stimulating factor receptors in disease states and different leukocytes. Exp Mol Med 2000;32:210-5.

29. Li TL, Gleeson M. The effect of single and repeated bouts of prolonged cycling on leukocyte redistribution, neutrophil degranulation, IL-6, and plasma stress hormone responses. Int J Sport Nutr Exerc Metab 2004;14:501-16.

30. Liles WC, Dale DC, Klebanoff SJ. Glucocorticoids inhibit apoptosis of human neutrophils. Blood 1995;86:3181-8.

31. Malcolm ID, Flegel KM, Katz M. Vacuolization of the neutrophil in bacteremia. Arch Intern Med 1979;139:675-6.

32. McCall CE, Katayama I, Cotran RS, Finland M. Lysosomal and ultrastructural changes in human "toxic" neutrophils during bacterial infection. J Exp Med 1969;129:267-93.

33. Novak R. Granulocytic (myeloid cells). In: Glassy E, ed. Color atlas of hematology. College of American Pathologists (CAP); 1998:22-7.

34. Quindry JC, Stone WL, King J, Broeder CE. The effects of acute exercise on neutrophils and plasma oxidative stress. Med Sci Sports Exerc 2003;35:1139-45.

35. Richardson RP, Rhyne CD, Fong Y, et al. Peripheral blood leukocyte kinetics following in vivo lipopolysaccharide (LPS) administration to normal human subjects. Influence of elicited hormones and cytokines. Ann Surg 1989;210:239-45.

36. Rogowski O, Sasson Y, Kassirer M, et al. Downregulation of the CD62L antigen as a possible mechanism for neutrophilia during inflammation. Br J Haematol 1998;101:666-9.

37. Schelonka RL, Yoder BA, Hall RB, et al. Differentiation of segmented and band neutrophils during the early newborn period. J Pediatr 1995;127:298-300.

38. Seebach JD, Morant R, Ruegg R, Seifert B, Fehr J. The diagnostic value of the neutrophil left shift in predicting inflammatory and infectious disease. Am J Clin Pathol 1997;107:582-91.

39. van der Meer W, van Gelder W, de Keijzer R, et al. Does the band cell survive the 21st century? Eur J Haematol 2006;76:251-4.

40. van Eeden SF, Hogg JC. The response of human bone marrow to chronic cigarette smoking. Eur Respir J 2000;15:915-21.

41. Van Tiel E, Peeters PH, Smit HA, et al. Quitting smoking may restore hematological characteristics within five years. Ann Epidemiol 2002;12:378-88.

42. Wang YC, Yang S, Tzen CY, Lin CC, Lin J. Renal cell carcinoma producing granulocyte colony-stimulating factor. J Formos Med Assoc 2006;105:414-7.

43. Wong RS, Wu A, To KF, et al. Haematological manifestations in patients with severe acute respiratory syndrome: retrospective analysis. BMJ 2003;326:1358-62.

44. Zieve PD, Haghshenass M, Blanks M, Krevans JR. Vacuolization of the neutrophil. An aid in the diagnosis of septicemia. Arch Intern Med 1966;118:356-7.

Neutrophilia: Growth Factor Effect in Bone Marrow

45. Adachi N, Yamaguchi K, Morikawa T, Suziki M, Matsuda I, Abe MK. Constitutive production of multiple colony-stimulating factors in patients with lung cancer associated with neutrophilia. Br J Cancer 1994;69:125-9.

46. Campbell LJ, Maher DW, Tay DL, et al. Marrow proliferation and the appearance of giant neutrophils in response to recombinant human granulocyte colony stimulating factor (rhG-CSF). Br J Haematol 1992;80:298-304.

47. Dale DC. Advances in the use of colony-stimulating factors for chemotherapy-induced neutropenia. J Support Oncol 2005;3:39-41.

48. Gonzalez SA, Jacobson IM. The role of hematopoietic growth factors in special populations with chronic hepatitis C: patients with HIV coinfection, end-stage renal disease, or liver transplantation. Cleve Clin J Med 2004;71(Suppl 3):S22-6.

49. Harris AC, Todd WM, Hackney MH, Ben-Ezra J. Bone marrow changes associated with recombinant granulocyte-macrophage and granulocyte colony-stimulating factors. Discrimination of granulocytic regeneration. Arch Pathol Lab Med 1994;118:624-9

50. Hubel K, Engert A. Clinical applications of granulocyte colony-stimulating factor: an update and summary. Ann Hematol 2003;82:207-13.

51. Innes DJ Jr, Hess CE, Bertholf MF, Wade P. Promyelocyte morphology. Differentiation of acute promyelocytic leukemia from benign myeloid proliferations. Am J Clin Pathol 1987;88:725-9.

52. Katayama Y, Deguchi S, Shinagawa K, et al. Bone marrow necrosis in a patient with acute myeloblastic leukemia during administration of G-CSF and rapid hematologic recovery after allotransplantation of peripheral blood stem cells. Am J Hematol 1998;57:238-40.

53. Kerrigan DP, Castillo A, Foucar K, Townsend K, Neidhart J. Peripheral blood morphologic changes after high-dose antineoplastic chemotherapy and recombinant human granulocyte colony-stimulating factor administration. Am J Clin Pathol 1989;92:280-5.

54. Lieschke GJ, Burgess AW. Granulocyte colony-stimulating factor and granulocyte-macrophage colony-stimulating factor (1). N Engl J Med 1992;327:28-35.

55. Lieschke GJ, Burgess AW. Granulocyte colony-stimulating factor and granulocyte-macrophage colony-stimulating factor (2). N Engl J Med 1992;327:99-106.

56. Liu CZ, Persad R, Inghirami G, et al. Transient atypical monocytosis mimic acute myelomonocytic leukemia in post-chemotherapy patients receiving G-CSF: report of two cases. Clin Lab Haematol 2004;26:359-62.

57. Maianski NA, Maianski AN, Kuijpers TW, Roos D. Apoptosis of neutrophils. Acta Haematol 2004;111:56-66.

58. McNeil C. NCCN guidelines advocate wider use of colony-stimulating factor. J Natl Cancer Inst 2005;97:710-1.

59. Meyerson HJ, Farhi DC, Rosenthal NS. Transient increase in blasts mimicking acute leukemia and progressing myelodysplasia in patients receiving growth factor. Am J Clin Pathol 1998;109:675-81.

60. Price TH, Chatta GS, Dale DC. Effect of recombinant granulocyte colony-stimulating factor on neutrophil kinetics in normal young and elderly humans. Blood 1996;88:335-40.

61. Relling MV, Boyett JM, Blanco JG, et al. Granulocyte colony-stimulating factor and the risk of secondary myeloid malignancy after etoposide treatment. Blood 2003;101:3862-7.

62. Ringden OT, Le Blanc K, Remberger M. Granulocyte and granulocyte-macrophage colony-stimulating factors in allografts: uses, misuses, misconceptions, and future applications. Exp Hematol 2005;33:505-12.

63. Ryder JW, Lazarus HM, Farhi DC. Bone marrow and blood findings after marrow transplantation and rhGM-CSF therapy. Am J Clin Pathol 1992;97:631-7.

64. Sato T, Omura M, Saito J, et al. Neutrophilia associated with anaplastic carcinoma of the thyroid: production of macrophage colony-stimulating factor (M-CSF) and interleukin-6. Thyroid 2000;10:1113-8.

65. Schmitz LL, McClure JS, Litz CE, et al. Morphologic and quantitative changes in blood and marrow cells following growth factor therapy. Am J Clin Pathol 1994;101:67-75.

66. Shi Y, Liu CH, Roberts AI, et al. Granulocyte-macrophage colony-stimulating factor (GM-CSF) and T-cell responses: what we do and don't know. Cell Res 2006;16:126-33.

67. Stav K, Leibovici D, Siegel YI, Lindner A. Leukemoid reaction associated with transitional cell carcinoma. Isr Med Assoc J 2002;4:223-4.

68. Tachibana M, Murai M. G-CSF production in human bladder cancer and its ability to promote autocrine growth: a review. Cytokines Cell Mol Ther 1998;4:113-20.

69. Wilson PA, Ayscue LH, Jones GR, Bentley SA. Bone marrow histiocytic proliferation in association with colony-stimulating factor therapy. Am J Clin Pathol 1993;99:311-3.

Neutrophilia: Leukemoid Reaction Versus Chronic Myelogenous Leukemia

70. Arguelles-Grande C, Leon F, Matilla J, Dominguez J, Montero J. Steroidal management and serum cytokine profile of a case of alcoholic hepatitis with leukemoid reaction. Scand J Gastroenterol 2002;37:1111-3.

71. Bohm J, Kock S, Schaefer HE, Fisch P. Evidence of clonality in chronic neutrophilic leukaemia. J Clin Pathol 2003;56:292-5.

72. Calhoun DA, Kirk JF, Christensen RD. Incidence, significance, and kinetic mechanism responsible for leukemoid reactions in patients in the neonatal intensive care unit: a prospective evaluation. J Pediatr 1996;129:403-9.

73. Imbert M, Bain B, Pierre R, et al. Chronic neutrophilic leukaemia. In: Jaffe E, Harris N, Stein H, et al, eds. WHO classification of tumours: pathology & genetics: tumours of haematopoietic and lymphoid tissues. Lyon, France: IARC Press; 2001:20-6.

74. McKee LC Jr. Excess leukocytosis (leukemoid reactions) associated with malignant diseases. South Med J 1985;78:1475-82.

75. Reilly JT. Chronic neutrophilic leukaemia: a distinct clinical entity? Br J Haematol 2002;116:10-8.

75a. Sakka V, Tsiodras S, Giamarellos-Bourboulis EJ, Giamarellou H. An update on the etiology and diagnostic evaluation of a leukemoid reaction. Eur J Intern Med 2006;17:394-8.

76. Steensma DP, Dewald GW, Lasho TL, et al. The JAK2 V617F activating tyrosine kinase mutation is an infrequent event in both "atypical" myeloproliferative disorders and myelodysplastic syndromes. Blood 2005;106:1207-9.

77. Vardiman JW, Pierre R, Thiele J. Chronic myelogenous leukaemia. In: Jaffe E, Harris N, Stein H, et al, eds. WHO classification of tumours: pathology & genetics: tumours of haematopoietic and lymphoid tissues. Lyon, France: IARC Press; 2001:20-6.

Neutrophilic Disorders that Imitate Neoplastic Processes in Children

78. Brink DS. Transient leukemia (transient myeloproliferative disorder, transient abnormal myelopoiesis) of Down syndrome. Adv Anat Pathol 2006;13:256-62.

79. Craig FE. Bone marrow evaluation in pediatric patients. Semin Diagn Pathol 2003;20:237-46.

80. Crispino JD. GATA1 mutations in Down syndrome: implications for biology and diagnosis of children with transient myeloproliferative disorder and acute megakaryoblastic leukemia. Pediatr Blood Cancer 2005;44:40-4.

81. Cushing T, Clericuzio CL, Wilson CS, et al. Risk for leukemia transformation in infants without Down syndrome who have transient myeloproliferative disorder. J Pediatr 2006;148:687-9.

82. Karandikar NJ, Aquino DB, McKenna RW, Kroft SH. Transient myeloproliferative disorder and acute myeloid leukemia in Down syndrome. An immunophenotypic analysis. Am J Clin Pathol 2001;116:204-10.

83. Pinkel D. Differentiating juvenile myelomonocytic leukemia from infectious disease. Blood 1998;91:365-7.

84. Toyoda H, Ido M, Hori H, et al. A case of juvenile myelomonocytic leukemia with concomitant cytomegalovirus infection. J Pediatr Hematol Oncol 2004;26:606-8.

Congential Neutrophilia

85. Etzioni A, Sturla L, Antonellis A, et al. Leukocyte adhesion deficiency (LAD) type II/carbohydrate deficient glycoprotein (CDG) IIc founder effect and genotype/phenotype correlation. Am J Med Genet 2002;110:131-5.

86. Haas N, Kuster W, Zuberbier T, Henz BM. Muckle-Wells syndrome: clinical and histological skin findings compatible with cold air urticaria in a large kindred. Br J Dermatol 2004;151:99-104.

87. Herring WB, Smith LG, Walker RI, Herion JC. Hereditary neutrophilia. Am J Med 1974;56:729-34.

87a. Newburger PE. Disorders of neutrophil number and function. Hematology Am Soc Hematol Educ Program 2006:104-10.

88. Shaw JM, Al-Shamkhani A, Boxer LA, et al. Characterization of four CD18 mutants in leucocyte adhesion deficient (LAD) patients with differential capacities to support expression and function of the CD11/CD18 integrins LFA-1, Mac-1 and p150,95. Clin Exp Immunol 2001;126:311-8.

Neutropenia

89. Bain BJ. Ethnic and sex differences in the total and differential white cell count and platelet count. J Clin Pathol 1996;49:664-6.

90. Bain BJ, Phillips D, Thomson K, Richardson D, Gabriel I. Investigation of the effect of marathon running on leucocyte counts of subjects of different ethnic origins: relevance to the aetiology of ethnic neutropenia. Br J Haematol 2000;108:483-7.

91. Berliner N, Horwitz M, Loughran TP Jr. Congenital and acquired neutropenia. Hematology Am Soc Hematol Educ Program 2004:63-79.

92. Capsoni F, Sarzi-Puttini P, Zanella A. Primary and secondary autoimmune neutropenia. Arthritis Res Ther 2005;7:208-14.

93. Carey PJ. Drug-induced myelosuppression: diagnosis and management. Drug Saf 2003;26:691-706.

94. Hershman D, Weinberg M, Rosner Z, et al. Ethnic neutropenia and treatment delay in African American women undergoing chemotherapy for early-stage breast cancer. J Natl Cancer Inst 2003;95:1545-8.

95. Iosub S, Naik M, Bhalani K, Gromisch DS. Leukocyte and neutrophil counts in healthy Puerto Rican children and children with acute appendicitis. Clin Pediatr (Phila) 1986;25:366-8.

96. Kaufman DW, Kelly JP, Jurgelon JM, et al. Drugs in the aetiology of agranulocytosis and aplastic anaemia. Eur J Haematol Suppl 1996;60:23-30.

97. Lima CS, Paula EV, Takahashi T, Saad ST, Lorand-Metze I, Costa FF. Causes of incidental neutropenia in adulthood. Ann Hematol 2006;85:705-9.

98. Phillips D, Rezvani K, Bain BJ. Exercise induced mobilisation of the marginated granulocyte pool in the investigation of ethnic neutropenia. J Clin Pathol 2000;53:481-3.

99. Rezvani K, Flanagan AM, Sarma U, Constantinovici N, Bain BJ. Investigation of ethnic neutropenia by assessment of bone marrow colony-forming cells. Acta Haematol 2001;105:32-7.

100. Starkebaum G. Chronic neutropenia associated with autoimmune disease. Semin Hematol 2002;39:121-7.

101. Wanachiwanawin W, Siripanyaphinyo U, Piyawattanasakul N, et al. A cohort study of the nature of paroxysmal nocturnal hemoglobinuria clones and PIG-A mutations in patients with aplastic anemia. Eur J Haematol 2006;76:502-9.

Acquired Neutropenia in Adults

102. Akamizu T, Ozaki S, Hiratani H, et al. Drug-induced neutropenia associated with anti-neutrophil cytoplasmic antibodies (ANCA): possible involvement of complement in granulocyte cytotoxicity. Clin Exp Immunol 2002;127:92-8.

103. Balint GP, Balint PV. Felty's syndrome. Best Pract Res Clin Rheumatol 2004;18:631-45.

104. Berliner N, Horwitz M, Loughran TP Jr. Congenital and acquired neutropenia. Hematology Am Soc Hematol Educ Program 2004:63-79.

105. Bloom BJ, Smith P, Alario AJ. Felty syndrome complicating juvenile rheumatoid arthritis. J Pediatr Hematol Oncol 1998;20:511-3.

106. Evans HL, Burks E, Viswanatha D, Larson RS. Utility of immunohistochemistry in bone marrow evaluation of T-lineage large granular lymphocyte leukemia. Hum Pathol 2000;31:1266-73.

107. Farr M, Tunn EJ, Symmons DP, Scott DG, Bacon PA. Sulphasalazine in rheumatoid arthritis: haematological problems and changes in haematological indices associated with therapy. Br J Rheumatol 1989;28:134-8.

107a. Garrido P, Ruiz-Cabello F, Barcena P, et al. Monoclonal TCR-Vbeta13.1+/CD4+/NKa+/CD8-/+dim T-LGL lymphocytois: evidence for an antigen-driven chronic T-cell stimulation origin. Blood 2007;109:4890-8.

108. Hsieh SC, Yu HS, Lin WW, et al. Anti-SSB/La is one of the antineutrophil autoantibodies responsible for neutropenia and functional impairment of polymorphonuclear neutrophils in patients with systemic lupus erythematosus. Clin Exp Immunol 2003;131:506-16.

109. Julia A, Olona M, Bueno J, et al. Drug-induced agranulocytosis: prognostic factors in a series of 168 episodes. Br J Haematol 1991;79:366-71.

110. Kaufman DW, Kelly JP, Jurgelon JM, et al. Drugs in the aetiology of agranulocytosis and aplastic anaemia. Eur J Haematol Suppl 1996;60:23-30.

111. Kothapalli R, Nyland SB, Kusmartseva I, Bailey RD, McKeown TM, Loughran TP. Constitutive production of proinflammatory cytokines RANTES, MIP-1beta and IL-18 characterizes LGL leukemia. Int J Oncol 2005;26:529-35.

112. Morice WG, Kurtin PJ, Tefferi A, Hanson CA. Distinct bone marrow findings in T-cell granular lymphocytic leukemia revealed by paraffin section immunoperoxidase stains for CD8, TIA-1, and granzyme B. Blood 2002;99:268-74.

113. Osuji N, Beiske K, Randen U, et al. Characteristic appearances of the bone marrow in T-cell large granular lymphocyte leukaemia. Histopathology 2007;50:547-54.

114. Palmblad J, Papadaki HA, Eliopoulos G. Acute and chronic neutropenias. What is new? J Intern Med 2001;250:476-91.

115. Papadaki HA, Chatzivassili A, Stefanaki K, Koumaki V, Kanavaros P, Eliopoulos GD. Morphologically defined myeloid cell compartments, lymphocyte subpopulations, and histological findings of bone marrow in patients with nonimmune chronic idiopathic neutropenia of adults. Ann Hematol 2000;79:563-70.

116. Papadaki HA, Eliopoulos AG, Kosteas T, et al. Impaired granulocytopoiesis in patients with chronic idiopathic neutropenia is associated with increased apoptosis of bone marrow myeloid progenitor cells. Blood 2003;101:2591-600.

117. Papadaki HA, Eliopoulos GD, Coulocheri SA, Spyropoulou M, Stavropoulos-Giokas C. Increased frequency of HLA-DRB1*1302 haplotype in patients with nonimmune chronic idiopathic neutropenia of adults. Blood 2001;97:580-1.

118. Papadaki HA, Psyllaki M, Eliopoulos DG, Tsiroyianni A, Eliopoulos GD. Increased frequency and specific reactivity of serum antinuclear antibodies in patients with nonimmune chronic idiopathic neutropenia of adults. Acta Haematol 2001;105:13-20.

119. Rizzi R, Pastore D, Liso A, et al. Autoimmune myelofibrosis: report of three cases and review of the literature. Leuk Lymphoma 2004;45:561-6.

120. Sokoloff P. Focus on clozapine: a new explanation for its atypical character. Int J Neuropsychopharmacol 2005;8:311-3.

121. Starkebaum G. Chronic neutropenia associated with autoimmune disease. Semin Hematol 2002;39:121-7.

122. van Staa TP, Boulton F, Cooper C, Hagenbeek A, Inskip H, Leufkens HG. Neutropenia and agranulocytosis in England and Wales: incidence and risk factors. Am J Hematol 2003;72:248-54.

123. Vandendries ER, Drews RE. Drug-associated disease: hematologic dysfunction. Crit Care Clin 2006;22:347-55, viii.

124. Yunis JJ, Corzo D, Salazar M, Lieberman JA, Howard A, Yunis EJ. HLA associations in clozapine-induced agranulocytosis. Blood 1995;86:1177-83.

Acquired Neutropenia in Infancy and Childhood

125. Bruin M, Dassen A, Pajkrt D, Buddelmeyer L, Kuijpers T, de Haas M. Primary autoimmune neutropenia in children: a study of neutrophil antibodies and clinical course. Vox Sang 2005;88:52-9.

126. Bruin MC, von dem Borne AE, Tamminga RY, Kleijer M, Buddelmeijer L, de Haas M. Neutrophil antibody specificity in different types of childhood autoimmune neutropenia. Blood 1999;94:1797-802.

127. Bux J, Behrens G, Jaeger G, Welte K. Diagnosis and clinical course of autoimmune neutropenia in infancy: analysis of 240 cases. Blood 1998;91:181-6.

128. Curtis BR, Reno C, Aster RH. Neonatal alloimmune neutropenia attributed to maternal immunoglobulin G antibodies against the neutrophil alloantigen HNA-1c (SH): a report of five cases. Transfusion 2005;45:1308-13.

129. Juul SE, Haynes JW, McPherson RJ. Evaluation of neutropenia and neutrophilia in hospitalized preterm infants. J Perinatol 2004;24:150-7.

130. Maheshwari A, Christensen RD, Calhoun DA. Immune-mediated neutropenia in the neonate. Acta Paediatr Suppl 2002;91:98-103.

131. Perdikogianni C, Dimitriou H, Stiakaki E, Markaki EA, Kalmanti M. Adhesion molecules, endogenous granulocyte colony-stimulating factor levels and replating capacity of progenitors in autoimmune neutropenia of childhood. Acta Paediatr 2003;92:1277-83.

Congenital Neutropenia

132. Ancliff PJ. Congenital neutropenia. Blood Rev 2003;17:209-16.

133. Aprikyan AA, Liles WC, Park JR, Jonas M, Chi EY, Dale DC. Myelokathexis, a congenital disorder of severe neutropenia characterized by accelerated apoptosis and defective expression of bcl- x in neutrophil precursors. Blood 2000;95:320-7.

134. Aprikyan AA, Liles WC, Rodger E, Jonas M, Chi EY, Dale DC. Impaired survival of bone marrow hematopoietic progenitor cells in cyclic neutropenia. Blood 2001;97:147-53.

135. Austin KM, Leary RJ, Shimamura A. The Shwachman-Diamond SBDS protein localizes to the nucleolus. Blood 2005;106:1253-8.

136. Bellanne-Chantelot C, Clauin S, Leblanc T, et al. Mutations in the ELA2 gene correlate with more severe expression of neutropenia: a study of 81 patients from the French Neutropenia Register. Blood 2004;103:4119-25.

137. Berliner N, Horwitz M, Loughran TP, Jr. Congenital and acquired neutropenia. Hematology Am Soc Hematol Educ Program 2004:63-79.

138. Boxer LA, Stein S, Buckley D, Bolyard AA, Dale DC. Strong evidence for autosomal dominant inheritance of severe congenital neutropenia associated with ELA2 mutations. J Pediatr 2006;148:633-6.

139. Carlsson G, Aprikyan AA, Tehranchi R, et al. Kostmann syndrome: severe congenital neutropenia associated with defective expression of Bcl-2, constitutive mitochondrial release of cytochrome c, and excessive apoptosis of myeloid progenitor cells. Blood 2004;103:3355-61.

140. Cham B, Bonilla MA, Winkelstein J. Neutropenia associated with primary immunodeficiency syndromes. Semin Hematol 2002;39:107-12.

141. Dale DC, Cottle TE, Fier CJ, et al. Severe chronic neutropenia: treatment and follow-up of patients in the Severe Chronic Neutropenia International Registry. Am J Hematol 2003;72:82-93.

142. Diaz GA, Gulino AV. WHIM syndrome: a defect in CXCR4 signaling. Curr Allergy Asthma Rep 2005;5:350-5.

143. Donadieu J, Leblanc T, Bader Meunier B, et al. Analysis of risk factors for myelodysplasias, leukemias and death from infection among patients with congenital neutropenia. Experience of the French Severe Chronic Neutropenia Study Group. Haematologica 2005;90:45-53.

144. Dong F, Brynes RK, Tidow N, Welte K, Lowenberg B, Touw TP. Mutations in the gene for the granulocyte colony-stimulating-factor receptor in patients with acute myeloid leukemia preceded by severe congenital neutropenia. N Engl J Med 1995;333:487-93.

144a. Donini M, Fontana S, Savoldi G, et al. G-CSF treatment of severe congenital neutropenia reverses neutropenia but does not correct the underlying functional deficiency of the neutrophil in defending against microorganisms. Blood 2007;109:4716-23.

145. Dror Y, Ginzberg H, Dalal I, et al. Immune function in patients with Shwachman-Diamond syndrome. Br J Haematol 2001;114:712-7.

146. Druhan LJ, Ai J, Massullo P, Kindwall-Keller T, Ranalli MA, Avalos BR. Novel mechanism of G-CSF refractoriness in patients with severe congenital neutropenia. Blood 2005;105:584-91.

147. Eapen M, DeLaat CA, Baker KS, et al. Hematopoietic cell transplantation for Chediak-Higashi syndrome. Bone Marrow Transplant 2007;39:411-5.

147a. Horwitz MS, Duan Z, Korkmaz B, Lee HH, Mealiffe ME, Salipante SJ. Neutrophil elastase in cyclic and severe congenital neutropenia. Blood 2007;109:1817-24.

148. Huynh C, Roth D, Ward DM, Kaplan J, Andrews NW. Defective lysosomal exocytosis and plasma membrane repair in Chediak-Higashi/beige cells. Proc Natl Acad Sci U S A 2004;101:16795-800.

149. Introne W, Boissy RE, Gahl WA. Clinical, molecular, and cell biological aspects of Chediak-Higashi syndrome. Mol Genet Metab 1999;68:283-303.

150. Kjeldsen L, Calafat J, Borregaard N. Giant granules of neutrophils in Chediak-Higashi syndrome are derived from azurophil granules but not from specific and gelatinase granules. J Leukoc Biol 1998;64:72-7.

151. Kolehmainen J, Wilkinson R, Lehesjoki AE, et al. Delineation of Cohen syndrome following a large-scale genotype-phenotype screen. Am J Hum Genet 2004;75:122-7.

151a. Kostmann R. Infantile genetic agranulocytosis; agranulocytosis infantilis hereditaria. Acta Paediatr Suppl 1956;45:1-78.

152. Kuijpers TW, Alders M, Tool AT, Mellink C, Roos D, Hennekam RC. Hematologic abnormalities in Shwachman Diamond syndrome: lack of genotype-phenotype relationship. Blood 2005;106:356-61.

153. Massullo P, Druhan LJ, Bunnell BA, et al. Aberrant subcellular targeting of the G185R neutrophil elastase mutant associated with severe congenital neutropenia induces premature apoptosis of differentiating promyelocytes. Blood 2005;105:3397-404.

154. Melis D, Fulceri R, Parenti G, et al. Genotype/phenotype correlation in glycogen storage disease type 1b: a multicentre study and review of the literature. Eur J Pediatr 2005;164:501-8.

155. Papadaki HA, Eliopoulos GD. The role of apoptosis in the pathophysiology of chronic neutropenias associated with bone marrow failure. Cell Cycle 2003;2:447-51.

156. Papadaki HA, Stamatopoulos K, Damianaki A, et al. Activated T-lymphocytes with myelosuppressive properties in patients with chronic idiopathic neutropenia. Br J Haematol 2005;128:863-76.

157. Popovic M, Goobie S, Morrison J, et al. Fine mapping of the locus for Shwachman-Diamond syndrome at 7q11, identification of shared disease haplotypes, and exclusion of TPST1 as a candidate gene. Eur J Hum Genet 2002;10:250-8.

158. Rezaei N, Farhoudi A, Pourpak Z, et al. Neutropenia in Iranian patients with primary immunodeficiency disorders. Haematologica 2005;90:554-6.

158a. Rosenberg PS, Alter BP, Bolyard AA, et al. The incidence of leukemia and mortality from sepsis in patients with severe congenital neutropenia receiving long-term G-CSF therapy. Blood 2006;107:4628-35.

159. Spiegel R, Shalev S, Huebner A, Horovitz Y. Association of chronic symptomatic neutropenia with the triple A syndrome. J Pediatr Hematol Oncol 2005;27:53-5.

159a. Tamary H, Alter BP. Current diagnosis of inherited bone marrow failure syndromes. Pediatr Hematol Oncol 2007;24:87-99.

160. Taniuchi S, Yamamoto A, Fujiwara T, Hasui M, Tsuji S, Kobayashi Y. Dizygotic twin sisters with myelokathexis: mechanism of its neutropenia. Am J Hematol 1999;62:106-11.

161. Wei ML. Hermansky-Pudlak syndrome: a disease of protein trafficking and organelle function. Pigment Cell Res 2006;19:19-42.

162. Woloszynek JR, Rothbaum RJ, Rawls AS, et al. Mutations of the SBDS gene are present in most patients with Shwachman-Diamond syndrome. Blood 2004;104:3588-90.

163. Zarzour W, Kleta R, Frangoul H, et al. Two novel CHS1 (LYST) mutations: clinical correlations in an infant with Chediak-Higashi syndrome. Mol Genet Metab 2005;85:125-32.

164. Zeidler C, Schwinzer B, Welte K. Congenital neutropenias. Rev Clin Exp Hematol 2003;7:72-83.

Abnormal Neutrophil Morphology

165. Asmis LM, Hadaya K, Majno P, Toso C, Triponez F, Starobinski M. Acquired and reversible Pelger-Huet anomaly of polymorphonuclear neutrophils in three transplant patients receiving mycophenolate mofetil therapy. Am J Hematol 2003;73:244-8.

166. Best S, Salvati F, Kallo J, et al. Lamin B-receptor mutations in Pelger-Huet anomaly. Br J Haematol 2003;123:542-4.

167. Constantino B. Pelger-Huet anomaly-morphology, mechanism, and significance in the peripheral blood film. ASCP Lab Med 2005;36:103-7.

168. Deutsch PH, Mandell GL. Reversible Pelger-Huet anomaly associated with ibuprofen therapy. Arch Intern Med 1985;145:166.

169. Eichacker P, Lawrence C. Steroid-induced hypersegmentation in neutrophiles. Am J Hematol 1985;18:41-5.

170. Etzell JE, Wang E. Acquired Pelger-Huet anomaly in association with concomitant tacrolimus and mycophenolate mofetil in a liver transplant patient: a case report and review of the literature. Arch Pathol Lab Med 2006;130:93-6.

171. Gehlot GS, Monga JN. Prevalence of Pelger-Huet anomaly of leucocytes in Adivasi population of western Madhya Pradesh. Indian J Med Res 1973;61:653-62.

172. Godwin JH. Howell-Jolly body-like inclusions. Am J Clin Pathol 1994;102:389-90.

173. Gondo H, Okamura C, Osaki K, Shimoda K, Asano Y, Okamura T. Acquired Pelger-Huet anomaly in association with concomitant tacrolimus and fluconazole therapy following allogeneic bone marrow transplantation. Bone Marrow Transplant 2000;26:1255-7.

174. Hansen H, Graucob E. Mucopolysaccharidoses. Hematologic Cytology of Storage Diseases. Berlin, Germany: Springer-Verlag; 1985:32.

175. Harless W, Crowell E, Abraham J. Anemia and neutropenia associated with copper deficiency of unclear etiology. Am J Hematol 2006;81:546-9.

176. Hoffmann K, Dreger CK, Olins AL, et al. Mutations in the gene encoding the lamin B receptor produce an altered nuclear morphology in granulocytes (Pelger-Huet anomaly). Nat Genet 2002;31:410-4.

177. Huff JD, Keung YK, Thakuri M, et al. Copper deficiency causes reversible myelodysplasia. Am J Hematol 2007;82:625-30.

178. Kahwash E, Gewirtz AS. Howell-Jolly body-like inclusions in neutrophils. Arch Pathol Lab Med 2003;127:1389-90.

179. Knecht H, Eichhorn P, Streuli RA. Granulocytes with ring-shaped nuclei in severe alcoholism. Acta Haematol 1985;73:184.

180. Kornberg A, Goldfarb A, Shalev O. Pseudo-Pelger-Huet anomaly in chronic lymphocytic leukemia. Acta Haematol 1981;66:127-8.

181. Krause JR. The bone marrow in nutritional deficiencies. Hematol Oncol Clin North Am 1988;2:557-66.

182. Pecci A, Canobbio I, Balduini A, et al. Pathogenetic mechanisms of hematological abnormalities of patients with MYH9 mutations. Hum Mol Genet 2005;14:3169-78.

183. Peterson L, Parkin J, Nelson A. Mucopolysaccharidosis type VII. A morphologic, cytochemical, and ultrastructural study of the blood and bone marrow. Am J Clin Pathol 1982;78:544-8.

184. Presentey B. Alder anomaly accompanied by a mutation of the myeloperoxidase structural gene. Acta Haematol 1986;75:157-9.

185. Pujol-Moix N, Kelley MJ, Hernandez A, et al. Ultrastructural analysis of granulocyte inclusions in genetically confirmed MYH9-related disorders. Haematologica 2004;89:330-7.

186. Rajeevan K, Anandan KR, Vinayan KP, Urmila KE, Aravindan KP. Jordans' anomaly. Indian J Pediatr 1999;66:626-8.

187. Reilly W. The granules in the leukocytes in gargoylism. Am J Dis Child. 1941;62:489-91.

188. Savage PJ, Dellinger RP, Barnes JV, Carruth CW. Pelger-Huet anomaly of granulocytes in a patient with tuberculosis. Chest 1984;85:131-2.

189. Seri M, Pecci A, Di Bari F, et al. MYH9-related disease: May-Hegglin anomaly, Sebastian syndrome, Fechtner syndrome, and Epstein syndrome are not distinct entities but represent a variable expression of a single illness. Medicine (Baltimore) 2003;82:203-15.

190. Shetty VT, Mundle SD, Raza A. Pseudo Pelger-Huet anomaly in myelodysplastic syndrome: hyposegmented apoptotic neutrophil? Blood 2001;98:1273-5.

191. Sipahi T, Tavil B, Unver Y. Neutrophil hypersegmentation in children with iron deficiency anemia. Pediatr Hematol Oncol 2002;19:235-8.

192. Slagel DD, Lager DJ, Dick FR. Howell-Jolly body-like inclusions in the neutrophils of patients with acquired immunodeficiency syndrome. Am J Clin Pathol 1994;101:429-31.

193. Taegtmeyer AB, Halil O, Bell AD, Carby M, Cummins D, Banner NR. Neutrophil dysplasia (acquired pseudo-pelger anomaly) caused by ganciclovir. Transplantation 2005;80:127-30.

194. Thompson WG, Cassino C, Babitz L, et al. Hypersegmented neutrophils and vitamin B12 deficiency. Hypersegmentation in B12 deficiency. Acta Haematol 1989;81:186-91.

195. Willis M, Monaghan S, Miller M, et al. Zinc-induced copper deficiency. Am J Clin Pathol 2005;123:125-31.

Eosinophilia

196. Allam JP, Paus T, Reichel C, Bieber T, Novak N. DRESS syndrome associated with carbamazepine and phenytoin. Eur J Dermatol 2004;14:339-42.

197. Baccarani M, Cilloni D, Rondoni M, et al. The efficacy of imatinib mesylate in patients with FIP1l1-PDGFRalpha-positive hypereosinophilic syndrome. Results of a multicenter prospective study. Haematologica 2007;92:1173-9.

198. Bacher U, Reiter A, Haferlach T, et al. A combination of cytomorphology, cytogenetic analysis, fluorescence in situ hybridization and reverse transcriptase polymerase chain reaction for establishing clonality in cases of persisting hypereosinophilia. Haematologica 2006;91:817-20.

199. Brito-Babapulle F. The eosinophilias, including the idiopathic hypereosinophilic syndrome. Br J Haematol 2003;121:203-23.

200. Butterfield JH. Diverse clinical outcomes of eosinophilic patients with T-cell receptor gene rearrangements: the emerging diagnostic importance of molecular genetics testing. Am J Hematol 2001;68:81-6.

201. Cara DC, Negrao-Correa D, Teixeira MM. Mechanisms underlying eosinophil trafficking and their relevance in vivo. Histol Histopathol 2000;15:899-920.

202. Certad G, Arenas-Pinto A, Pocaterra L, et al. Isosporiasis in Venezuelan adults infected with human immunodeficiency virus: clinical characterization. Am J Trop Med Hyg 2003;69:217-22.

203. Cragun WC, Yamshchikov GV, Bissonette EA, et al. Low-dose IL-2 induces cytokine cascade, eosinophilia, and a transient Th2 shift in melanoma patients. Cancer Immunol Immunother 2005;54:1095-105.

204. Dorman SC, Sehmi R, Gauvreau GM, et al. Kinetics of bone marrow eosinophilopoiesis and associated cytokines after allergen inhalation. Am J Respir Crit Care Med 2004;169:565-72.

205. Falcone FH, Loukas A, Quinnell RJ, Pritchard DI. The innate allergenicity of helminth parasites. Clin Rev Allergy Immunol 2004;26:61-72.

206. Fletcher S, Bain B. Diagnosis and treatment of hyperosinophilic syndromes. Curr Opin Hematol 2007;14:37-42.

207. Gotlib J, Cools J, Malone JM 3rd, Schrier SL, Grilliland DG, Coutre SE. The FIP1L1-PDGFRalpha fusion tyrosine kinase in hypereosinophilic syndrome and chronic eosinophilic leukemia: implications for diagnosis, classification, and management. Blood 2004;103:2879-91.

208. Granter SR, Barnhill RL, Duray PH. Borrelial fasciitis: diffuse fasciitis and peripheral eosinophilia associated with Borrelia infection. Am J Dermatopathol 1996;18:465-73.

209. Gutierrez A, Solano C, Ferrandez A, et al. Peripheral T-cell lymphoma associated consecutively with hemophagocytic lymphohistiocytosis and hypereosinophilic syndrome. Eur J Haematol 2003;71:303-6.

210. Hellmich B, Ehlers S, Csernok E, Gross WL. Update on the pathogenesis of Churg-Strauss syndrome. Clin Exp Rheumatol 2003;21:S69-77.

211. Henry NL, Law M, Nutman TB, Klion AD. Onchocerciasis in a nonendemic population: clinical and immunologic assessment before treatment and at the time of presumed cure. J Infect Dis 2001;183:512-6.

212. JabbarAl-Obaidi M, Rymes N, White P, et al. A fourth case of 8p11 myeloproliferative disorder transforming to B-lineage acute lymphoblastic leukaemia. A case report. Acta Haematol 2002;107:98-100.

213. Klion AD, Law MA, Riemenschneider W, et al. Familial eosinophilia: a benign disorder? Blood 2004;103:4050-5.

214. Klion AD, Nutman TB. The role of eosinophils in host defense against helminth parasites. J Allergy Clin Immunol 2004;113:30-7.

215. Klion AD, Robyn J, Akin C, et al. Molecular remission and reversal of myelofibrosis in response to imatinib mesylate treatment in patients with the myeloproliferative variant of hypereosinophilic syndrome. Blood 2004;103:473-8.

216. Kralovics R, Skoda RC. Molecular pathogenesis of Philadelphia chromosome negative myeloproliferative disorders. Blood Rev 2005;19:1-13.

217. Mitsuyama H, Matsuyama W, Watanabe M, et al. Increased expression of TRAIL receptor 3 on eosinophils in Churg-Strauss syndrome. Arthritis Rheum 2007;56:662-73.

218. Pardanani A, Brockman SR, Paternoster SF, et al. FIP1L1-PDGFRA fusion: prevalence and clinicopathologic correlates in 89 consecutive patients with moderate to severe eosinophilia. Blood 2004;104:3038-45.

219. Patnaik MM, Rindos M, Kouides PA, Tefferi A, Pardanani A. Systemic mastocytosis: a concise clinical and laboratory review. Arch Pathol Lab Med 2007;131:784-91.

220. Preiss U, Ockert G, Broemme S, Otto A. On the clinical importance of Dientamoeba fragilis infections in childhood. J Hyg Epidemiol Microbiol Immunol 1991;35:27-34.

221. Renauld JC. New insights into the role of cytokines in asthma. J Clin Pathol 2001;54:577-89.

222. Roche-Lestienne C, Lepers S, Soenen-Cornu V, et al. Molecular characterization of the idiopathic hypereosinophilic syndrome (HES) in 35 French patients with normal conventional cytogenetics. Leukemia 2005;19:792-8.

223. Rodgers S, Rees RC, Hancock BW. Changes in the phenotypic characteristics of eosinophils from patients receiving recombinant human interleukin-2 (rhIL-2) therapy. Br J Haematol 1994;86:746-53.

224. Tefferi A. Blood eosinophilia: a new paradigm in disease classification, diagnosis, and treatment. Mayo Clin Proc 2005;80:75-83.

225. Tefferi A, Patnaik MM, Pardanani A. Eosinophilia: secondary, clonal and idiopathic. Br J Haematol 2006;133:468-92.

226. Tefferi A, Vardiman JW. The diagnositc interface between histology and molecular tests in myeloproliferative disorders. Curr Opin Hematol 2007;14:115:22.

227. Turk M, Kaptan F, Turker N, et al. Clinical and laboratory aspects of a trichinellosis outbreak in Izmir, Turkey. Parasite 2006;13:65-70.

227a. Vaklavas C, Tefferi A, Butterfield J, et al. 'Idiopathic' eosinophilia with an occult T-cell clone: prevalence and clinical course. Leuk Res 2007;31:691-4.

228. Wilson F, Tefferi A. Acute lymphocytic leukemia with eosinophilia: two case reports and a literature review. Leuk Lymphoma 2005;46:1045-50.

229. Wolfe MS. Eosinophilia in the returning traveler. Med Clin North Am 1999;83:1019-32, vii.

230. Zuliani E, Zwahlen H, Gilliet F, Marone C. Vancomycin-induced hypersensitivity reaction with acute renal failure: resolution following cyclosporine treatment. Clin Nephrol 2005;64:155-8.

Basophilia

231. Anthony HM. Blood basophils in lung cancer. Br J Cancer 1982;45:209-16.

232. Arnalich F, Lahoz C, Larrocha C, et al. Incidence and clinical significance of peripheral and bone marrow basophilia. J Med 1987;18:293-303.

233. Arock M, Schneider E, Boissan M, Tricottet V, Dy M. Differentiation of human basophils: an overview of recent advances and pending questions. J Leukoc Biol 2002;71:557-64.

234. Bloebaum RM, Dharajiya N, Grant JA. Mechanisms of IgE-mediated allergic reactions. Clin Allergy Immunol 2004;18:65-84.

235. Bodger MP, Newton LA. The purification of human basophils: their immunophenotype and cytochemistry. Br J Haematol 1987;67:281-4.

236. Buhring HJ, Simmons PJ, Pudney M, et al. The monoclonal antibody 97A6 defines a novel surface antigen expressed on human basophils and their multipotent and unipotent progenitors. Blood 1999;94:2343-56.

237. Falcone FH, Haas H, Gibbs BF. The human basophil: a new appreciation of its role in immune responses. Blood 2000;96:4028-38.

238. Graham DY, Osato MS, Olson CA, Zhang J, Figura N. Effect of H. pylori infection and CagA status on leukocyte counts and liver function tests: extra-gastric manifestations of H. pylori infection. Helicobacter 1998;3:174-8.

239. Grattan CE, Dawn G, Gibbs S, Francis DM. Blood basophil numbers in chronic ordinary urticaria and healthy controls: diurnal variation, influence of loratadine and prednisolone and relationship to disease activity. Clin Exp Allergy 2003;33:337-41.

240. Matsushima T, Handa H, Yokohama A, et al. Prevalence and clinical characteristics of myelodysplastic syndrome with bone marrow eosinophilia or basophilia. Blood 2003;101:3386-90.

241. May ME, Waddell CC. Basophils in peripheral blood and bone marrow. A retrospective review. Am J Med 1984;76:509-11.

242. Mitre E, Nutman TB. Basophils, basophilia and helminth infections. Chem Immunol Allergy 2006;90:141-56.

243. Mitre E, Taylor RT, Kubofcik J, Nutman TB. Parasite antigen-driven basophils are a major source of IL-4 in human filarial infections. J Immunol 2004;172:2439-45.

243a. Obata K, Mukai K, Tsujimura Y, et al. Basophils are essential initiators of a novel type of chronic allergic inflammation. Blood 2007;110:913-20.

244. Phillips C, Coward WR, Pritchard DI, Hewitt CR. Basophils express a type 2 cytokine profile on exposure to proteases from helminths and house dust mites. J Leukoc Biol 2003;73:165-71.

245. Takao K, Tanimoto Y, Fujii M, et al. In vitro expansion of human basophils by interleukin-3 from granulocyte colony-stimulating factor-mobilized peripheral blood stem cells. Clin Exp Allergy 2003;33:1561-7.

246. Tikkanen J, Lemstrom K, Halme M, Pakkala S, Taskinen E, Koskinen P. Cytological monitoring of peripheral blood, bronchoalveolar lavage fluid, and transbronchial biopsy specimens during acute rejection and cytomegalovirus infection in lung and heart-lung allograft recipients. Clin Transplant 2001;15:77-88.

247. Togias AG. Systemic immunologic and inflammatory aspects of allergic rhinitis. J Allergy Clin Immunol 2000;106:S247-50.

248. Uston PI, Lee CM. Characterization and function of the multifaceted peripheral blood basophil. Cell Mol Biol (Noisy-le-grand) 2003;49:1125-35.

Monocytosis

249. Bux J, Kissel K, Nowak K, Spengel U, Mueller-Eckhardt C. Autoimmune neutropenia: clinical and laboratory studies in 143 patients. Ann Hematol 1991;63:249-52.

250. Chen YC, Chou JM, Ketterling RP, Letendre L, Li CY. Histologic and immunohistochemical study of bone marrow monocytic nodules in 21 cases with myelodysplasia. Am J Clin Pathol 2003;120:874-81.

251. Dinauer MC. The phagocyte system and disorders of granulopoiesis and granulocyte function. In: Nathan DG, Orkin SH, eds. Nathan and Oski's hematology of infancy and childhood, 5th ed, Vol 1. Philadelphia: WB Saunders Company; 1998:889-967.

252. Dunphy CH, Orton SO, Mantell J. Relative contributions of enzyme cytochemistry and flow cytometric immunophenotyping to the evaluation of acute myeloid leukemias with a monocytic component and of flow cytometric immunophenotyping to the evaluation of absolute monocytoses. Am J Clin Pathol 2004;122:865-74.

253. Foucar K. Constitutional and reactive myeloid disorders. Bone marrow pathology, 2nd ed. Chicago: ASCP Press; 200:146-72.

254. Galanakis E, Bourantas KL, Leveidiotou S, Lapatsanis PD. Childhood brucellosis in north-western Greece: a retrospective analysis. Eur J Pediatr 1996;155:1-6.

255. Gasche C, Reinisch W, Schwarzmeier JD. Evidence of colony suppressor activity and deficiency of hematopoietic growth factors in hairy cell leukemia. Hematol Oncol 1993;11:97-104.

256. Herbst B, Kohler G, Mackensen A, Veelken H, Lindemann A. GM-CSF promotes differentiation of a precursor cell of monocytes and Langerhans-type dendritic cells from CD34+ haemopoietic progenitor cells. Br J Haematol 1998;101:231-41.

257. Kampalath B, Cleveland RP, Chang CC, Kass L. Monocytes with altered phenotypes in posttrauma patients. Arch Pathol Lab Med 2003;127:1580-5.

258. Kawakami A, Fukunaga T, Usui M, et al. Visceral leishmaniasis misdiagnosed as malignant lymphoma. Intern Med 1996;35:502-6.

259. Kehrl JH, Fauci AS. The clinical use of glucocorticoids. Ann Allergy 1983;50:2-8.

260. Kraut EH. Clinical manifestations and infectious complications of hairy-cell leukaemia. Best Pract Res Clin Haematol 2003;16:33-40.

261. Li CY, Yam LT. Cytochemistry and immunochemistry in hematologic diagnoses. Hematol Oncol Clin North Am 1994;8:665-81.

262. Lichtman M. Monocytosis and monocytopenia. Williams Hematology, 7th ed. New York, NY: McGraw Hill Medical; 2006:983-7.

263. Maekawa Y, Anzai T, Yoshikawa T, et al. Prognostic significance of peripheral monocytosis after reperfused acute myocardial infarction:a possible role for left ventricular remodeling. J Am Coll Cardiol 2002;39:241-6.

264. Nakajima H, Mori S, Takeuchi T, et al. Monocytosis and high serum macrophage colony-stimulating factor in Waldenstrom's macroglobulinemia. Blood 1995;86:2863-4.

265. Rosmarin AG, Yang Z, Resendes KK. Transcriptional regulation in myelopoiesis: Hematopoietic fate choice, myeloid differentiation, and leukemogenesis. Exp Hematol 2005;33:131-43.

266. Santangelo S, Gamelli RL, Shankar R. Myeloid commitment shifts toward monocytopoiesis after thermal injury and sepsis. Ann Surg 2001;233:97-106.

267. Tokioka T, Shimamoto Y, Motoyoshi K, Yamaguchi M. Clinical significance of monocytosis and human monocytic colony-stimulating factor in patients with adult T-cell leukaemia/lymphoma. Haematologia (Budap) 1994;26:1-9.

268. Wendland T, Herren S, Yawalkar N, Cerny A, Pichler WJ. Strong alpha beta and gamma delta TCR response in a patient with disseminated Mycobacterium avium infection and lack of NK cells and monocytopenia. Immunol Lett 2000;72:75-82.

269. Xu Y, McKenna RW, Karandikar NJ, Pildain AJ, Kroft SH. Flow cytometric analysis of monocytes as a tool for distinguishing chronic myelomonocytic leukemia from reactive monocytosis. Am J Clin Pathol 2005;124:799-806.

270. Yetgin S, Cetin M, Yenicesu I, Ozaltin F, Uckan D. Acute parvovirus B19 infection mimicking juvenile myelomonocytic leukemia. Eur J Haematol 2000;65:276-8.

6 NON-NEOPLASTIC MEGAKARYOCYTIC LINEAGE DISORDERS

GENERAL CONCEPTS

In this chapter, platelet and megakaryocyte disorders are reviewed, with an emphasis on the bone marrow morphology of these pathologic processes. The major hematologic manifestation of a megakaryocytic disorder is an alteration in the peripheral blood platelet count or in the morphologic features of the circulating platelets. Numerical platelet abnormalities include thrombocytopenia (platelet count below 150,000/µL) or thrombocytosis/ thrombocythemia (platelet count elevated above 400,000/µL). Unlike other lineages, normal ranges for platelet counts do not show significant age-related variations.

Most cases of thrombocytopenia are the consequence of platelet survival defects rather than any intrinsic bone marrow pathology, and bone marrow examination may not be required to diagnose and manage these patients. Similarly, cases of reactive thrombocytosis are often diagnosed by integrating complete blood count findings with the clinical information, such as a history of recent trauma, surgery, or other acute stresses. A review of previous complete blood count data may be valuable in confirming an antecedent normal platelet count. Bone marrow examination is generally necessary only in cases of thrombocytosis in which a neoplastic hematopoietic disorder cannot be excluded by clinical and laboratory assessment.

Some megakaryocytic disorders manifest with both numerical and morphologic abnormalities of platelets. These disorders are infrequent and include rare constitutional megakaryocytic and platelet disorders as well as relatively more common myeloid neoplasms. Bone marrow examination is typically necessary in patients with either suspected constitutional disorders or suspected primary hematopoietic neoplasms.

NORMAL MEGAKARYOCYTE DEVELOPMENT AND PLATELET HOMEOSTASIS

Peripheral blood platelet homeostasis is maintained by normal megakaryocyte growth and maturation (fig. 6-1). As with all hematopoietic elements, megakaryocytes arise from pluripotential stem cells that give rise to committed megakaryocytic progenitor cells (17). Various

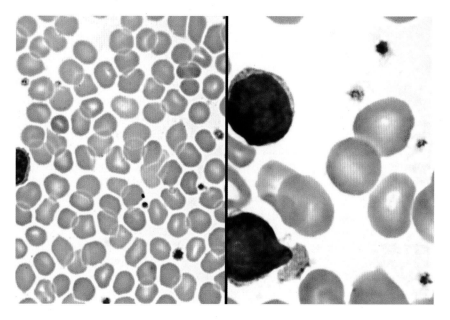

Figure 6-1

NORMAL PLATELETS

Intermediate- (left) and high-power (right) magnification of normal platelets within the peripheral blood shows minimal variation in platelet size as well as abundant granularity (Wright stain).

Table 6-1

MEGAKARYOCYTE PRODUCTION AND MATURATION[a,b]

Cell Type	Morphology	Immunophenotype	Comments
Precursor cells (stem cell/ progenitor cells)	No distinctive morphologic features	CD34+, CDw109+ in earliest stages, CD117+, gradual aquisition of HLA-DR, CD41, and Mpl 1 (thrombopoietin receptor)	Cells defined by features in cell culture systems and by immunophenotype Bipotent erythromegakaryocytic progenitor cell identified in normal human bone marrow
Promegakaryoblast (transitional cell)	Not morphologically distinct	Immature cell (CD34+) that expresses many megakaryocyte-associated antigens such as CD41, von Willebrand factor (vWF), Mpl 1	Platelet peroxidase (PPO) can be detected by electron microscopy
Megakaryoblast	Difficult to recognize by morphology alone—tends to be large blast with high nuclear to cytoplasmic ratio Basophilic cytoplasm; variable cytoplasmic blebbing	Variable CD34+ in conjunction with HLA-DR+, CD41+, CD42b+, CD61+, vWF+, PPO+, Mpl 1+	Not typically identified in normal bone marrow specimens Switch from mitosis to endomitosis linked to acquisition of lineage-specific antigens
Promegakaryocytes	Spectrum of large cells with various degrees of nuclear lobulation; progressive increase in overall size; variable cytoplasmic granules	Loss of CD34 but retention of the full complement of megakaryocyte-associated antigens; Mpl 1+	Readily identifiable in normal bone marrow specimens; concentrated in particles on aspirate smears
Platelet-shedding megakaryocyte	Large multilobulated megakaryocytes with highly condensed nuclear chromatin reside adjacent to bone marrow sinuses Voluminous amounts of cytoplasm with abundant cytoplasmic granules	Retention of full complement of megakaryocyte-associated antigens Expression of some megakaryocyte-associated antigens such as CD31, CD41, vWF increases with maturation; Mpl 1+	Direct shedding of platelets into circulation: 200 billion/day

[a]Data from references 2, 4–7, 10, 13, 16, 17, and 19.
[b]See chapter 1 for a more detailed discussion of hematopoiesis.

multilineage early-acting cytokines such as granulocyte-monocyte–colony-stimulating factor (GM-CSF), interleukin (IL)3, IL6, IL11, and stem cell factor (c-kit ligand) bind to receptors, thus stimulating the proliferation of pluripotential and early committed progenitors, while more lineage-specific cytokines, notably thrombopoietin, drive megakaryocyte-specific proliferation and maturation (2,3,6,7,11,13,15,16). Genes that encode transcription factors that regulate downstream gene expression in megakaryocytic precursor cells include *GATA1, FOG1, NF-E2, FLI1,* and *RUNX1* (14).

The morphologic features of pluripotential stem cells and committed progenitor cells are nonspecific; instead, these cells are defined by either properties in cell culture systems or immunophenotypic profiles (Table 6-1). Progressive maturation of these immature cells is characterized by the acquisition of both morphologic and immunophenotypic features that are specific for the megakaryocyte lineage. The binding of thrombopoietin to its ligand, c-Mpl, initiates a cascade of events that is ultimately responsible for the unique megakaryocytic properties.

Within normal bone marrow, megakaryoblasts are not readily identifiable morphologically, although large blastic forms with distinct cytoplasmic shedding are likely to be megakaryoblasts (fig. 6-2). The definitive detection of megakaryoblasts requires the identification of lineage-specific antigens, including CD41, CD42b, CD61, von Willebrand factor, CD31, and Mpl 1, which can be assessed by either flow cytometric or immunohistochemical techniques (Table 6-1; figs. 6-3, 6-4) (10).

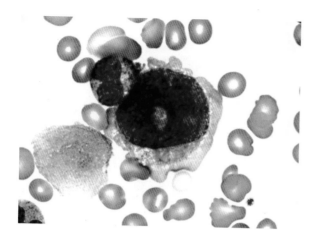

Figure 6-2

MEGAKARYOBLAST

Megakaryoblast from bone marrow aspirate of a young child. Zoning of the cytoplasm as well as blebbing are seen (Wright stain).

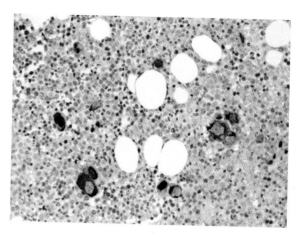

Figure 6-3

MEGAKARYOCYTE IMMUNOHISTOCHEMISTRY (CD42b)

Immunoperoxidase stain for CD42b highlights both nonlobulated and mature megakaryocytes in this bone marrow core biopsy.

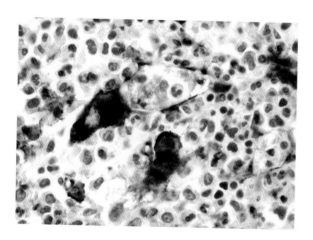

Figure 6-4

MEGAKARYOCYTE IMMUNOHISTOCHEMISTRY (CD31)

Immunoperoxidase stain for CD31 illustrates the perisinusoidal localization of normal megakaryocytes.

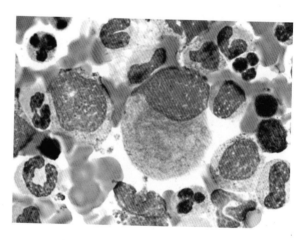

Figure 6-5

SO-CALLED MONONUCLEAR MEGAKARYOCYTE

A mononuclear (nonlobulated) megakaryocyte with early cytoplasmic maturation is present in a bone marrow aspirate smear from a 6-year-old boy (Wright stain).

Megakaryocytes are unique among hematopoietic elements in that DNA synthesis is not linked to mitosis, but rather to a progressive increase in nuclear size and DNA content along with multilobulation, a process termed endomitosis (5,8,12,19,20). With successive multilobulation, megakaryocytes become readily identifiable on both aspirate and biopsy specimens since megakaryocytes are by far the largest cell in normal bone marrow (figs. 6-5–6-11). Nuclear lobation, the consequence of endomitosis, results in highly folded but still connected lobulations rather than separate discrete multinucleation (fig. 6-12). Multilobulated megakaryocytes may reach 64N ploidy, although the average megakaryocyte has 16N ploidy and approximately eight lobes (1). Mature megakaryocytes have abundant intracellular organelles for platelet function as well as demarcation membranes and proplatelet processes for platelet shedding (see figs. 6-9, 6-10) (5).

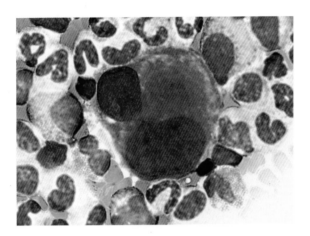

Figure 6-6

BILOBED MEGAKARYOCYTE

A bilobed megakaryocyte in a bone marrow aspirate smear from a 6-year-old boy (Wright stain).

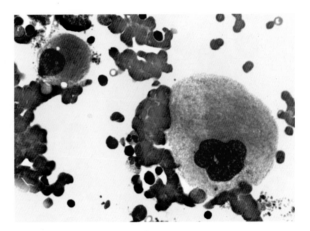

Figure 6-7

MEGAKARYOCYTE MATURATION

Two megakaryocytes at different stages of maturation are present in a bone marrow aspirate smear. The size and degree of nuclear lobulation vary (Wright stain).

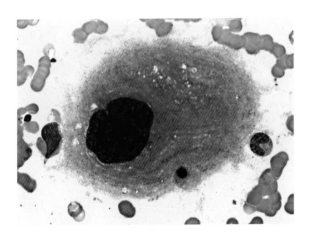

Figure 6-8

MATURE MEGAKARYOCYTE

A mature megakaryocyte with voluminous amounts of cytoplasm with fine uniform granularity. An adjacent myeloid cell highlights size comparison (Wright stain).

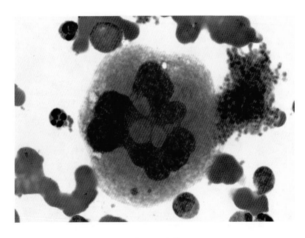

Figure 6-9

MATURE HYPERLOBULATED MEGAKARYOCYTE

A mature hyperlobulated megakaryocyte has an adherent clump of platelets (Wright stain).

Although often inapparent on routinely processed tissue sections, megakaryocytes typically reside immediately adjacent to the bone marrow sinus network; megakaryocyte pseudopodia extend into the sinus lumens, and platelets are shed directly into the circulation (figs. 6-13–6-16) (7). Because of this perisinusoidal localization, other mature hematopoietic cells, such as neutrophils, may need to pass through megakaryocytes to enter the circulation, a process termed emperipolesis (fig. 6-17). After megakaryocytes have shed their cytoplasm, residual senescent nuclei with scanty residual cytoplasm are presumably phagocytosed by bone marrow macrophages.

Megakaryocytes are readily apparent within the particles on bone marrow aspirate smear preparations (fig. 6-18). However, megakaryocytic number, morphology, and distribution are best assessed on hematoxylin and eosin (H&E)-stained clot and core biopsy specimens. Clot or core biopsy sections generally contain 1 to 3, relatively evenly distributed megakaryocytes with nuclear

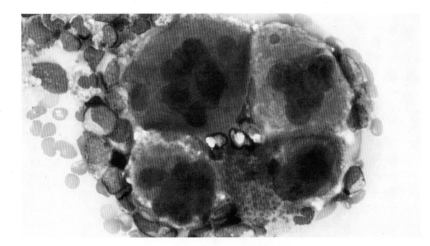

Figure 6-10

MEGAKARYOCYTE MATURATION

A spectrum of multilobulated mature megakaryocytes is evident in this bone marrow aspirate smear from a child (Wright stain).

Figure 6-11

INCREASED MEGAKARYOCYTES

This bone marrow clot section from a patient with immune thrombocytopenic purpura shows increased megakaryocytes with mature nuclear lobulation (hematoxylin and eosin [H&E] stain).

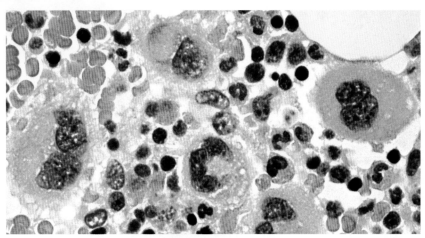

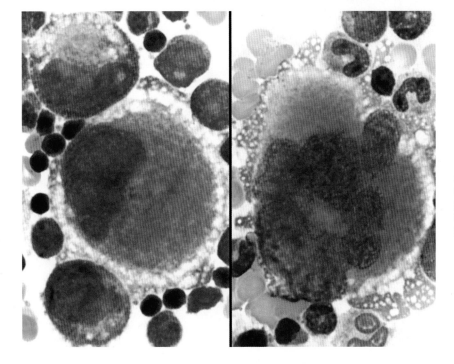

Figure 6-12

MEGAKARYOCYTES

The spectrum of megakaryocyte maturation is seen, including a broad range in size (left) and prominent hyperlobulation of a mature megakaryocyte (right) (Wright stain).

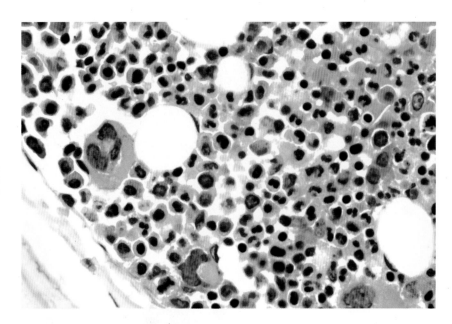

Figure 6-13

PERISINUSOIDAL MEGAKARYOCYTES

The perisinusoidal localization of mature megakaryocytes is evident on this bone marrow core biopsy section (H&E stain).

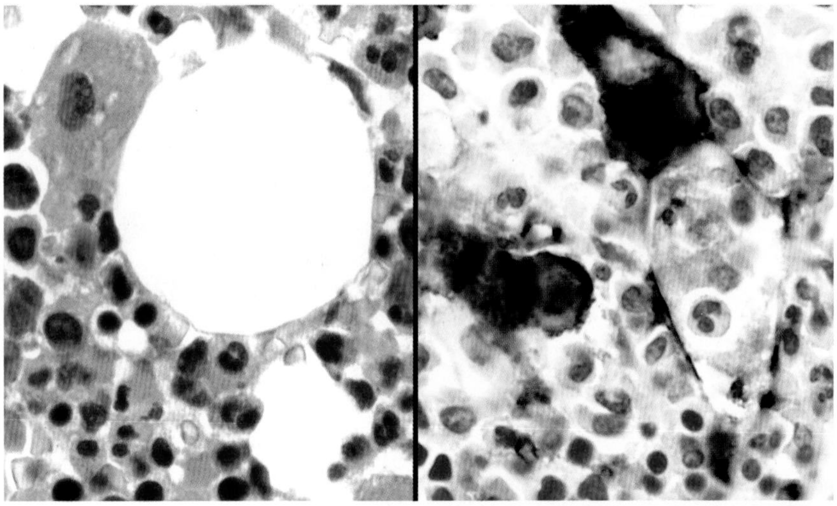

Figure 6-14

PERISINUSOIDAL MEGAKARYOCYTES

The perisinusoidal localization of normal mature megakaryocytes in the bone marrow core biopsy is seen (H&E, immunoperoxidase stain for CD31).

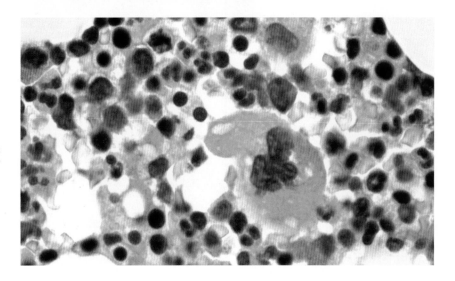

Figure 6-15

MEGAKARYOCYTE PROJECTION INTO SINUS

A megakaryocyte projects into a sinus in the bone marrow (H&E stain).

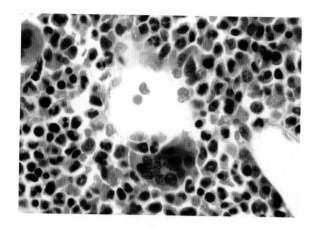

Figure 6-16

MEGAKARYOCYTE SHEDDING PLATELETS

A megakaryocyte sheds platelets into a bone marrow sinus (H&E stain).

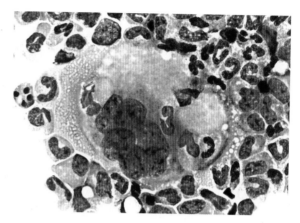

Figure 6-17

NEUTROPHILS WITHIN MEGAKARYOCYTE

Numerous neutrophils are passing through this megakaryocyte cytoplasm, so-called emperipolesis (Wright stain).

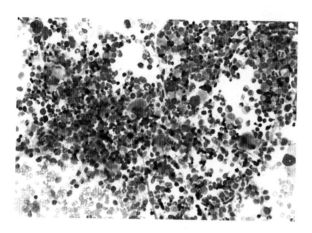

Figure 6-18

**ABUNDANT MEGAKARYOCYTES
IN BONE MARROW PARTICLE**

This low magnification photomicrograph of a bone marrow aspirate smear from a 4-day-old infant undergoing staging for Langerhans cell histiocytosis shows abundant megakaryocytes (Wright stain).

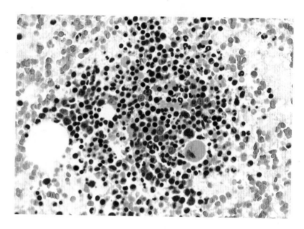

Figure 6-19

**SINGLE MEGAKARYOCYTE
IN BONE MARROW PARTICLE**

Bone marrow clot section in an adult shows a single megakaryocyte (H&E stain).

multilobulation per 40X high-power fields; somewhat higher numbers of megakaryocytes may be evident in specimens from neonates (figs. 6-19, 6-20). Nonlobulated megakaryocytes comprise a minority of the megakaryocytes and are presumably more immature than hyperlobulated megakaryocytes (fig. 6-21). If nonlobulated megakaryocytes are prominent, a pathologic process should be considered (such as infection with human immunodeficiency virus [HIV]-1 or myelodysplasia).

On core biopsy sections, megakaryocytes appear randomly dispersed individually with no predilection for a paratrabecular localization (fig. 6-22). The perisinusoidal residence of megakaryocytes is better appreciated on plastic-embedded sections than on routine paraffin-embedded tissue. Megakaryocyte clustering is not typically evident in normal bone marrow specimens, but may be evident during bone marrow regeneration following myelosuppressive/ablative therapy or other bone marrow insults (fig. 6-23). Megakaryocyte clustering is also a feature of primary myeloid neoplasms (fig. 6-23).

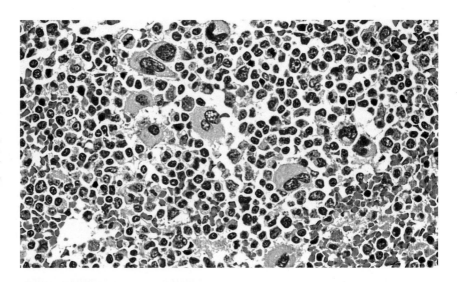

Figure 6-20

MEGAKARYOCYTES IN NORMAL NEONATE

Bone marrow clot section from a healthy newborn shows abundant, largely individually dispersed megakaryocytes (H&E stain). (Courtesy of Dr. L. Rimsza, Tucson, AZ.)

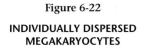

Figure 6-21

HYPOLOBULATED MEGAKARYOCYTES IN FAMILIAL AUTOSOMAL DOMINANT THROMBOCYTOPENIA

Hypolobulated megakaryocytes are evident in this bone marrow aspirate from a young adult female with familial autosomal dominant thrombocytopenia (Wright stain).

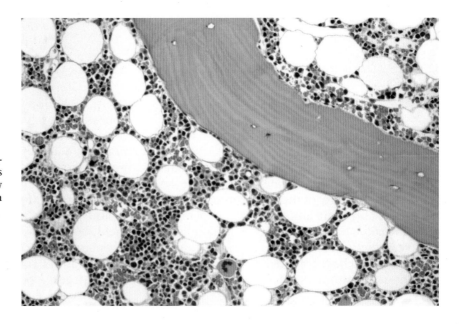

Figure 6-22

INDIVIDUALLY DISPERSED MEGAKARYOCYTES

Individually dispersed, non-paratrabecular megakaryocytes are evident in this bone marrow core biopsy specimen from a normal adult (H&E stain).

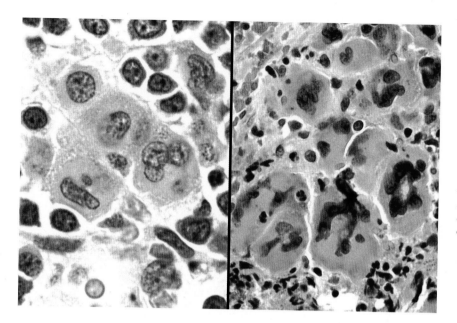

Figure 6-23

**MEGAKARYOCYTE
CLUSTERING**

The degree of megakaryocyte clustering that typifies early regeneration (left) is compared with the marked megakaryocyte clustering that characterizes chronic myeloproliferative disorders (right) (H&E stain).

Homeostatic platelet production rates are very high, approximating 200 billion platelets/day in normal subjects. Platelet production can be increased 8- to 10-fold in response to acute platelet survival disorders such as immune thrombocytopenic purpura (ITP) (2,5). Normal platelet counts range from 150,000 to 400,000/µL and age-related variations are not apparent, although platelet counts tend to be somewhat lower in premature infants (18). Thrombopoietin likely plays a major role in platelet homeostasis, and age-related normal ranges for thrombopoietin levels have been established (3,9). The liver is the primary source of thrombopoietin, and production rates are fairly stable (5). The highest physiological levels are noted in the perinatal period. Plasma levels are largely regulated by absorption by cells that express the thrombopoietin receptor, c-Mpl (5). Since platelets express c-Mpl, they consequently bind thrombopoietin. In conditions with elevated platelet counts, excess thrombopoietin is bound to platelets, and the thrombopoietin available to bind to bone marrow precursor cells is reduced, thereby reducing platelet production. In thrombocytopenic conditions, thrombopoietin is available to drive progenitor cell proliferation and increase platelet production (15). Thus, the circulating platelet mass directly determines the plasma level of thrombopoietin, and, consequently, the amount of thrombopoi-

etin available to drive megakaryocyte production in the bone marrow (11).

MORPHOLOGIC ABNORMALITIES OF PLATELETS AND MEGAKARYOCYTES

Qualitative abnormalities of platelets and megakaryocytes provide morphologic clues to various non-neoplastic disorders (Table 6-2). During peripheral blood smear review, it is important to assess platelets for both size and granularity (fig. 6-24). Although rare constitutional disorders, such as gray platelet syndrome, are characterized by platelets with inconspicuous granules, profoundly hypogranular platelets are more commonly encountered in myeloid neoplasms (figs. 6-25–6-27). Specimen age must also be considered, since platelet degranulation may occur when venipuncture specimen processing has been delayed.

Enlarged, well-granulated platelets are notable in platelet survival defect disorders (e.g., ITP), while enlarged, hypogranular platelets typify neoplastic myeloid processes (fig. 6-27). Both constitutional macrothrombocytic and microthrombocytic disorders have been described; these disorders are reviewed later in this chapter. Circulating megakaryocytes are more commonly encountered in neoplastic processes, especially chronic myeloproliferative disorders, although they are also seen in normal neonates and even adults (figs. 6-28–6-31) (36). By automated cell

Table 6-2

MORPHOLOGIC ABNORMALITIES OF PLATELETS AND MEGAKARYOCYTES[a]

Feature	Comments
Hypogranular platelets	Defects in platelet granule formation may be the consequence of a constitutional disorder (e.g., gray platelet syndrome), degranulation of platelets in specimens with processing delays, or, more commonly, primary myeloid neoplasms (e.g., myelodysplasia/AML)[b]
Enlarged platelets	Platelets demonstrating increased mean platelet volume may be the consequence of accelerated release from bone marrow (e.g., ITP) or defective platelet production (e.g., myelodysplastic syndromes in chronic myeloproliferative disorders)
	Platelets that are both enlarged and hypogranular are more often associated with myeloid neoplasms
	Variety of constitutional macrothrombocyte disorders described including May-Hegglin anomaly, Bernard-Soulier syndrome, gray platelet syndrome, and Fechner syndrome
Small platelets	Wiskott-Aldrich syndrome, X-linked thrombocytopenia
Platelet satellitism	Laboratory anomaly that is due to EDTA-induced antiplatelet antibody, resulting in adherence of platelets to neutrophils in specimens collected in EDTA but not other anticoagulants
Circulating megakaryocytes	Fragments of megakaryocyte cytoplasm or intact nuclei may be seen on blood smears, especially in patients with chronic myeloid neoplasms; normal finding in neonates; occasionally seen in normal adult specimens
Micromegakaryocytes/ nonlobulated[c] or hypolobulated megakaryocytes	Increased numbers of small nonlobulated megakaryocytes with condensed chromatin is a bone marrow feature of CML and MDS
	Left-shifted megakaryocyte maturation is common in the bone marrow of patients with platelet survival defects, notably ITP
	Megakaryocyte hypolobulation is noted in specimens from hematologically normal elderly patients
Megakaryocytes with separate nuclei	Seen in myeloid neoplasms such as MDS and AML; rather than multilobulation, nuclei are separate and disconnected; often seen in conjunction with other dysplastic findings
	Transient stage of normal megakaryocyte maturation may show apparent separate nuclei
Pyknotic, "denuded" megakaryocytes	Increased numbers of dark, pyknotic megakaryocytic nuclei with inconspicuous, apparently absent, cytoplasm is a bone marrow morphologic correlate of HIV-1 infection
Megakaryocytic emperipolesis	Prominent neutrophils within megakaryocytic cytoplasm is an accentuation of the physiologic process of neutrophil migration to the systemic circulation that occurs when megakaryocytes are abundant along the bone marrow sinus walls; frequently observed in bone marrow specimens from patients with thrombocytosis, either reactive or neoplastic
Enlarged, hyperlobulated megakaryocytes	Excessive nuclear lobulations in enlarged megakaryocytes is a feature of chronic myeloproliferative disorders and is not typically encountered in any striking degree in non-neoplastic conditions
Clustering of megakaryocytes	Small clusters of megakaryocytes can be seen in early regenerative conditions, especially following myeloablative therapy
	Rarely, striking benign megakaryocytic hyperplasia with atypia is a transient benign feature following induction therapy for AML
	Large clusters and sheets of megakaryocytes are more typically encountered in neoplastic myeloid disorders (MDS, CMPD, AML)
Intrasinusoidal megakaryocytes	The ready identification of megakaryocytes within dilated bone marrow sinuses is a feature of CMPD and not usually noted in non-neoplastic processes
Paratrabecular localization of megakaryocytes	Abnormal localization of megakaryocytes is a feature of myeloid neoplasm; often occurs in conjunction with clustering and abnormal morphologic features

[a]Data from references 21–23, 27–35, 37, and 38.

[b]AML = acute myeloid leukemia; ITP = immune thrombocytopenic purpura; MDS = myelodysplastic syndrome; CML = chronic myelogenous leukemia; HIV = human immunodeficiency virus; CMPD = chronic myeloproliferative disorder; EDTA = ethylenediaminetetraacidic acid.

[c]The designation "nonlobulated" megakaryocyte is used instead of the more common term "mononuclear" megakaryocyte since megakaryocytes at all stages of maturation are mononuclear, i.e., even highly lobulated megakaryocytes still have only one nucleus.

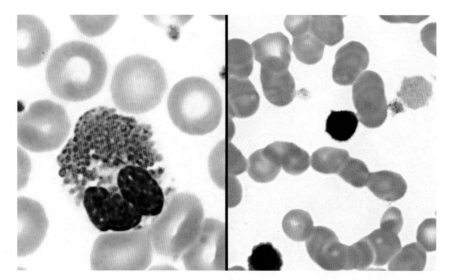

Figure 6-24

NORMAL PLATELETS/LARGE HYPOGRANULAR PLATELETS

Normal platelets (left) are compared to large hypogranular platelets (right) in a patient with an advanced chronic myeloproliferative disorder (Wright stain).

Figure 6-25

GRAY PLATELET SYNDROME

A peripheral blood smear from a patient with gray platelet syndrome illustrates an enlarged, poorly granulated platelet adjacent to a normal lymphocyte (Wright stain). (Courtesy of Dr. C. Sever, Albuquerque, NM.)

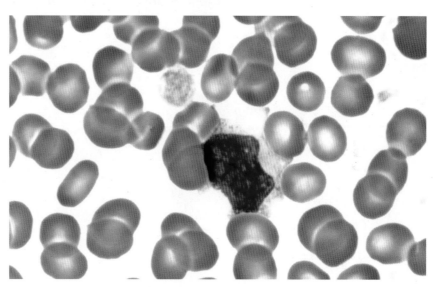

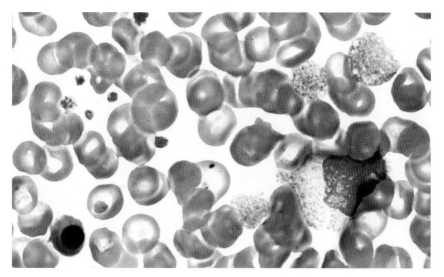

Figure 6-26

MEGAKARYOCYTE FRAGMENTS

Both normal-sized and markedly enlarged platelet/megakaryocyte fragments are evident in this peripheral blood smear from a patient with chronic idiopathic myelofibrosis (Wright stain).

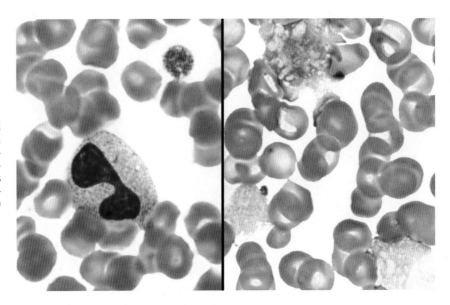

Figure 6-27

PLATELET COMPARISON

Enlarged, well-granulated platelets, which are evident in patients with immune thrombocytopenic purpura (left) are compared to large, atypical platelets that characterize chronic myeloproliferative disorders (right) (Wright stain).

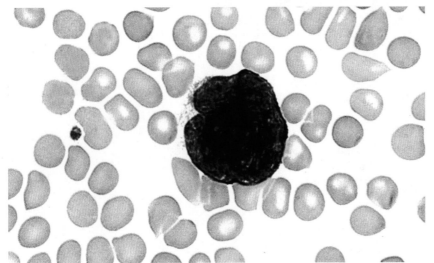

Figure 6-28

CIRCULATING MEGAKARYOCYTE NUCLEUS

A circulating megakaryocyte nucleus is evident in this peripheral blood smear from a normal term newborn (Wright stain).

Figure 6-29

CIRCULATING MEGAKARYOCYTE NUCLEUS

A circulating megakaryocyte nucleus is evident postoperatively in the peripheral blood of an adult male (Wright stain).

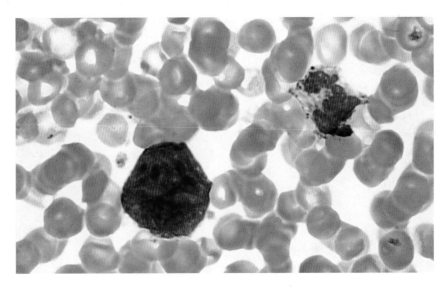

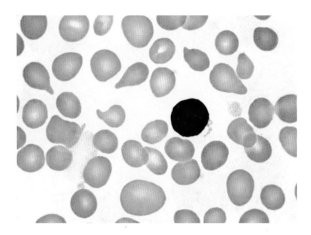

Figure 6-30

CIRCULATING MICROMEGAKARYOCYTE

A circulating micromegakaryocyte nucleus in conjunction with a large hypogranular platelet is evident in this peripheral blood smear from a patient with a chronic myeloproliferative disease (Wright stain).

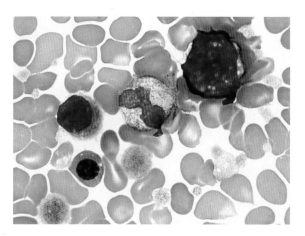

Figure 6-31

CIRCULATING MEGAKARYOCYTES IN TRANSIENT MYELOPROLIFERATIVE DISORDER

Circulating megakaryocytes along with enlarged platelets and nucleated red blood cells are evident in this peripheral blood smear from a Down syndrome newborn with a transient myeloproliferative disorder (Wright stain).

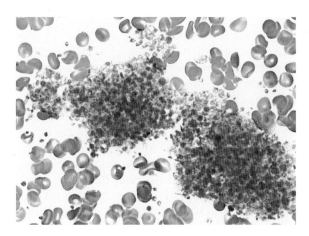

Figure 6-32

PLATELET CLUMPS

Massive clumps of platelets are evident in this peripheral blood smear (Wright stain).

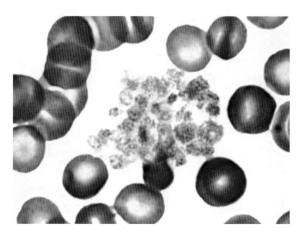

Figure 6-33

PLATELET CLUMP

A small clump of platelets is evident in this peripheral blood smear from a child (Wright stain).

counting techniques, spurious thrombocytopenia can be the consequence of platelet clumping or adherence to neutrophils (satellitism), an immune-mediated laboratory anomaly induced by the ethylenediaminetetraacidic acid (EDTA) anticoagulant (figs. 6-32–6-34) (34,36). In some cases of satellitism, platelet ingestion by neutrophils is evident (figs. 6-35, 6-36).

The disorders associated with numerical, morphologic, and distribution aberrations of

megakaryocytes are delineated on Table 6-2. The most common megakaryocytic abnormalities in the non-neoplastic setting are left-shifted megakaryocytic maturation (mildly increased nonlobulated forms) in platelet survival disorders, pyknotic and denuded megakaryocytes in HIV-1 infection, and mild megakaryocytic clustering during bone marrow regeneration following myelosuppressive/myeloablative therapy or other bone marrow insults (21,27–29,31,38). Recent

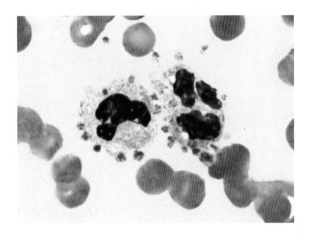

Figure 6-34

PLATELET SATELLITISM

Platelet satellitism, also called platelet leukocyte adherence phenomenon, is evident in this peripheral blood smear (Wright stain).

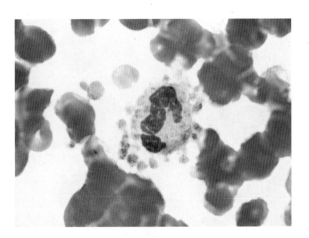

Figure 6-35

PLATELET SATELLITISM WITH INGESTION

Platelet satellitism is evident in this peripheral blood smear. Platelets are ingested by the neutrophil cytoplasm (Wright stain).

studies indicate that bone marrow specimens obtained prior to cardiac surgery from hematologically normal elderly patients (older than 60 years) exhibit mildly atypical features of megakaryocytes (30). These abnormal morphologic features were noted in only a small proportion of megakaryocytes and consisted of small nonlobulated micromegakaryocytes, multinucleated rather than multilobulated megakaryocytes, and enlarged nonlobulated megakaryocytes.

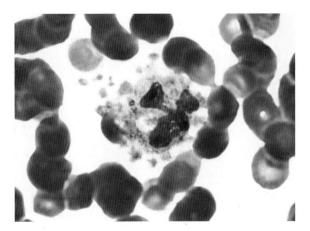

Figure 6-36

PLATELET SATELLITISM WITH INGESTION

Prominent ingestion of platelets in conjunction with platelet satellitism is evident in this neutrophil (Wright stain).

PLATELET/MEGAKARYOCYTIC DISORDERS IN CHILDREN AND ADULTS

The first step in the evaluation of a patient for a possible megakaryocytic disorder includes correlation of the instrument-generated platelet count with the morphologic features of the platelets. Since thrombocytopenia is more common in clinical practice than thrombocytosis, a greater emphasis is placed on the assessment of patients in whom platelet counts are below 150,000/µL (Tables 6-3 and 6-4).

Thrombocytopenia is the consequence of either an acquired or constitutional disorder; spurious thrombocytopenia can result from platelet clumping or platelet satellitism/platelet leukocyte adherence phenomenon (PLAP) (figs. 6-35, 6-36) (40,43). The pathophysiologic mechanisms responsible for bona fide thrombocytopenia include a failure of production (usually due to inadequate numbers of megakaryocytes within the bone marrow) or excessive platelet destruction/consumption disorders (i.e., platelet survival defects), which are associated with abundant bone marrow megakaryocytes (Table 6-3). Although less common, thrombocytopenia may also be the consequence of intramedullary cell death/excessive apoptosis, as seen in megaloblastic anemia and myelodysplastic syndromes (figs. 6-37, 6-38).

Age-related variations in the incidence of specific disorders associated with thrombocytopenia are predictable to some extent, in

Table 6-3

NON-NEOPLASTIC PLATELET/MEGAKARYOCYTIC DISORDERS WITH THROMBOCYTOPENIA

Constitutional Platelet Production Defect Disorders
(see Table 6-6)
Fanconi anemia
Down syndrome-associated clonal transient myelo-proliferative disorder (some cases)
Thrombocytopenia with absent radii
Congenital amegakaryocytic thrombocytopenia
Autosomal dominant thrombocytopenia with incomplete megakaryocyte differentiation
Congenital dysmegakaryocytic thrombocytopenia with 11q23 deletions
X-linked thrombocytopenia with *GATA1* (Xp11) mutations
Familial platelet disorder with predisposition to acute myeloid leukemia (AML)
Wiskott-Aldrich syndrome
Dyskeratosis congenita (some cases)
Shwachman-Diamond syndrome (some cases)
Cyclic amegakaryocytic thrombocytopenia
Bernard-Soulier syndrome
May-Hegglin anomaly
Gray platelet syndrome
Constitutional bone marrow effacement disorders (osteopetrosis, oxalosis, lysosomal storage disease)

Acquired Platelet Production Defect Disorders
Aplastic anemia
Bone marrow effacement[a]/fibrosis
Myeloablative therapy/toxin exposure/radiation
Severe infection with bone marrow suppression
Immunoregulatory defects
Megaloblastic anemia
Paroxysmal nocturnal hemoglobinuria (some cases)
Acquired amegakaryocytic disorders (infections, neoplasms, immune dysfunction, toxin/medication-associated)

Constitutional Platelet Survival Defect Disorders
(see Table 6-6)
Type 2B von Willebrand disease
Congenital thrombocytopenic purpura due to ADAMTS13 deficiency

Acquired Platelet Survival Defect Disorders
Immune-mediated thrombocytopenic purpura (1°, 2°)
Disseminated intravascular coagulation, sepsis
Thrombotic thrombocytopenic purpura
Hemolytic uremic syndrome (HUS)
Pregnancy-associated HUS-like disorders/eclampsia
Neonatal alloimmune thrombocytopenia
Hypersplenism
Post-transfusion purpura
Heparin-induced thrombocytopenia
Turbulent blood flow (hemangiomas, cardiac valve anomalies)

[a]The differential diagnosis includes effacement from primary hematopoietic neoplasms or secondary tumors.

Table 6-4

NON-NEOPLASTIC THROMBOCYTOPENIC DISORDERS BY PATIENT AGE[a]

Infants
Congenital infections/sepsis
Maternal factors (e.g., alloimmunization)
Down syndrome-associated transient myeloproliferative disorder (some cases manifest with thrombocytopenia)
Impaired megakaryocytopoiesis in preterm infants with placental insufficiency or chronic hypoxia
Kasabach-Merritt syndrome (turbulent blood flow)
Other constitutional disorders (e.g., thrombocytopenia with absent radii)

Children
Immune thrombocytopenic purpura (often 1°)
Systemic infections
Bone marrow effacement/fibrosis[b]
Immunoregulatory defects
Megaloblastic anemia
Hemolytic uremic syndrome
Constitutional disorders
Aplastic anemia

Adults
Immune thrombocytopenic purpura (1°, 2°)
Disseminated intravascular coagulation
Thrombotic thrombocytopenic purpura
Systemic infections
Bone marrow suppressive therapy/radiation/toxic exposure
Bone marrow effacement/fibrosis[b]
Immunoregulatory defects
Post-transfusion purpura
Heparin-induced thrombocytopenia
Aplastic anemia
Pregnancy-associated platelet disorders
Hypersplenism
Paroxysmal nocturnal hemoglobinuria
Gray platelet syndrome

[a]Listed in order of estimated frequency
[b]The differential diagnosis includes primary and secondary neoplasms.

that constitutional disorders are more likely to manifest in early childhood, while both acquired platelet production and survival defect disorders are relatively more common in older children and older adults (Table 6-4).

Thrombocytosis (more than 400,000/μL) may also be the consequence of either a constitutional or an acquired disorder, although constitutional thrombocytotic disorders are exceedingly rare and are typically described in family kindreds (Table 6-5) (41). Heritable mutations in either the thrombopoietin (*TPO*) or *MPL* genes are postulated in some of these kindreds (41,42,45).

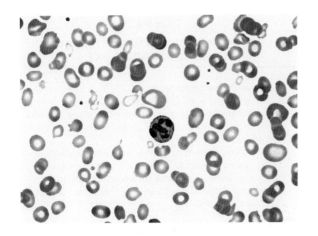

Figure 6-37

MEGALOBLASTIC ANEMIA

Pancytopenia with hypersegmented neutrophils and oval macrocytes is evident in this peripheral blood smear from a patient with florid megaloblastic anemia (Wright stain).

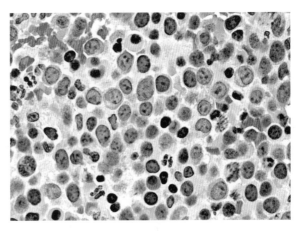

Figure 6-38

MEGALOBLASTIC ANEMIA

Despite the pancytopenia, the bone marrow is 100 percent cellular in this patient with advanced megaloblastic anemia (H&E stain).

Table 6-5
NON-NEOPLASTIC PLATELET/MEGAKARYOCYTIC DISORDERS WITH THROMBOCYTOSIS (THROMBOCYTHEMIA)[a,b]
Constitutional Thrombocytotic Disorders Down syndrome-associated clonal transient myelo-proliferative disorder (some cases manifest with thrombocytosis) Familial essential thrombocythemia-like disorders
Acquired Thrombocytotic Disorders Reactive thrombocytosis secondary to stress, trauma, myocardial infarction, surgery, thermal injury, blood loss, infection, inflammation, immune disorders, malignancy, exercise, drug-induced, other conditions Postsplenectomy (functional asplenia) Iron deficiency anemia (modest thrombocytosis) Chronic hemolytic anemias, hemoglobinopathies (occasional cases) Rebound following bone marrow suppression, blood loss, or therapy for nutritional deficiency
[a]Data from references 39 and 45–50. [b]The differential diagnosis includes primary clonal myeloid neoplasms especially chronic myeloproliferative disorders.

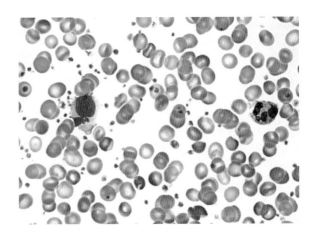

Figure 6-39

MARKED THROMBOCYTOSIS

Marked thrombocytosis is evident in this peripheral blood smear from a postoperative patient (Wright stain).

Acquired thrombocytosis is much more frequently encountered in clinical practice; in one large study, approximately 88 percent of cases of acquired thrombocytosis in adults were secondary, while about 12 percent were linked to clonal hematopoietic neoplasms such as essential thrombocythemia and chronic myelogenous leukemia (figs. 6-39–6-41) (44). In children, acquired thrombocytosis is much more likely to be secondary, with an incidence of over 600/million children compared to 1/million children with primary thrombocytosis (41).

Most patients with secondary (reactive) thrombocytosis do not require bone marrow examination. In these patients, the elevated platelet count may be an isolated hemogram abnormality, or another hematologic aberration such as neutrophilia or anemia may be present. Clinical correlation is generally all that is

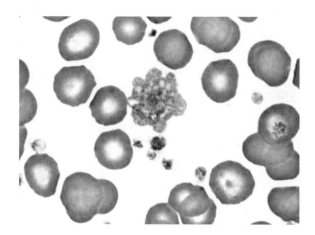

Figure 6-40

**MEGAKARYOCYTE FRAGMENT
AND MARKED THROMBOCYTOSIS**

Marked thrombocytosis in conjunction with circulating megakaryocyte fragments is evident in this peripheral blood smear in a patient with reactive thrombocytosis (Wright stain).

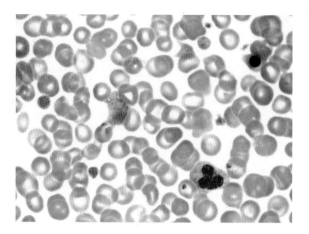

Figure 6-41

**PLATELET AND MEGAKARYOCYTE ABNORMALITIES
IN CHRONIC MYELOPROLIFERATIVE DISORDER**

Thrombocytosis in conjunction with markedly enlarged and hypogranular platelets is evident in this peripheral blood smear from a patient with chronic myeloproliferative disease (Wright stain).

needed if all hematologic abnormalities can be attributed to specific clinical findings in patients with secondary thrombocytosis. In contrast, bone marrow examination is a standard component in the diagnostic workup of patients with suspected clonal hematopoietic neoplasms.

Constitutional Megakaryocytic Disorders with Thrombocytopenia

A variety of types of constitutional (familial) thrombocytopenia have been described (Tables 6-3, 6-6). As with other constitutional disorders, *hereditary thrombocytopenia* is only rarely encountered in clinical practice. Indeed, most cases of neonatal thrombocytopenia are attributed to various acquired fetal or maternal disorders such as infection, disseminated intravascular coagulation, or immune disorders.

The prototypic constitutional disorder linked to isolated thrombocytopenia is *thrombocytopenia with absent radii* (TAR) (Table 6-6; fig. 6-42). This autosomal recessive disorder is characterized by defective megakaryopoiesis at an early stage of maturation, and bone marrow megakaryocytes are typically, although not invariably, absent (52,58,76). Spontaneous recovery is common with normalization of the platelet count and the appearance of more normal numbers of bone marrow megakaryocytes. Rare cases of subsequent myeloid neoplasms, notably

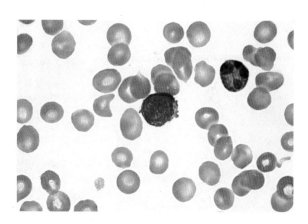

Figure 6-42

THROMBOCYTOPENIA WITH ABSENT RADII

A peripheral blood smear from a child with thrombocytopenia with absent radii (TAR) shows profound thrombocytopenia with enlarged platelets (Wright stain). (Courtesy of P. Izadi, Los Angeles, CA.)

acute myeloid leukemia, have been described in TAR patients (61).

Another constitutional thrombocytopenic disorder, *congenital amegakaryocytic thrombocytopenia*, is also associated with absent or markedly reduced bone marrow megakaryocytes (fig. 6-43). This autosomal recessive disorder is caused by mutations in the thrombopoietin receptor, c-Mpl (53,72).

Table 6-6

CONSTITUTIONAL MEGAKARYOCYTIC DISORDERS WITH THROMBOCYTOPENIA[a]

Disorders	Key Features	Morphologic Findings/Other Features
Thrombocytopenia with absent radii (see chapter 7)	Autosomal recessive; absent radii, usually bilateral Block in megakaryopoiesis at early stage of differentiation Severe thrombocytopenia at birth with gradual improvement Favorable long-term prognosis	Absent bone marrow megakaryocytes at birth; may see gradual recovery of megakaryopoiesis Small micromegakaryocytes described in one case Increased incidence of bone marrow neoplasms (AML)[b] Associated with shortened/absent radii bilaterally
Congenital amega-karyocytic throm-bocytopenia (see chapter 7)	Autosomal recessive, rarely X-linked types; mutations in thrombopoietin receptor (*c-MPL*) gene Isolated thrombocytopenia in infancy with later development of pancytopenia	Absent or markedly reduced bone marrow megakaryocytes Subsequent multilineage bone marrow failure usually by second decade
Fanconi anemia[c]	Autosomal recessive, diagnosed by excessive exposure to diepoxybutane in cell culture Multiple genetic subtypes; multiple DNA repair defects Other congenital anomalies in 75%, short stature in 60%	Progressive bone marrow failure; may have lineage aplasia initially, but subsequent development of multilineage loss (i.e., aplasia) Increased incidence of bone marrow neoplasms (AML/MDS)
Wiskott-Aldrich syndrome	X-linked recessive, mutations in *WAS* gene Thrombocytopenia due to increased platelet turnover	Normal numbers of bone marrow megakaryocytes Microthrombocytopenia Underlying immunodeficiency dominates clinical picture Associated with eczema and subsequent lymphoma
Cyclic thrombocy-topenia[d]	Usually occurs in adults; female predom-inance Intermittent thrombocytopenia with rebound thrombocytosis Cytokine variation linked to platelet levels; clonal T-cell postulated in some cases	Cyclical decrease in megakaryocytes in some cases; other cases more ITP-like with abun-dant bone marrow megakaryocytes Small megakaryocytes (varied from normal to to reduced numbers) noted in single infant with cyclic thrombocytopenia since birth
Additional autosomal dominant disorders	May-Hegglin anomaly, gray platelet syndrome, Sebastian syndrome, Velocardiofacial/DiGeorge syndrome, Epstein syndrome, Mediterranean thrombocytopenia	Macrothrombocytopenia is characteristic finding in disorders linked to *MYH9* mutations includ-ing May-Hegglin anomaly, Fechner syndrome, Epstein syndrome, and Sebastian syndrome. In gray platelet syndrome, the enlarged platelets are hypogranular due to α-granule deficiency; myelofibrosis and splenomegaly noted in some cases Thrombocytopenia and bleeding manifestations are generally mild
Bernard-Soulier syndrome	Autosomal recessive	Macrothrombocytopenia; no other associated abnormalities
X-linked thrombo-cytopenia	X-linked, mutations in *WAS* gene	Milder form of Wiskott-Aldrich syndrome Microthrombocytes Stable thrombocytopenia
Congenital thrombotic thrombocytopenic purpura (TTP)	Autosomal recessive Two pathologic mechanisms: homozygous or compound heterozygous mutations of *ADAMTS13* or inhibition of ADAMTS13 by autoantibodies (more typical of acquired TTP)	Microangiopathic hemolytic anemia with thrombocytopenia

[a]Data from references 52,53, 55, 57–59, 61, 62, 64, 68, 70–74, 76, 78, 83, 84, 86, 87, and 92.

[b]AML = acute myeloid leukemia; MDS = myelodysplastic syndrome; ITP = immune-mediated thrombocytopenic purpura.

[c]Other bone marrow failure disorders include Shwachman-Diamond syndrome and dyskeratosis congenita.

[d]Unclear if cyclic thrombocytopenia is truly a constitutional disorder; many, if not all, cases may be acquired; may be a variant of acquired amegakaryocytic thrombocytopenia.

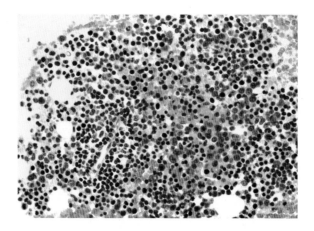

Figure 6-43

AMEGAKARYOCYTIC THROMBOCYTOPENIA

A bone marrow clot section shows absence of megakaryocytes in this child with amegakaryocytic thrombocytopenia (H&E stain).

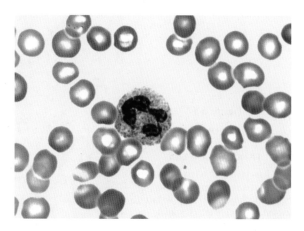

Figure 6-44

SMALL PLATELET IN WISKOTT-ALDRICH SYNDROME

Peripheral blood smear shows a minute platelet in a patient with Wiskott-Aldrich syndrome (Wright stain).

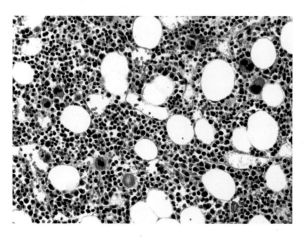

Figure 6-45

POORLY LOBULATED MEGAKARYOCYTES IN WISKOTT-ALDRICH SYNDROME

Bone marrow core biopsy shows increased megakaryocytes, which are small and show reduced nuclear lobulation (H&E stain).

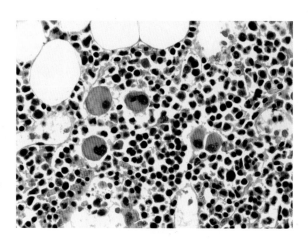

Figure 6-46

POORLY LOBULATED MEGAKARYOCYTES IN WISKOTT-ALDRICH SYNDROME

Increased, small, poorly lobulated megakaryocytes are evident on high-power magnification of a bone marrow core biopsy from a patient with Wiskott-Aldrich syndrome (H&E stain).

Many other types of constitutional isolated thrombocytopenia have been described (59). The features of the platelets and megakaryocytes are distinctive in many of these disorders. *Wiskott-Aldrich syndrome* is characterized by both microthrombocytes in blood and small, poorly lobulated megakaryocytes in bone marrow (figs. 6-44–6-46) (64). The various constitutional multilineage bone marrow failure disorders, including

Fanconi anemia, Shwachman-Diamond syndrome, and *dyskeratosis congenita,* are characterized by single/multilineage cytopenias in conjunction with the gradual development of multilineage hypoplasia (fig. 6-47) (see chapter 7) (52). There is a strong association between these multilineage bone marrow failure disorders and subsequent bone marrow malignancies, such as acute myeloid leukemia and myelodysplasia.

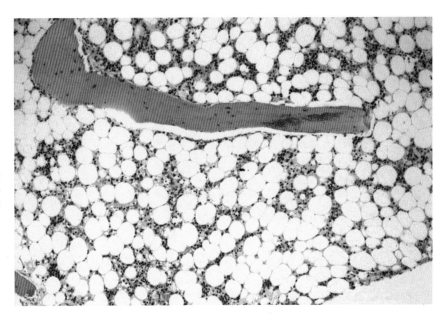

Figure 6-47

HYPOCELLULAR BONE MARROW IN FANCONI ANEMIA

This patient with Fanconi anemia has progressive hypocellularity and markedly reduced megakaryocytes (H&E stain).

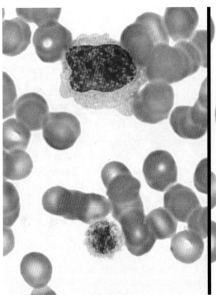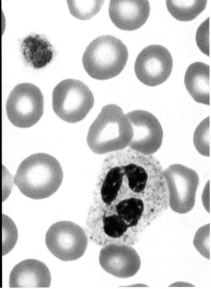

Figure 6-48

ENLARGED PLATELETS IN FAMILIAL AUTOSOMAL DOMINANT THROMBOCYTOPENIA AND MAY-HEGGLIN ANOMALY

Two peripheral blood smears show a macrothrombocyte in a patient with familial autosomal dominant thrombocytopenia (left) and an enlarged platelet as well as a neutrophil with a pseudo-Döhle body in a patient with May-Hegglin anomaly (right) (Wright stain).

A variety of hereditary giant platelet (macrothrombocyte) thrombocytopenic disorders have been described, including *Bernard-Soulier syndrome, gray platelet syndrome, May-Hegglin anomaly, Fechner syndrome,* and other less characterized disorders (Table 6-6; fig. 6-48) (54,63, 67,69,74,75,77,81,88,90). Various defects in platelet function, including adhesion and granule secretion defects, have been linked to these morphologically abnormal platelets. Bone marrow examination generally reveals normal to increased numbers of megakaryocytes. Abnormal forms may be striking, exhibiting nuclear hypolobulation (59,88). Defects in platelet shedding may contribute to the enlarged platelet size. The distinctive features of gray platelet syndrome include enlarged, hypogranular platelets due to alpha-granule deficiency; both myelofibrosis and abnormal megakaryocytes may be evident on bone marrow core biopsy sections (figs. 6-49–6-52) (55,69).

The newly described constitutional megakaryocytic disorders are even more uncommon. These include congenital dysmegakaryocytic

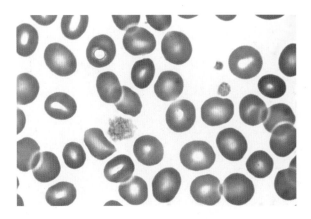

Figure 6-49

GRAY PLATELET SYNDROME

A peripheral blood smear shows representative platelets from a patient with gray platelet syndrome. There is a tendency for large overall size in conjunction with reduced cytoplasmic granularity of the platelets (Wright stain). (Courtesy of Dr. C. Sever, Albuquerque, NM.)

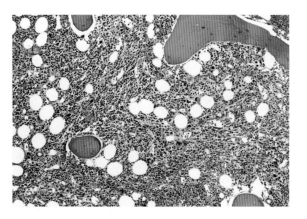

Figure 6-50

GRAY PLATELET SYNDROME

A bone marrow core biopsy from 47-year-old woman with gray platelet syndrome. The overall cellularity is mildly increased (H&E stain). (Courtesy of Dr. C. Sever, Albuquerque, NM.)

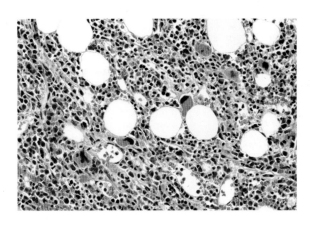

Figure 6-51

GRAY PLATELET SYNDROME

Intermediate magnification of a bone marrow core biopsy from a 47-year-old woman with gray platelet syndrome shows increased megakaryocytes that are relatively large and poorly lobulated (H&E stain). (Courtesy of Dr. C. Sever, Albuquerque, NM.)

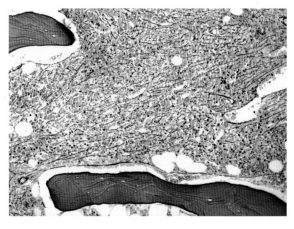

Figure 6-52

RETICULIN FIBROSIS IN GRAY PLATELET SYNDROME

Diffuse moderate reticulin fibrosis is evident in the bone marrow core biopsy from a 47-year-old woman with gray platelet syndrome and associated splenomegaly (reticulin stain). (Courtesy of Dr. C. Sever, Albuquerque, NM.)

thrombocytopenia with 11q23 deletions, X-linked thrombocytopenia with *GATA1* (Xp11) mutations, autosomal dominant thrombocytopenia with incomplete megakaryocyte differentiation, and the so-called familial platelet disorder with predisposition to acute myeloid leukemia with *AML1* (*RUNX1*) mutations (figs. 6-53–6-55) (56,60,66,78,79). Although descriptions of bone marrow morphology are limited, morphologi-

cally abnormal megakaryocytes have been linked to most of these rare disorders. Defects in megakaryocyte lobulation with nonlobulated/hypolobulated forms or micromegakaryocytes have been described in congenital dysmegakaryocytic thrombocytopenia, X-linked thrombocytopenia, and autosomal dominant thrombocytopenia (figs. 6-56–6-58).

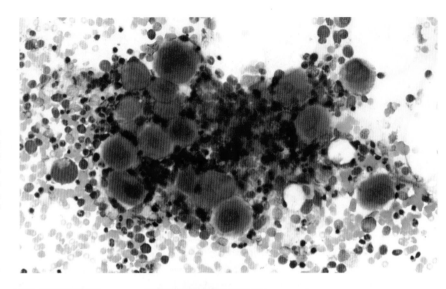

Figure 6-53

FAMILIAL AUTOSOMAL DOMINANT THROMBOCYTOPENIA

Markedly increased megakaryocytes are evident in this bone marrow aspirate smear from a young adult with familial autosomal dominant thrombocytopenia. The megakaryocytes have decreased nuclear lobulations (Wright stain).

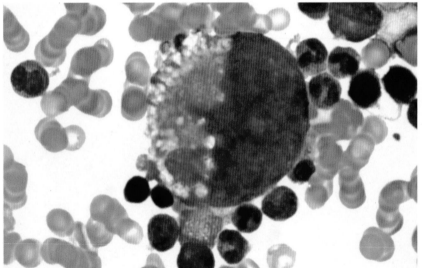

Figure 6-54

FAMILIAL AUTOSOMAL DOMINANT THROMBOCYTOPENIA

Defective nuclear lobulation is evident in this mature-appearing megakaryocyte in a bone marrow aspirate smear from a young adult female with familial autosomal dominant thrombocytopenia (Wright stain).

Figure 6-55

FAMILIAL AUTOSOMAL DOMINANT THROMBOCYTOPENIA

This bone marrow biopsy section shows increased megakaryocytes with a tendency toward hypolobulation (H&E stain).

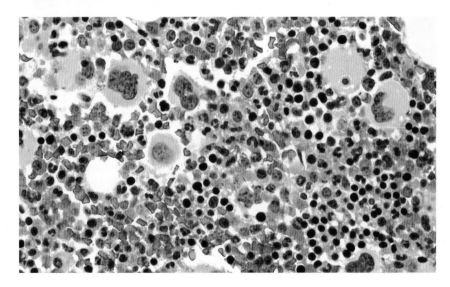

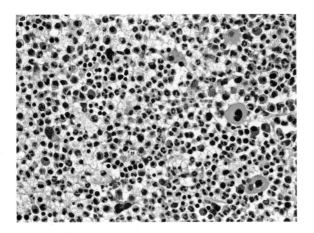

Figure 6-56

**POORLY DELINEATED FAMILIAL
MEGAKARYOCYTIC DISORDER**

The bone marrow biopsy section shows increased and
hypolobulated megakaryocytes (H&E stain).

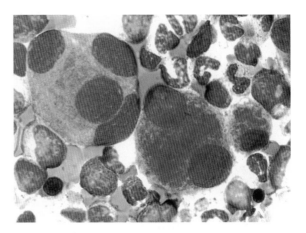

Figure 6-57

**POORLY DELINEATED FAMILIAL
MEGAKARYOCYTIC DISORDER**

Defective megakaryocyte lobulation is evident on this bone
marrow aspirate smear from a child with a poorly delineated
familial megakaryocyte disorder (Wright stain).

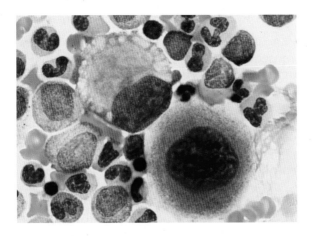

Figure 6-58

**POORLY DELINEATED FAMILIAL
MEGAKARYOCYTIC DISORDER**

Both immature and mature megakaryocytes are
nonlobulated in this bone marrow aspirate smear from
a pediatric patient with a poorly delineated familial
megakaryocyte disorder (Wright stain).

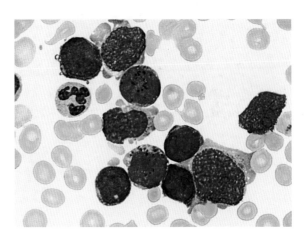

Figure 6-59

**CIRCULATING MEGAKARYOBLASTS IN
TRANSIENT MYELOPROLIFERATIVE DISORDER**

The peripheral blood smear shows profound leukocytosis
with numerous circulating blasts with megakaryoblast morphologic features in a Down syndrome neonate with a transient
myeloproliferative disorder (Wright stain). (Courtesy of Dr.
R. McKenna, Minneapolis, MN.)

Although not considered as a typical constitutional megakaryocyte disorder, both platelet
and megakaryocyte abnormalities are prominent
features in the neonatal transient myeloproliferative disorders that occur in patients with Down
syndrome (figs. 6-59–6-61). Mutations in *GATA1*
genes have been described recently in patients
with Down syndrome who have transient myeloproliferative disorders or overt acute megakaryoblastic leukemia (51,65,80,89,93).

Failure of adequate platelet production is
the most common pathogenic mechanism in
constitutional disorders with isolated thrombocytopenia. However, constitutional thrombocytopenic disorders due to increased platelet destruction have been recently described (82,85). These

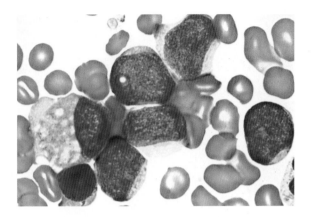

Figure 6-60

**CIRCULATING MEGAKARYOBLASTS IN
TRANSIENT MYELOPROLIFERATIVE DISORDER**

This peripheral blood smear from a 4-week-old infant with Down syndrome shows a predominance of blasts. At least one blast (left) shows megakaryocytic differentiation (Wright stain).

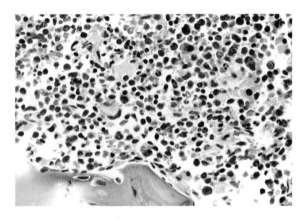

Figure 6-61

**BONE MARROW CORE BIOPSY IN
TRANSIENT MYELOPROLIFERATIVE DISORDER**

A bone marrow core biopsy from a 4-week-old infant with Down syndrome–associated transient myeloproliferative disorder shows a prominent megakaryocytic component as evidenced by the large cells with abundant eosinophilic cytoplasm diffusely distributed throughout the core biopsy (H&E stain).

thrombotic thrombocytopenic purpura (TTP)-like disorders have been described primarily in the neonatal period, but also in adulthood (86). The proposed mechanism for the platelet destruction is functional ADAMTS13 deficiency (82–86). Inhibitory antibodies have been described in some cases, while mutations in the *ADAMTS13* gene have been noted in other cases (83,84,86).

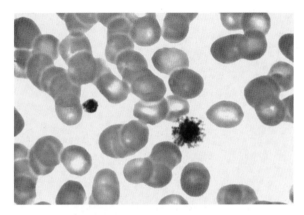

Figure 6-62

**MACROTHROMBOCYTE IN IMMUNE
THROMBOCYTOPENIA PURPURA**

Macrothrombocyte from the peripheral blood of a 15-year-old female with immune thrombocytopenic purpura (Wright stain).

Acquired Megakaryocytic Disorders with Thrombocytopenia

Acquired thrombocytopenias are typically the consequence of either a platelet survival defect or reduced platelet production within the bone marrow (see Table 6-3). Platelet survival defects are substantially more common in clinical practice and consist of immune-mediated platelet destruction disorders, nonimmune-mediated platelet destruction, and platelet sequestration within the spleen.

Immune-mediated thrombocytopenic purpura (ITP) is the prototypic platelet survival defect disorder and affects patients of all ages, even neonates. The salient epidemiologic, clinical, and morphologic features of ITP are delineated in Table 6-7 (95,96,99,102,103,107,109,122, 126,129,130,134–136,138,142,145). Morphologic features include isolated thrombocytopenia, typically with enlarged platelets on the blood smear, while both megakaryocytic hyperplasia and left-shifted megakaryocytes are evident in the bone marrow (figs. 6-62–6-66). A bone marrow examination is not generally required in patients with straightforward clinical and laboratory features. Although still somewhat controversial, consensus guidelines suggest that bone marrow examination is recommended in patients with atypical features, patients over 60 years of age, patients who fail frontline therapy, and those with prior splenectomy (102).

Table 6-7

IMMUNE-MEDIATED THROMBOCYTOPENIC PURPURA[a]

General features	Occurs in all ages, more common in patients >60 yrs Incidence of 4.0–5.3/100,000 per year in children Incidence of 5.8–6.6/100,000 per year in adults Female predominance in young adult patients Association with viral infection and immunizations in children Controversial association with *Helicobacter* infection in adults
Definition	Thrombocytopenia due to autoantibody binding to platelets with subsequent premature destruction by macrophage/histiocytic cells; likely due to T-cell regulatory defect with associated cytokine aberrations; other defects proposed and exact mechanisms unknown
Primary and secondary types	Primary ITP[b] is diagnosis of exclusion Secondary ITP is the result of autoantibody production that is linked to underlying disorders such as collagen vascular diseases, lymphoid neoplasms, medications, post-transfusion, infections including HIV-1
Morphology	Isolated thrombocytopenia with enlarged platelets (other CBC abnormalities may be present in patients with secondary ITP; anemia secondary to blood loss may be present) Increased megakaryocytes in bone marrow with left shift in megakaryocyte maturation resulting in proportionally increased numbers of smaller megakaryocytes that are mononuclear or have only a few nuclear lobulations[c]
Clinical course	Spontaneous resolution very common in pediatric patients, especially those with platelet counts exceeding 30,000/µL Bleeding manifestations generally mild and consist primarily of oral and gastrointestinal bleeding, easy bruisability, and lower extremity petechiae Childhood ITP often follows viral infection or immunization Many treatment options available for those patients who require therapy: gamma globulin, corticosteroids, anti-D immunoglobulin (WinRho), anti-CD20 antibody (rituximab), immunosuppressive agents, splenectomy

[a]Data from references 95, 96, 99, 102, 103, 107, 109, 122, 123, 126, 129, 130, 134–136, 138, 142, and 145.
[b]ITP = immune-mediated thrombocytopenic purpura; HIV = human immunodeficiency virus; CBC = complete blood count.
[c]Bone marrow examination is not generally required at diagnosis in children and young adults with straightforward clinical and laboratory features. Bone marrow examination is indicated for older patients (>60 years), those with atypical features, prior to splenectomy, and those who fail frontline therapy.

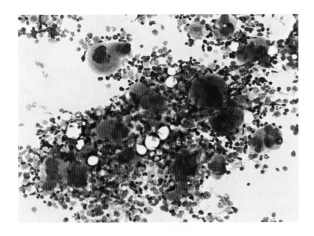

Figure 6-63

INCREASED MEGAKARYOCYTES IN IMMUNE THROMBOCYTOPENIA PURPURA

Bone marrow aspirate smear shows markedly increased megakaryocytes in 15-year-old female with immune thrombocytopenic purpura (Wright stain).

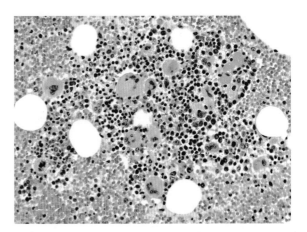

Figure 6-64

INCREASED MEGAKARYOCYTES IN IMMUNE THROMBOCYTOPENIA PURPURA

Bone marrow clot section shows particles with increased megakaryocytes (H&E stain).

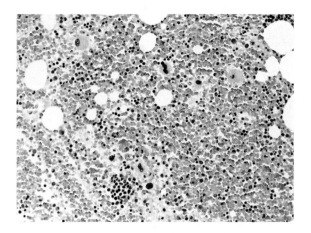

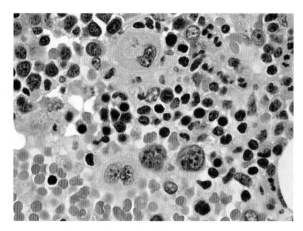

Figure 6-65

INCREASED MEGAKARYOCYTES WITH IMMATURE FORMS IN IMMUNE THROMBOCYTOPENIA PURPURA

Increased megakaryocytes with a left shift toward hypolobulated forms on clot section (H&E stain).

Figure 6-66

INCREASED MEGAKARYOCYTES WITH IMMATURE FORMS IN IMMUNE THROMBOCYTOPENIA PURPURA

Spectrum of megakaryocyte maturity is evident on this clot section from a 15-year-old female (H&E stain).

Figure 6-67

MICROANGIOPATHIC HEMOLYTIC ANEMIA AND THROMBOSED VESSEL IN THROMBOTIC THROMBOCYTOPENIC PURPURA

A microangiopathic hemolytic anemia picture with thrombocytopenia is evident in this peripheral blood smear from a patient with thrombotic thrombocytopenic purpura. An organizing thrombus is seen on bone marrow core biopsy (Wright, H&E stains).

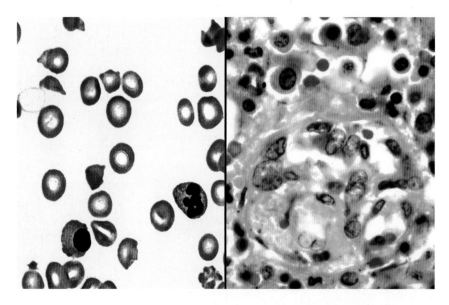

Other causes of acquired thrombocytopenia secondary to platelet survival defects include heparin- and drug-induced thrombocytopenias, other types of secondary ITP (associated with collagen vascular disease, lymphoid neoplasms, and chronic infections), disseminated intravascular coagulation, TTP, hemolytic uremic syndrome, thermal injury, and turbulent blood flow conditions (97,98,104,108,110,112,120,123,127,131, 133,137,144). The erythrocyte fragmentation that accompanies the thrombocytopenia in these disorders is linked to endothelial cell activation, small vessel damage/thrombi, or large vessel/heart valve anomalies (fig. 6-67) (104,116). Recent studies indicate that antibodies directed against ADAMTS13 are linked to the development of von Willebrand factor–rich platelet thrombi in capillaries and arterioles (110,133). The successful diagnosis of patients with these acquired thrombocytopenias is generally based on clinical and laboratory findings and blood smear review; bone marrow examination is not generally necessary.

Table 6-8

SPECIAL CONSIDERATIONS: NEONATAL AND PREGNANCY-ASSOCIATED THROMBOCYTOPENIA[a]

Neonatal Thrombocytopenia

Review blood smear for other abnormalities

Consider constitutional thrombocytopenic disorders and assess for associated anomalies and family history (see Table 6-6)

Check mother for evidence of thrombocytopenia as well as underlying conditions/medications; assess for history of maternal/infant thrombocytopenia in previous pregnancies

Consider fetal/neonatal alloimmune thrombocytopenia due to maternal alloimmunization against fetal platelet antigens

Clinical/laboratory examination for evidence of hemorrhage, infection, and vascular anomalies (e.g., Kasabach-Merritt syndrome), splenomegaly, other abnormalities

In setting of TTP[b]-like disorder with hyperbilirubinemia, consider ADAMTS13 deficiency

Pregnancy-Associated Thrombocytopenia (10% of pregnancies)

Many causes of thrombocytopenia in pregnancy: benign gestational thrombocytopenia, preeclampsia/HELLP syndrome, autoimmune such as primary or secondary ITP, DIC, HUS/TTP disorders of pregnancy, acute fatty liver of pregnancy, folate deficiency, and coincidental bone marrow disorders

The clearcut majority of cases of thrombocytopenia in healthy gravid women at term are due to benign gestational thrombocytopenia; there is no effect on the fetus and no increased risk of perinatal hemorrhage.

ITP can be primary or secondary and can occur throughout the pregnancy; ITP is the most common cause of first trimester thrombocytopenia (autoantibodies may cross placenta)

Pregnancy-associated HUS/TTP occurs in perinatal/postpartum period and may be catastrophic; RBC fragmentation common

RBC fragmentation is typical in HUS/TTP, DIC, and HELLP syndrome

[a]Data from references 101, 102, 105, 113, 115, 117, 128, 132, 138–140, and 143.

[b]TTP = thrombotic thrombocytopenic purpura; HELLP = hemolysis, elevated liver function tests, low platelet syndrome; ITP = immune-mediated thrombocytopenic purpura; DIC = disseminated intravascular coagulation; HUS/TTP = hemolytic uremic syndrome/thrombotic thrombocytopenic purpura; RBC = red blood cell.

The documentation of thrombocytopenia in either neonates or gravid females is linked to fairly unique clinical and pathologic considerations (Table 6-8). In cases of fetal/neonatal thrombocytopenia, both maternal and fetal conditions must be considered since many cases of fetal/neonatal thrombocytopenia are linked to maternal infections, hypertension, collagen vascular disease, or medications. In addition, maternal sensitization to fetal platelet antigens can result in fetal/neonatal alloimmune thrombocytopenia (101,117). Other distinctive causes of thrombocytopenia in neonates include constitutional disorders, fetal infections, vascular anomalies resulting in turbulent blood flow, and splenomegaly (105,113,132,139,143). Although rare, the constitutional thrombocytopenias described earlier in this chapter are also diagnostic considerations, including the newly recognized constitutional TTP-like disorders associated with prominent RBC fragmentation, thrombocytopenia, and hyperbilirubinemia (140,141).

The majority of cases of thrombocytopenia in healthy gravid females near term are determined to be of no consequence to either mother or fetus and are designated as *benign gestational thrombocytopenia* (128). There are, however, a variety of pregnancy-associated thrombocytopenias (Table 6-8; fig. 6-68). While many of these disorders manifest in late pregnancy, others, such as primary or secondary ITP, occur at any time during the pregnancy (102,128). A special consideration is the risk of hemorrhagic complications during labor and delivery in addition to the fetal/neonatal thrombocytopenia. Transplacental passage of maternal antiplatelet immunoglobulin (Ig)G in women with primary or secondary ITP is a significant issue. In addition, the risk to the fetus from maternal therapy for the diverse causes of maternal thrombocytopenia is a major clinical concern confounding treatment decision making.

Although much less common, some cases of acquired thrombocytopenia are the consequence of defective bone marrow production of platelets (see Table 6-3). In general, the reduced platelet production occurs in conjunction with multilineage bone marrow failure. Causes include aplastic anemia, bone marrow suppression from drugs/toxins/radiation/infection, paroxysmal nocturnal hemoglobinuria, and various bone marrow effacement/fibrotic disorders, including both primary and secondary neoplasms. In these diverse disorders, reduced bone marrow megakaryocytes

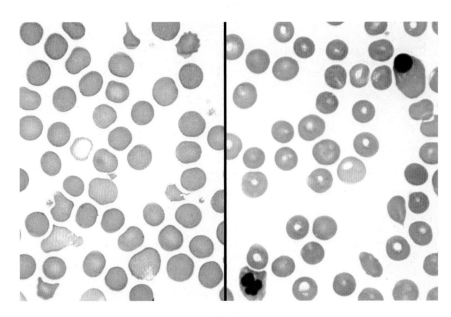

Figure 6-68

POSTPARTUM THROMBOTIC THROMBOCYTOPENIC PURPURA

A peripheral blood smear from a patient who developed severe thrombotic thrombocytopenic purpura-like features in the immediate postpartum period. Red blood cell fragmentation, polychromasia, microspherocytes, and nucleated red blood cells are seen (Wright stain).

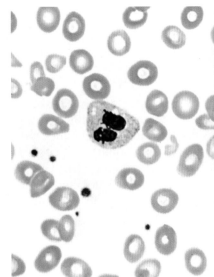
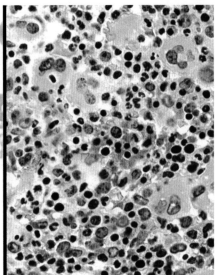

Figure 6-69

BLOOD CYTOPENIAS AND BONE MARROW HYPERCELLULARITY IN MYELODYSPLASIA

Pancytopenia in the peripheral blood (left) is compared to a markedly hypercellular bone marrow core biopsy with increased megakaryocytes (right) in a patient with myelodysplastic syndrome (Wright stain of blood, H&E stain of bone marrow biopsy).

are typically evident in conjunction with other hematopoietic lineage hypoplasias or aplasias.

Acquired isolated amegakaryocytosis is rare; some cases are secondary to infection, most notably viral infections such as parvovirus, Epstein-Barr virus (EBV), cytomegalovirus (CMV), and HIV-1 infections (94,100,111). The distinctive bone marrow abnormality in these cases is the virtual complete absence of megakaryocytes; other lineage abnormalities are variable. Other causes of acquired amegakaryocytosis are linked to idiosyncratic drug reactions, toxins, alcohol consumption, immune aberrations, and underlying neoplasms such as T-cell large

granular lymphocytic leukemia (94,111). Autoantibody-induced (anti-c-Mpl autoantibody) amegakaryocytosis occurs in rare patients with systemic sclerosis (114,118,119,125). In some patients, the initial isolated amegakaryocytosis is either cyclical or progresses to aplastic anemia (106,118,121).

Both megaloblastic anemias and primary hematologic neoplasms, especially myelodysplastic syndromes, may exhibit a paradoxical picture of thrombocytopenia despite increased bone marrow megakaryocytes (figs. 6-69, 6-70). Intramedullary apoptosis is the presumed explanation for this blood/bone marrow disparity.

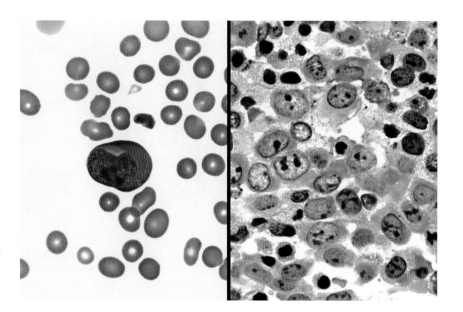

Figure 6-70

PROFOUND PANCYTOPENIA AND HYPERCELLULAR BONE MARROW IN MEGALOBLASTIC ANEMIA

Left: Profound pancytopenia with circulating nucleated red blood cell is evident in this peripheral blood smear from a patient with advanced megaloblastic anemia.

Right: A markedly hypercellular bone marrow core biopsy specimen from the same patient (Wright stain of blood, H&E stain of bone marrow biopsy).

Constitutional and Acquired Megakaryocytic Disorders with Thrombocytosis

Constitutional thrombocytotic disorders are only rarely encountered in clinical practice, and most descriptions of familial essential thrombocytosis-like disorders are individual case reports or kindred studies. Point mutations in the *TPO* gene have been described in some patients, while a point mutation in the *c-MPL* gene has been described recently in a single family kindred (148,149,153,156,158,159). Increased megakaryocytes with generally intact maturation have been noted in some cases.

Acquired thrombocytosis is much more common than its constitutional counterpart. In general, the cause of secondary/reactive thrombocytosis is readily apparent clinically (see Table 6-5) (148). The platelets are morphologically unremarkable, and bone marrow examination is not generally necessary (fig. 6-71). The cause of the secondary thrombocytosis in patients with underlying etiologic conditions ranging from infections to neoplasms has been linked to increased thrombopoietin production, excess IL-6, or increased production of other stimulatory cytokines (148,150–152,154,155).

Occasional patients with secondary thrombocytosis undergo bone marrow examination for other reasons, such as tumor staging. In these cases, bone marrow megakaryocytes are typically normal in number or mildly increased,

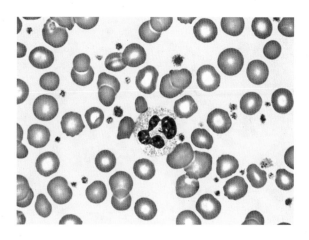

Figure 6-71

REACTIVE THROMBOCYTOSIS

This peripheral blood smear shows marked reactive thrombocytosis in an adult female with iron deficiency anemia (Wright stain).

morphologically mature, and individually dispersed rather than clustered. Overall, bone marrow cellularity is normal, and reticulin fibrosis is either absent or minimal. This contrasts with the prototypic findings in patients with thrombocytotic chronic myeloproliferative disorders in which bone marrow megakaryocytes are increased, prominently clustered, and morphologically atypical (see fig. 6-23) (146,147,157). Bone marrow fibrosis is also a finding in many chronic myeloproliferative disorders.

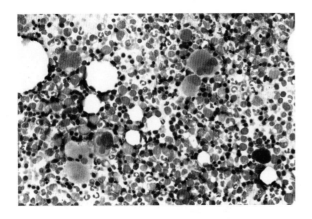

Figure 6-72

MEGAKARYOCYTES IN ACQUIRED IMMUNODEFICIENCY SYNDROME (AIDS)

This bone marrow aspirate smear shows increased mononuclear and pyknotic megakaryocytes in a patient with AIDS (Wright stain).

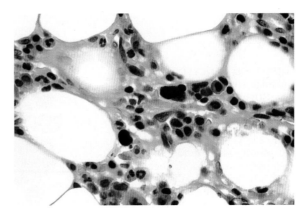

Figure 6-74

DENUDED MEGAKARYOCYTES IN ACQUIRED IMMUNODEFICIENCY SYNDROME (AIDS)

High magnification of pyknotic and denuded mega-karyocytes in a bone marrow biopsy section from a patient with AIDS (H&E stain).

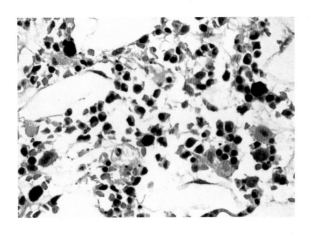

Figure 6-73

MEGAKARYOCYTES IN ACQUIRED IMMUNODEFICIENCY SYNDROME (AIDS)

This bone marrow biopsy section shows numerous pyknotic and denuded megakaryocytes in a patient with AIDS (H&E stain).

Megakaryocytic Abnormalities in Infectious and Noninfectious Systemic Diseases

Nonspecific numerical abnormalities of megakaryocytes are common in patients with systemic disorders, including megakaryocytic hyperplasia in response to various regulatory aberrations. These megakaryocytes are generally morphologically unremarkable. In HIV-1 infection, however, distinctive morphologically atypical megakaryocytes may be evident. These abnormal megakaryocytes often exhibit dense, pyknotic nuclear chromatin, and the cytoplasm may be scant (so-called denuded megakaryocytes) (figs. 6-72–6-74) (160,162,170). Apoptosis following HIV-1 infection is the presumed cause of these morphologic megakaryocyte aberrations. Denuded megakaryocytes are occasionally seen in non-HIV-1-infected patients, a possible reflection of some other immunoregulatory or apoptotic defect. Other unique infection-associated megakaryocytic disorders are reactive thrombocytosis and rare cases of acquired amegakaryocytosis.

Rare patients with collagen vascular diseases such as systemic lupus erythematosus, systemic sclerosis, or primary autoimmune myelofibrosis develop thrombocytopenia secondary to amegakaryocytosis (166). Most cases of thrombocytopenia in this setting, however, are due to antiplatelet autoantibody production, and the bone marrow findings in these cases are indistinguishable from those of primary ITP (163,165). Rarely, patients with rheumatologic disorders develop blood and bone marrow features that mimic those of a chronic myeloproliferative disorder with increased and clustered megakaryocytes (figs. 6-75–6-77).

Although not typically discussed with noninfectious systemic disorders, the distinctive megakaryocytic abnormalities in patients with Down syndrome warrant discussion. Abnormal megakaryoblastic proliferation is a key component

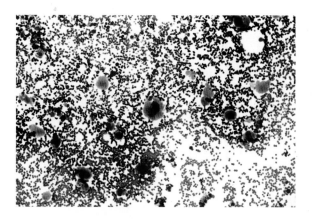

Figure 6-75

MYELOPROLIFERATIVE-LIKE PATTERN IN RHEUMATOID ARTHRITIS

Increased megakaryocytes are present on this bone marrow aspirate smear from a patient with longstanding rheumatoid arthritis who developed a chronic myeloproliferative disorder-like pattern in blood and bone marrow (Wright stain). (Courtesy of Dr. C. Sever, Albuquerque, NM.)

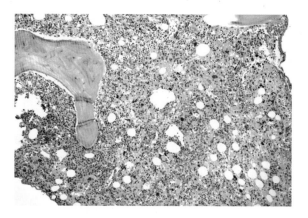

Figure 6-76

MYELOPROLIFERATIVE-LIKE PATTERN IN RHEUMATOID ARTHRITIS

Low magnification of bone marrow core biopsy shows increased overall cellularity and dilated sinuses in a patient with rheumatoid arthritis who developed a chronic myelo-proliferative disorder-like pattern in blood and bone marrow (H&E stain). (Courtesy of Dr. C. Sever, Albuquerque, MN.)

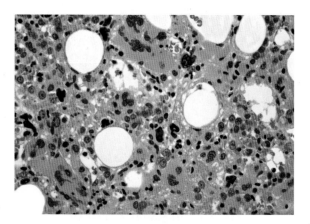

Figure 6-77

MYELOPROLIFERATIVE-LIKE PATTERN IN RHEUMATOID ARTHRITIS

High magnification of bone marrow core biopsy from a patient with longstanding rheumatoid arthritis shows increased and atypical megakaryocytes with marked pleo-morphism mimicking a chronic myeloproliferative disorder (H&E stain). (Courtesy of Dr. C. Sever, Albuquerque, NM.)

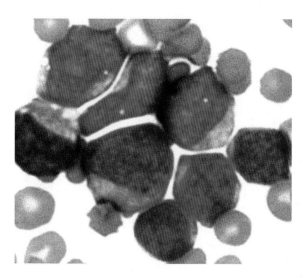

Figure 6-78

MEGAKARYOBLASTIC DIFFERENTIATION IN TRANSIENT MYELOPROLIFERATIVE DISORDER

This peripheral blood smear shows a predominance of blasts with a tendency toward megakaryoblastic differentiation as evidenced by the more abundant cytoplasm and more condensed nuclear chromatin in the immature cell population. This peripheral smear is from a 4-week-old Down syndrome infant with a transient myeloproliferative disorder (Wright stain).

of the transient myeloproliferative disorders of the neonatal and early infancy periods in these patients (figs. 6-78, 6-79). Many of the circulating immature cells are of megakaryocytic origin in these spontaneously remitting, yet clonal, processes linked to acquired *GATA1* mutations (161,164,167–169). Patients with Down syn-drome are also at considerable increased risk for the subsequent development of overt acute megakaryocytic leukemia, notably during the

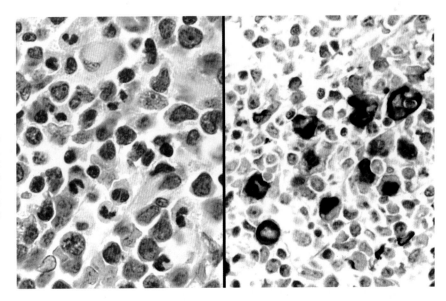

Figure 6-79

TRANSIENT MYELOPROLIFERATIVE DISORDER

This bone marrow core biopsy from a 4-week-old Down syndrome infant with transient myeloproliferative disorder is stained with H&E (left) and CD42b immunoperoxidase (right). The megakaryocytic component is prominent.

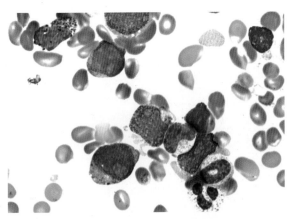

Figure 6-80

ACUTE MEGAKARYOBLASTIC LEUKEMIA IN DOWN SYNDROME

Bone marrow aspirate smear from a 22-month-old boy with Down syndrome and previous transient myeloproliferative disorder who developed acute megakaryoblastic leukemia (Wright stain).

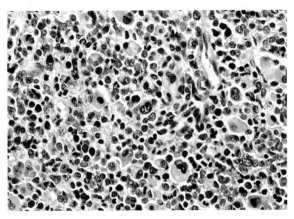

Figure 6-81

ACUTE MEGAKARYOBLASTIC LEUKEMIA IN DOWN SYNDROME

High magnification of a bone marrow core biopsy from a 7-month-old with Down syndrome and previous transient myeloproliferative disorder. The acute megakaryoblastic leukemia that developed shows a prominent population of immature blastic cells admixed with highly atypical and markedly increased megakaryocytes. The size of the megakaryoctyes is reduced and there is a predominance of nonlobulated megakaryocytes (H&E stain).

first 4 years of life (164,167,169). Both increased numbers and increased immaturity of mega-karyocytes are an expected bone marrow feature in overt acute megakaryoblastic leukemia (figs. 6-80–6-82).

Therapy-Related Megakaryocytic Abnormalities

Multilineage hypocellularity with stromal damage is the predicted bone marrow morphology following potent multiagent myeloabla-tive chemotherapy such as induction therapy for acute leukemia (fig. 6-83). Megakaryocyte regeneration following myeloablative therapy is generally somewhat delayed compared to erythroid and myeloid lineage regeneration. Early megakaryocyte regeneration is associated with megakaryocyte clustering (figs. 6-84, 6-85). In rare patients with acute leukemia, a striking

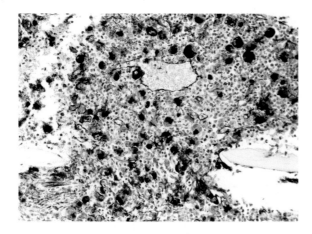

Figure 6-82

**ACUTE MEGAKARYOBLASTIC
LEUKEMIA IN DOWN SYNDROME**

Immunoperoxidase stain for CD31 highlights the hypolobulated megakaryocytes in a 7-month-old boy with Down syndrome who developed acute megakaryoblastic leukemia. (Courtesy of Dr. K. Monnin, Sacramento, CA.)

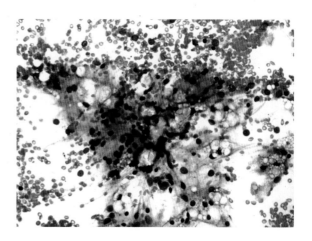

Figure 6-83

DAY 15 OF INDUCTION CHEMOTHERAPY

This profoundly hypocellular bone marrow is from day 15 of induction chemotherapy. All hematopoietic elements are reduced (Wright stain).

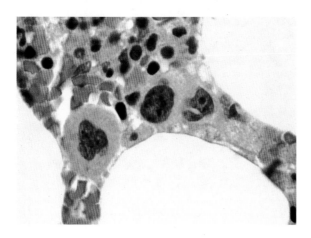

Figure 6-84

MEGAKARYOCYTE REGENERATION

Minimal megakaryocyte clustering with abnormal lobulation is evident upon regeneration following induction chemotherapy in this core biopsy specimen (H&E stain).

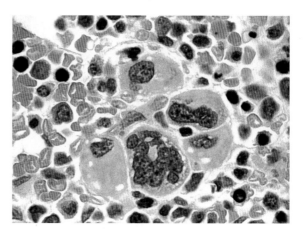

Figure 6-85

MEGAKARYOCYTE REGENERATION

Megakaryocyte clustering with atypia (both hypolobulation and hyperlobulation) is evident on this bone marrow core biopsy section following potent chemotherapy (H&E stain).

non-neoplastic proliferation of megakaryocytes is seen during early postinduction chemotherapy regeneration (175). The cause of this unique regeneration phenomenon is unclear, and its distinction from overt megakaryocytic neoplasia is problematic, although the absence of a megakaryoblastic component in the original acute leukemia is a helpful feature (figs. 6-86, 6-87).

A variety of other medication-related megakaryocytic abnormalities have been described. Dysplastic and clustered megakaryocytes have been noted in patients receiving valproic acid therapy (fig. 6-88) (173). Thrombocytopenia, and rarely pancytopenia, may develop in patients being treated with recombinant thrombopoietin. Several patients developed

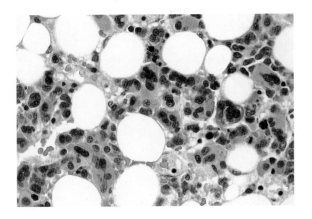

Figure 6-86

**POSTCHEMOTHERAPY
MEGAKARYOCYTE PROLIFERATION**

Marked megakaryocytic hyperplasia with hypolobulation is evident following induction chemotherapy in this patient with acute myeloid leukemia. The patient eventually achieved complete remission (H&E stain).

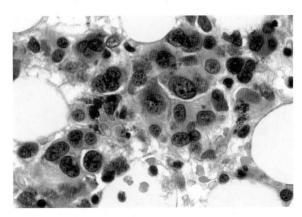

Figure 6-87

**POSTCHEMOTHERAPY
MEGAKARYOCYTE PROLIFERATION**

Marked megakaryocytic hyperplasia with hypolobulation is evident following induction chemotherapy in this patient with acute myeloid leukemia. The original leukemia did not have a megakaryocytic component (H&E stain).

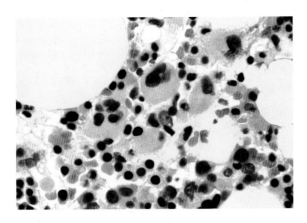

Figure 6-88

MEDICATION EFFECTS ON MEGAKARYOCYTES

This bone marrow biopsy section shows megakaryocytic hyperplasia with mild pyknosis and hypolobulation in a patient who was receiving valproic acid therapy (H&E stain). (Courtesy Dr. T. Elghetany, Galveston, TX.)

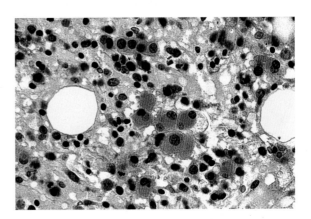

Figure 6-89

ABNORMAL MEGAKARYOCYTES IN MYELODYSPLASIA

Clustered hypolobulated megakaryocytes are evident in the bone marrow biopsy specimen from a patient with high-grade myelodysplasia (H&E stain).

amegakaryocytosis while on recombinant thrombopoietin therapy when antibodies produced against the recombinant thrombopoietin cross-reacted with endogenous thrombopoietin (174). A similar phenomenon has been described in which all hematopoietic elements were affected, producing aplastic anemia-like features associated with neutralizing antibodies to thrombopoietin (171). Another complication of recombinant therapy is the development of blood and bone marrow features closely

mimicking those of a chronic myeloproliferative disorder, with significant megakaryocyte abnormalities (172).

DIFFERENTIAL DIAGNOSIS OF NON-NEOPLASTIC MEGAKARYOCYTIC DISORDERS

The differential diagnosis of megakaryocytic disorders includes distinguishing between non-neoplastic and neoplastic megakaryocyte disorders and excluding megakaryocyte "look-alikes,"

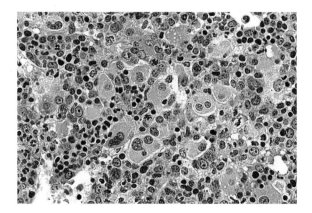

Figure 6-90

ABNORMAL MEGAKARYOCYTES IN MYELODYSPLASIA

Striking megakaryocytic proliferation, clustering, and dysplasia are evident in this bone marrow biopsy section from a patient with high-grade myelodysplasia (H&E stain).

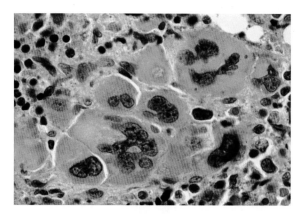

Figure 6-91

ABNORMAL MEGAKARYOCYTES IN MYELOFIBROSIS

Striking megakaryocytic clustering with marked pleomorphism is evident in the bone marrow biopsy section from a patient with chronic idiopathic myelofibrosis (H&E stain).

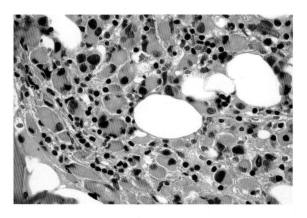

Figure 6-92

DYSPLASTIC MEGAKARYOCYTES

A bone marrow biopsy shows effacement by hypolobulated, dysplastic megakaryocytes (H&E stain).

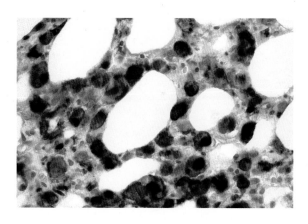

Figure 6-93

DYSPLASTIC MEGAKARYOCYTES (CD42b)

Immunoperoxidase stain for CD42b highlights immature and hypolobulated megakaryocytes in this core biopsy.

i.e., other large, multinucleated/multilobulated cells in the bone marrow that mimic megakaryocytes (176). In both chronic myeloproliferative and myelodysplastic disorders, all hematopoietic lineages are derived from the neoplastic clone. Consequently, both quantitative and qualitative abnormalities of all hematopoietic elements may be manifested. Multilineage dysplasia with cytopenia typifies myelodysplastic syndromes, whereas multilineage proliferation with excess cell production characterizes chronic myeloproliferative disorders. In both of these clonal disorders, megakaryocytes are often increased, morphologically abnormal, and clustered (figs. 6-89, 6-90). Either reduced or increased nuclear lobulation may be evident in conjunction with substantial clustering or intrasinusoidal localization (figs. 6-91–6-93). Consequently, the evaluation of all lineages, in conjunction with possible genetic testing, helps to distinguish a reactive megakaryocyte disorder from these neoplastic processes.

A variety of large cells may exhibit morphologic features simulating megakaryocytes. In non-neoplastic disorders, both osteoclasts and multinucleated histiocytes can mimic

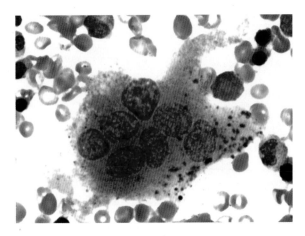

Figure 6-94

OSTEOCLAST

An osteoclast with discrete round nuclei is evident in this bone marrow aspirate smear from a child (Wright stain).

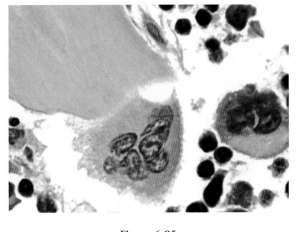

Figure 6-95

OSTEOCLAST

This bone marrow core biopsy section from a child shows a normal osteoclast (left) adjacent to a normal megakaryocyte (right) (H&E stain).

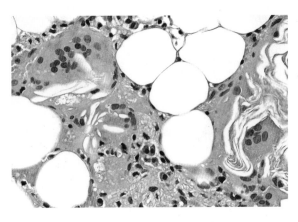

Figure 6-96

FOREIGN BODY GRANULOMAS WITH KERATIN

This sternal clot section shows multinucleated foreign body histiocytes and keratinous material in an adult patient with a history of previous cardiac surgery (H&E stain). (Courtesy of Dr. B. Cabello-Inchausti, Plantation, FL.)

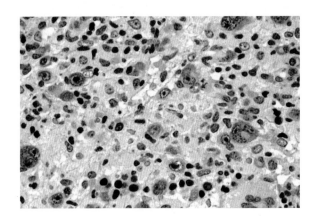

Figure 6-97

ANAPLASTIC LARGE CELL LYMPHOMA MIMICKING MYELOPROLIFERATIVE DISORDER

The extensive infiltration of anaplastic large cell lymphoma on a bone marrow biopsy mimics megakaryocytes (H&E stain). (Courtesy of Dr. R. Macaulay, Glenwood Springs, CO.)

megakaryocytes (figs. 6-94–6-96). Likewise, multinucleated tumor giant cells can mimic megakaryocytes in bone marrow specimens involved by Hodgkin and non-Hodgkin lymphomas, myeloma, and metastatic carcinomas (figs. 6-97–6-101) (176,177). The integration of morphology with clinical features and immunohistochemical stains generally readily distinguishes megakaryocytes from these look-alikes (figs. 6-98, 6-100).

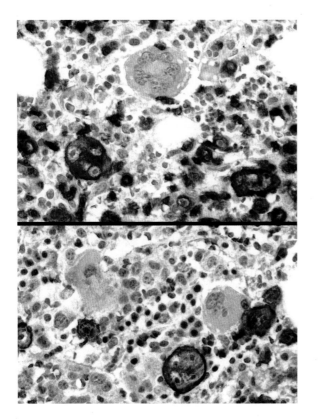

Figure 6-98

**ANAPLASTIC LYMPHOMA MIMICKING
MYELOPROLIFERATIVE DISORDER**

Immunoperoxidase stains for CD3 (top) and CD30 (bottom) show positivity of multinucleated anaplastic large cell lymphoma cells while admixed, benign megakaryocytes are negative. (Courtesy of Dr. R. Macaulay, Glenwood Springs, CO.)

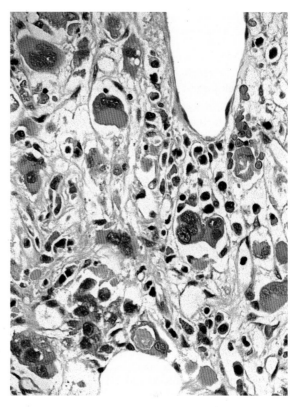

Figure 6-99

MULTINUCLEATED METASTATIC CARCINOMA CELLS

Multinucleated metastatic carcinoma cells mimic megakaryocytes within sinusoids in patient with metastatic carcinoma (H&E stain).

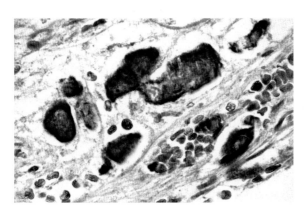

Figure 6-100

**METASTATIC CARCINOMA
MIMICKING MEGAKARYOCYTES (KERATIN)**

The immunoperoxidase stain for keratin is strongly positive in intrasinusoidal metastatic carcinoma, mimicking megakaryoctyes.

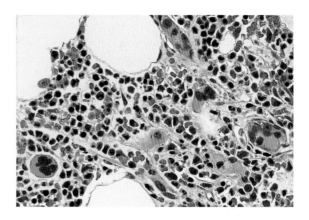

Figure 6-101

**METASTATIC NEUROBLASTOMA
MIMICKING MEGAKARYOCYTES**

Metastatic neuroblastoma within sinuses mimics megakaryocytes in this bone marrow biopsy section from a child. Normal megakaryocytes (left corner and upper central region) can be compared to the multinucleated tumor cells plugging sinuses (H&E stain).

213

REFERENCES

Normal Megakaryocyte Development and Platelet Homeostasis

1. Agosti S, Cornbleet P, Galagan K, et al. Megakaryocyte maturation. In: Glassy E, ed. Color atlas of hematology. Northfield, IL: College of American Pathologists; 1998:190-1.

2. Bruno E, Hoffman R. Human megakaryocyte progenitor cells. Semin Hematol 1998;35:183-91.

3. Dame C, Sutor AH. Primary and secondary thrombocytosis in childhood. Br J Haematol 2005;129:165-77.

4. Debili N, Coulombel L, Croisille L, et al. Characterization of a bipotent erythro-megakaryocytic progenitor in human bone marrow. Blood 1996;88:1284-96.

5. Drachman JG. Inherited thrombocytopenia: when a low platelet count does not mean ITP. Blood 2004;103:390-8.

6. Elagib KE, Racke FK, Mogass M, Khetawat R, Delehanty LL, Goldfarb AN. RUNX1 and GATA-1 coexpression and cooperation in megakaryocytic differentiation. Blood 2003;101:4333-41.

7. Foucar K. Reactive and neoplastic disorders of megakaryocytes. In: Bone marrow pathology. Chicago: ASCP Press; 2001:324-43.

8. Geddis AE, Kaushansky K. Megakaryocytes express functional Aurora-B kinase in endomitosis. Blood 2004;104:1017-24.

9. Ishiguro A, Nakahata T, Matsubara K, et al. Age-related changes in thrombopoietin in children: reference interval for serum thrombopoietin levels. Br J Haematol 1999;106:884-8.

10. Juneja S, Trute L, Westerman D, Venter D, Seymour JF, Prince HM. Paraffin section immunotyping of leukaemias. Br J Haematol 2000;109:267-71.

11. Kuter DJ, Begley CG. Recombinant human thrombopoietin: basic biology and evaluation of clinical studies. Blood 2002;100:3457-69.

12. Levine RF, Olson TA, Shoff PK, Miller MK, Weisman LE. Mature micromegakaryocytes: an unusual developmental pattern in term infants. Br J Haematol 1996;94:391-9.

13. Long MW. Megakaryocyte differentiation events. Semin Hematol 1998;35:192-9.

14. Lorsbach RB. Megakaryoblastic disorders in children. Am J Clin Pathol 2004;122(Suppl):S33-46.

15. Poncz M. Inherited platelet disorders. In: Nathan DG, Orkin S, Ginsburg D, et al., eds. Nathan and Oski's hematology of infancy and childhood, 6th ed. Philadelphia: WB Saunders; 2003:1527-41.

16. Sato T, Ono M, Fujita H, et al. Development of a liquid culture system for megakaryocyte terminal differentiation: fibrinogen promotes megakaryocytopoiesis but not thrombopoiesis. Br J Haematol 2003;121:315-23.

17. Tomer A. Human marrow megakaryocyte differentiation: multiparameter correlative analysis identifies von Willebrand factor as a sensitive and distinctive marker for early (2N and 4N) megakaryocytes. Blood 2004;104:2722-7.

18. Van den Hof MC, Nicolaides KH. Platelet count in normal, small, and anemic fetuses. Am J Obstet Gynecol 1990;162:735-9.

19. Vitrat N, Cohen-Solal K, Pique C, et al. Endomitosis of human megakaryocytes are due to abortive mitosis. Blood 1998;91:3711-23.

20. Zhang Y, Nagata Y, Yu G, et al. Aberrant quantity and localization of Aurora-B/AIM-1 and survivin during megakaryocyte polyploidization and the consequences of Aurora-B/AIM-1-deregulated expression. Blood 2004;103:3717-26.

Morphologic Abnormalities of Platelets and Megakaryocytes

21. Bauer S, Khan A, Klein A, Starasoler L. Naked megakaryocyte nuclei as an indicator of human immunodeficiency virus infection. Arch Pathol Lab Med 1992;116:1025-9.

22. Bellucci S. Megakaryocytes and inherited thrombocytopenias. Baillieres Clin Haematol 1997;10:149-62.

23. Cashell AW, Buss DH. The frequency and significance of megakaryocytic emperipolesis in myeloproliferative and reactive states. Ann Hematol 1992;64:273-6.

24. Criswell KA, Breider MA, Bleavins MR. EDTA-dependent platelet phagocytosis. A cytochemical, ultrastructural, and functional characterization. Am J Clin Pathol 2001;115:376-84.

25. Ding J, Komatsu H, Wakita A, et al. Familial essential thrombocythemia associated with a dominant-positive activating mutation of the c-MPL gene, which encodes for the receptor for thrombopoietin. Blood 2004;103:4198-200.

26. Fiorin F, Steffan A, Pradella P, Steffan A, Potenza R, De Angelis V. IgG platelet antibodies in EDTA-dependent pseudothrombocytopenia bind to platelet membrane glycoprotein IIb. Am J Clin Pathol 1998;110:178-83.

27. Foucar K. Bone marrow manifestation of non-infectious systemic diseases. In: Bone marrow pathology, 2nd ed. Chicago: ASCP Press; 2001: 640-53.

28. Foucar K. Bone marrow manifestations of systemic infections. In: Bone marrow pathology. 2nd ed. Chicago: ASCP Press; 2001:616-38.

29. Foucar K. Reactive and neoplastic disorders of megakaryocytes. In: Bone marrow pathology. Chicago: ASCP Press; 2001:324-43.

30. Girodon F, Favre B, Carli PM, et al. Minor dysplastic changes are frequently observed in the bone marrow aspirate in elderly patients without haematological disease. Clin Lab Haematol 2001;23:297-300.

31. Hatfill SJ, Fester ED, Steytler JG. Apoptotic megakaryocyte dysplasia in the myelodysplastic syndromes. Hematol Pathol 1992;6:87-93.

32. Jantunen E, Hanninen A, Naukkarinen A, Vomanen M, Lahtinen R. Gray platelet syndrome with splenomegaly and signs of extramedullary hematopoiesis: a case report with review of the literature. Am J Hematol 1994;46:218-24.

33. Kunishima S, Matsushita T, Yoshihara T, et al. First description of somatic mosaicism in MYH9 disorders. Br J Haematol 2005;128:360-5.

34. Kunishima S, Saito H. Congenital macrothrombocytopenias. Blood Rev 2006;20:111-21.

35. Lopez JA, Andrews RK, Afshar-Kharghan V, Berndt MC. Bernard-Soulier syndrome. Blood 1998;91:4397-418.

36. Murray NA, Roberts IA. Circulating megakaryocytes and their progenitors (BFU-MK and CFU-MK) in term and pre-term neonates. Br J Haematol 1995;89:41-6.

37. Rosenthal NS, Farhi DC. Dysmegakaryopoiesis resembling acute megakaryoblastic leukemia in treated acute myeloid leukemia. Am J Clin Pathol 1991;95:556-60.

38. Zucker-Franklin D. The effect of viral infections on platelets and megakaryocytes. Semin Hematol 1994;31:329-37.

Platelet/Megakaryocytic Disorders in Children and Adults

39. Buss DH, Cashell AW, O'Connor ML, Richards F 2nd, Case LD. Occurrence, etiology, and clinical significance of extreme thrombocytosis: a study of 280 cases. Am J Med 1994;96:247-53.

40. Criswell KA, Breider MA, Bleavins MR. EDTA-dependent platelet phagocytosis. A cytochemical, ultrastructural, and functional characterization. Am J Clin Pathol 2001;115:376-84.

41. Dame C, Sutor AH. Primary and secondary thrombocytosis in childhood. Br J Haematol 2005;129:165-77.

42. Ding J, Komatsu H, Wakita A, et al. Familial essential thrombocythemia associated with a dominant-positive activating mutation of the c-MPL gene, which encodes for the receptor for thrombopoietin. Blood 2004;103:4198-200.

43. Fiorin F, Steffan A, Pradella P, Steffan A, Potenza R, De Angelis V. IgG platelet antibodies in EDTA-dependent pseudothrombocytopenia bind to platelet membrane glycoprotein IIb. Am J Clin Pathol 1998;110:178-83.

44. Griesshammer M, Bangerter M, Sauer T, Wennauer R, Bergmann L, Heimpel H. Aetiology and clinical significance of thrombocytosis: analysis of 732 patients with an elevated platelet count. J Intern Med 1999;245:295-300.

45. Kondo T, Okabe M, Sanada M, et al. Familial essential thrombocythemia associated with one-base deletion in the 5'-untranslated region of the thrombopoietin gene. Blood 1998;92:1091-6.

46. Sasaki Y, Takahashi T, Miyazaki H, et al. Production of thrombopoietin by human carcinomas and its novel isoforms. Blood 1999;94:1952-60.

47. Schafer AI. Thrombocytosis. N Engl J Med 2004;350:1211-9.

48. Stuhrmann M, Bashawri L, Ahmed MA, et al. Familial thrombocytosis as a recessive, possibly X-linked trait in an Arab family. Br J Haematol 2001;112:616-20.

49. Tefferi A, Silverstein MN, Hoagland HC. Primary thrombocythemia. Semin Oncol 1995;22:334-40.

50. Wiestner A, Schlemper RJ, van der Maas AP, Skoda RC. An activating splice donor mutation in the thrombopoietin gene causes hereditary thrombocythaemia. Nat Genet 1998;18:49-52.

Constitutional Megakaryocytic Disorders with Thrombocytopenia

51. Ahmed M, Sternberg A, Hall G, et al. Natural history of GATA1 mutations in Down syndrome. Blood 2004;103:2480-9.

52. Alter BP. Arms and the man or hands and the child: congenital anomalies and hematologic syndromes. J Pediatr Hematol Oncol 1997;19:287-91.

53. Ballmaier M, Germeshausen M, Schulze H, et al. c-mpl mutations are the cause of congenital amegakaryocytic thrombocytopenia. Blood 2001;97:139-46.

54. Becker PS, Clavell LA, Beardsley DS. Giant platelets with abnormal surface glycoproteins: a new familial disorder associated with mitral valve insufficiency. J Pediatr Hematol Oncol 1998;20:69-73.

55. Bolton-Maggs PH, Chalmers EA, Collins PW, et al. A review of inherited platelet disorders with guidelines for their management on behalf of the UKHCDO. Br J Haematol 2006;135:603-33.

56. Breton-Gorius J, Favier R, Guichard J, et al. A new congenital dysmegakaryopoietic thrombocytopenia (Paris-Trousseau) associated with giant platelet alpha-granules and chromosome 11 deletion at 11q23. Blood 1995;85:1805-14.

57. Bruin M, Tijssen MR, Bierings M, de Haas M. Juvenile cyclic amegakaryocytic thrombocytopenia: a novel entity. J Pediatr Hematol Oncol 2005;27:148-52.

58. de Alarcon PA, Graeve JA, Levine RF, McDonald TP, Beal DW. Thrombocytopenia and absent radii syndrome: defective megakaryocytopoiesis-thrombocytopoiesis. Am J Pediatr Hematol Oncol 1991;13:77-83.

59. Drachman JG. Inherited thrombocytopenia: when a low platelet count does not mean ITP. Blood 2004;103:390-8.

60. Drachman JG, Jarvik GP, Mehaffey MG. Autosomal dominant thrombocytopenia: incomplete megakaryocyte differentiation and linkage to human chromosome 10. Blood 2000;96:118-25.

61. Fadoo Z, Naqvi SM. Acute myeloid leukemia in a patient with thrombocytopenia with absent radii syndrome. J Pediatr Hematol Oncol 2002;24:134-5.

62. Fureder W, Mitterbauer G, Thalhammer R, et al. Clonal T cell-mediated cyclic thrombocytopenia. Br J Haematol 2002;119:1059-61.

63. Gilman AL, Sloand E, White JG, Sacher R. A novel hereditary macrothrombocytopenia. J Pediatr Hematol Oncol 1995;17:296-305.

64. Go RS. Idiopathic cyclic thrombocytopenia. Blood Rev 2005;19:53-9.

65. Groet J, McElwaine S, Spinelli M, et al. Acquired mutations in GATA1 in neonates with Down's syndrome with transient myeloid disorder. Lancet 2003;361:1617-20.

66. Heller PG, Glembotsky AC, Gandhi MJ, et al. Low Mpl receptor expression in a pedigree with familial platelet disorder with predisposition to acute myelogenous leukemia and a novel AML1 mutation. Blood 2005;105:4664-70.

67. Hyman T, Huizing M, Blumberg PM, Falik-Zaccai TC, Anikster Y, Gahl WA. Use of a cDNA microarray to determine molecular mechanisms involved in grey platelet syndrome. Br J Haematol 2003;122:142-9.

68. Inoue H, Kurosawa H, Nonoyama S, et al. X-linked thrombocytopenia in a girl. Br J Haematol 2002;118:1163-5.

69. Jantunen E. Inherited giant platelet disorders. Eur J Haematol 1994;53:191-6.

70. Jantunen E, Hanninen A, Naukkarinen A, Vornanen M, Lahtinen R. Gray platelet syndrome with splenomegaly and signs of extramedullary hematopoiesis: a case report with review of the literature. Am J Hematol 1994;46:218-24.

71. Kimura F, Nakamura Y, Sato K, et al. Cyclic change of cytokines in a patient with cyclic thrombocytopenia. Br J Haematol 1996;94:171-4.

72. King S, Germeshausen M, Strauss G, Welte K, Ballmaier M. Congenital amegakaryocytic thrombocytopenia: a retrospective clinical analysis of 20 patients. Br J Haematol 2005;131:636-44.

73. Kirito K, Fox N, Kaushansky K. Thrombopoietin stimulates Hoxb4 expression: an explanation for the favorable effects of TPO on hematopoietic stem cells. Blood 2003;102:3172-8.

74. Kunishima S, Matsushita T, Yoshihara T, et al. First description of somatic mosaicism in MYH9 disorders. Br J Haematol 2005;128:360-5.

75. Kunishima S, Saito H. Congenital macrothrombocytopenias. Blood Rev 2006;20:111-21.

76. Letestu R, Vitrat N, Masse A, et al. Existence of a differentiation blockage at the stage of a megakaryocyte precursor in the thrombocytopenia and absent radii (TAR) syndrome. Blood 2000;95:1633-41.

77. Lopez JA, Andrews RK, Afshar-Kharghan V, Berndt MC. Bernard-Soulier syndrome. Blood 1998;91:4397-418.

78. Mehaffey MG, Newton AL, Gandhi MJ, Crossley M, Drachman JG. X-linked thrombocytopenia caused by a novel mutation of GATA-1. Blood 2001;98:2681-8.

79. Michaud J, Wu F, Osato M, et al. In vitro analyses of known and novel RUNX1/AML1 mutations in dominant familial platelet disorder with predisposition to acute myelogenous leukemia: implications for mechanisms of pathogenesis. Blood 2002;99:1364-72.

80. Rainis L, Bercovich D, Strehl S, et al. Mutations in exon 2 of GATA1 are early events in megakaryocytic malignancies associated with trisomy 21. Blood 2003;102:981-6.

81. Sachs UJ, Kroll H, Matzdorff AC, Berghofer H, Lopez JA, Santoso S. Bernard-Soulier syndrome due to the homozygous Asn-45Ser mutation in GPIX: an unexpected, frequent finding in Germany. Br J Haematol 2003;123:127-31.

82. Schiff DE, Roberts WD, Willert J, Tsai HM. Thrombocytopenia and severe hyperbilirubinemia in the neonatal period secondary to congenital thrombotic thrombocytopenic purpura and ADAMTS13 deficiency. J Pediatr Hematol Oncol 2004;26:535-8.

83. Soejima K, Nakagaki T. Interplay between ADAMTS13 and von Willebrand factor in inherited and acquired thrombotic microangiopathies. Semin Hematol 2005;42:56-62.

84. Studt JD, Hovinga JA, Antoine G, et al. Fatal congenital thrombotic thrombocytopenic purpura with apparent ADAMTS13 inhibitor: in vitro inhibition of ADAMTS13 activity by hemoglobin. Blood 2005;105:542-4.

85. Studt JD, Hovinga JA, Radonic R, et al. Familial acquired thrombotic thrombocytopenic purpura: ADAMTS13 inhibitory autoantibodies in identical twins. Blood 2004;103:4195-7.

86. Uchida T, Wada H, Mizutani M, et al. Identification of novel mutations in ADAMTS13 in an adult patient with congenital thrombotic thrombocytopenic purpura. Blood 2004;104:2081-3.

87. van den Oudenrijn S, Bruin M, Folman CC, Bussel J, de Haas M, von dem Borne AE. Three parameters, plasma thrombopoietin levels, plasma glycocalicin levels and megakaryocyte culture, distinguish between different causes of congenital thrombocytopenia. Br J Haematol 2002;117:390-8.

88. Willig TB, Breton-Gorius J, Elbim C, et al. Macrothrombocytopenia with abnormal demarcation membranes in megakaryocytes and neutropenia with a complete lack of sialyl-Lewis-X antigen in leukocytes—a new syndrome? Blood 2001;97:826-8.

89. Xu G, Nagano M, Kanezaki R, et al. Frequent mutations in the GATA-1 gene in the transient myeloproliferative disorder of Down syndrome. Blood 2003;102:2960-8.

90. Young G, Luban N, White JG. Giant platelet disorders in African-American children misdiagnosed as idiopathic thrombocytopenic purpura. J Pediatr Hematol Oncol 1999;21:231-6.

91. Yu C, Niakan KK, Matsushita M, Stamatoyannopoulos G, Orkin SH, Raskind WH. X-linked thrombocytopenia with thalassemia from a mutation in the amino finger of GATA-1 affecting DNA binding rather than FOG-1 interaction. Blood 2002;100:2040-5.

92. Zent CS, Ratajczak J, Ratajczak MZ, Anastasi J, Hoffman PC, Gerwitz AM. Relationship between megakaryocyte mass and serum thrombopoietin levels as revealed by a case of cyclic amegakaryocytic thrombocytopenic purpura. Br J Haematol 1999;105:452-8.

93. Zipursky A. Transient leukaemia—a benign form of leukaemia in newborn infants with trisomy 21. Br J Haematol 2003;120:930-8.

Acquired Megakaryocytic Disorders with Thrombocytopenia

94. Agarwal N, Spahr JE, Werner TL, Newton DL, Rogers GM. Acquired amegakaryocytic thrombocytopenic purpura. Am J Hematol 2006;81:132-5.

95. Ahmed S, Siddiqui AK, Shahid RK, Kimpo M, Sison CP. Prognostic variables in newly diagnosed childhood immune thrombocytopenia. Am J Hematol 2004;77:358-62.

96. Aledort LM, Hayward CP, Chen MG, Nichol JL, Bussel J; ITP Study Group. Prospective screening of 205 patients with ITP, including diagnosis, serological markers, and the relationship between platelet counts, endogenous thrombopoietin, and circulating antithrombopoietin antibodies. Am J Hematol 2004;76:205-13.

97. Allford SL, Hunt BJ, Rose P, Machin SJ; Haemostasis and Thrombosis Task Force, British Committee for Standards in Haematology. Guidelines on the diagnosis and management of the thrombotic microangiopathic haemolytic anaemias. Br J Haematol 2003;120:556-73.

98. Aster RH. Drug-induced immune thrombocytopenia: an overview of pathogenesis. Semin Hematol 1999;36:2-6.

99. Atabay B, Oren H, Irken G, et al. Role of transforming growth factor-beta 1 gene polymorphisms in childhood idiopathic thrombocytopenic purpura. J Pediatr Hematol Oncol 2003;25:885-9.

100. Bhattacharyya J, Kumar R, Tyagi S, Kishore J, Mahapatra M, Choudhry VP. Human parvovirus B19-induced acquired pure amegakaryocytic thrombocytopenia. Br J Haematol 2005;128:128-9.

101. Birchall JE, Murphy MF, Kaplan C, Kroll H; European Fetomaternal Alloimmune Thrombocytopenia Study Group. European collaborative study of the antenatal management of fetomaternal alloimmune thrombocytopenia. Br J Haematol 2003;122:275-88.

102. British Committee for Standards in Haematology General Haematology Task Force. Guidelines for the investigation and management of idiopathic thrombocytopenic purpura in adults, children and in pregnancy. Br J Haematol 2003;120:574-96.

103. Bruin M, Bierings M, Uiterwaal C, et al. Platelet count, previous infection and FCGR2B genotype predict development of chronic disease in newly diagnosed idiopathic thrombocytopenia in childhood: results of a prospective study. Br J Haematol 2004;127:561-7.

104. Burns ER, Lou Y, Pathak A. Morphologic diagnosis of thrombotic thrombocytopenic purpura. Am J Hematol 2004;75:18-21.

105. Burrows RF, Kelton JG. Perinatal thrombocytopenia. Clin Perinatol 1995;22:779-801.

106. Chaudhary UB, Eberwine SF, Hege KM. Acquired amegakaryocytic thrombocytopenia purpura and eosinophilic fasciitis: a long relapsing and remitting course. Am J Hematol 2004;75:146-50.

107. Cooper N, Bussel J. The pathogenesis of immune thrombocytopaenic purpura. Br J Haematol 2006;133:364-74.

108. Davoren A, Aster RH. Heparin-induced thrombocytopenia and thrombosis. Am J Hematol 2006;81:36-44.

109. Fabris F, Scandellari R, Ruzzon E, Randi ML, Luzzatto G, Girolami A. Platelet-associated autoantibodies as detected by a solid-phase modified antigen capture ELISA test (MACE) are a useful prognostic factor in idiopathic thrombocytopenic purpura. Blood 2004;103:4562-4.

110. Fakhouri F, Vernant JP, Veyradier A, et al. Efficiency of curative and prophylactic treatment with rituximab in ADAMTS13-deficient thrombotic thrombocytopenic purpura: a study of 11 cases. Blood 2005;106:1932-7.

111. Foucar K. Reactive and neoplastic disorders of megakaryocytes. In: Bone marrow pathology. Chicago: ASCP Press; 2001:324-43.

112. George JN, Vesely SK, Terrell DR. The Oklahoma Thrombotic Thrombocytopenic Purpura-Hemolytic Uremic Syndrome (TTP-HUS) Registry: a community perspective of patients with clinically diagnosed TTP-HUS. Semin Hematol 2004;41:60-7.

113. Hall GW. Kasabach-Merritt syndrome: pathogenesis and management. Br J Haematol 2001;112:851-62.

114. Hoffman R. Acquired pure amegakaryocytic thrombocytopenic purpura. Semin Hematol 1991;28:303-12.

115. Hohlfeld P, Forestier F, Kaplan C, Tissot JD, Daffos F. Fetal thrombocytopenia: a retrospective survey of 5,194 fetal blood samplings. Blood 1994;84:1851-6.

116. Hosler GA, Cusumano AM, Hutchins GM. Thrombotic thrombocytopenic purpura and hemolytic uremic syndrome are distinct pathologic entities. A review of 56 autopsy cases. Arch Pathol Lab Med 2003;127:834-9.

117. Kaplan C. Alloimmune thrombocytopenia of the fetus and the newborn. Blood Rev 2002;16:69-72.

118. Kashyap R, Choudhry VP, Pati HP. Danazol therapy in cyclic acquired amegakaryocytic thrombocytopenic purpura: a case report. Am J Hematol 1999;60:225-8.

119. Katsumata Y, Suzuki T, Kuwana M, et al. Anti-c-Mpl (thrombopoietin receptor) autoantibody-induced amegakaryocytic thrombocytopenia in a patient with systemic sclerosis. Arthritis Rheum 2003;48:1647-51.

120. Kelton JG. Heparin-induced thrombocytopenia: an overview. Blood Rev 2002;16:77-80.

121. King JA, Elkhalifa MY, Latour LF. Rapid progression of acquired amegakaryocytic thrombocytopenia to aplastic anemia. South Med J 1997;90:91-4.

122. Klaassen RJ, Doyle JJ, Krahn MD, Blanchette VS, Naglie G. Initial bone marrow aspiration in childhood idiopathic thrombocytopenia: decision analysis. J Pediatr Hematol Oncol 2001;23:511-8.

123. Koefoed K, Ditzel HJ. Identification of talin head domain as an immunodominant epitope of the antiplatelet antibody response in patients with HIV-1-associated thrombocytopenia. Blood 2004;104:4054-62.

124. Kokame K, Miyata T. Genetic defects leading to hereditary thrombotic thrombocytopenic purpura. Semin Hematol 2004;41:34-40.

125. Kouides PA, Rowe JM. Large granular lymphocyte leukemia presenting with both amegakaryocytic thrombocytopenic purpura and pure red cell aplasia: clinical course and response to immunosuppressive therapy. Am J Hematol 1995;49:232-6.

126. Kumar M, Vik TA, Johnson CS, Southwood ME, Croop JM. Treatment, outcome, and cost of care in children with idiopathic thrombocytopenic purpura. Am J Hematol 2005;78:181-7.

127. Levi M. Current understanding of disseminated intravascular coagulation. Br J Haematol 2004;124:567-76.

128. McCrae KR. Thrombocytopenia in pregnancy: differential diagnosis, pathogenesis, and management. Blood Rev 2003;17:7-14.

129. McMillan R, Durette C. Long-term outcomes in adults with chronic ITP after splenectomy failure. Blood 2004;104:956-60.

130. Michel M, Cooper N, Jean C, Frissora C, Bussel JB. Does Helicobater pylori initiate or perpetuate immune thrombocytopenic purpura? Blood 2004;103:890-6.

131. Moake JL. von Willebrand factor, ADAMTS-13, and thrombotic thrombocytopenic purpura. Semin Hematol 2004;41:4-14.

132. Mulliken JB, Anupindi S, Ezekowitz RA, Mihm MC Jr. Case records of the Massachusetts General Hospital. Weekly clinicopathological exercises. Case 13-2004. A newborn girl with a large cutaneous lesion, thrombocytopenia, and anemia. N Engl J Med 2004;350:1764-75.

133. Murrin RJ, Murray JA. Thrombotic thrombocytopenic purpura: aetiology, pathophysiology and treatment. Blood Rev 2006;20:51-60.

134. Neylon AJ, Saunders PW, Howard MR, Proctor SJ, Taylor PR; Northern Region Haematology Group. Clinically significant newly presenting autoimmune thrombocytopenic purpura in adults: a prospective study of a population-based cohort of 245 patients. Br J Haematol 2003;122:966-74.

135. Nugent DJ. Childhood immune thrombocytopenic purpura. Blood Rev 2002;16:27-9.

136. Panitsas FP, Theodoropoulou M, Kouraklis A, et al. Adult chronic idiopathic thrombocytopenic purpura (ITP) is the manifestation of a type-1 polarized immune response. Blood 2004;103:2645-7.

137. Peterson JA, Nyree CE, Newman PJ, Aster RH. A site involving the "hybrid" and PSI homology domains of GPIIIa (beta 3-integrin subunit) is a common target for antibodies associated with quinine-induced immune thrombocytopenia. Blood 2003;101:937-42.

138. Provan D, Newland A. Idiopathic thrombocytopenic purpura in adults. J Pediatr Hematol Oncol 2003;25(Suppl 1):S34-8.

139. Roberts IA, Murray NA. Management of thrombocytopenia in neonates. Br J Haematol 1999;105:864-70.

140. Schiff DE, Roberts WD, Willert J, Tsai HM. Thrombocytopenia and severe hyperbilirubinemia in the neonatal period secondary to congenital thrombotic thrombocytopenic purpura and ADAMTS13 deficiency. J Pediatr Hematol Oncol 2004;26:535-8.

141. Studt JD, Hovinga JA, Radonic R, et al. Familial acquired thrombotic thrombocytopenic purpura: ADAMTS13 inhibitory autoantibodies in identical twins. Blood 2004;103:4195-7.

142. Thiele J, von Ammers E, Wagner S, Degel C, Fischer R. Megakaryocytopoiesis in idiopathic thrombocytopenic purpura: a morphometric and immunohistochemical study on bone marrow biopsies with special emphasis on precursor cells. Hematol Pathol 1991;5:75-82.

143. Udom-Rice I, Bussel JB. Fetal and neonatal thrombocytopenia. Blood Rev 1995;9:57-64.

144. Wada H, Gabazza EC, Asakura H, et al. Comparison of diagnostic criteria for disseminated intravascular coagulation (DIC): diagnostic criteria of the International Society of Thrombosis and Hemostasis and of the Japanese Ministry of Health and Welfare for overt DIC. Am J Hematol 2003;74:17-22.

145. Zimmer J, Andres E, Noel E, Koumarianou A, Blickle JF, Maloisel F. Current management of adult idiopathic thrombocytopenic purpura in practice: a cohort study of 201 patients from a single center. Clin Lab Haematol 2004;26:137-42.

Constitutional and Acquired Megakaryocytic Disorders with Thrombocytosis

146. Buhr T, Georgii A, Schuppan O, Amor A, Kaloutsi V. Histologic findings in bone marrow biopsies of patients with thrombocythemic cell counts. Ann Hematol 1992;64:286-91.

147. Buss DH, O'Connor ML, Woodruff RD, Richards F 2nd, Brockschmidt JK. Bone marrow and peripheral blood findings in patients with extreme thrombocytosis. A report of 63 cases. Arch Pathol Lab Med 1991;115:475-80.

148. Dame C, Sutor AH. Primary and secondary thrombocytosis in childhood. Br J Haematol 2005;129:165-77.

149. Ding J, Komatsu H, Wakita A, et al. Familial essential thrombocythemia associated with a dominant-positive activating mutation of the c-MPL gene, which encodes for the receptor for thrombopoietin. Blood 2004;103:4198-200.

150. Folman CC, Ooms M, Kuenen BB, et al. The role of thrombopoietin in post-operative thrombocytosis. Br J Haematol 2001;114:126-33.

151. Grumbeck E, Aiginger P, Gisslinger B, Geissler K, Thalhammer-Scherrer R, Gisslinger H. Macrocytic anemia and thrombocytosis associated with thymoma: a case report. Am J Hematol 2000;63:38-41.

152. Ishiguro A, Suzuki Y, Mito M, et al. Elevation of serum thrombopoietin precedes thrombocytosis in acute infections. Br J Haematol 2002;116:612-8.

153. Kondo T, Okabe M, Sanada M, et al. Familial essential thrombocythemia associated with one-base deletion in the 5'-untranslated region of the thrombopoietin gene. Blood 1998;92:1091-6.

154. Sasaki Y, Takahashi T, Miyazaki H, et al. Production of thrombopoietin by human carcinomas and its novel isoforms. Blood 1999;94:1952-60.

155. Schafer AI. Thrombocytosis. N Engl J Med 2004;350:1211-9.

156. Stuhrmann M, Bashawri L, Ahmed MA, et al. Familial thrombocytosis as a recessive, possibly X-linked trait in an Arab family. Br J Haematol 2001;112:616-20.

157. Tefferi A, Silverstein MN, Hoagland HC. Primary thrombocythemia. Semin Oncol 1995;22:334-40.

158. Wiestner A, Padosch SA, Ghilardi N, et al. Hereditary thrombocythaemia is a genetically heterogeneous disorder: exclusion of TPO and MPL in two families with hereditary thrombocythaemia. Br J Haematol 2000;110:104-9.

159. Wiestner A, Schlemper RJ, van der Maas AP, Skoda RC. An activating splice donor mutation in the thrombopoietin gene causes hereditary thrombocythaemia. Nat Genet 1998;18:49-52.

Megakaryocytic Abnormalities in Infectious and Noninfectious Systemic Diseases

160. Bauer S, Khan A, Klein A, Starasoler L. Naked megakaryocyte nuclei as an indicator of human immunodeficiency virus infection. Arch Pathol Lab Med 1992;116:1025-9.

161. Groet J, McElwaine S, Spinelli M, et al. Acquired mutations in GATA1 in neonates with Down's syndrome with transient myeloid disorder. Lancet 2003;361:1617-20.

162. Hatfill SJ, Fester ED, Steytler JG. Apoptotic megakaryocyte dysplasia in the myelodysplastic syndromes. Hematol Pathol 1992;6:87-93.

163. Katsumata Y, Suzuki T, Kuwana M, et al. Anti-c-Mpl (thrombopoietin receptor) autoantibody-induced amegakaryocytic thrombocytopenia in a patient with systemic sclerosis. Arthritis Rheum 2003;48:1647-51.

164. Lorsbach RB. Megakaryoblastic disorders in children. Am J Clin Pathol 2004;122(Suppl): S33-46.

165. Nagasawa T, Sakurai T, Kashiwagi H, Abe T. Cell-mediated amegakaryocytic thrombocytopenia associated with systemic lupus erythematosus. Blood 1986;67:479-83.

166. Pullarkat V, Bass RD, Gong JZ, Feinstein DI, Brynes RK. Primary autoimmune myelofibrosis: definition of a distinct clinicopathologic syndrome. Am J Hematol 2003;72:8-12.

167. Rainis L, Bercovich D, Strehl S, et al. Mutations in exon 2 of GATA1 are early events in megakaryocytic malignancies associated with trisomy 21. Blood 2003;102:981-6.

168. Xu G, Nagano M, Kanezaki R, et al. Frequent mutations in the GATA-1 gene in the transient myeloproliferative disorder of Down syndrome. Blood 2003;102:2960-8.

169. Zipursky A. Transient leukaemia—a benign form of leukaemia in newborn infants with trisomy 21. Br J Haematol 2003;120:930-8.

170. Zucker-Franklin D. The effect of viral infections on platelets and megakaryocytes. Semin Hematol 1994;31:329-37.

Therapy-Related Megakaryocytic Abnormalities

171. Basser RL, O'Flaherty E, Green M, et al. Development of pancytopenia with neutralizing antibodies to thrombopoietin after multi-cycle chemotherapy supported by megakaryocyte growth and development factor. Blood 2002;99:2599-602.

172. Douglas VK, Tallman MS, Cripe LD, Peterson LC. Thrombopoietin administered during induction chemotherapy to patients with acute myeloid leukemia induces transient morphologic changes that may resemble chronic myeloproliferative disorders. Am J Clin Pathol 2002;117:844-50.

173. Gesundheit B, Kirby M, Lau W, Koren G, Abdelhaleem M. Thrombocytopenia and megakaryocyte dysplasia: an adverse effect of valproic acid treatment. J Pediatr Hematol Oncol 2002;24:589-90.

174. Li J, Yang C, Xia Y, et al. Thrombocytopenia caused by the development of antibodies to thrombopoietin. Blood 2001;98:3241-8.

175. Rosenthal NS, Farhi DC. Dysmegakaryopoiesis resembling acute megakaryoblastic leukemia in treated acute myeloid leukemia. Am J Clin Pathol 1991;95:556-60.

Differential Diagnosis of Non-Neoplastic Megakaryocytic Disorders

176. Foucar K. Reactive and neoplastic disorders of megakaryocytes. In: Bone marrow pathology. Chicago: ASCP Press; 2001:324-43.

177. Wang C, Amato D. Megakaryocyte-like giant myeloma cells. Am J Hematol 2004;77:311-2.

7 BONE MARROW FAILURE DISORDERS

GENERAL CONCEPTS

The term "bone marrow failure" encompasses a large spectrum of diseases that is broadly divided into disorders affecting predominantly single lineage hematopoiesis versus those affecting multiple lineages. These entities can be further subcategorized as congenital or acquired (Table 7-1) (1,2). Although some disorders considered as single lineage production failures (e.g., Diamond-Blackfan anemia, Shwachman-Diamond syndrome) may eventuate in more extensive bone marrow hypoplasia and pancytopenia, this general framework for classification is clinically useful when evaluating a patient for possible bone marrow failure.

The diagnostic approach to a suspected marrow failure syndrome requires consideration of several important aspects, especially in children, to assess the likelihood of an underlying constitutional syndrome. Congenital disorders are diagnosed by a combination of dysmorphic or other physical anomalies, early onset of abnormal blood and bone marrow findings, positive family history suggesting a specific ethnic association or pattern of inheritance, and increasingly, the results of specialized genetic investigations (Table 7-2). Although germline disease-specific molecular genetic mutations are becoming better characterized for many constitutional bone marrow failure syndromes, a comprehensive molecular classification remains incomplete due to the variability in disease phenotypes, the complex pathophysiology, and the as yet unknown causative genetic aberrations in many patients.

National and international groups have evolved to document the incidence, features, and variations of the major congenital bone marrow disorders in order to facilitate research and to provide support and counseling for

---

Table 7-1

CATEGORIZATION OF BONE MARROW PRODUCTION DISORDERS

Constitutional Disorders Affecting Multilineage Hematopoiesis	Constitutional Disorders Affecting Predominantly Single Lineage Hematopoiesis[a]	Acquired Disorders Affecting Multilineage Hematopoiesis	Acquired Disorders Affecting Predominantly Single Lineage Hematopoiesis
Fanconi anemia	Diamond-Blackfan anemia[b]	Idiopathic aplastic anemia	Iron deficiency anemia
Dyskeratosis congenita	Congenital dyserythropoietic anemias	Paroxysmal nocturnal hemoglobinuria	Anemia of chronic disease
Familial aplastic anemias	Congenital sideroblastic anemias	Nutritional deficiency (e.g., vitamin B_{12}/folate)	Transient erythroblastopenia of childhood
Congenital amegakaryocytic thrombocytopenia	Shwachman-Diamond syndrome[b]	Idiosyncratic drug or toxin effects	Pure red cell aplasia associated with thymoma
Pearson syndrome	Severe congenital neutropenia/Kostmann syndrome	Viral infections (e.g., (hepatitis, HIV[c])	Neutropenia or red cell aplasia associated with chronic T-cell large granular lymphocyte leukemia
Familial hemophagocytic lymphohistiocytosis	Cyclic neutropenia		Idiosyncratic drug or toxin effects
Metabolic storage disorders	Thrombocytopenia with absent radii		Viral infections (e.g., parvovirus B19)
Osteopetrosis			

[a]Single lineage disorders are also included in respective lineage chapters.
[b]Can progress to multilineage cytopenias and bone marrow failure in subsets of patients.
[c]HIV = human immunodeficiency virus.

Table 7-2

COMPARISON OF MAJOR CONGENITAL BONE MARROW FAILURE DISORDERS

Disorder	Incidence	Inheritance Pattern	Physical Abnormalities	Typical Age at Presentation	Hematologic Findings	Genetic Basis	Treatment	Outcome
Fanconi anemia	Very rare	AR[a]	Facial dysmorphism, upper limb/hand anomalies, visceral organ defects; 1/3 may not show physical findings	Most in first decade (median 8 years)	Progressive pancytopenia; marrow hypoplasia/aplasia	Mutations in *FANC* genes; defects in DNA repair and genome integrity; hallmark feature is chromosome breakage on exposure to clastogenic agents (e.g., diepoxybutane)	Androgens, hematopoietic growth factors, transfusions; HSCT in selected patients	Median survival ~30 years; death due to marrow failure; longer survivors have increased risk for MDS, AML, and solid tumors
Dyskeratosis congenita	Very rare	X-linked; AR and AD less common	Classic triad of skin hyperpigmentation, dystrophic nails, and leukoplakia; other anomalies described	~50% develop aplastic anemia similar to FA by second decade (median 16 years)	Progressive pancytopenia; marrow hypoplasia/aplasia	X-linked form has mutations in dyskerin (*DKC1*) on Xq28; AD form has mutations in *TERC* (*DKC2*); genetic basis for many others with AR, sporadic occurrence and some AD not known	Androgens, hematopoietic growth factors; transfusions; HSCT in selected patients	Median survival ~30 years for X-linked and AR; AD has significantly longer survival; increased risk mainly for solid tumors
Congenital amegakaryocytic thrombocytopenia	Very rare	AR	2/3 patients lack anomalies; 1/3 with various malformations	Infancy (<6 months)	Decreased platelets; marked decrease in megakaryocytes; pancytopenia with marrow aplasia in nearly 50%	*c-MPL* gene mutations (receptor for thrombopoietin) in patients without physical anomalies	Hematopoietic growth factors, HSCT	Median survival <10 years
Diamond-Blackfan anemia	Rare	AD and AR described, but most are sporadic de novo mutations	Minority of patients with upper limb deficits, other skeletal anomalies, short stature or eye abnormalities	Infancy (<6 months)	Progressive macrocytic anemia, increased red cell ADA, reticulocytopenia; marrow erythroid hyperplasia	Mutations in *RPS19* on 19(q13.2) in 25%; second subset of patients have linkage to 8(p23.2-p22); other gene loci implicated	Red cell transfusion, steroids, possibly HSCT	Median survival 40-50 years; small increased risk of cancer; spontaneous remission in 20-25%
Shwachman-Diamond syndrome	Very rare	AR	~50% with short stature, metaphyseal dysostosis; exocrine pancreatic insufficiency	Infancy (<1 year)	Predominantly progressive neutropenia, but ~40% have other cytopenias; myeloid hypoplasia with left-shifted "maturation arrest"	Mutations in *SBDS* gene on 7(q11)	Androgens, G-CSF; HSCT	Median survival of 35 years, increased risk of AML and MDS

Table 7-2 (continued)

Disorder	Incidence	Inheritance Pattern	Physical Abnormalities	Age at Presentation	Hematologic Findings	Genetic Basis	Treatment	Outcome
Severe congenital neutropenia (Kostmann syndrome)	Very rare	Most are AD and sporadic; rare AR families	None	Infancy (<6 months)	Severe early onset neutropenia with infections; marked granulocytic hypoplasia in marrow with only immature forms present	Mutations in ELA2 gene encoding neutrophil elastase[b]	Antibiotics; G-CSF	Median survival ~20-25 years; some increased risk of AML[c]
Thrombocytopenia with absent radii (TAR)	Very rare	AR	Absent radii with preservation of thumbs; other skeletal anomalies (hands, lower extremity) and small % cardiac defects	Infancy (<1 month)	Severe thrombocytopenia in perinatal or newborn period; few immature or absent marrow megakaryocytes	Unknown (no abnormalities of c-MPL)	Supportive (e.g., platelet transfusions)	Risk of bleeding decreases over first year of life with spontaneous recovery in majority of patients; median survival >50 years

[a]AR = autosomal recessive inheritance; AD = autosomal dominant inheritance; HSCT = hematopoietic stem cell transplant; G-CSF = granulocyte colony-stimulating factor therapy; MDS = myelodysplastic syndrome; AML = acute myeloid leukemia; ADA = adenosine deaminase, FA = Fanconi anemia.
[b]ELA2 is also mutated in cyclic neutropenia, but in a different region of the gene.
[c]Currently unclear if AML risk is a primary (intrinsic) predisposition, effect of prolonged G-CSF, or both.

affected individuals and their families (1,2). Significantly, the study of these rare congenital bone marrow failure syndromes has provided remarkable insights concerning normal cell and molecular biology and has helped to illuminate the genetic and biochemical derangements present in some types of sporadically occurring hematologic malignancies.

Some features of bone marrow failure disorders are noteworthy: 1) Although peripheral blood changes may be present (e.g., red blood cell [RBC] macrocytosis, abnormal neutrophil morphology), circulating cells are often qualitatively unremarkable. 2) Many congenital bone marrow failure syndromes (and also some of the acquired multilineage disorders) are associated with an increased risk of developing acute leukemia or other types of cancer. 3) While telltale dysmorphism or other physical anomalies associated with congenital syndromes may be present at birth or in early infancy, many patients lack such features; these patients may present in later years with progressive cytopenias and bone marrow failure thought to be due to myelodysplasia or "idiopathic" aplastic anemia. Given the variable genetic expressivity or phenotypic penetrance in some types of inherited bone marrow failure disorders, an unexpected presentation of a congenital syndrome should be considered in young adults with unexplained cytopenias or certain malignancies.

This chapter summarizes the constitutional syndromes of bone marrow failure and the major forms of acquired bone marrow failure. Several other congenital and acquired disorders resulting in single or multiple cytopenias, with otherwise relatively intact bone marrow hematopoiesis, are covered in detail in chapters 4, 5, and 6.

CONSTITUTIONAL DISORDERS AFFECTING MULTILINEAGE HEMATOPOIESIS

Fanconi Anemia

Definition. *Fanconi anemia* (FA) is a rare autosomal recessive disorder with an incidence approximating $1/10^6$, although the exact incidence is difficult to precisely determine. The disease occurs in many ethnic groups and the frequency of heterozygote carriers is about 1/300 individuals in Western countries. Specific ethnic subgroups, such as Ashkenazi Jews, are known

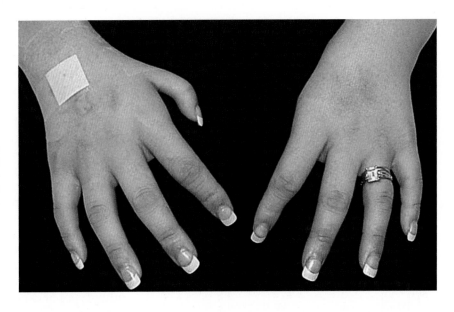

Figure 7-1

HANDS IN PATIENT WITH FANCONI ANEMIA

There is left thumb aplasia and rudimentary development of the right thumb. Finger development and proportion also appear abnormal. (Courtesy Dr. C. Clericuzio, Albuquerque, NM.)

to harbor founder mutations. FA is characterized by a combination of physical anomalies and the development of progressive bone marrow failure (3,29); these patients also have an increased risk of developing several types of malignant neoplasms (see Table 7-2) (19,25).

Clinical Features. The median age at diagnosis is the latter half of the first decade for both males and females, although infants are also rarely affected. The classic physical abnormalities include facial dysmorphism (hypertelorism, microcephaly), upper limb anomalies (absent radii and thumbs) (fig. 7-1), short stature, skin abnormalities (café au lait spots, other pigmentation anomalies), and visceral organ defects (renal, genitourinary, gastrointestinal, or cardiac malformations) (3,29). The presence of physical anomalies correlates with the early development of hematopoietic compromise. Nearly one third of patients, however, have been described as being physically normal and the first indication of FA is the development of progressive cytopenias and bone marrow failure (3). Due to incompletely understood variability in disease expression, occasional patients are identified beyond the childhood period, suggesting that FA should be included in the differential diagnosis of apparently idiopathic presentations of aplastic anemia in adolescents and young adults. The predisposition to bone marrow hypoplasia can be exacerbated by environmental factors or exposures (e.g., idiosyncratic drug reactions, viral infections).

Pathologic Findings. The hematologic changes in FA typically begin with thrombocytopenia and/or leukopenia, with progression to pancytopenia as the bone marrow failure becomes more established. RBCs are often macrocytic, and fetal hemoglobin (HgbF) is increased in a heterocellular distribution. The bone marrow examination reveals variable hypoplasia or aplasia of hematopoietic lineages, depending on the timing of the biopsy and the degree of the bone marrow failure (fig. 7-2). At the extremes of clinical manifestation, patients may initially present with severe pancytopenia, myelodysplasia, acute myeloid leukemia, or epithelial cancer (23).

Pathogenesis. The molecular pathogenesis of FA is complex, but increasingly better understood (3,4,7,28,34a). Currently, 12 putative abnormal proteins in FA have been elucidated, mainly through cell-fusion complementation studies. Of these, 11 corresponding disease-related genes have been identified: *FANCA, FANCB, FANCC, FANCD1* (now known to be *BRCA2*), *FANCD2, FANCE, FANCF, FANCG, FANCJ* (recognized as *BRCA1*-interacting DNA helicase, *BRIP-1*), *FANCL,* and *FANCM*. The remaining complementation group, FA-I, is implicated in a small number of FA patients, but the corresponding gene and protein product are less well characterized (34a). Of the known genes, *FANCA* is the most commonly mutated, followed by *FANCC* and *FANCG*; the other FA-associated genes are less frequently involved.

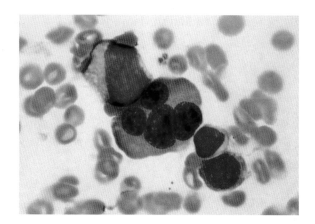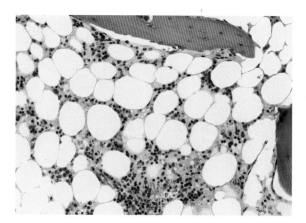

Figure 7-2

FANCONI ANEMIA

Left: Hypocellular bone marrow aspirate smear shows a dyspoietic multinucleated erythroid precursor (Wright stain).
Right: Core biopsy section in a patient with advanced Fanconi anemia (FA). The bone marrow space is markedly hypocellular. The remaining cellular elements are constituted predominantly by erythroid precursors, small lymphocytes, and plasma cells (hematoxylin and eosin [H&E] stain).

Molecular Findings. Several genotype-phenotype correlations have been noted among the FA complementation groups, as determined by analyses of large patient series. Patients with the *FANCC* gene exhibit a lower incidence of physical abnormalities overall, except for a subset in Ashkenazi Jews with a founder mutation (IVS4+4→T) associated with multiple birth defects. Certain *FANCC* mutations predispose to early onset bone marrow failure and poorer overall survival (19). Patients with *FANCG* mutations or homozygous *FANCA* "null" mutations tend to have more severe cytopenias and a higher incidence of acute myeloid leukemia (AML) (11,29). Biallelic *FANCD1* (*BRCA2*) mutations produce a possibly distinct FA presentation with early onset of AML, as well as an association with brain tumors and Wilms tumor (24). Individuals who carry heterozygous germline *BRCA2* mutations do not develop FA, but are susceptible to hereditary breast and ovarian cancer syndrome in early to middle adulthood.

The FA-associated genes cloned to date have been mapped to various chromosomal sites and are not significantly homologous. Although the nature of these gene products is diverse, they produce similar clinical and phenotypic features in patients with defective FA complementation groups, implying that these proteins interact in a common biochemical pathway. The normal FA system cooperates with additional proteins (e.g.,

Atm, Atr, Nbs1, BRCA1) to detect and facilitate repair of damaged DNA (7,25a,28,29,34b). Moreover, the FANCD2 and Nbs1 proteins are critical elements in the normal cellular response to DNA damage from chemotoxic agents and ionizing radiation.

The FA protein family is also linked to the BRCA-mediated response to DNA damage both directly (since FANCD1 is in fact BRCA2), and through other protein-protein interactions in this pathway (7,31). The salient features of the FA protein system and its relationship to other DNA repair proteins are depicted schematically in figure 7-3. In contrast, cells from FA patients are highly sensitized to chemotoxic DNA cross-linking agents, such as mitomycin-C, and display variable hypersensitivity to ionizing radiation-induced damage; BRCA-, Nbs1-, and Atm-deficient cells (characteristic of hereditary breast cancer, Nijmegen breakage syndrome, and ataxia-telangiectasia, respectively) also share overlapping features with the FA cellular phenotypes. A major cell physiologic function of the FA protein system is, therefore, the maintenance of genome stability via interactions with DNA damage sensor and repair systems; as such, the normal FA proteins can be considered to be part of the general group of "caretaker" gene products subserving the maintenance of DNA integrity (20). Defective FA proteins in the marrow stem and progenitor cells of affected

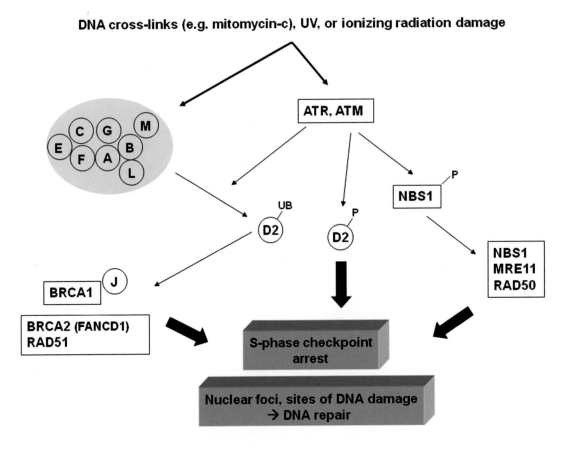

DNA cross-links (e.g. mitomycin-c), UV, or ionizing radiation damage

Figure 7-3

THE NORMAL FANCONI ANEMIA PROTEIN FAMILY AND FUNCTIONAL INTERACTIONS

This diagram represents a broad overview of the major functional responses and interactions of the FA protein family. Although 12 members of the FA protein system are recognized, currently 11 have identified genes and proteins, as shown in this illustration. FA gene products are depicted as capitalized letters within circles, except for FANCD1, which is also known as the DNA repair protein BRCA2.

The upstream "core" complex of FA proteins (shown in the large gray disc), functions as a ubiquitin ligase serving to monoubiquitinate FANCD2. Activated FANCD2 colocalizes in nuclear foci, with DNA repair proteins mediating homologous recombination, including BRCA1, BARD1, BRCA2 (FANCD1), and RAD51. FANCJ (also known as BRIP-1) interacts directly with BRCA1. The ataxia-telangiectasia mutated (ATM)-related protein ATR also appears to have a function in promoting FANCD2 ubiquitination. Ionizing radiation–induced DNA damage mainly invokes the ATM protein sensor, which results in activation of the NBS1 damage response pathway. Nonetheless, proper function of the NBS1-MRE11-RAD50 DNA repair axis apparently requires an intact FA core complex. Together, these protein responses induce S-phase arrest and promote repair of damaged DNA. The normal FA protein system thus serves to maintain DNA integrity, in conjunction with a number of additional interacting proteins.

patients thereby produce a state of genomic instability, ultimately resulting in ineffective intramedullary hematopoiesis, cell death by apoptosis, and progressive bone marrow failure. This abnormal cellular background is also thought to underlie the predisposition to malignancies later in life.

Chromosome breakage analysis, which is based upon the hypersensitivity of FA cells to DNA damaging agents, is the key initial diagnostic study for patients with suspected FA. While spontaneous chromosome fragility of FA cells is uncommonly observed in standard cytogenetic cell preparations, bone marrow cells stimulated by a mitogenic factor like phytohemagglutinin and cultured in the presence of so-called clastogenic agents (e.g., mitomycin-C or diepoxybutane) readily reveal chromosomal breakage, including radial chromosome forms and other abnormal interchromatid exchanges (fig. 7-4). In some

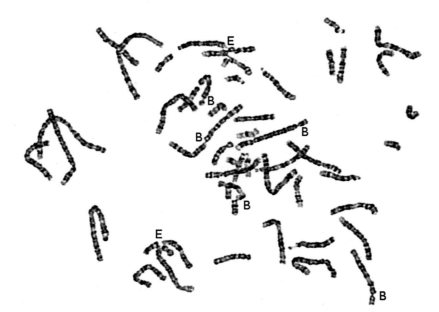

Figure 7-4

SPONTANEOUS CHROMOSOME BREAKAGE IN FANCONI ANEMIA

Metaphase preparations of chromosomes in FA may demonstrate spontaneous chromosome breakage; however, this phenomenon is significantly enhanced by exposure of the cells of the patient to so-called clastogenic agents, such as diepoxybutane (DEB) or mitomycin-C. In this example, a DEB-treated metaphase cell from a patient with FA is shown. Chromosome/chromatid breaks are identified by the letter "B," while atypical non-homologous chromatid exchange figures are identified by the letter "E." (Courtesy Dr. J. Mascarello, Santa Fe, NM and S. Haines MT-ASCP, Albuquerque, NM.)

cases, skin fibroblast cultures may be required to demonstrate this phenomenon.

Additional laboratory assays to determine specific FA gene mutations have been described. Point mutations in FA genes have been documented in many patients, although the individual genes are generally large and direct DNA sequencing may not be practical. In addition, unusual genetic lesions that occur in a minority of FA individuals, such as somatic cell mosaicism or large genomic deletions, can produce false negative or erroneous results by sequencing analysis. Functional molecular diagnostic approaches have been developed in the research setting to better delineate disease genotypes, including in vitro complementation of FA cells using retroviral constructs harboring specific FA gene products (14,26), immunoblotting for FANCD2 protein ubiquitination status (27), and denaturing high performance liquid chromatography (D-HPLC) analysis.

Treatment and Prognosis. The management of FA patients begins with the pharmacologic stimulation of flagging hematopoiesis with androgens (e.g., oxymetholone), either with or without hematopoietic growth factors (3,27). Allogeneic hematopoietic stem cell transplantation (HSCT) is currently considered definitive therapy; however, FA patients are at risk for significant clinical complications and HSCT may not be possible for patients lacking a matched human leukocyte antigen (HLA) donor. The advent of nonmyeloablative "minitransplants" may be of benefit in some patients. The long-term outcome for FA patients is unfavorable and many die in childhood or adolescence from complications of bone marrow failure or malignancies (primarily AML). Even patients with successful HSCT continue to have a high risk for developing solid tumors, often in the head and neck region.

Dyskeratosis Congenita

Definition. *Dyskeratosis congenita* (DC) is a rare inherited bone marrow failure syndrome characterized by the triad of cutaneous hyperpigmentation, dystrophic nails, and mucosal leukoplakia (see Table 7-2). A relatively large proportion of patients with DC develop pancytopenia due to progressive bone marrow failure and these patients also have an increased risk of developing cancer (3,5,8). The clinical presentation and severity in DC is determined by the nature of the specific genetic mutation. A subset of male patients have an X-linked recessive inheritance; additionally, autosomal recessive, autosomal dominant, and sporadic occurrences are described and affect both sexes. A particularly severe form of X-linked DC, known as *Hoyeraal-Hreidarsson syndrome*, is characterized by early bone marrow aplasia, microcephaly, mental and growth retardation, and cerebellar hypoplasia (8).

Clinical Features. The median age at diagnosis is typically in the teenage years, although the autosomal dominant form often manifests during the 3rd decade of life. Skin changes are nearly uniform among the genetic types of DC and involve the head and neck region, shoulders, and trunk as a reticulated hyperpigmentation. The presence of nail dystrophy and mucosal leukoplakia is seen mostly in the X-linked and autosomal recessive types of DC. Other common physical findings include ocular abnormalities (blocked tear ducts), dental caries, and visceral organ anomalies (e.g., esophageal webs, genitourinary defects) (3). A significant minority of DC patients develop an unusual restrictive type of pulmonary disorder.

Pathologic Findings. Progressive bone marrow failure resulting in blood cytopenias is the hallmark hematologic finding. Entities in the differential diagnosis with this hematologic finding are other familial syndromes such as FA; conversely, the hematologic features may be the first presentation of DC if physical signs are subtle or absent. Bone marrow failure affects approximately one third of X-linked and 60 percent of autosomal recessive type DC patients before adulthood (5). Hematologic findings in DC typically manifest as worsening anemia and/or thrombocytopenia, followed by pancytopenia. RBCs may be macrocytic, and HgbF is increased. The bone marrow usually shows a compensatory hypercellularity early on, but then becomes gradually and progressively more severely hypocellular.

Molecular Findings. The X-linked form of DC involves the *DKC1* gene, which has been mapped to chromosome band Xq28 (8,9,15,21). *DKC1* encodes a 58-kDa ribonucleoprotein termed dyskerin, thought to be involved in ribosomal assembly; however, dyskerin is also associated with the RNA template for telomerase (TERC), and so may also be involved in the process of normal chromosomal telomere maintenance. Significantly, the gene implicated in many individuals with the autosomal dominant pattern of DC is, in fact, *TERC* (also known as *DKC2*) (32). The latter patients actually have haplo-insufficiency for TERC due to heterozygous allelic mutations, and tend to have less severe disease, which may not be identified until later in life. In addition, patients with the autosomal dominant type DC display the phenomenon of "disease anticipation" in which successive generations of a DC kindred experience earlier onset of symptoms (33). In many other families with DC, including most of those with autosomal recessive inheritance and those sporadically affected, the underlying genetic associations remain unknown (34).

In classic DC, shortened chromosomal telomeres are thought to result in the genetic instability that leads to progressive bone marrow failure and a predisposition to the development of malignancies (21,22). However, the clinical spectrum of telomere maintenance gene abnormalities now appears broader with the discovery that a small number of patients with apparently acquired aplastic anemia in adulthood have mutations in either *TERC* (12), or in the gene encoding telomerase itself, i.e., *TERT* (35), but lack the clinical features of DC. These rare mutations are present in the germline of affected patients and can also be found in family members who do not have hematologic disease or features of DC. These observations indicate that classic DC and small subsets of apparent idiopathic and familial aplastic anemia may best be considered as disorders of defective telomere maintenance, with genotypic effects and variable disease penetrance underlying the differences in onset and clinical severity among patients.

The diagnosis of DC should be considered in children, but also in adults with unexplained bone marrow hypoplasia or aplasia. Diagnostic suspicion is particularly heightened in those individuals who show components of the classic triad of cutaneous, nail, and mucosal abnormalities, and particularly when an X-linked or dominant pattern of familial bone marrow failure syndrome can be demonstrated. The results of chromosome breakage studies are normal, serving to distinguish DC from FA. The molecular confirmation of X-linked and autosomal dominant type DC includes sequencing of genomic DNA for mutations in *DKC1* (15 exons) and *TERC* (primarily first exon), respectively (5). Point mutation abnormalities are most common and may include missense single base substitutions or splice site changes. A recent study revealed that combined flow cytometry and fluorescence in situ hybridization analysis for very short telomeres in peripheral blood lymphocytes helps identify individuals suspected to have DC (3a).

Treatment and Prognosis. The management of patients with DC involves hematologic support with blood products as needed for cytopenias (3,5,8). Androgen therapy to stimulate bone marrow production has achieved success in some patients, along with administration of granulocyte-monocyte–colony-stimulating factor (GM-CSF) or granulocyte (G)-CSF for severe neutropenia. HSCT has been attempted, but the morbidity and mortality of this approach can be unpredictable for these patients. Over two thirds of DC patients die from the effects of bone marrow failure at an early age (median, 20 to 25 years). Those surviving longer, with a less severe disease phenotype, have an increased risk of cancer, with 10 to 15 percent developing carcinomas and a smaller number developing myelodysplasia.

Familial Aplastic Anemias

Rare hereditary bone marrow failure syndromes are recognized that do not conform to the current definitions of FA, DC, or other recognized disorders (3). These disorders may be autosomal dominant, autosomal recessive, or X-linked, and may be associated with various physical manifestations (e.g., skeletal anomalies) and an increased risk of hematologic malignancies. Immunodeficiency may also be an accompanying manifestation. The severity and expression of these *familial aplastic anemias* can be variable, with cytopenias and bone marrow failure occurring in childhood or into adulthood. The hematologic findings include RBC macrocytosis, progressive pancytopenia, and eventual bone marrow aplasia. The genetic basis of these variant syndromes is not well known, but an abnormal karyotype may be present.

The diagnosis of a familial aplastic anemia is based on the presence of a family history of bone marrow failure and negative chromosome breakage studies. Physical anomalies (if present), documentation of immunodeficiency, and a nonrandom bone marrow cytogenetic abnormality are additional supportive features and may help distinguish a familial syndrome from idiopathic or secondary aplastic anemia. The treatment is mainly supportive and most individuals succumb to the effects of bone marrow failure at an early age. As noted in the discussion of DC, a small subset of familial aplastic anemias (and some sporadically occurring bone marrow aplasias) involve genetic lesions in components of the telomerase complex, suggesting that these cases may constitute a spectrum of a distinct bone marrow failure predisposition with variable clinical features.

Congenital Amegakaryocytic Thrombocytopenia

Definition. While most heritable platelet disorders are seldom associated with additional cytopenias or a significant bone marrow production deficiency (10), rare syndromes of multilineage hematopoietic and primary megakaryocytic marrow failure are recognized. *Congenital amegakaryocytic thrombocytopenia* (CAT) is a hereditary autosomal recessive cause of infant or early childhood thrombocytopenia, associated with reduced and abnormal megakaryocytes (see Table 7-2). The syndrome may or may not be associated with congenital anomalies (a feature of significant distinction) and eventually leads to pancytopenia and complete trilineage bone marrow failure in nearly half of the patients (3). The diagnosis of CAT requires the exclusion of neonatal alloimmune thrombocytopenia, immune-mediated thrombocytopenia (ITP), and other congenital syndromes, including FA, DC, and thrombocytopenia with absent radii (TAR, discussed below) (see chapter 6).

Clinical Features. Patients with CAT are typically identified in the neonatal period or in infancy as a result of marked thrombocytopenia, often producing skin ecchymoses, or mucosal and gastrointestinal tract bleeding. Most patients lack congenital physical anomalies; however, a smaller number have such findings, including microcephaly, micrognathia, intracranial malformations, low birth weight, congenital heart disease, or failure to thrive.

Pathologic Findings. Laboratory findings confirm a low platelet count, with qualitatively unremarkable morphology. RBCs may be macrocytic with increased HgbF. The bone marrow examination shows normal cellularity and decreased to nearly absent megakaryocytes, which are small and atypical. Many patients go on to develop pancytopenia from multilineage bone marrow failure; this occurs mainly in the subset lacking congenital anomalies.

Molecular Findings. The genetic basis for CAT without physical anomalies has been traced to mutations in the *c-MPL* gene at chromosome 1q34, which encodes the receptor for the megakaryocyte growth factor, thrombopoietin (6,17,30). Mutations occur in a homozygous (biallelic) manner, consistent with the autosomal recessive manner of inheritance. The genetic basis for the subgroup of patients with thrombocytopenic presentations and abnormal physical features is presently unknown, although the inheritance pattern is also recessive.

Differential Diagnosis. The diagnosis of CAT should be suspected in neonates and infants who present with bleeding and/or severe thrombocytopenia. Although a positive family history may be present, bone marrow examination is required to reveal the marked reduction in megakaryocytes. Exclusion of causes of peripheral platelet destruction and other syndromic disorders characterized by early onset thrombocytopenia (e.g., TAR) are required. Chromosome breakage studies are normal in CAT. Confirmatory analysis involves the detection of c-*MPL* gene mutations by polymerase chain reaction (PCR) and DNA sequencing or related methods.

Treatment and Prognosis. The management of patients with CAT is largely supportive in the form of platelet transfusions. HSCT has shown promise in a small number of patients. The overall outlook for CAT patients lacking physical anomalies is nonetheless poor, with most individuals progressing to worsening pancytopenia and death due to bone marrow failure. Malignant disease complications are rare. The median survival period is about 9 years, but children with CAT and associated congenital anomalies have an even shorter survival period (about 3 years).

Other Congenital Disorders Associated with Multilineage Hematopoietic Failure

Several additional complex congenital disorders are associated with peripheral cytopenias and may eventuate in bone marrow failure.

Pearson Syndrome. *Pearson syndrome* (see also chapter 4) consists of inherited sideroblastic anemia with vacuolated bone marrow precursors, exocrine pancreatic insufficiency, and metabolic acidosis (3). Although sideroblastic anemia is the major hematologic manifestation, approximately half of the patients develop moderate neutropenia and thrombocytopenia. Patients typically present in infancy with anemia; however, hematologic manifestations are

generally not severe. In addition to pancreatic disease and metabolic acidosis, complications include organ failure and heart disease. The bone marrow pathology is remarkable for increased sideroblasts (including many ringed sideroblasts); the granulocytic and erythroid precursors also show cytoplasmic vacuoles.

Pearson syndrome is best considered a congenital form of anemia with an abnormal RBC iron distribution, and it is recognized as a mitochondrial DNA (mtDNA) disorder. Specifically, large deletions of maternally derived mtDNA are thought to affect cellular oxidative phosphorylation and metabolism, although affected individuals actually have variable subsets of cells with both normal and deleted mtDNA. The diagnosis is established in an infant or young child with sideroblastic anemia and vacuolated bone marrow precursors, along with other key features such as pancreatic exocrine insufficiency, acidosis, renal tubular disease, and liver disease. Genetic testing for mtDNA deletions can provide confirmation of the diagnosis.

The treatment is supportive and includes blood transfusions, administration of hematopoietic growth factors, and correction of the acidosis. Spontaneous amelioration of hemoglobin levels occurs in most patients; this clinical improvement may be related to the emergence of expanded subsets of progenitor cells with a normal complement of mtDNA over time.

Familial Hemophagocytic Lymphohistiocytosis. *Familial hemophagocytic lymphohistiocytosis* (FHL) is a rare disorder of presumed autosomal recessive inheritance, characterized by high fever, hepatosplenomegaly, pancytopenia, and marked bone marrow hemophagocytosis (see chapter 9) (18). Additional clinical features include central nervous system involvement with seizures or cranial nerve palsies, and various laboratory abnormalities (e.g., elevated liver enzymes). This disease occurs in infancy or early childhood, and if untreated, carries a very high rate of mortality. FHL must be distinguished from secondary or acquired infection-associated hemophagocytosis, which occurs over a wider age range. Tissue infiltration by T cells and macrophages is a prominent histologic finding. The exuberant hemophagocytosis in the bone marrow leads to hematopoietic production failure through increased intramedullary destruction.

The genetic basis for FHL has been resolved, in part (16,18), and involves mutations in the perforin gene (*PRF1*) on chromosome 10(q21-q22) in 20 to 40 percent of cases (known as FHL type 2). Another 10 percent of individuals with FHL have a lesion mapping to a second genetic locus on chromosome 9(q21-q22) (FHL type 1). Slightly more than half of the patients have undetermined genetic alterations, although mutations in other immune/inflammatory mediator genes are emerging. Defects in perforin production in type 2 FHL cause impaired cytotoxic T-cell and natural killer (NK)-cell function in the setting of infection. The resultant deregulation of cellular immunity leads to the accumulation of T cells and numerous phagocytic histiocytes, with the ensuing destruction of bone marrow cells.

FHL can be considered a type of immune deficiency disease characterized by defective apoptosis (13), and thus shares pathogenetic similarities to autoimmune lymphoproliferative syndrome. The treatment includes administration of appropriate antimicrobial agents; however, management of the abnormal immune response with epipodophyllotoxins and steroids is required or the disease is eventually fatal. HSCT may be curative and potentially prolong survival.

Osteopetrosis. *Osteopetrosis* is a rare disease with a variable inheritance pattern and clinical severity (see chapter 9) (3). The more severe infantile and intermediate variants are autosomal recessive (often associated with consanguinity), whereas an autosomal dominant form is associated with less pronounced disease and essentially no hematologic abnormalities.

The manifestations of aggressive osteopetrosis include sclerotic dense bones, hepatosplenomegaly, blindness, deafness, and cranial nerve palsies. Bone marrow failure develops due to relentless marked bony sclerosis and thickening, leading to the elimination of hematopoietic tissue. The peripheral blood thus reveals leukoerythroblastic features, while extramedullary hematopoiesis accounts for the enlargement of liver and spleen.

The pathogenesis of osteopetrosis is related to abnormal osteoclast function in the process of bony remodeling. The bone marrow biopsy thus demonstrates thickened sclerotic bone trabeculae with increased osteoclasts and osteoblasts. The

recessive variant of the disease appears to be multigenic. In general, the prognosis for these patients is very poor.

CONSTITUTIONAL DISORDERS AFFECTING PREDOMINANTLY SINGLE LINEAGE HEMATOPOIESIS

Diamond-Blackfan Anemia

Definition. *Diamond-Blackfan anemia* (DBA), also described in chapter 4, is a congenital disorder characterized by macrocytic anemia and failure of bone marrow erythropoiesis (see Table 7-2) (36,37,41,51,57). While the mode of inheritance can be autosomal dominant or recessive in a significant number of affected families, most cases arise sporadically due to de novo mutations (56). Patients are typically recognized in infancy and most manifest with persistent or worsening anemia within the first 2 years of life, although severe early onset anemia may occur if precipitated by concomitant nutritional deficiencies or infections (e.g., parvovirus B19). Rare cases occur in adults, either sporadically or in older members of DBA kindreds with known childhood occurrences.

Clinical Features. Patients with DBA may have accompanying physical abnormalities: facial dysmorphism, cleft lip and/or palate, or micrognathia (25 percent); occasional upper limb and hand abnormalities (flattened thenar eminence, triphalangeal thumbs, other hand and radial arm findings); and short stature (10 percent) (36). Developmental and visceral organ anomalies are also infrequently described.

Pathologic Findings. Hematologic findings are essentially confined to the erythroid lineage and include macrocytic (or less commonly, normocytic) anemia without compensatory reticulocytosis. White blood cells (WBCs) are typically unremarkable, but may be mildly decreased, and platelets are quantitatively normal. HbF is often increased and RBC adenosine deaminase (ADA) levels are characteristically elevated. Importantly, laboratory evaluation reveals normal serum iron, ferritin, vitamin B_{12}, and folate levels, and antibodies to erythropoietin are not present. The bone marrow in DBA patients is normocellular and reveals normal myeloid and megakaryocytic development; however, erythroid hypoplasia is nearly always present (fig. 7-5). Increased

Figure 7-5

DIAMOND-BLACKFAN ANEMIA

A: Peripheral blood from an infant with Diamond-Blackfan anemia shows severe, slightly macrocytic anemia without polychromasia (Wright stain).

B: A cellular bone marrow aspirate shows severely diminished erythroid precursors and abundant granulocytic cells and megakaryocytes (Wright stain).

C: Only a rare erythroblast is present without evidence of further maturation (note abundant hematogones) (Wright stain). (Courtesy of P. Izadi, Los Angeles, CA.)

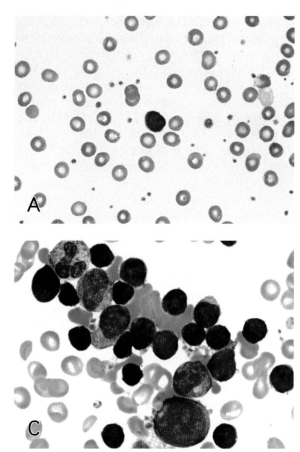

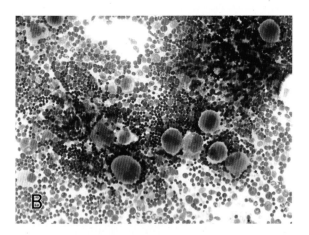

small lymphocytes and hematogones may be observed in the bone marrow.

Molecular Findings. Approximately 25 percent of DBA patients have a constitutional genetic abnormality localized to chromosome 19(q13.2), affecting a gene known as *RPS19*, which encodes a 16-kDa ribosomal subunit protein (48). Mutations in *RPS19* cause nonsense, frameshift, missense, or splice site changes in the coding sequence. A second subset of patients have a chromosomal abnormality mapped to 8(p23.2-p22), designated the *DBA2* gene (53). The remainder of patients do not show linkage to either of these loci, implicating the presence of a third or additional gene(s) associated with this disease. The exact pathophysiology of how *RPS19* mutations lead to selective defects in erythropoiesis is presently unclear, but the presence of functional RPS19 protein is required for normal ribosomal biogenesis (50a,50b).

Differential Diagnosis. A diagnosis of DBA is strongly suspected in an infant or young child with classic macrocytic anemia, lack of reticulocy-

tosis, and hypoplastic bone marrow erythropoiesis. Additional supportive findings, such as elevated HgbF and an increased RBC ADA level, are helpful, as is the presence of any physical dysmorphic features. While a family history of anemia may be very useful in this setting, a hereditary background is lacking in the many individuals who develop DBA from sporadically occurring mutations. The diagnosis of DBA further requires a negative chromosome breakage study in order to exclude FA. It is also critical to exclude transient erythroblastopenia of childhood (TEC) and parvovirus B19 infection as these entities are acquired and typically self-limited causes of pure red cell aplasia in this age group. Mutation screening of all five exons of the *RPS19* gene can be performed for confirmation of DBA, although as noted, this is only informative in 25 percent of the patients.

Treatment and Prognosis. Therapeutic management of DBA consists initially of glucocorticoid administration (e.g., prednisone); responses, however, are highly variable (36,41,58). Less than 5 percent of patients have a rapid response to treatment, with no subsequent requirement for steroids; another 20 percent eventually recover and tolerate the withdrawal of steroids. In contrast, 30 to 40 percent of DBA patients do not respond to steroid administration, and the rest of the patients show intermediate or poor response characterized by ongoing steroid dependence. In the latter situation, therapy may have to be individually tailored or stopped, given the growth and metabolic concerns for children on high-dose steroids. Adding to this complexity, 15 to 25 percent of patients have spontaneous hematologic recovery regardless of the degree of steroid responsiveness. The individual variability in the requirement for steroids and therapeutic outcome cannot be reliably predicted in DBA. Patients who are unresponsive to steroids are managed supportively with RBC transfusions and can be considered for HSCT with a sibling matched donor; excellent survival rates (80 percent) have been attained with this approach, but not so if the donor is unrelated.

The long-term outlook for DBA patients is variable. "Good steroid responders" or spontaneous remitters have an excellent prognosis. Although somewhat controversial, progression to complete bone marrow failure has been described in rare patients with severe anemia (54); however, in general, DBA is considered an isolated erythroid lineage anemia with better outcome compared to the multilineage congenital bone marrow failure disorders. Overall, the projected median survival time for DBA patients is into the 5th decade of life. The predisposition to developing hematologic or nonhematologic malignancies is low.

Congenital Dyserythropoietic Anemias

The *congenital dyserythropoietic anemias* (CDAs) are not considered true bone marrow failure disorders, but rather are syndromes of ineffective erythropoiesis resulting in mildly to moderately severe anemia. This related group of entities is briefly presented here as an example of a congenital single lineage anemia, and they are described in greater detail in chapter 4.

The three major types of CDA (I, II, III) are defined by relatively distinct clinical, morphologic, and laboratory findings. Type I CDA is characterized by mild anemia, megaloblastoid erythroid cells in the bone marrow, minimal

binucleation of erythroid precursors (2 to 5 percent of cells), and the presence of chromatin bridges. Type II CDA shows binucleation or multinucleation (10 to 40 percent of cells) and karyorrhexis; this type of CDA is also known as the "hereditary erythroblastic multinuclearity with positive acidified serum" variant, or HEMPAS. The RBCs in type II CDA are positive for i and I antigens. Type III CDA is characterized by erythroid gigantoblasts (10 to 40 percent of cells). In addition to these defined categories, a type IV CDA is also recognized with features of type II but a negative acidified serum test.

The hereditary pattern of types I and II CDA is autosomal recessive, with genetic loci localized to chromosomes 15(q15.1-15.3) and 20(q11.2), encoding the *CDA1* and *CDA2* genes, respectively. Type III CDA is an autosomal dominant disorder, with the *CDA3* gene localized to chromosome 15(q21-25). In general, the congenital dyserythropoietic anemias are not associated with profound anemia. Patients with type II and III CDA may benefit from splenectomy.

Shwachman-Diamond Syndrome

Definition. *Shwachman-Diamond syndrome* (SDS), also known as *Bodian-Shwachman syndrome*, is an autosomal recessive congenital disorder characterized by myeloid hypoproliferation and neutropenia, bone marrow failure, exocrine pancreatic insufficiency, and metaphyseal dysostosis leading to short stature in nearly half of the patients (see Table 7-2 and chapter 5) (36,41,49,50). This disorder is also described in chapter 5. Patients have an increased risk of developing myelodysplasia and AML. Although considered here as predominantly a single lineage bone marrow failure syndrome affecting the myeloid series, SDS involves other bone marrow lineages in about 40 percent of patients; however, even in the setting of more extensive bone marrow production impairment, terminal hematopoietic aplasia is not a predominant outcome for many patients. Additional findings in SDS include mental retardation in a subset of patients, facial dysmorphism (e.g., cleft lip/palate), dental anomalies, ichthyosis, and skeletal deformities of the thoracic rib cage.

Pathologic Findings. The diagnosis of SDS is usually considered in early childhood due to the infectious complications of neutropenia, gastrointestinal malabsorption (e.g., steatorrhea), and,

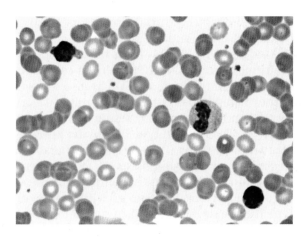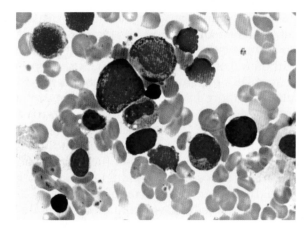

Figure 7-6

SHWACHMAN-DIAMOND SYNDROME

Left: Peripheral blood smear displays a relatively normal morphologic picture in a patient with Shwachman-Diamond syndrome and severe neutropenia (Wright stain).

Right: A marrow aspirate from this patient reveals slightly diminished neutrophilic myeloid precursors with left-shifted maturation (Wright stain). (Courtesy of P. Izadi, Los Angeles, CA.)

if present, physical anomalies. Key laboratory findings include neutropenia of variable severity and, in a significant proportion of patients, concomitant anemia or thrombocytopenia (fig. 7-6, left). The bone marrow shows hypoplasia of the granulocytic series, possibly with features of left-shifted maturation (fig. 7-6). Increased bone marrow blood vessel density has been described in the absence of abnormal vascular endothelial growth factor (VEGF) levels (55). The erythroid and megakaryocytic lineages are typically preserved early on, although as indicated, multilineage deficits occur in some patients. Evidence of pancreatic insufficiency can be demonstrated by low levels of serum amylase and trypsinogen. As with all congenital bone marrow failure assessments, FA must be excluded by a negative chromosome breakage study.

Molecular Findings. The genetic basis of SDS has been traced to inactivating mutations of the *SBDS* gene on chromosome 7(q11) (44). Two common gene mutations account for 75 percent of familial SDS due to gene conversion events involving a pseudogene with 97 percent homology to the functional *SBDS* gene. The normal SBDS gene product is thought to be involved with RNA processing with RNA processing, a hypothesis supported by recent data demonstrating that SRDS associates with ribosomal RNA (52a). Confirmatory genetic testing of blood or buccal swab DNA samples involves sequencing the five exons of *SBDS*; 90 percent of patients carry at least one converted allele and 60 percent have two, mainly involving exons 2 and 3 of the gene.

Treatment and Prognosis. The treatment of SDS patients consists largely of supportive care with G-CSF, blood product transfusions, and pancreatic enzyme replacement (41). The management of skeletal deformities may also be an important consideration. HSCT is a potentially curative therapeutic option, although as with FA and DC, the prospect of substantial morbidity and treatment-related mortality mandates careful patient selection (45).

The clinical course for SDS patients is variable. While exocrine pancreatic disease may improve with time, bone marrow failure tends to be progressive. The most serious consequences of SDS include the development of aplastic anemia, myelodysplasia, or AML. Patients with less severe hematologic complications have a relatively prolonged survival period.

Severe Congenital Neutropenia/ Kostmann Syndrome

Severe chronic neutropenia (see also chapter 5) constitutes a heterogeneous set of disorders linked by maturational defects in neutrophilic myelopoiesis (36,50). The term most broadly encompasses *severe congenital neutropenia* (SCN), *cyclic neutropenia* (CN), and *idiopathic neutro-penia*. Kindreds with a background of consanguinity and an autosomal recessive inheritance pattern were initially described by Kostmann (*Kostmann syndrome*). However, most cases of SCN (and CN) are in fact now known to be caused by mutations in the neutrophil elastase gene (*ELA2*) and are sporadically occurring or autosomal dominant. Nevertheless, the terms tend to be used interchangeably in this clinical setting, even though Kostmann syndrome more specifically defines a familial disorder with an autosomal recessive mode of inheritance and at present, an unknown genetic basis.

Patients with SCN present in early infancy with the consequences of marked neutropenia, including life-threatening pyogenic infections. The peripheral blood shows isolated severe neutropenia (less than 500/μL) or agranulocytosis, and there may be compensatory monocytosis. The bone marrow is of normal cellularity, but reveals a marked decrease in myelopoiesis, often limited to rare myeloblasts and promyelocytes ("maturation arrest").

Heterozygous point mutations in the *ELA2* gene on chromosome 19(p13.3) encoding neutrophil elastase are encountered in most cases of SCN (38,39,42,43,46). The mutant elastase protein is thought to act in a dominant negative manner to the normal enzyme, inhibiting the processes of normal neutrophilic development and maturation, with resultant intramedullary cell death (39,40,54a). Some investigations have suggested that patients with SCN and *ELA2* mutations have a more severe form of disease compared to those without detectable mutations; furthermore, the *ELA2* mutation site may have modulating effects on disease expression (42). As noted, *ELA2* mutations also underlie the pathogenesis of CN, although the locations of the point mutations in the gene are different than those found in SCN. Of note, a subset of patients with SCN phenotype and normal *ELA2* alleles harbor mutations in the *GFI1* gene, a regulator of *ELA2* as well as other genes involved in neutrophil development (36).

The diagnosis of SCN is established by the presence of severe persistent neutropenia in infancy with associated clinical sequelae; confirmation is obtained in most cases by the demonstration of disease-specific *ELA2* mutations. Prior to the advent of G-CSF therapy, the prognosis was very poor for SCN patients, with early deaths due to infection. Pharmacologic doses of G-CSF induce neutrophil responses in over 90 percent of patients and the median survival period has significantly improved. Nonetheless, SCN patients have an increased risk of AML and myelodysplasia despite intensive G-CSF treatment. The issue of whether this risk of malignancy is an iatrogenic consequence of G-CSF treatment versus a true inherent biologic complication of SCN seen with prolonged patient survival, remains currently unresolved (52).

Thrombocytopenia with Absent Radii

Definition. *Thrombocytopenia with absent radii* (TAR) is a congenital syndrome consisting of the bilateral absence of the radii associated with neonatal thrombocytopenia (see Table 7-2 and chapter 6) (36,47). Despite the presence of radial aplasia, thumbs are present, serving to distinguish TAR from other congenital anemias, particularly FA, which can also be associated with marked forearm skeletal abnormalities. TAR is characterized by autosomal recessive inheritance, possibly due to the acquisition of double heterozygous genetic mutations, as the degree of consanguinity is low in affected families.

Clinical Features. The physical defects are commonly bilateral and many patients have short stature. Additional upper limb skeletal anomalies can be seen and include syndactyly, clinodactyly, or hypoplastic thumbs. The list of described physical manifestations in TAR is extensive and patients may also present with ulnar shortening or absence, upper arm defects of the humerus, web neck or hypoplastic scapulae, and abnormalities affecting the lower limbs (e.g., deformity of hips, knees, and feet or absence of tibiae/fibulae). Some individuals have other developmental defects, such as congenital heart disease.

Pathologic Findings. Patients with TAR demonstrate early onset moderate to severe thrombocytopenia, frequently with accompanying neutrophilic leukocytosis, or "leukemoid" reaction. The bone marrow in these infants is normocellular, with the preservation of myeloid and erythroid lineages. In the majority of patients, megakaryocytes are essentially absent and in the remainder, severe megakaryocytic

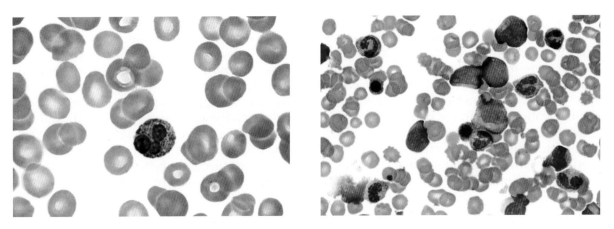

Figure 7-7

THROMBOCYTOPENIA WITH ABSENT RADII

Left: Thrombocytopenia is evident in the peripheral blood from an infant with thrombocytopenia with absent radii (TAR) (Wright stain).

Right: A bone marrow aspirate from this patient reveals normally maturing neutrophilic myeloid and erythroid precursors, with an absence of megakaryocytes (Wright stain). (Courtesy of P. Izadi, Los Angeles, CA.)

hypoplasia is present, with abnormal small and immature forms (fig. 7-7).

Molecular Findings. The molecular genetic basis for TAR is not understood at present. No abnormalities of the *c-MPL* gene (which is mutated in congenital amegakaryocytic thrombocytopenia [CAT]) have been identified in TAR. Affected individuals are recognized early in the neonatal period due to the characteristic skeletal deformities and thrombocytopenic bleeding manifestations such as petechiae.

Differential Diagnosis. Immune thrombocytopenic purpura (ITP) must be ruled out as a differential diagnostic consideration; however, the bone marrow in ITP shows compensatory megakaryocyte proliferation. Exclusion of FA by a negative chromosome breakage study and CAT by the absence of *c-MPL* gene mutations is important in the diagnostic evaluation. Patients with CAT usually lack physical abnormalities and if malformations are present, these do not include the classic bilateral absence of radii of TAR.

Treatment and Prognosis. Therapeutic management of infants with TAR is based on platelet transfusions for symptomatic thrombocytopenia. Although catastrophic bleeding is the prime concern in these individuals, overall survival is excellent if this serious complication can be successfully avoided or treated. Platelet counts and bleeding tendency improve with time and

permit orthopedic correction of skeletal abnormalities. In the long term, patients with TAR do not exhibit an increased risk of bone marrow failure and aplastic anemia. Similarly, there does not appear to be an appreciably increased incidence of neoplastic disease over time.

ACQUIRED DISORDERS AFFECTING MULTILINEAGE HEMATOPOIESIS

Idiopathic Aplastic Anemia

Definition. *Acquired aplastic anemia* (AA) is characterized by hematopoietic stem cell failure, bone marrow hypoproliferation, and progressive pancytopenia. While AA can arise idiosyncratically following bone marrow injury from a variety of agents, including drugs, toxins, infections (e.g., viral hepatitis), and radiation (70,72,83,90), the diagnosis of *idiopathic* or *primary AA* (constituting the majority of patients) is reserved for cases in which no definitive inciting event can be discerned relative to the development of the bone marrow failure.

Clinical Features. The frequency of AA overall is between 1 and 4/million and the disease occurs throughout all age groups. Individuals of Asian origin appear to have a relatively higher incidence (69,70,81). In contrast to the onset of *secondary AA*, which is often rapid and clearly related to a causative exposure, idiopathic AA typically progresses more insidiously, resulting in gradually

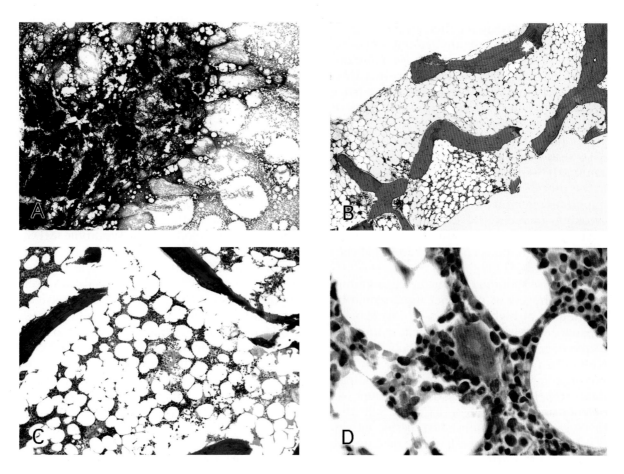

Figure 7-8

IDIOPATHIC APLASTIC ANEMIA COMPARED TO HYPOCELLULAR MYELODYSPLASIA

A: A hypocellular bone marrow aspirate particle in a patient with idiopathic aplastic anemia (Wright stain).

B: These findings are confirmed by the core biopsy histology, which shows cellularity approximating 5 percent (H&E stain).

C: A case of hypocellular myelodysplasia in an adult is characterized by a severely hypoplastic-appearing bone marrow core biopsy (H&E stain).

D: Additional laboratory investigations, such as CD34 immunoperoxidase stain, can be very useful for differentiating hypocellular myeloid malignancies from idiopathic aplastic anemia.

more severe peripheral cytopenias and eventuating in hypoplastic bone marrow failure.

The clinical symptoms in AA are related to the presence of marked cytopenias: infections, bleeding, and anemia with high output cardiac failure. The diagnosis is established when two of the following three criteria are present: an absolute neutrophil count of less than 500/μL, platelets less than 20,000/μL, or reticulocytes less than 20,000/μL (60,78). The bone marrow biopsy reveals marked hypocellularity (under 25 percent) (fig. 7-8). Regardless of whether a probable precipitating cause for AA is identified in a given patient, the exclusion of an underly-ing constitutional multilineage anemia can be important for patient evaluation (79).

Pathologic Findings and Pathogenesis. Among idiopathic AA cases, a presumed, but as yet unknown, infectious trigger has been proposed (89–91). There is a striking relation-ship between rare cases of fulminant hepatitis and the subsequent development of profound and sustained bone marrow aplasia; however, these individuals are seronegative for the major known hepatitis viruses, suggesting a novel etio-logic agent or autoimmune mechanism.

The pathophysiology of the large majority of AA cases is increasingly focused on the abnormal biology and destruction of hematopoietic stem cells (HSC), diminishing the self-renewal or repopulating capacity of these cells for maintaining normal bone marrow hematopoiesis. CD34-positive cells in AA show an increased tendency to apoptosis. Several experimental lines of evidence implicate the upregulation of the proapoptotic cell surface receptor for Fas ligand (CD95), as well as increased levels of interferon-gamma (IFN-G) and tumor necrosis factor-alpha in this process (62,64,66). T lymphocytes are an important reservoir for the production of many cytokines including IFN-G, and some studies have demonstrated the induction of apoptotic and immune response pathways in CD34 cells exposed to IFN-G (92).

The role of abnormal cell-mediated immunity in AA pathogenesis is further underscored by the finding of highly selected or oligoclonally expanded subsets of cytotoxic T cells in the bone marrow (75,76,82). Similarly, HLA-DR2/HLA-DR15 is found in a subgroup of AA patients, potentially linking components of the major histocompatibility complex to the process of autoimmune recognition and destruction of HSCs (85). Still other investigators have demonstrated specific autoantibody responses against cell surface proteins like kinectin or moeisin (67,86a). Early hematopoietic cells in AA have been associated with shortened survival due to defects in telomere maintenance, which leads to mitotic catastrophe and premature intramedullary cell death.

As noted in the section on DC, a few patients with apparently acquired, idiopathic AA harbor heterozygous mutations in either *TERT* (the gene of telomerase reverse transcriptase) or *TERC* (the RNA template component of telomerase) (87,88). In some instances, these mutations are in the germline of the affected individuals and can also be detected in family members unaffected by hematologic disease or the physical evidence of DC. The latter observations suggest that it may be possible to subclassify some AA patients as part of a "DC spectrum," or more aptly, a broader hematologic syndrome of telomerase deficiency. Finally, rare patients with acquired idiopathic AA have been shown to harbor heterozygous mutations in the *SBDS* or perforin (*PRF1*) genes in their peripheral blood cells, and these mutations apparently increase the risk of developing AA (61a,85a).

Molecular Findings. Clonal cytogenetic aberrancies have been described in some patients with AA, most commonly trisomy 8, monosomy 7, abnormalities of chromosome 13, and trisomy 6 (73). Various studies have associated trisomy 8 or deletion 13q with favorable responses to immunosuppression, whereas the presence of monosomy 7 or trisomy 6 connotes an aggressive disease with an increased risk of transformation to myelodysplasia or AML (68,71,77,84).

Differential Diagnosis. The finding of clonal karyotypic anomalies in de novo presentations of AA raises the differential diagnosis of hypocellular myelodysplastic syndrome (MDS), which shares some of the same genetic aberrations. In this context, quantitative assessment of bone marrow CD34-positive cells has been advocated as a helpful discriminator between AA and hypoplastic MDS (80). Application of CD34 immunohistochemistry can also help establish the diagnosis of hypocellular MDS in these cases by highlighting atypical clusters of blasts in the bone marrow biopsy or clot section (fig. 7-8). If blasts are not prominent and there is minimal evidence of bone marrow maturational dyspoiesis, distinguishing MDS from AA is difficult. Nonetheless, these considerations may, in part, be semantic since both AA and a subset of MDS patients may initially respond well to immunosuppressive therapies, whereas the presence of monosomy 7 in either disease is associated with an aggressive course.

Rare patients with chronic T-cell large granular lymphocytic leukemia present with pancytopenia and AA (65), rather than the more typical association with isolated red cell aplasia. Evaluation for an aberrant T-cell immunophenotype and/or evidence of T-cell monoclonality is important in this setting. These uncommon cases of AA associated with T-cell large granular lymphocyte (LGL) lymphoproliferative disorder may represent an extreme manifestation of the cytotoxic T-cell immune attack on bone marrow HSC, and therapy with immunosuppressive agents is often successful.

Patients with AA have a greater propensity to develop other hematologic disorders, including MDS, AML, and paroxysmal nocturnal hemoglobinuria (PNH). The actuarial risk of developing MDS or AML is estimated at 15 to 20 percent at 6 to 10 years following treatment for AA (90).

AML arising in this setting is typically highly aggressive. As indicated, the presence of monosomy 7 in AA is an adverse factor for the development of AML. The relationship of PNH to AA is particularly enigmatic, as PNH can either follow or precede AA, and minor populations of "PNH-like" cells are noted in a large proportion of AA patients at diagnosis. Some investigators have linked the presence of PNH cell subsets in AA to a favorable response to immunosuppression (86). PNH and its relationship to AA are discussed in detail in the following sections.

Treatment. Treatment of patients with AA seeks to restore normal bone marrow function either through allogeneic HSC reconstitution or immunosuppression, most commonly with antithymocyte globulin (ATG) and cyclosporine A (CsA) (59–61,61b,72,74,78,90). HLA-matched sibling donor HSCT can produce survival rates as high as 75 to 90 percent in AA patients; however, this treatment modality is not readily available to most patients due to the lack of a suitable donor. Complications of HSCT include peritransplant mortality, chronic graft versus host disease (CGVHD), and the potential for secondary malignancies in successfully transplanted patients. Immunosuppression with ATG and CsA can also induce prolonged survival in AA patients who are not candidates for HSCT. One large prospective series of childhood AA revealed better complete and durable response rates to immunosuppressive therapy in patients with more severe aplastic disease at presentation (63). In general, however, relapse rates after immunosuppressive therapy remain substantial and patients may require repeated courses of these potentially toxic agents (60,90), or develop treatment-refractory disease. The initial decision between HSCT and immunosuppression is determined by patient factors (age less than 40 years, disease severity) and the availability of an acceptable transplant donor. Efforts at stimulating hematopoiesis with synthetic androgens are of limited efficacy, although appropriate intervention with pharmacologic doses of hematopoietic growth factors (e.g., G-CSF) may be beneficial in some patients (86b).

Paroxysmal Nocturnal Hemoglobinuria

Definition. *Paroxysmal nocturnal hemoglobinuria* (PNH) is a disorder of clonal hematopoiesis characterized by the triad of intravascular hemolysis (with classic nocturnal hemoglobinuria), increased tendency for venous thrombosis, and increased risk of bone marrow failure (96,100,104,106). This disease, which is also described in chapter 4, affects patients of all age and ethnic groups, although it is far less common in children (107).

Clinical Features. Patients with PNH can present with many findings, including direct antiglobulin (Coombs)-negative hemolytic anemia, recurrent infections, thromboembolic episodes, unexplained (refractory) anemia, or gradually progressive pancytopenia. The clinical syndrome of PNH has been recognized for over 100 years; however, the disease manifestations are often variable and can be subtle. Patients exhibiting primarily hemolytic features account for a minority of diagnostic cases.

It is helpful to distinguish PNH patients who have predominantly hemolytic and/or thrombotic features (but relatively stable hematopoietic bone marrow function) from patients who have cytopenias and a more progressive course toward bone marrow failure. It is now recognized that essentially all patients with PNH have some degree of bone marrow insufficiency. Examination of the peripheral blood can be unremarkable, or more frequently, shows single or multiple lineage cytopenias of varying severity. The bone marrow may be of normal or even increased cellularity, with preservation of hematopoiesis. Cases with established hypoproliferation show panhypoplasia, possibly disproportionately affecting some lineages (e.g., megakaryocytes) more than others. The diagnosis of PNH is often considered following the exclusion of a variety of neoplastic and non-neoplastic differential diagnostic conditions, including myelodysplasia, other causes of RBC hemolysis, primary hypercoagulable states, and evolving aplastic anemia.

Pathogenesis. The propensity for intravascular hemolysis in PNH is related to an increased sensitivity of RBCs to complement-mediated lysis (95). This abnormal property can be demonstrated in the special hematology laboratory by the acidified serum (Ham) test or sucrose lysis test. The understanding of PNH pathogenesis and a corresponding improvement in diagnostic accuracy for this disease have emerged with the discovery that the susceptibility of RBCs to complement-mediated lysis in vivo results from a lack of specific cell surface proteins, including a class of cellular "defensins." These seemingly diverse cell membrane proteins are variably reduced or absent on subsets of RBCs, granulocytes, monocytes, platelets, and some lymphocytes in PNH patients, consistent with the concept of PNH as a stem cell disorder.

The underlying genetic and biochemical defect has its basis in acquired small insertion or deletion type DNA mutations of the phosphatidylinositol-glycan complementation class A gene (*PIG-A*) located on chromosome X(p22.1), which encodes an enzyme component critical for the production of a glycosylphosphatidylinositol (GPI) moiety (96,100). GPI is normally covalently linked to its target proteins by post-translational modification, and this step is critical for the attachment of these proteins to the cell membrane. Thus, the inability of PNH cells to properly express a large set of surface proteins is a direct result of the lack of this GPI anchor, conferring the noted vulnerability to complement-mediated lysis. Accordingly, PNH cells can now be sensitively and specifically identified by flow cytometry using monoclonal antibodies to detect the degree of loss or lack of certain GPI anchor-dependent surface markers on RBCs and leukocytes; common epitopes detected by immunophenotypic studies include CD14, CD55, and CD59, among many others (see fig. 4-31).

Modifications of the flow technique and the ability to gate or preferentially evaluate individual cell subsets (e.g., neutrophils) have resulted in the ability to identify PNH clonal subpopulations even when present in very low numbers (less than 0.01 percent). These approaches have revealed the presence of minor PNH-like subsets of cells in patients with other bone marrow failure disorders such as AA and MDS, especially when the sensitivity of the Ham test is insufficient. Notably, the size of the abnormal GPI-deficient cell population among PNH patients is variable, most often coexisting with some proportion of normal hematopoietic cells. In addition, the level of expression of GPI-linked proteins on PNH cells in a given individual can vary, leading to the definitions of type I (normal GPI expression), type II (partial GPI loss), and type III (complete GPI loss) abnormalities, which in turn correlate with the

degree of susceptibility to in vitro complement-mediated RBC lysis (96). A large percentage of PNH-positive cells, as detected by flow cytometry, appears to be related to the development of overt clinical manifestations, most significantly the risk of thrombosis (96,102); however, detailed aspects of the underlying pathogenesis remain to be fully explained. At the DNA level, the location of *PIG-A* mutations is also variable between individuals, with no obvious relationship to disease severity (100). Leukocytes from PNH patients who show progression to bone marrow failure may harbor several mutations, suggestive of an ongoing mutation process in these cells (101); similar findings are present in the PNH-like cells in AA.

The pathophysiology of PNH is complex and shares some features postulated for the current model of idiopathic AA. The "dual pathogenesis" hypothesis postulates that following an acquired *PIG-A* gene mutation, abnormal bone marrow conditions favor either selective growth of PNH cells over normal bone marrow counterparts, or confer a survival advantage to the PNH cell compartment (98). These mechanisms are likely not mutually exclusive, based on experimental evidence supporting both possibilities (100,103). The PNH clone apparently does not possess a significant intrinsic proliferative advantage, as evidenced by the lack of ongoing clonal cell expansion over time in most patients (93). This concept is also consistent with the finding of stable subsets of PNH-like cells in many patients with AA and some individuals with MDS, as well as the presence of minute PNH-cell populations even among healthy controls.

In individuals with PNH, immune-mediated destruction of normal (GPI-positive) hematopoietic precursors is thought to lead to the preferential emergence of the PNH clone ("immunologic escape"), following which additional putative mutations confer the genetic background for greater proliferative stability relative to normal counterparts (97). The presence of an autoimmune component in the pathogenesis of PNH has been supported by the findings of restricted (oligoclonal) T-cell repertoires in some PNH patients (95a,99); the overexpression of proapoptotic Fas receptor on normal hematopoietic counterparts in PNH patients; and the demonstration that PNH cells may be better able

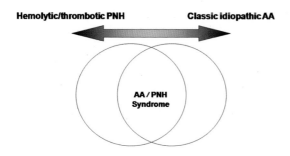

Figure 7-9

RELATIONSHIP BETWEEN PAROXYSMAL
NOCTURNAL HEMOGLOBINURIA (PNH)
AND IDIOPATHIC APLASTIC ANEMIA (AA)

A distinct relationship exists between the entities PNH and idiopathic AA. A substantial proportion of patients with idiopathic AA have minor populations of PNH-like cells, detectable by flow cytometry. Conversely, a subset of individuals presenting with classic hemolytic/thrombotic PNH eventuate in bone marrow aplasia. This overlap of clinical and pathologic features is considered to be the spectrum of AA/PNH syndrome.

to avoid cytotoxic T- and NK-cell destruction, in contrast to normal stem cells (100).

Treatment and Prognosis. Given the spectrum of PNH disease severity, the clinical course and outcome for these patients is variable, with a median overall survival period of 10 years (94,96,104). Some individuals have relatively indolent disease with well-tolerated minor cytopenias (e.g., anemia), whereas others experience symptomatic effects from multilineage cytopenias or relentless progression to aplastic bone marrow failure. Overall, 30 to 50 percent of patients have thromboembolic events, which may be catastrophic in nature.

The therapeutic management includes supportive care, with blood and platelet transfusions, or growth factor administration. Those at risk for repeated thrombotic events may require anticoagulation. Patients who proceed to bone marrow failure (AA endpoint) may respond to immunosuppressive therapy. Allogeneic HSCT has been described as potentially curative (105), but the relatively high treatment-related mortality rate is a primary consideration in light of the ability to conservatively manage many complications and therefore mandates careful patient selection. Newer agents to inhibit components of the activated complement pathway (e.g., eculizumab) may hold substantial promise for treating hemolytic PNH (105,106).

Despite the remarkable advances made in understanding this rare hematologic disorder, many unanswered questions remain, including why the PNH population is quantitatively different among individuals even with similar *PIG-A* genetic mutations and what determines the various clinical outcomes of the disease, such as a relatively stable maintenance of PNH to normal hematopoiesis in some patients, versus the development of progressive bone marrow failure in others.

Relationship of Aplastic Anemia and Paroxysmal Nocturnal Hemoglobinuria: the AA/PNH Syndrome

From the foregoing descriptions, it is apparent that some similarity and overlap exist in the pathogenesis of PNH and AA. The findings that 10 to 25 percent of PNH patients may eventuate in AA and that up to one third of de novo AA patients have a variable proportion of PNH-like cells at diagnosis provide strong empirical evidence for a common pathogenetic link (111,115). Using highly sensitive flow cytometry modifications, very small numbers of GPI-deficient cells have been reported in up to 90 percent of AA cases (112,113). Conversely, approximately 5 to 10 percent of AA patients managed successfully develop hemolytic PNH, in some cases sufficient enough to maintain a partial recovery from the aplastic state, albeit with abnormal clonal hematopoiesis.

These observations, coupled with accumulated evidence for autoimmune targeting of normal hematopoietic stem cells in both disorders, have prompted a reevaluation of the previous concept of AA and PNH as separate entities. While "pure" hemolytic/thrombotic PNH is clinically distinct in presentation from classic idiopathic AA, PNH with variable features of bone marrow failure, as well as cases of AA with PNH-positive cells, constitute the spectrum of the so-called *AA/PNH syndrome* (fig. 7-9) (108,110,112,114). Further strengthening this model is the association with HLA-DR2 and a relatively favorable response to immunosuppressive therapy for patients with the AA/PNH syndrome (109,115). Intriguingly, a small number of cases classified pathologically as low-grade MDS (e.g., refractory anemia) also demonstrate the presence of PNH-like cells as well as HLA-DR2 over-representation, and these individuals also respond to immunosuppression. It is therefore apparent that occasional cases of hypocellular MDS may be difficult to differentiate from AA/PNH syndrome, further illustrating the degree of overlap in pathogenesis at the intersection of these disorders.

Other Acquired Disorders Associated with Multilineage Hematopoietic Failure

Secondary, multilineage bone marrow production insufficiency or aplasia can result from a large number of causes, including infections (e.g., hepatitis C virus, HIV) and idiosyncratic effects from exogenous agents such as antibiotics, other medications, or toxins. The combination of clinical history and appropriate laboratory investigations nearly always identifies the etiologic factor(s). These pathologic disorders are discussed in detail in chapters 4 to 6, 10, and 11. The extrinsic causes of bone marrow failure and pancytopenia usually require exclusion of a primary acquired bone marrow failure syndrome (AA, PNH, or MDS), or a constitutional disorder. While secondary causes of bone marrow compromise are often reversible either spontaneously or following withdrawal of the inciting agent(s), some patients develop irreversible bone marrow aplasia, as classically described following chloramphenicol or hepatitis virus exposure.

ACQUIRED DISORDERS AFFECTING SINGLE LINEAGE HEMATOPOIESIS

Table 7-1 summarizes the varied causes of single cytopenias resulting from acquired disorders affecting hematopoiesis. Some conditions, such as iron deficiency anemia and anemia of chronic disease, are not truly due to a failure of hematopoietic capability, but rather are secondary to metabolic and biochemical derangements resulting in impaired bone marrow production with consequent peripheral cytopenia. These disorders, as well as the great number of causes of peripheral cell destruction with associated hyperplastic bone marrow responses (e.g., immune-mediated hemolytic anemia and thrombocytopenia) are discussed in chapters 4 and 6. Isolated neutropenia is commonly encountered as an adverse and typically reversible event following drug administration. In this setting, secondary immune destruction of neutrophils and precursors results in granulocytic hypoplasia in the bone

marrow, often with the morphologic appearance of a "maturation arrest." During bone marrow recovery, the initial marked expansion of left-shifted neutrophil lineage cells can occasionally mimic the features of a neoplasm (AML).

Transient erythroblastopenia of childhood (TEC) due to the selective loss of erythroid bone marrow precursors (pure red cell aplasia) can be seen in a subset of unrelated, but intriguing disorders (see also chapter 4) (121,123). TEC is an enigmatic disease affecting young children, typically from 6 months to 3 years of age (116,119,122,124). This self-limiting condition produces moderate to severe anemia without compensatory reticulocytosis. In some patients, neutropenia is also seen (119). Morphologic examination of the bone marrow reveals near absence of the erythroid lineage and a marked left shift of remaining RBC precursors; however, erythroid regeneration may be noted if the bone marrow is sampled during the recovery phase. Although the demographics and clinical features of this illness strongly suggest an infectious etiology, no specific association with a particular viral infection has been demonstrated thus far (131).

The diagnosis of TEC is established by the clinical presentation and the exclusion of plausible etiologic agents, such as parvovirus B19 infection (described below). In patients under 1 year of age, the distinction of TEC from DBA is important (130,132). Helpful features supporting TEC include normocytic normochromic anemia (as opposed to RBC macrocytosis in most instances of DBA), normal RBC ADA level, and lack of increased HgbF expression. Regardless, occasional patients require additional confirmatory studies to help exclude DBA and other syndromes of congenital bone marrow failure. Most significantly, TEC is spontaneously remitting within weeks, whereas DBA is characterized by progressive erythropoietic bone marrow failure.

Parvovirus B19 infection may share a similar clinical presentation with TEC; however, the age range for individuals acquiring symptomatic parvovirus infection is much broader. Parvovirus affects healthy individuals, as well as those with underlying diseases (117). In otherwise healthy persons, parvovirus infection may induce a period of transient bone marrow erythroid aplasia with reticulocytopenia; however, given the normal life span of circulating RBCs, symptomatic anemia is seldom the outcome since recovery from the infection and bone marrow erythroid reconstitution occur relatively quickly. In patients who have either intrinsic disorders of RBCs or abnormal globin synthesis resulting in reduced mature RBC longevity, parvovirus can produce a sudden and potentially severe anemia, which may require therapeutic intervention with packed RBC transfusions. Even in this situation, recovery from the infection leads to a return to the individual's baseline state of bone marrow erythropoiesis.

The most profound effects of parvovirus infection are seen in patients with a chronic immunodeficiency state, as seen in the post-transplantation setting or in patients with acquired immunodeficiency syndrome (AIDS) (120,128). In these cases, infection of RBC progenitors by parvovirus can cause a prolonged anemia requiring treatment. There is also evidence that parvovirus may affect the megakaryocyte lineage, thereby further diminishing bone marrow production in immunocompromised patients.

During active infection with parvovirus, the morphologic examination of the bone marrow shows marked erythroid lineage depletion with only rare pronormoblasts. Large amorphous nuclear inclusions are occasionally detected in these cells on aspirate smears. The abnormal cells are typically observed in fixed hematoxylin and eosin (H&E)-stained bone marrow core biopsy or clot sections as large, homogeneous pink intranuclear inclusions, also referred to as "lantern cells" (see chapter 10). The presence of parvovirus can be specifically shown by immunohistochemistry on bone marrow core biopsy sections. Additional diagnostic procedures include serologic studies for elevated antiparvovirus IgM titers and PCR analysis to detect the viral DNA.

Although predisposing clinical conditions for symptomatic parvovirus infection are usually apparent in most patients, the diagnosis of parvovirus in a bone marrow biopsy specimen may on occasion represent the initial recognition of an underlying chronic disease process, such as viral immunodeficiency or a hemoglobinopathy. The possibility of parvovirus infection must be excluded in all cases of apparently isolated bone marrow red cell aplasia.

Pure red cell aplasia has been well described in conjunction with several neoplastic disorders. Most commonly, it has been associated with non-Hodgkin lymphomas, chronic B-cell leukemias, thymoma, and chronic T-cell large granular lymphocytic leukemia (T-LGL lymphoproliferative disorder) (125–127,129). In each of these disorders, induction of bone marrow red cell aplasia is hypothesized to be due to an autoimmune attack on erythroid progenitor cells, although the pathogenetic mechanisms are incompletely understood. In general, treatment of the underlying neoplasm is required to alleviate the red cell aplasia. Support for an immune mechanism in some cases derives from its rare occurrence in patients with chronic renal failure treated with erythropoietin who develop antierythropoietin antibodies leading to a functional erythroid lineage "knockout" in the bone marrow (118). Similar mechanisms may be operative in patients with classic autoimmune disorders (e.g., systemic lupus erythematosus), in whom selective red cell aplasia uncommonly occurs.

REFERENCES

General Concepts

1. Alter B. Inherited bone marrow failure syndromes. In: Nathan D, Orkin S, Ginsburg D, et al., eds. Nathan and Oski's hematology of infancy and childhood, 6th ed. Philadelphia: W.B. Saunders; 2003:280-364.
2. Bagby G, Lipton J, Sloand E, Schiffer CA. Marrow failure. Hematology Am Soc Hematol Educ Program 2004;:318-36.

Constitutional Disorders Affecting Multilineage Hematopoiesis

3. Alter B. Inherited bone marrow failure syndromes. In: Nathan D, Orkin S, Ginsburg D, et al., eds. Nathan and Oski's hematology of infancy and childhood, 6th ed. Philadelphia: W.B. Saunders; 2003:280-364.
3a. Alter BP, Baerlocher GM, Savage SA, et al. Very short telomere length by flow fluorescence in situ hybridization identifies patients with dyskeratosis congenita. Blood 2007;110:1439-47.
4. Alter BP. Bone marrow failure: a child is not just a small adult (but an adult can have a childhood disease). Hematology Am Soc Hematol Educ Program 2005;:96-103.
5. Bagby G, Lipton J, Sloand E, Schiffer. Marrow failure. Hematology Am Soc Hematol Educ Program 2004;:318-36.
6. Ballmaier M, Germeshausen M, Schulze H, et al. c-mpl mutations are the cause of congenital amegakaryocytic thrombocytopenia. Blood 2001;97:139-46.
7. D'Andrea AD, Grompe M. The Fanconi anaemia/BRCA pathway. Nat Rev Cancer 2003;3:23-34.
8. Dokal I. Dyskeratosis congenita in all its forms. Br J Haematol 2000;110:768-79.
9. Dokal I, Vulliamy T. Dyskeratosis congenita: its link to telomerase and aplastic anaemia. Blood Rev 2003;17:217-25.
10. Drachman JG. Inherited thrombocytopenia: when a low platelet count does not mean ITP. Blood 2004;103:390-8.
11. Faivre L, Guardiola P, Lewis C, et al. Association of complementation group and mutation type with clinical outcome in Fanconi anemia. European Fanconi Anemia Research Group. Blood 2000;96:4064-70.
12. Fogarty PF, Yamaguchi H, Wiestner A, et al. Late presentation of dyskeratosis congenita as apparently acquired aplastic anaemia due to mutations in telomerase RNA. Lancet 2003;362:1628-30.
13. Grunebaum E, Roifman CM. Gene abnormalities in patients with hemophagocytic lymphohistiocytosis. Isr Med Assoc J 2002;4:366-9.
14. Hanenberg H, Batish SD, Pollok KE, et al. Phenotypic correction of primary Fanconi anemia T cells with retroviral vectors as a diagnostic tool. Exp Hematol 2002;30:410-20.
15. Heiss NS, Knight SW, Vulliamy TJ, et al. X-linked dyskeratosis congenita is caused by mutations in a highly conserved gene with putative nucleolar functions. Nat Genet 1998;19:32-8.
16. Henter JI. Biology and treatment of familial hemophagocytic lymphohistiocytosis: importance of perforin in lymphocyte-mediated cytotoxicity and triggering of apoptosis. Med Pediatr Oncol 2002;38:305-9.
17. Ihara K, Ishii E, Eguchi M, et al. Identification of mutations in the c-mpl gene in congenital amegakaryocytic thrombocytopenia. Proc Natl Acad Sci U S A 1999;96:3132-6.
18. Katano H, Cohen JI. Perforin and lymphohistiocytic proliferative disorders. Br J Haematol 2005;128:739-50.
19. Kutler DI, Singh B, Satagopan J, et al. A 20-year perspective on the International Fanconi Anemia Registry (IFAR). Blood 2003;101:1249-56.
20. Levitt NC, Hickson ID. Caretaker tumour suppressor genes that defend genome integrity. Trends Mol Med 2002;8:179-86.
21. Marrone A, Dokal I. Dyskeratosis congenita: molecular insights into telomerase function, ageing and cancer. Expert Rev Mol Med 2004;6:1-23.
22. Mason PJ. Stem cells, telomerase and dyskeratosis congenita. Bioessays 2003;25:126-33.
23. Meyer S, Barber LM, White DJ, et al. Spectrum and significance of variants and mutations in the Fanconi anaemia group G gene in children with sporadic acute myeloid leukaemia. Br J Haematol 2006;133:284-92.
24. Offit K, Levran O, Mullaney B, et al. Shared genetic susceptibility to breast cancer, brain tumors, and Fanconi anemia. J Natl Cancer Inst 2003;95:1548-51.
25. Rosenberg PS, Greene MH, Alter BP. Cancer incidence in persons with Fanconi anemia. Blood 2003;101:822-6.
25a. Shimamura A. Inherited bone marrow failure syndromes: molecular features. Hematology Am Soc Hematol Educa Program 2006:63-71.
26. Shimamura A, D'Andrea AD. Subtyping of Fanconi anemia patients: implications for clinical management. Blood 2003;102:3459.
27. Shimamura A, Montes de Oca R, Svenson JL, et al. A novel diagnostic screen for defects in the Fanconi anemia pathway. Blood 2002;100:4649-54.
28. Taniguchi T, D'Andrea AD. Molecular pathogenesis of Fanconi anemia: recent progress. Blood 2006;107:4223-33.

29. Tischkowitz M, Dokal I. Fanconi anaemia and leukaemia—clinical and molecular aspects. Br J Haematol 2004;126:176-91.

30. van den Oudenrijn S, Bruin M, Folman CC, et al. Mutations in the thrombopoietin receptor, Mpl, in children with congenital amegakaryocytic thrombocytopenia. Br J Haematol 2000;110:441-8.

31. Venkitaraman AR. Tracing the network connecting BRCA and Fanconi anaemia proteins. Nat Rev Cancer 2004;4:266-76.

32. Vulliamy T, Marrone A, Goldman F, et al. The RNA component of telomerase is mutated in autosomal dominant dyskeratosis congenita. Nature 2001;413:432-5.

33. Vulliamy T, Marrone A, Szydlo R, Walne A, Mason PJ. Disease anticipation is associated with progressive telomere shortening in families with dyskeratosis congenita due to mutations in TERC. Nat Genet 2004;36:447-9.

34. Vulliamy TJ, Marrone A, Knight SW, Walne A, Mason PJ, Dokal I. Mutations in dyskeratosis congenita: their impact on telomere length and the diversity of clinical presentation. Blood 2006;107:2680-5.

34a. Wang W. Emergence of a DNA-damage response network consisting of Fanconi anaemia and BRCA proteins. Nat Rev Genet 2007;8:735-48.

35. Yamaguchi H, Baerlocher GM, Lansdorp PM, et al. Mutations of the human telomerase RNA gene (TERC) in aplastic anemia and myelodysplastic syndrome. Blood 2003;102:916-8.

Constitutional Disorders Affecting Predominantly Single Lineage Hematopoiesis

36. Alter B. Inherited bone marrow failure syndromes. In: Nathan D, Orkin S, Ginsburg D, et al., eds. Nathan and Oski's hematology of infancy and-childhood, 6th ed. Philadelphia: W.B. Saunders; 2003:280-364.

37. Alter BP. Modern review of congenital hypoplastic anemia. J Pediatr Hematol Oncol 2001;23:383-4.

38. Ancliff PJ. Congenital neutropenia. Blood Rev 2003;17:209-16.

39. Ancliff PJ, Gale RE, Liesner R, Hann IM, Linch DC. Mutations in the ELA2 gene encoding neutrophil elastase are present in most patients with sporadic severe congenital neutropenia but only in some patients with the familial form of the disease. Blood 2001;98:2645-50.

40. Aprikyan AA, Liles WC, Boxer LA, et al. Mutant elastase in pathogenesis of cyclic and severe congenital neutropenia. J Pediatr Hematol Oncol 2002;24:784-6.

41. Bagby G, Lipton J, Sloand E, Schiffer CA. Marrow failure. Hematology Am Soc Hematol Educ Program 2004;:318-36.

42. Bellanne-Chantelot C, Clauin S, Leblanc T, et al. Mutations in the ELA2 gene correlate with more severe expression of neutropenia: a study of 81 patients from the French Neutropenia Register. Blood 2004;103:4119-25.

43. Berliner N, Horwitz M, Loughran TP Jr. Congenital and acquired neutropenia. Hematology Am Soc Hematol Educ Program 2004;:63-79.

44. Boocock GR, Morrison JA, Popovic M, et al. Mutations in SBDS are associated with Shwachman-Diamond syndrome. Nat Genet 2003;33:97-101.

45. Cesaro S, Oneto R, Messina C, et al. Haematopoietic stem cell transplantation for Shwachman-Diamond disease: a study from the European Group for blood and marrow transplantation. Br J Haematol 2005;131:231-6.

46. Dale DC, Person RE, Bolyard AA, et al. Mutations in the gene encoding neutrophil elastase in congenital and cyclic neutropenia. Blood 2000;96:2317-22.

47. Drachman JG. Inherited thrombocytopenia: when a low platelet count does not mean ITP. Blood 2004;103:390-8.

48. Draptchinskaia N, Gustavsson P, Andersson B, et al. The gene encoding ribosomal protein S19 is mutated in Diamond-Blackfan anaemia. Nat Genet 1999;21:169-75.

49. Dror Y, Freedman MH. Shwachman-Diamond syndrome: an inherited preleukemic bone marrow failure disorder with aberrant hematopoietic progenitors and faulty marrow microenvironment. Blood 1999;94:3048-54.

50. Dror Y, Sung L. Update on childhood neutropenia: molecular and clinical advances. Hematol Oncol Clin North Am 2004;18:1439-58, x.

50a. Flygare J, Aspesi A, Bailey JC, et al. Human RPS19, the gene mutated in Diamond-Blackfan anemia, encodes a ribosomal protein required for the maturation of 40S ribosomal subunits. Blood 2007;109:980-6.

50b. Flygare J, Karlsson S. Diamond-Blackfan anemia: erythropoiesis lost in translation. Blood 2007;109:3152-4.

51. Foucar K. Erythroblastopenic disorders. Bone marrow pathology, 2nd ed. Chicago: ASCP Press; 2001:124-36.

52. Freedman MH, Bonilla MA, Fier C, et al. Myelodysplasia syndrome and acute myeloid leukemia in patients with congenital neutropenia receiving G-CSF therapy. Blood 2000;96:429-36.

52a. Ganapathi KA, Austin KM, Lee CS, et al. The human Schwachman-Diamond syndrome protein, SBDS, associates with ribosomal RNA. Blood 2007;110:1458-65.

53. Gazda H, Lipton JM, Willig TN, et al. Evidence for linkage of familial Diamond-Blackfan anemia to chromosome 8p23.3-p22 and for non-19q non-8p disease. Blood 2001;97:2145-50.

54. Giri N, Kang E, Tisdale JF, et al. Clinical and laboratory evidence for a trilineage haematopoietic defect in patients with refractory Diamond-Blackfan anaemia. Br J Haematol 2000;108:167-75.

54a. Horwitz MS, Duan Z, Korkmaz B, Lee HH, Mealiffe ME, Salipante SJ. Neutrophil elastase in cyclic and severe congenital neutropenia. Blood 2007;109:1817-24.

55. Leung EW, Rujkijyanont P, Beyene J, et al. Shwachman-Diamond syndrome: an inherited model of aplastic anaemia with accelerated angiogenesis. Br J Haematol 2006;133:558-61.

56. Orfali KA, Ohene-Abuakwa Y, Ball SE. Diamond Blackfan anaemia in the UK: clinical and genetic heterogeneity. Br J Haematol 2004;125:243-52.

57. Vlachos A, Klein GW, Lipton JM. The Diamond-Blackfan Anemia Registry: tool for investigating the epidemiology and biology of Diamond-Blackfan anemia. J Pediatr Hematol Oncol 2001;23:377-82.

58. Willig TN, Niemeyer CM, Leblanc T, et al. Identification of new prognosis factors from the clinical and epidemiologic analysis of a registry of 229 Diamond-Blackfan anemia patients. DBA group of Societe d'Hematologie et d'Immunologie Pediatrique (SHIP), Gesellshaft fur Padiatrische Onkologie und Hamatologie (GPOH), and the European Society for Pediatric Hematology and Immunology (ESPHI). Pediatr Res 1999;46:553-61.

Idiopathic Anaplastic Anemia

59. Bacigalupo A, Brand R, Oneto R, et al. Treatment of acquired severe aplastic anemia: bone marrow transplantation compared with immunosuppressive therapy—The European Group for Blood and Marrow Transplantation experience. Semin Hematol 2000;37:69-80.

60. Bagby G, Lipton J, Sloand E, Schiffer CA. Marrow failure. Hematology Am Soc Hematol Educ Program 2004;:318-36.

61. Ball SE. The modern management of severe aplastic anaemia. Br J Haematol 2000;110:41-53.

61a. Calado RT, Graf SA, Wilkerson KL, et al. Mutations in the SBDS gene in acquired aplastic anemia. Blood 2007;110:1141-6.

61b. Davies JK, Guinan EC. An update on the management of severe idiopathic aplastic anaemia in children. Br J Haematol 2007;136:549-64.

62. Dufour C, Corcione A, Svahn J, Haupt R, Battilana N, Pistoia V. Interferon g and tumour necrosis factor a are overexpressed in bone marrow T lymphocytes from paediatric patients with aplastic anaemia. Br J Haematol.2001;115:1023-31.

63. Fuhrer M, Rampf U, Baumann I, et al. Immunosuppressive therapy for aplastic anemia in children: a more severe disease predicts better survival. Blood 2005;106:2102-4.

64. Giannakoulas NC, Karakantza M, Theodorou GL, et al. Clinical relevance of balance between type 1 and type 2 immune responses of lymphocyte subpopulations in aplastic anaemia patients. Br J Haematol 2004;124:97-105.

65. Go RS, Lust JA, Phyliky RL. Aplastic anemia and pure red cell aplasia associated with large granular lymphocyte leukemia. Semin Hematol 2003;40:196-200.

66. Hara T, Ando K, Tsurumi H, Moriwaki H. Excessive production of tumor necrosis factor-alpha by bone marrow T lymphocytes is essential in causing bone marrow failure in patients with aplastic anemia. Eur J Haematol 2004;73:10-6.

67. Hirano N, Butler MO, Von Bergwelt-Baildon MS, et al. Autoantibodies frequently detected in patients with aplastic anemia. Blood 2003;102:4567-75.

68. Ishiyama K, Karasawa M, Miyawaki S, et al. Aplastic anaemia with 13q-: a benign subset of bone marrow failure responsive to immunosuppressive therapy. Br J Haematol 2002;117:747-50.

69. Kaufman DW, Kelly JP, Issaragrisil S, et al. Relative incidence of agranulocytosis and aplastic anemia. Am J Hematol 2006;81:65-7.

70. Kaufman DW, Kelly JP, Jurgelon JM, et al. Drugs in the aetiology of agranulocytosis and aplastic anaemia. Eur J Haematol Suppl 1996;60:23-30.

71. Kearns WG, Sutton JF, Maciejewski JP, Young NS, Liu JM. Genomic instability in bone marrow failure syndromes. Am J Hematol 2004;76:220-4.

72. Keohane EM. Acquired aplastic anemia. Clin Lab Sci 2004;17:165-71.

73. Keung YK, Pettenati MJ, Cruz JM, Powell BL, Woodruff RD, Buss DH. Bone marrow cytogenetic abnormalities of aplastic anemia. Am J Hematol 2001;66:167-71.

74. Killick SB, Marsh JC. Aplastic anaemia: management. Blood Rev 2000;14:157-71.

75. Kook H, Zeng W, Guibin C, Kirby M, Young NS, Maciejewski JP. Increased cytotoxic T cells with effector phenotype in aplastic anemia and myelodysplasia. Exp Hematol 2001;29:1270-7.

76. Lu J, Basu A, Melenhorst JJ, Young NS, Brown KE. Analysis of T-cell repertoire in hepatitis-associated aplastic anemia. Blood 2004;103:4588-93.

77. Maciejewski JP, Risitano A, Sloand EM, Nunez O, Young NS. Distinct clinical outcomes for cytogenetic abnormalities evolving from aplastic anemia. Blood 2002;99:3129-35.

78. Marsh JC. Management of acquired aplastic anaemia. Blood Rev 2005;19:143-51.

79. Marsh JC, Ball SE, Darbyshire P, et al. Guidelines for the diagnosis and management of acquired aplastic anaemia. Br J Haematol 2003;123:782-801.

80. Matsui WH, Brodsky RA, Smith BD, Borowitz MJ, Jones RI. Quantitative analysis of bone marrow CD34 cells in aplastic anemia and hypoplastic myelodysplastic syndromes. Leukemia 2006;20:458-62.

81. McCahon E, Tang K, Rogers PC, McBride ML, Schultz KR. The impact of Asian descent on the incidence of acquired severe aplastic anaemia in children. Br J Haematol 2003;121:170-2.

82. Melenhorst JJ, Fibbe WE, Struyk L, van der Elsen PJ, Willemze R, Landegent JE. Analysis of T-cell clonality in bone marrow of patients with acquired aplastic anaemia. Br J Haematol 1997;96:85-91.

83. Muir KR, Chilvers CE, Harriss C, et al. The role of occupational and environmental exposures in the aetiology of acquired severe aplastic anaemia: a case control investigation. Br J Haematol 2003;123:906-14.

84. Ohga S, Ohara A, Hibi S, et al. Treatment responses of childhood aplastic anaemia with chromosomal aberrations at diagnosis. Br J Haematol 2002;118:313-9.

85. Saunthararajah Y, Nakamura R, Nam JM, et al. HLA-DR15 (DR2) is overrepresented in myelodysplastic syndrome and aplastic anemia and predicts a response to immunosuppression in myelodysplastic syndrome. Blood 2002;100:1570-4.

85a. Solomou EE, Gibellini F, Steward B, et al. Perforin gene mutations in patients with acquired aplastic anemia. Blood 2007;109:5234-7.

86. Sugimori C, Chuhjo T, Feng X, et al. Minor population of CD55-CD59- blood cells predicts response to immunosuppressive therapy and prognosis in patients with aplastic anemia. Blood 2006;107:1308-14.

86a. Takamatsu H, Feng X, Chuhjo T, et al. Specific antibodies to moesin, a membrane-cytoskeleton linker protein, are frequently detected in patients with acquired aplastic anemia. Blood 2007;109:2514-20.

86b. Teramura M, Kimura A, Iwase S, et al. Treatment of severe aplastic anemia with antithymocyte globulin and cyclosporin A with or without G-CSF in adults: a multicenter randomized study in Japan. Blood 2007;110:1765-61.

87. Yamaguchi H, Baerlocher GM, Lansdorp PM, et al. Mutations of the human telomerase RNA gene (TERC) in aplastic anemia and myelodysplastic syndrome. Blood 2003;102:916-8.

88. Yamaguchi H, Calado RT, Ly H, et al. Mutations in TERT, the gene for telomerase reverse transcriptase, in aplastic anemia. N Engl J Med 2005;352:1413-24.

89. Young NS. Hematopoietic cell destruction by immune mechanisms in acquired aplastic anemia. Semin Hematol 2000;37:3-14.

90. Young NS. Acquired aplastic anemia. Ann Intern Med 2002;136:534-46.

91. Young NS, Abkowitz JL, Luzzatto L. New insights into the pathophysiology of acquired cytopenias. Hematology Am Soc Hematol Educ Program 2000;:18-38.

92. Zeng W, Miyazato A, Chen G, Kajigaya S, Young NS, Maciejewski JP. Interferon-gamma-induced gene expression in CD34 cells: identification of pathologic cytokine-specific signature profiles. Blood 2006;107:167-75.

Paroxysmal Nocturnal Hemoglobinuria

93. Araten DJ, Bessler M, McKenzie S, et al. Dynamics of hematopoiesis in paroxysmal nocturnal hemoglobinuria (PNH): no evidence for intrinsic growth advantage of PNH clones. Leukemia 2002;16:2243-8.

94. Bagby G, Lipton J, Sloand E, Schiffer CA. Marrow failure. Hematology Am Soc Hematol Educ Program 2004;:318-36.

95. Dacie JV, Lewis SM. Paroxysmal nocturnal haemoglobinuria: clinical manifestations, haematology, and nature of the disease. Ser Haematol 1972;5:3-23.

95a. Gargiulo L, Lastraioli S, Cerruti G, et al. Highly homologous T-cell receptor beta sequences support a common target for autoreactive T cells in most patients with paroxysmal nocturnal hemoglobinuria. Blood 2007;109:5036-42.

96. Hillmen P, Richards JJ. Implications of recent insights into the pathophysiology of paroxysmal nocturnal haemoglobinuria. Br J Haematol 2000;108:470-9.

97. Inoue N, Murakami Y, Kinoshita T. Molecular genetics of paroxysmal nocturnal hemoglobinuria. Int J Hematol 2003;77:107-12.

98. Karadimitris A, Luzzatto L. The cellular pathogenesis of paroxysmal nocturnal haemoglobinuria. Leukemia 2001;15:1148-52.

99. Karadimitris A, Manavalan JS, Thaler HT, et al. Abnormal T-cell repertoire is consistent with immune process underlying the pathogenesis of paroxysmal nocturnal hemoglobinuria. Blood 2000;96:2613-20.

100. Meletis J, Terpos E. Recent insights into the pathophysiology of paroxysmal nocturnal hemoglobinuria. Med Sci Monit 2003;9:RA161-72.

101. Mortazavi Y, Merk B, McIntosh J, et al. The spectrum of PIG-A gene mutations in aplastic anemia/paroxysmal nocturnal hemoglobinuria (AA/PNH): a high incidence of multiple mutations and evidence of a mutational hot spot. Blood 2003;101:2833-41.

102. Moyo VM, Mukhina GL, Garrett ES, Brodsky RA. Natural history of paroxysmal nocturnal haemoglobinuria using modern diagnostic assays. Br J Haematol 2004;126:133-8.

103. Nakakuma H. Mechanism of intravascular hemolysis in paroxysmal nocturnal hemoglobinuria (PNH). Am J Hematol 1996;53:22-9.

104. Packman CH. Pathogenesis and management of paroxysmal nocturnal haemoglobinuria. Blood Rev 1998;12:1-11.

105. Parker C, Omine M, Richards S, et al. Diagnosis and management of paroxysmal nocturnal hemoglobinuria. Blood 2005;106:3699-709.

106. Rosse WF, Hillmen P, Schreiber AD. Immune-mediated hemolytic anemia. Hematology Am Soc Hematol Educ Program 2004;:48-62.

107. van den Heuvel-Eibrink MM, Bredius RG, te Winkel ML, et al. Childhood paroxysmal nocturnal haemoglobinuria (PNH), a report of 11 cases in the Netherlands. Br J Haematol 2005;128:571-7.

Relationship of AA and PNH: the AA/PNH Syndrome

108. Dunn DE, Tanawattanacharoen P, Boccuni P, et al. Paroxysmal nocturnal hemoglobinuria cells in patients with bone marrow failure syndromes. Ann Intern Med 1999;131:401-8.

109. Maciejewski JP, Follmann D, Nakamura R, et al. Increased frequency of HLA-DR2 in patients with paroxysmal nocturnal hemoglobinuria and the PNH/aplastic anemia syndrome. Blood 2001;98:3513-9.

110. Maciejewski JP, Rivera C, Kook H, Dunn D, Young NS. Relationship between bone marrow failure syndromes and the presence of glycophosphatidyl inositol-anchored protein-deficient clones. Br J Haematol 2001;115:1015-22.

111. Marsh JC, Elebute MO. Stem cells in paroxysmal nocturnal haemoglobinuria and aplastic anaemia: increasing evidence for overlap of haemopoietic defect. Transfus Med 2003;13:377-86.

112. Mukhina GL, Buckley JT, Barber JP, Jones RJ, Brodsky RA. Multilineage glycosylphosphatidylinositol anchor-deficient haematopoiesis in untreated aplastic anaemia. Br J Haematol 2001;115:476-82.

113. Wang H, Chuhjo T, Yamazaki H, et al. Relative increase of granulocytes with a paroxysmal nocturnal haemoglobinuria phenotype in aplastic anaemia patients: the high prevalence at diagnosis. Eur J Haematol 2001;66:200-5.

114. Wang H, Chuhjo T, Yasue S, Omine M, Nakao S. Clinical significance of a minor population of paroxysmal nocturnal hemoglobinuria-type cells in bone marrow failure syndrome. Blood 2002;100:3897-902.

115. Young NS, Maciejewski JP, Sloand E, et al. The relationship of aplastic anemia and PNH. Int J Hematol 2002;76(Suppl 2):168-72.

Other Acquired Disorders Associated with Multilineage Hematopoietic Failure

116. Alter B. Inherited bone marrow failure syndromes. In: Nathan D, Orkin S, Ginsburg D, et al., eds. Nathan and Oski's hematology of infancy and childhood, 6th ed. Philadelphia: W.B. Saunders; 2003:280-364.

117. Brown KE, Young NS. Parvovirus B19 infection and hematopoiesis. Blood Rev 1995;9:176-82.

118. Casadevall N, Nataf J, Viron B, et al. Pure red-cell aplasia and antierythropoietin antibodies in patients treated with recombinant erythropoietin. N Engl J Med 2002;346:469-75.

119. Cherrick I, Karayalcin G, Lanzkowsky P. Transient erythroblastopenia of childhood. Prospective study of fifty patients. Am J Pediatr Hematol Oncol 1994;16:320-4.

120. Crook T, Rogers BB, McFarland R, et al. Unusual bone marrow manifestations of parvovirus B19 infection in immunocompromised patients. Hum Pathol 2000;31:161-8.

121. Erslev AJ. Clinical erythrokinetics: a critical review. Blood Rev 1997;11:160-7.

122. Farhi DC, Luebbers EL, Rosenthal NS. Bone marrow biopsy findings in childhood anemia: prevalence of transient erythroblastopenia of childhood. Arch Pathol Lab Med 1998;122:638-41.

123. Fisch P, Handgretinger R, Schaefer HE. Pure red cell aplasia. Br J Haematol 2000;111:1010-22.

124. Foucar K. Erythroblastopenic disorders. In: Bone marrow pathology, 2nd ed. Chicago: ASCP Press; 2001:124-36.

125. Go RS, Lust JA, Phyliky RL. Aplastic anemia and pure red cell aplasia associated with large granular lymphocyte leukemia. Semin Hematol 2003;40:196-200.

126. Go RS, Tefferi A, Li CY, Lust JA, Phyliky RL. Lymphoproliferative disease of granular T lymphocytes presenting as aplastic anemia. Blood 2000;96:3644-6.

127. Lacy MQ, Kurtin PJ, Tefferi A. Pure red cell aplasia: association with large granular lymphocyte leukemia and the prognostic value of cytogenetic abnormalities. Blood 1996;87:3000-6.

128. Liu W, Ittmann M, Liu J, et al. Human parvovirus B19 in bone marrows from adults with acquired immunodeficiency syndrome: a comparative study using in situ hybridization and immunohistochemistry. Hum Pathol 1997;28:760-6.

129. Masuda M, Arai Y, Okamura T, MIzoguchi H. Pure red cell aplasia with thymoma: evidence of T-cell clonal disorder. Am J Hematol 1997;54:324-8.

130. Miller R, Berman B. Transient erythroblastopenia of childhood in infants < 6 months of age. Am J Pediatr Hematol Oncol 1994;16:246-8.

131. Skeppner G, Kreuger A, Elinder G. Transient erythroblastopenia of childhood: prospective study of 10 patients with special reference to viral infections. J Pediatr Hematol Oncol 2002;24:294-8.

132. Ware RE, Kinney TR. Transient erythroblastopenia in the first year of life. Am J Hematol 1991;37:156-8.

8 NON-NEOPLASTIC LYMPHOID AND PLASMA CELL DISORDERS

LYMPHOCYTES IN BLOOD

The age-related variations in the peripheral blood absolute lymphocyte count are well recognized, and these variations are especially

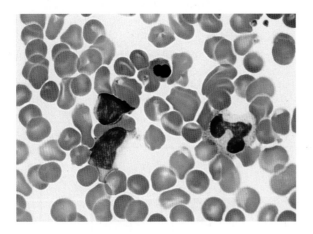

Figure 8-1

PERIPHERAL BLOOD FROM NEWBORN

A physiologically elevated white blood cell count consists of lymphocytes and predominantly neutrophils. A nucleated red blood cell is seen (Wright stain).

pronounced in pediatric patients (2). Although neutrophils predominate in the peripheral blood at birth, lymphocytes are the most numerous peripheral blood white blood cell (WBC) element by about 2 weeks of age (figs. 8-1, 8-2). In infancy and early childhood, the upper limit of normal range for the absolute lymphocyte count is 10,000/μL, while the normal range in adults is 1,000 to 3,000/μL (2). In young children, the circulating normal lymphocytes may exhibit morphologic features of immaturity including nucleoli, more dispersed chromatin, and irregular nuclear contours (figs. 8-3, 8-4). Consequently, patient age and other hematologic parameters such as platelet count, hematocrit, and absolute neutrophil count must be taken into account when assessing peripheral blood for a possible lymphocyte disorder.

The majority of circulating lymphoid cells are mature T cells (60 to 72 percent of lymphocytes), with a helper to suppressor ratio of approximately 2-4 to 1 in adults; in neonates, infants, and young children, this ratio is typically higher due to a physiological preponderance of

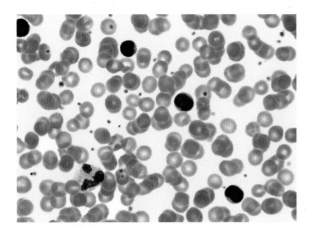

Figure 8-2

PERIPHERAL BLOOD FROM 2-MONTH-OLD

The normal peripheral blood smear from a 2-month-old infant shows a predominance of mature lymphocytes (Wright stain).

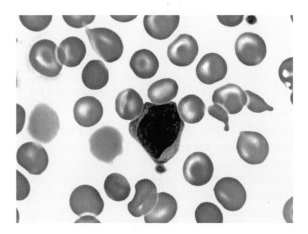

Figure 8-3

LYMPHOCYTE FROM NEWBORN

A circulating lymphocyte with immature nuclear features in a 19-day-old infant (Wright stain).

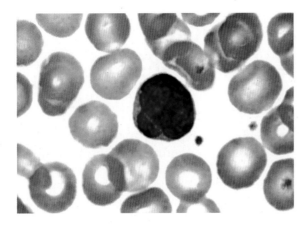

Figure 8-4

LYMPHOID CELL FROM NEWBORN

Both nuclear irregularity and dispersed chromatin are apparent in this normal lymphoid cell in the peripheral blood of a 3-month-old baby (Wright stain).

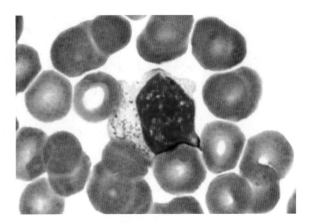

Figure 8-5

LARGE GRANULAR LYMPHOCYTE

Prototypic large granular lymphocyte with moderate amounts of cytoplasm and distinct cytoplasmic granules (Wright stain).

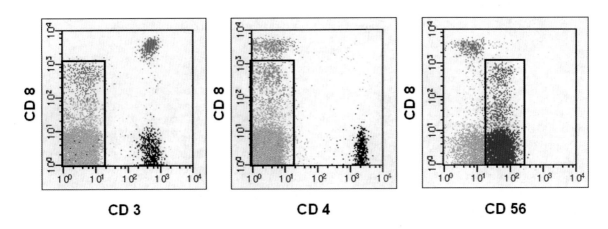

Figure 8-6

TRUE NATURAL KILLER CELLS

An immunophenotypic profile of a true natural killer (NK) cell population demonstrates expression of CD8 (subset) and CD56, while CD3 and CD4 are negative (multicolor flow cytometry). (Box denotes NK cell population.)

helper T cells in these subjects (2,5,11,13). The normal range for absolute CD4 counts declines with age (5). Mature B lymphocytes comprise approximately 10 to 30 percent of circulating lymphoid cells, with a kappa to lambda ratio of about 3 to 1.

Natural killer (NK) cells comprise the smallest normal lymphocyte subset and typically account for 500/μL or less (fig. 8-5) (12,14). True NK cells have the morphology of large granular lymphocytes and express NK-associated antigens (CD56, CD16), while surface CD3

is absent (fig. 8-6) (12,14). These true NK cells often express CD2 and CD8 on the cell surface membrane, while cytoplasmic T-cell intracellular antibody (TIA)-1, granzyme, and perforin stains highlight the cytoplasmic granules, which are essential for NK function.

Lymphocytosis (exceeding the upper limit of normal range for absolute lymphocyte count based on patient age) is a common finding in clinical practice. Because the majority of patients with absolute lymphocytosis do not require bone marrow examination, benign lymphocyte

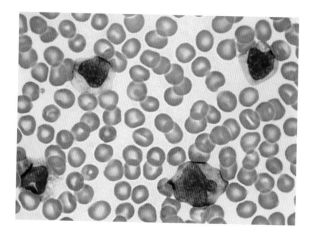

Figure 8-7

**LYMPHOCYTE MORPHOLOGY
IN INFECTIOUS MONONUCLEOSIS**

The peripheral blood smear shows the spectrum of activated lymphocytes in acute infectious mononucleosis infection (Wright stain).

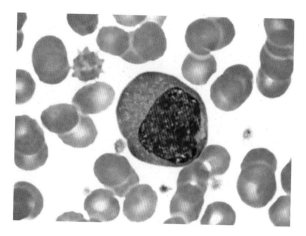

Figure 8-8

IMMUNOBLAST IN INFECTIOUS MONONUCLEOSIS

Activated lymphocyte/immunoblast in a patient with infectious mononucleosis (Wright stain).

Table 8-1

**CAUSES OF NON-NEOPLASTIC
LYMPHOCYTOSIS IN BLOOD[a]**

Morphologic Features of Activation
  Infectious mononucleosis (Epstein-Barr virus)
  Cytomegalovirus infection
  Viral hepatitis
  Acute human immunodeficiency virus-1 infection
  Other viral infections
  Toxoplasmosis
  Drug treatments (e.g., diphenylhydantoin)
  Postvaccination

Nonactivated Morphology
  Pertussis
  Smoking
  Transient stress lymphocytosis
  Thymoma
  Polyclonal B lymphocytosis

[a]Data from references 7, 11, 18, 19, and 21.

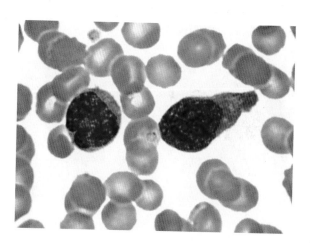

Figure 8-9

**ACTIVATED LYMPHOCYTES
IN INFECTIOUS MONONUCLEOSIS**

The activated lymphocytes have an immunoblast-like appearance. Cytoplasmic granules indicate transformed large granular lymphocytes (Wright stain).

disorders associated with lymphocytosis are only briefly reviewed in this chapter.

The most common causes of reactive lymphocytosis in the blood are listed in Table 8-1. With few exceptions (pertussis, smoking, and acute stress), reactive lymphocytes exhibit a broad morphologic spectrum associated with activation, and the cause of this lymphocyte activation is frequently determined to be a viral infection (fig. 8-7). A hallmark of a benign activated lymphocytosis is the morphologic spectrum of the lymphoid cells, which exhibit a range of nuclear activation (open chromatin, nucleoli) and variable amounts of pale to deeply basophilic cytoplasm (fig. 8-8). In acute viral infections, a substantial portion of these activated lymphocytes exhibit cytoplasmic granules indicative of cytotoxic suppressor T cells or true NK cells (fig. 8-9). Similarly, the presence of circulating immunoblasts is a feature of hantavirus pulmonary syndrome (fig. 8-10). In patients with systemic viral infections, clinical

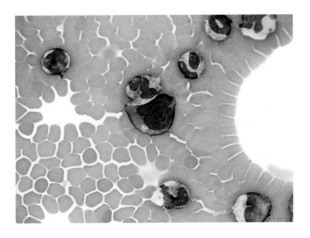

Figure 8-10

**IMMUNOBLAST IN HANTAVIRUS
PULMONARY SYNDROME**

Hantavirus pulmonary syndrome is characterized by a constellation of blood findings which include immunoblasts, thrombocytopenia, hemoconcentration, and left shift (Wright stain).

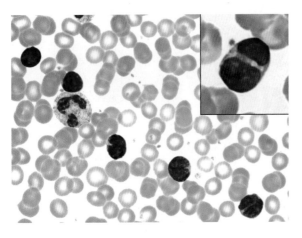

Figure 8-11

LYMPHOCYTOSIS WITH CLEFTING IN PERTUSSIS

Markedly clefted mature lymphocytes in the peripheral blood of a child with pertussis (Wright stain).

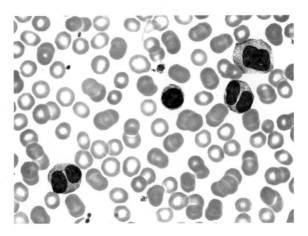

Figure 8-12

POLYCLONAL B LYMPHOCYTOSIS

Sustained absolute lymphocytosis in an adult female smoker (Wright stain). (Courtesy Dr. C. Y. Li, Rochester, MN.)

L-selectin on lymphocytes is the postulated cause of this migratory defect, which results in marked absolute lymphocytosis (10). The circulating lymphocytes in patients with pertussis do not exhibit the prominent spectrum of size due to nuclear and cytoplasmic changes that is linked to an active immune response. Instead, the lymphocytes are generally small, with scanty amounts of cytoplasm, although both nuclear irregularity and clefting are common (fig. 8-11). The diagnosis in these children is often suspected clinically and can be confirmed by nasal swab culture. Consequently, neither bone marrow examination nor flow cytometric immunophenotyping of blood is required in this patient population.

Other causes of sustained lymphocytosis are rare, one of which is persistent polyclonal B lymphocytosis, a human leukocyte antigen (HLA)-DR7-associated disorder described in young women who are typically heavy smokers (6,9). The lymphocyte morphology may be distinctive, and binucleated forms may be evident (figs. 8-12, 8-13) (16). Despite a prolonged indolent and stable course, bcl-2/immunoglobulin heavy chain gene rearrangements and chromosome 3 abnormalities have been detected in these cases, and an underlying constitutional B-cell defect has been proposed (3,4,9). Nonetheless, studies have failed to document an increased risk for the development of overt hematologic malignancies in these patients (6). The overexpression of

correlation and serologic testing are generally sufficient for a definitive diagnosis (see chapter 10 for more details). Flow cytometric immunophenotyping of circulating cells and bone marrow examination are not typically required.

Primarily in children, but also in adults, pertussis infection (whooping cough), secondary to a bacterial infection with *Bordetella pertussis*, is a cause of nonactivated lymphocytosis due to a migration defect of T cells (8). Decreased expression of

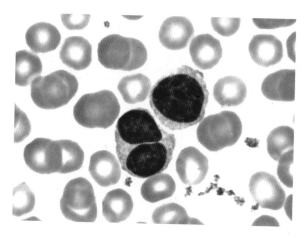

Figure 8-13

POLYCLONAL B LYMPHOCYTOSIS

Sustained absolute lymphocytosis in adult female smoker (Wright stain). (Courtesy of Dr. C. Y. Li, Rochester, MN.)

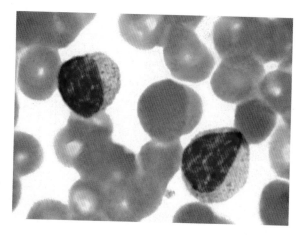

Figure 8-14

LARGE GRANULAR LYMPHOCYTES

Absolute lymphocytosis with a predominance of large granular lymphocytes was confirmed to be NK cells by flow cytometric immunophenotyping in an adult with underlying carcinoma (Wright stain).

bcl-2 and the inhibition of apoptosis may play a role in the increased B-cell accumulation in this disorder. Similarly, reduced expression of adhesion molecules may be linked to the peripheral blood accumulation of B cells (6).

Increased numbers of large granular lymphocytes are seen in a variety of conditions. In many acute viral infections, large granular lymphocytes are increased and show the morphologic features of activation (see fig. 8-9) (17). Some blood smears demonstrate sustained increased numbers of mature, nonactivated, large granular lymphocytes that are either true NK cells or cytotoxic/suppressor T cells (fig. 8-14). In some of these cases, an underlying rheumatologic disorder or a neoplasm is identified, but the cause of the sustained increase in large granular lymphocytes may not be clinically apparent (13,15). These proliferations of large granular lymphocytes may be clonal or nonclonal (fig. 8-15). Although molecular analysis of blood may be used to identify clonal cytotoxic/suppressor T-cell large granular lymphocyte populations, the diagnostician must be aware that these clonal expansions may be transient and may not represent overt neoplastic disorders, especially in asymptomatic patients or patients without associated cytopenias (1). Nonetheless, in symptomatic individuals with a T-cell large granular lymphocytic proliferation, molecular T-cell

clonality analysis is an important diagnostic adjunct to morphologic and phenotypic evaluation. Evaluation of increased large granular lymphocytes of true NK cell derivation can be challenging, since neither flow cytometric immunophenotyping nor T-cell receptor molecular assays are useful in establishing clonality.

In cases in which the cause of the absolute lymphocytosis is not straightforward, multicolor flow cytometric immunophenotyping may be required to characterize these cells and facilitate the identification of clonal, B-cell neoplastic processes or the determination of possible causes of non-neoplastic lymphocytoses. For example, acute viral infections are characterized by a surge in cytotoxic/suppressor T cells, resulting in a dramatic skewing of the helper to suppressor ratio (fig. 8-15) (17). These activated cytotoxic/suppressor T cells express HLA-DR and CD38. Recent reports describe the downregulation of CD7 on activated T cells in acute infectious mononucleosis (20). Increases in true NK cells characterize acute Epstein-Barr virus (EBV) infection (17). Flow cytometric immunophenotyping in patients with polyclonal B lymphocytosis demonstrates increased mature B cells with a normal kappa to lambda light chain ratio. Bone marrow examination is generally required only for suspected or confirmed clonal disorders.

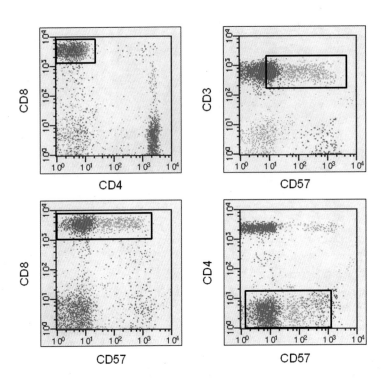

Figure 8-15

**CYTOTOXIC
SUPRESSOR T CELLS**

A flow cytometric histogram of cytotoxic/suppressor (CD3 positive, CD8 positive) large granular T lymphocytes shows partial expression of CD57 (multicolor flow cytometry). (Box denotes T-cytotoxic suppressor population.)

Table 8-2

LYMPHOCYTES AND PLASMA CELLS IN NORMAL BONE MARROW[a]

	Neonates, Infants, Young Children	Children (to puberty)	Adults
% Lymphocytes	May exceed 40%	~ 15-20%	5-15%
Morphology of lymphocytes	Hematogones may be abundant	Variable proportion of hematogones	Usually mature
Distribution of lymphocytes	Diffuse, small clusters	Diffuse, small clusters	Diffuse, small clusters
IP[b] of lymphocytes	B cells predominate	Variable	T cells more numerous (T:B = 4-5:1)
H:S ratio	H = S	S > H	S > H
NK cells	2-4%	2-4%	2-4%
Plasma cells	1-4%	1-4%	1-4%
Morphology, localization of plasma cells	Mature, primarily perivascular; occasional individual interstitial p.c	Mature, primarily perivascular; occasional individual interstitial p.c.	Mature, primarily perivascular; occasional individual interstitial p.c.

[a]Data from references 23, 24, 28, 29, 31, and 33–35.
[b]IP = immmunophenotype; H = helper T cell; S = cytotoxic/suppressor T cell; NK = natural killer cell; p.c. = plasma cell.

NORMAL LYMPHOCYTE AND PLASMA CELL PARAMETERS IN BONE MARROW

Except in infants and young children, lymphocytes are generally relatively inconspicuous in bone marrow specimens from normal patients (Table 8-2). In adolescents and adults, these lymphocytes are cytologically mature, diffusely admixed with normal hematopoietic elements, and comprise 15 percent or fewer of the cells in differential counts (26). Small aggregates of lymphocytes may be appreciated in normal subjects; more sizable lymphoid aggregates are more common in bone marrow specimens from hematologically normal elderly patients. For patients over 60 years of age, benign lymphoid

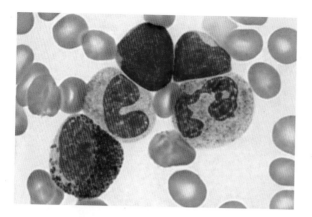

Figure 8-16

HEMATOGONE COMPARED TO NORMAL LYMPHOCYTE

The bone marrow from an infant shows a hematogone with dense homogenous nuclear chromatin and a normal lymphoid cell (Wright stain).

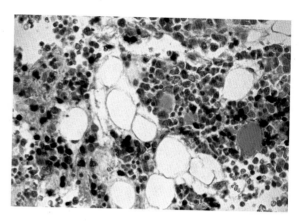

Figure 8-17

NORMAL T CELLS (CD3)

Immunoperoxidase staining for CD3 highlights interstitial patches and individually dispersed mature T cells from a young adult patient with negative bone marrow staging for lymphoma.

aggregates are noted in 10 percent of males and 20 percent of females (27).

Hematogones

In infants and young children, benign lymphoid precursor cells, termed hematogones, are typically abundant and account for 40 percent or more of the cells in a differential count (35). Hematogones are characterized by a high nuclear to cytoplasmic ratio, homogeneously condensed nuclear chromatin with absent to inconspicuous nucleoli, and variable nuclear size (fig. 8-16) (26). Lymphocytes with this morphology are typically B cells that exhibit a range in immunophenotypic maturity, including cells with terminal deoxynucleotidyltransferase (TdT), CD10, and CD34 positivity (see later in this chapter). Although lymphoid cells with these immunophenotypic features of hematogones may be detected in bone marrow specimens from adults, morphologically distinctive hematogones are generally inconspicuous in adult specimens.

Lymphocyte Immunophenotype

Both flow cytometric immunophenotyping and paraffin immunoperoxidase studies have been used to characterize normal lymphocyte subsets in bone marrow from patients of various ages (Table 8-2). Although both the sensitivity and multicolor antigen assessment results achieved by flow cytometric immunophenotyping are desirable, the extent of peripheral

blood contamination varies substantially in bone marrow aspirate specimens and can skew flow results significantly (33). Except in cases with abundant hematogones, mature T cells predominate in normal bone marrow, with a T cell to B cell ratio of about 4-5 to 1 (28). Unlike peripheral blood, cytotoxic/suppressor (CD8-positive) T cells tend to outnumber helper T cells (CD4-positive) in normal bone marrow specimens. Except in pediatric cases with abundant hematogones, bone marrow B cells are generally cytologically and immunophenotypically mature and have a kappa to lambda ratio that parallels that of the peripheral blood.

Paraffin immunoperoxidase studies of normal bone marrow from adults show both T and B lymphocytes that are either diffusely dispersed or present in small interstitial clusters on core biopsy sections (figs. 8-17–8-19) (28,31). The more numerous T cells may also concentrate along blood vessels, while B cells are primarily individually dispersed.

Plasma Cells

Plasma cells are cytologically mature in normal bone marrow specimens and typically comprise only 1 to 4 percent of the total number of cells (fig. 8-20) (25). Normal plasma cells have a distinct perivascular location and have a kappa to lambda ratio of 1.2–3.4 to 1 (figs. 8-21–8-23) (29). Heavy chain expression studies reveal relatively

Figure 8-18

NORMAL T CELLS (CD3)

A tendency for normal mature T cells to concentrate near blood vessels in an adult with negative bone marrow staging for lymphoma.

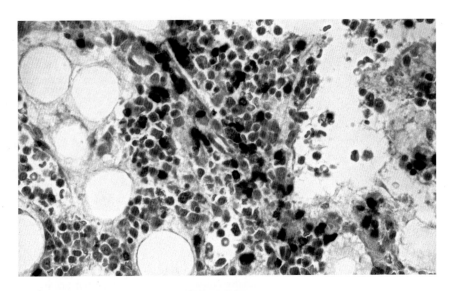

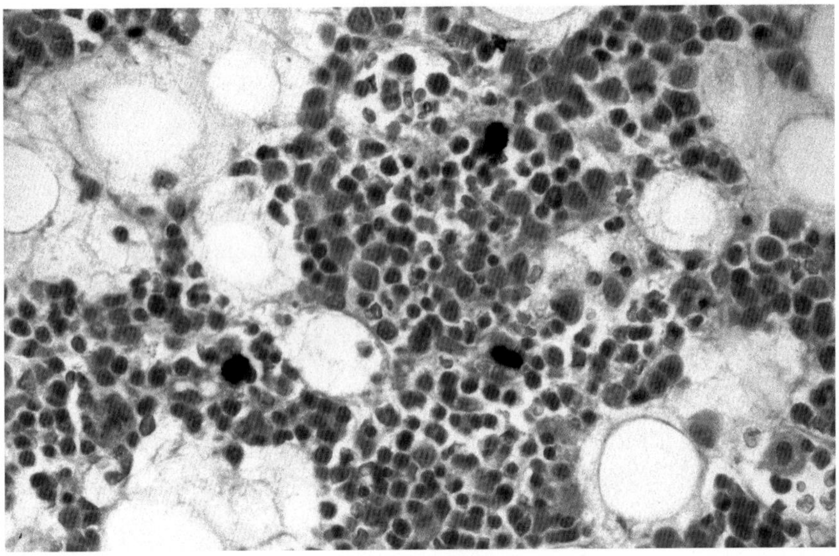

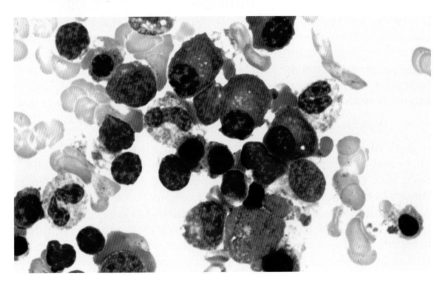

Figure 8-19

NORMAL B CELLS (CD20)

Sparse, individually dispersed mature B cells are evident by immunoperoxidase staining for CD20 in normal adult bone marrow obtained for lymphoma staging.

Figure 8-20

PLASMACYTOSIS

Abundant plasma cells on bone marrow aspirate smear from a pediatric patient (Wright stain).

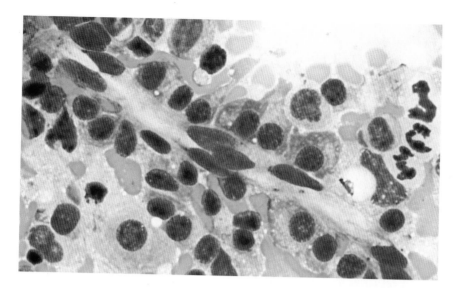

Figure 8-21

**PERIVASCULAR
PLASMA CELLS**

The perivascular distribution of plasma cells is evident on a bone marrow aspirate particle crush preparation containing capillaries (Wright stain).

Figure 8-22

**NORMAL PLASMA
CELLS (KAPPA)**

Immunoperoxidase staining for kappa light chain highlights individually dispersed plasma cells, several of which are located adjacent to vascular spaces from a normal adult.

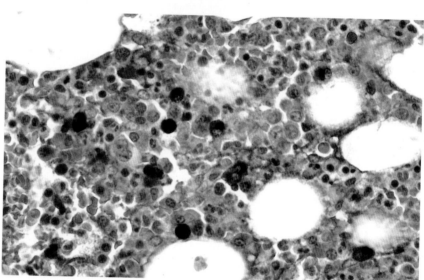

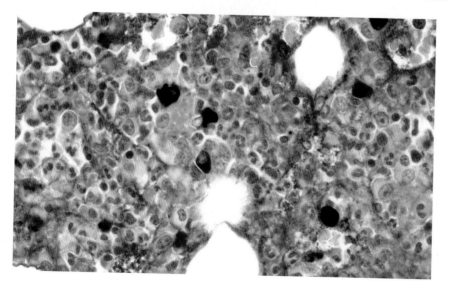

Figure 8-23

**NORMAL PLASMA
CELLS (LAMBDA)**

Immunoperoxidase staining for lambda light chain demonstrates individually dispersed plasma cells, some of which are perivascular, from a normal adult.

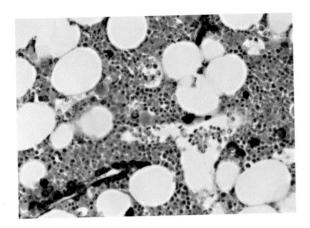

Figure 8-24

PERIVASCULAR PLASMA CELLS (CD138)

Immunoperoxidase staining for CD138 highlights the perivascular distribution of plasma cells in normal adult bone marrow.

equal numbers of immunoglobulin (Ig)G- and IgA-positive plasma cells in normal bone marrow; IgM- and IgD-positive plasma cells are infrequent (29). Plasma cells can be highlighted by immunoperoxidase CD138 or CD38 staining (fig. 8-24) (22,25). By flow cytometric immunophenotyping, the intensity of the CD38 expression must be assessed along with other markers (e.g., CD45, cytoplasmic light chains), since activated T cells and other proliferating cells may exhibit moderate CD38 expression, while plasma cells exhibit brighter positivity. Normal plasma cells are characteristically CD56 negative and CD45 positive, features useful in the distinction from a plasma cell dyscrasia (30,32). In a recent immunohistochemical study utilizing a monoclonal antibody to CD56, expression of this antigen was evident on over 90 percent of overt myelomas but only 20 percent of reactive plasmacytoses (30).

CONSTITUTIONAL DISORDERS WITH ABNORMAL LYMPHOCYTES

Although only rarely encountered in clinical practice, distinctive lymphocyte morphologic features are an important clue to various constitutional lysosomal storage disorders including the mucopolysaccharidoses and mucolipidoses (36–39). These lymphocyte aberrations are best appreciated on peripheral blood smears, but may also be seen in the bone marrow. Abundant sharp cytoplasmic vacuoles, large cytoplasmic

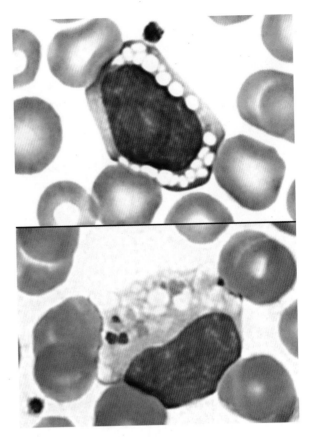

Figure 8-25

LYMPHOCYTES IN SIALIDOSIS

Distinct cytoplasmic vacuolization with abnormal granulation is evident in peripheral blood lymphocytes in an infant with sialidosis (Wright stain).

inclusions, and cytoplasmic granules different from those of normal large granular lymphocytes are characteristic (figs. 8-25, 8-26). The distinct cytoplasmic granules may be surrounded by halos. In patients with mucopolysaccharidoses or mucolipidoses, abnormal cytoplasmic inclusions may be evident in plasma cells, histiocytes, reticular cells, and osteoblasts of bone marrow (37). (See chapter 9 for a discussion of lipidoses including Niemann-Pick and Gaucher disease.) A definitive diagnosis should not be made based on the morphologic features of the lymphocytes; various confirmatory genetic or enzymatic assays must be performed on appropriate specimens to confirm the diagnosis of these rare constitutional disorders (38,39). In general, the other multisystem abnormalities, especially neurologic manifestations, dominate and the hematologic manifestations are relatively insignificant.

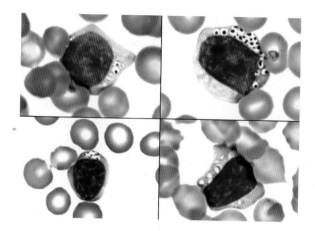

Figure 8-26

ABNORMAL LYMPHOCYTES

Abnormal lymphocyte granules/inclusions (some with halos) in children with various metabolic disorders, including Hurler syndrome (top left), Hunter-Hurler syndrome (bottom left), Maroteaux-Lamy syndrome (top right), and Sanfilippo disease (bottom right) (Wright stain). (Courtesy of Dr. C. Hanson, Rochester, MN.)

NON-NEOPLASTIC DIFFUSE LYMPHOID INFILTRATES IN BONE MARROW

Increased Hematogones in Bone Marrow

As noted above, bone marrow specimens from children, especially infants and young children, typically contain abundant hematogones, benign B cells that exhibit a spectrum of morphologic and immunophenotypic maturation (Table 8-3) (42,43,46,47,54,56,59). In some patients, hematogones may be strikingly increased, mimicking acute leukemia; in preterm infants, hematogone populations may account for 60 percent of the cells (51). In order to successfully distinguish these non-neoplastic precursor cells from overt leukemia, the diagnostician must be aware of not only the morphologic and immunophenotypic features of these cells, but also the clinical settings in which increased bone marrow hematogones are likely (Table 8-3).

Hematogones exhibit a broad range in size, while nuclear and cytoplasmic features are fairly homogeneous (figs. 8-27, 8-28). On bone marrow biopsy sections, hematogones generally demonstrate round nuclear contours and condensed chromatin. Notably, hematogones do not exhibit the convoluted and blastic features of typical acute lymphoblastic leukemia cells on

Table 8-3

KEY FEATURES OF HEMATOGONES[a]

Benign bone marrow B-cell precursors showing maturation

Dense homogeneous nuclear chromatin, absent or inconspicuous nucleoli, scant cytoplasm

Diffuse infiltration in bone marrow

Cells with morphologic features of hematogones not generally evident on blood smears

Spectrum of B-cell maturation; only small proportion are TdT[b], CD34 positive; majority show loss of Ig light chain with gradual loss of intensity of CD10 positivity and gain in CD20 expression

By multicolor flow cytometry, immunophenotypic hematogones identified in very low numbers in blood from children and adults

Absence of significant CD34, TdT clustering on clot/biopsy sections; individual positive cells present

Most prominent in neonates, infants, and in settings of bone marrow recovery (after infection, chemotherapy, transplantation) or in association with constitutional disorders, ITP, or nonhematopoietic neoplasms

Account for up to 60% of cells bone marrow in preterm infants

Nonclonal, diploid cells

[a]Data from references 40–43, 45–54, 56–58, 60–62.
[b]TdT = terminal deoxynucleotidyltransferase; Ig = immunoglobulin; ITP = immune thrombocytopenic purpura.

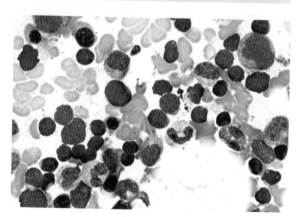

Figure 8-27

INCREASED BONE MARROW HEMATOGONES

Increased lymphocytes including hematogones show a range in nuclear size in a bone marrow aspirate smear from a child recovering from multiagent chemotherapy for acute myelogenous leukemia (Wright stain).

tissue sections (figs. 8-29, 8-30). These cells are diffusely dispersed throughout the bone marrow and may account for 40 percent or more of

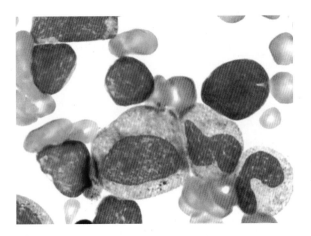

Figure 8-28

INCREASED BONE MARROW HEMATOGONES

High-power magnification of a bone marrow aspirate smear from an infant shows prototypic nuclear features of hematogones with uniformly condensed nuclear chromatin, occasional irregular nuclear contours, and scant cytoplasm (Wright stain).

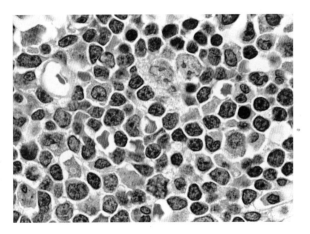

Figure 8-30

INCREASED BONE MARROW HEMATOGONES

Hematogones on a paraffin section exhibit relatively condensed nuclear chromatin, round nuclear contours, and inconspicuous mitotic activity (H&E stain). (Courtesy of Dr. Dennis O'Malley, Irvine, CA.)

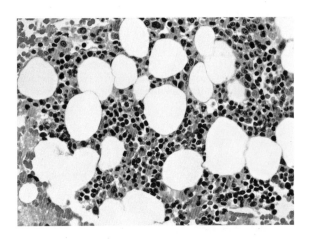

Figure 8-29

INCREASED BONE MARROW HEMATOGONES

A bone marrow clot section shows numerous dense hematogones in conjunction with early hematopoietic regeneration following potent multiagent chemotherapy (hematoxylin and eosin [H&E] stain).

the bone marrow cells. Lymphoid cells with the morphologic features of hematogones are not generally appreciated on blood smears.

Bone marrow hematogones can be especially numerous after bone marrow suppression and in infants and young children with various constitutional hematologic disorders, immune thrombocytopenic purpura, and nonhematopoietic solid tumors (47,48,53). Although also identified immunophenotypically in specimens from adults, especially in patients with either significant bone marrow suppression or B-cell dysfunction, these hematogones are neither as conspicuous morphologically nor as cytologically immature as those encountered in pediatric specimens (41,49,58,62). The types of bone marrow suppression linked to increased hematogones include multiagent chemotherapy, bone marrow transplantation, and infections, especially viral. In these settings, the surge in bone marrow hematogones is presumed to parallel immunologic recovery (62). Indeed, hematogones tend to be most numerous within the first 6 months of the cessation of antileukemic therapy (57,60,61).

The integration of morphology with immunophenotypic findings is essential in distinguishing hematogones from acute lymphoblastic leukemia (49,50). Hematogones typically exhibit a broad spectrum of maturation highlighted by multicolor immunophenotyping. In acute lymphoblastic leukemia, the neoplastic cells are both immunophenotypically homogeneous and show frequent aberrant patterns of antigen expression (44). Consequently, a range in expression of CD45, CD34, TdT, CD20, and CD10 is detected in bone marrow specimens with increased hematogones, reflecting ongoing lymphoid maturation (figs. 8-31, 8-32) (44). Recent

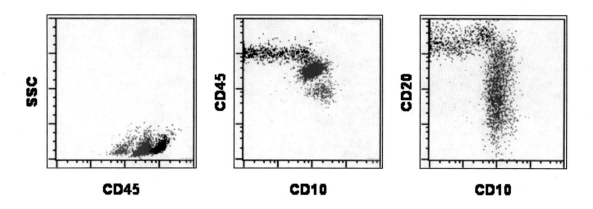

Figure 8-31

IMMUNOPHENOTYPIC PROFILE OF HEMATOGONES

There is a spectrum of expression of CD45, CD10, and CD20 by flow cytometric immunophenotyping (multicolor flow cytometry).

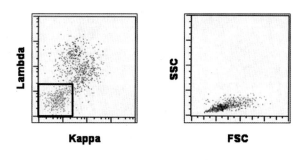

Figure 8-32

IMMUNOPHENOTYPIC PROFILE OF MATURE B CELLS AND HEMATOGONES

Polyclonal mature B cells are evident along with immature surface immunoglobulin-negative B cells in a bone marrow with increased hematogones (multicolor flow cytometry). (Hematogone population in box.)

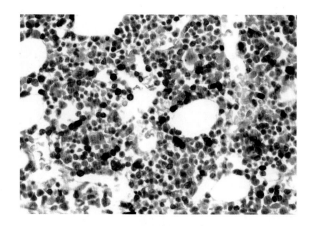

Figure 8-33

HEMATOGONES (CD79a)

Immunoperoxidase staining for CD79a highlights increased B cells in 2-year-old child with immune thrombocytopenic purpura and increased bone marrow hematogones.

studies describe a spectrum of CD43 expression in hematogones. The expression of this antigen can be integrated with CD10, CD20, and CD34 antigen coexpression profiles to distinguish hematogones from acute lymphoblastic leukemia (55). Importantly, aberrant or dyssynchronous antigen expression is not found in non-neoplastic hematogone populations but is common in acute lymphoblastic leukemia (45,49).

Paraffin immunoperoxidase assessment of bone marrow clot or core biopsy sections is also useful for identifying hematogones and distinguishing them from acute lymphoblastic leukemia (52). Even though a subset of hematogones express CD34 and/or TdT, these immature cells do not characteristically exhibit the significant clustering or the effacing sheets of cells on tissue sections that typify acute lymphoblastic leukemia at presentation (sheets) or early relapse (clusters) (figs. 8-33–8-35) (52,62). Multicolor flow cytometric immunophenotypic studies of peripheral blood reveal few immunophenotypic hematogones in either pediatric or adult subjects (40,45).

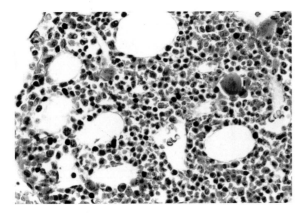

Figure 8-34

HEMATOGONES (TdT)

Nuclear positivity in the bone marrow and increased hematogones in a 2-year-old boy with immune thrombocytopenic purpura (immunoperoxidase for TdT).

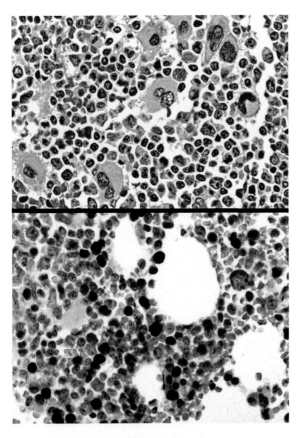

Figure 8-35

**PREMATURE NEWBORN
WITH INCREASED HEMATOGONES**

Composite of H&E (top) and TdT (bottom) stains in a premature infant with increased bone marrow hematogones. (Courtesy of Dr. L. Rimsza, Tucson, AZ.)

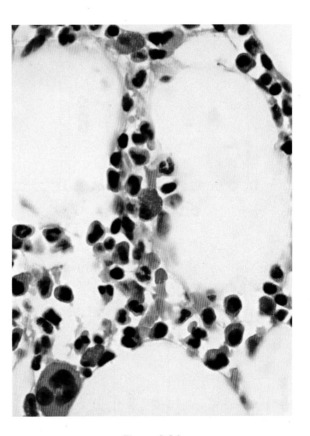

Figure 8-36

**HYPOCELLULAR BONE MARROW WITH
INCONSPICUOUS LYMPHOID INFILTRATE**

An inconspicuous diffuse increase in lymphocytes is seen on bone marrow biopsy section (H&E stain).

Diffuse Non-Neoplastic
T-Cell Infiltrates in Bone Marrow

In adults, a bone marrow core biopsy specimen with a marked diffuse interstitial increase in T cells represents a distinct diagnostic challenge. Often, the patient has undergone bone marrow examination for an unexplained cytopenia or nonspecific, yet alarming, symptoms such as fatigue, weight loss, or fever. In these cases, the lymphoid cells on both aspirate smears and core biopsy sections may be relatively inconspicuous, with nondescript cytologic features (fig. 8-36); however, with paraffin immunoperoxidase assessment, a substantial increase in CD3-positive T cells is highlighted (fig. 8-37). Additional workup in these cases should include assessment of T-cell subsets (CD4 and CD8), TIA-1 (or other cytotoxic markers), and TdT and CD34 if nuclear immaturity is appreciated (fig. 8-37).

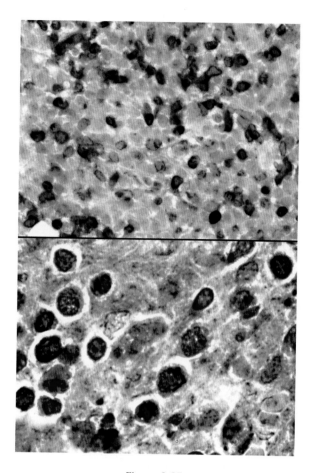

Figure 8-37

INTERSTITIAL T CELLS

A diffuse interstitial increase in T cells is highlighted by CD3 staining (top) and TIA-1 staining (bottom).

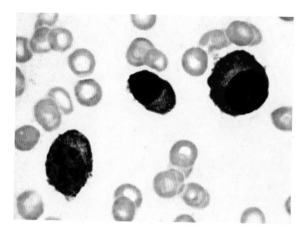

Figure 8-38

SYSTEMIC POLYCLONAL IMMUNOBLASTIC REACTION

The immunoblastic and plasma cell infiltrate of the bone marrow is extensive in a child with systemic polyclonal immunoblastic reaction (Wright stain).

In the setting of a diffuse increase in mature T cells, a diagnosis of occult T-cell large granular lymphocytic leukemia (positivity for CD3, CD8, TIA-1, and CD57) must be excluded. Correlation with the morphologic assessment of the peripheral blood for the proportion of large granular lymphocytes is essential. Confirmation of T-cell receptor gene rearrangement by molecular assessment is important in cases of suspected T-cell large granular lymphocytic leukemia (67). Because substantial T-cell infiltrates can be morphologically inconspicuous, a low threshold for performing immunoperoxidase assessment for T cells (CD3) is recommended, and should always be performed in conjunction with an assessment for B cells (CD20). If an aspirate specimen is available, multicolor flow cytometric assessment of bone marrow for B- and T-cell subsets is an optimal modality to evaluate "aspirable" lymphocyte populations.

In cases with increased, yet nonclonal T cells, several differential diagnostic considerations need to be entertained. Disorders associated with T-cell proliferations in blood and/or bone marrow include thymoma, other immune disorders, various infections (human immunodeficiency virus [HIV]-1, human T-cell leukemia-lymphoma virus [HTLV]-1, and *Ehrlichia*), and even post vaccination (63–66,68–70,72–74). Apparent T-cell clonality (sometimes transient) may be detected in some of these cases, even those that spontaneously remit (64,65,71). Although a common etiology may not apply to all of these unique situations, a florid T-cell proliferation (often cytotoxic/suppressor type) may be the consequence of an underlying immunoregulatory aberration or immunodeficiency (63,64,68,74).

Systemic Polyclonal Immunoblastic Proliferations Involving Bone Marrow

Rare patients present with an acute systemic illness characterized by widespread polyclonal immunoblastic infiltration of blood, bone marrow, lymph node, and other sites (75–79). In some cases, a relatively uniform population of large immunoblasts is present in multiple sites; these immunoblasts have large nuclei, distinct

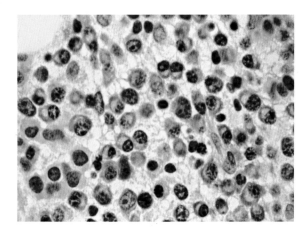

Figure 8-39

SYSTEMIC POLYCLONAL IMMUNOBLASTIC REACTION

Extensive infiltrate of plasma cells and immunoblasts in a child with polyclonal systemic immunoblastic reaction (H&E stain).

nucleoli, and moderate amounts of basophilic cytoplasm. Admixed plasma cells may be evident, and a morphologic progression between plasma cells and immunoblasts may be seen (figs. 8-38, 8-39). In the bone marrow, the immunoblastic infiltrate may be interstitial, admixed with hematopoietic elements, or solidly effacing (fig. 8-39). Despite extensive tissue infiltration, these large cells are polyclonal by immunophenotypic assessment (fig. 8-40). In some cases, immune aberrations such as hemolytic anemia and polyclonal hypergammaglobulinemia are detected (77). Although underlying infections occasionally trigger this type of exuberant, aberrant immune response, a specific etiology is not detected in most cases (75,77).

BENIGN LYMPHOID AGGREGATES IN BONE MARROW

Lymphoid aggregates are well-delineated, dense aggregates of small lymphocytes best appreciated on bone marrow clot or core biopsy sections (fig. 8-41). Lymphoid aggregates are a relatively common finding in bone marrow specimens, most notably from older patients (especially females) and patients with underlying immune disorders or systemic infections (82,86,89,91). Benign bone marrow lymphoid aggregates are also associated with aplastic anemia, chronic myeloid disorders, and multiple myeloma (fig. 8-41) (90,94).

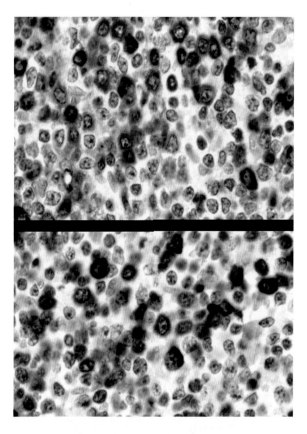

Figure 8-40

POLYCLONAL PLASMA CELLS

Polyclonal staining of immunoblasts and plasma cells for kappa and lambda in the bone marrow demonstrates a systemic immunoblastic reaction.

They may also be evident following myeloablative chemotherapy (fig. 8-42).

Although small mature lymphocytes generally predominate in these aggregates, other minor cell types include mature plasma cells, histiocytes, mast cells, and occasional eosinophils (fig. 8-43). Cytologic atypia is absent to minimal; however, some degree of nuclear irregularity is seen in small to intermediate-sized aggregated lymphocytes in patients with HIV-1 infection (fig. 8-44) (82,89).

The localization of the lymphoid aggregate in the bone marrow is a key feature to evaluate because benign and neoplastic lymphoid aggregates tend to reside in different areas of the core biopsy. For example, three-dimensional reconstruction of benign lymphoid aggregates in bone marrow core biopsies show a central, nonparatrabecular localization (fig. 8-45) (92). In addition, the majority

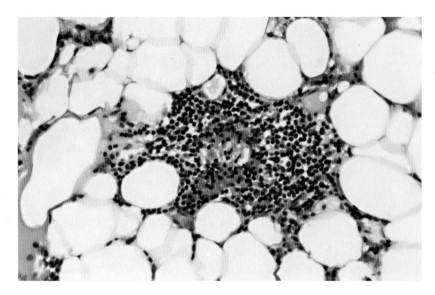

Figure 8-41

BENIGN LYMPHOID AGGREGATE

Bone marrow core biopsy section shows a lymphoid aggregate in a patient with aplastic anemia (H&E stain).

Figure 8-42

LYMPHOID AGGREGATE FOLLOWING CHEMOTHERAPY

A small lymphoid aggregate is evident in an otherwise hypocellular bone marrow following myeloablative chemotherapy (H&E stain).

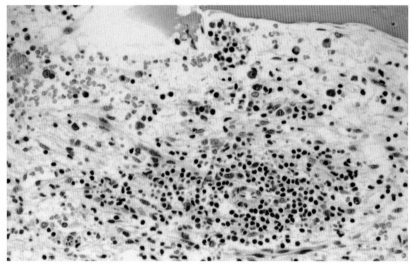

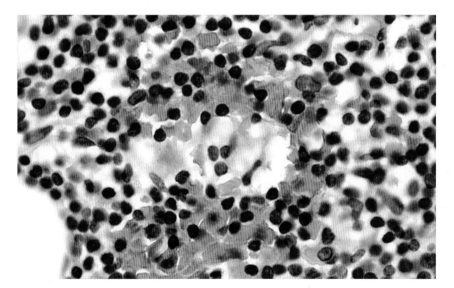

Figure 8-43

BENIGN LYMPHOID AGGREGATE

Mature lymphocytes predominate in a benign lymphoid aggregate. Admixed macrophages and plasma cells are also evident (H&E stain).

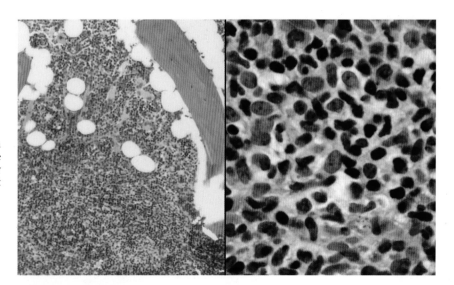

Figure 8-44

ATYPICAL LYMPHOID AGGREGATE IN AIDS

Low and high magnification of an atypical lymphoid aggregate in a human immunodeficiency virus (HIV)-1-positive patient (H&E stain).

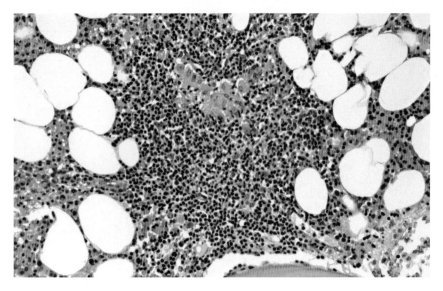

Figure 8-45

NONPARATRABECULAR LYMPHOID AGGREGATE

Epithelioid granuloma within a benign lymphoid aggregate in a bone marrow biopsy section from an adult. The lymphoid aggregate is close to the bony trabecula although not molded to it (H&E stain).

of benign lymphoid aggregates are perivascular or adjacent to dilated sinuses (figs. 8-46–8-49). Lymphoid aggregates may be associated with either lipogranulomas or epithelioid granulomas (figs. 8-45, 8-50–8-52). Germinal center formation may be evident within benign lymphoid aggregates, especially in patients with underlying autoimmune disorders (figs. 8-53–8-55) (82,86,91).

Distinguishing benign lymphoid aggregates from overt non-Hodgkin lymphoma can be problematic and requires the integration of cytologic, morphologic, immunophenotypic, and clinical findings (Table 8-4). Immunophenotyping may be particularly helpful since T cells typically predominate in benign lymphoid aggregates while B cells predominate in many non-Hodgkin lymphomas that involve bone marrow; light chain restriction can be determined if fresh cells are available (figs. 8-56–8-62). The B-cell neoplasms that are composed of small mature-appearing lymphoid cells may aberrantly coexpress antigens such as CD5 and CD43, which are not characteristically present on normal mature B cells except in very minor normal subpopulations; however, hematogones may be CD43 positive (95). Consequently, aberrant antigen expression patterns can distinguish neoplastic from reactive processes. Neoplastic lymphoid infiltrates in bone marrow often demonstrate distinctive patterns of infiltration, including paratrabecular and sinusoidal, neither of which is typical of a non-neoplastic infiltrate

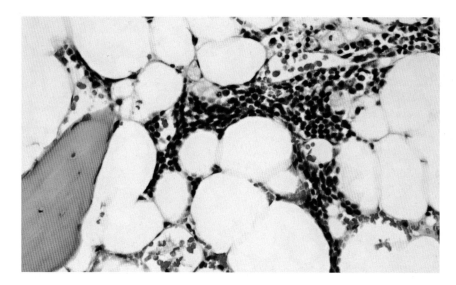

Figure 8-46

PERIVASCULAR LYMPHOID AGGREGATE

Perivascular benign lymphoid aggregate in a patient with aplastic anemia (H&E stain).

Figure 8-47

LYMPHOID AGGREGATE IN VIRAL INFECTION

A small lymphoid aggregate in the bone marrow in a patient with acute parvovirus infection (H&E stain).

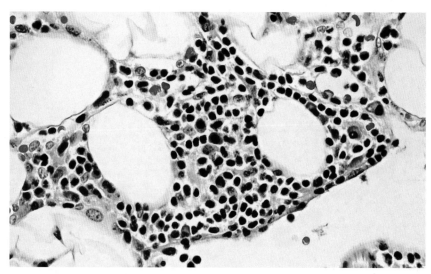

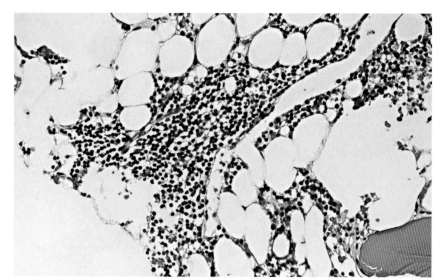

Figure 8-48

LYMPHOID AGGREGATE ADJACENT TO BONE MARROW SINUS

A small benign lymphoid aggregate is adjacent to a dilated bone marrow sinus in a bone marrow core biopsy section from an adult (H&E stain).

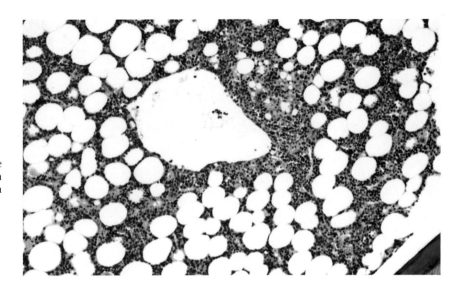

Figure 8-49

LYMPHOID AGGREGATE ADJACENT TO BONE MARROW SINUS

A benign lymphoid aggregate is adjacent to a dilated sinus on a bone marrow biopsy section (H&E stain).

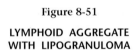

Figure 8-50

LYMPHOID AGGREGATE WITH EPITHELIOID GRANULOMA

A benign lymphoid aggregate and an epithelioid granuloma are present on a bone marrow core biopsy specimen (H&E stain).

Figure 8-51

LYMPHOID AGGREGATE WITH LIPOGRANULOMA

The lymphoid aggregate has a prominent lipogranulomatous component on a bone marrow biopsy section (H&E stain).

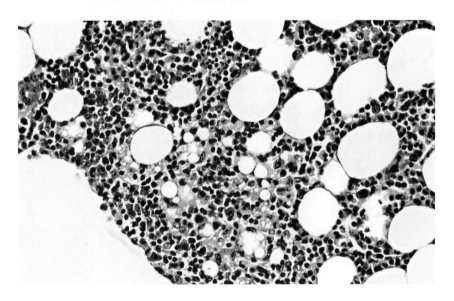

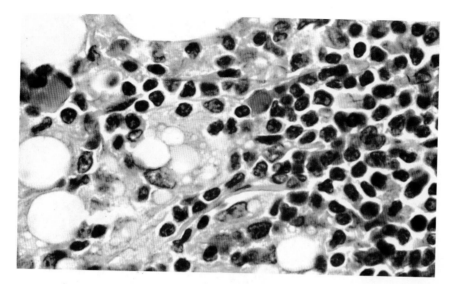

Figure 8-52

LIPOGRANULOMA

Foamy macrophages comprise a lipogranuloma associated with a benign perivascular lymphoid aggregate (H&E stain).

Figure 8-53

LYMPHOID AGGREGATE WITH SMALL GERMINAL CENTER

A lymphoid aggregate with a small germinal center in a 21-month-old child (H&E stain).

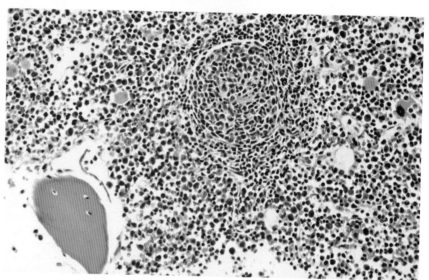

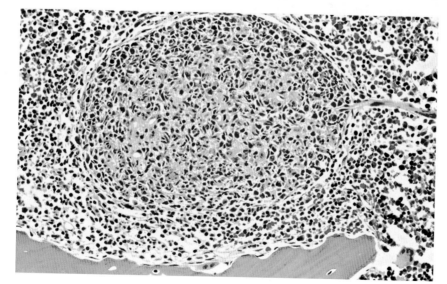

Figure 8-54

LYMPHOID AGGREGATE WITH PROMINENT GERMINAL CENTER

Discrete germinal center formation within a benign lymphoid aggregate in child with immune thrombocytopenic purpura (H&E stain).

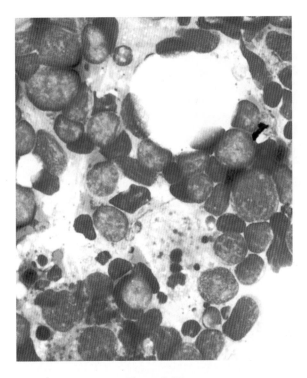

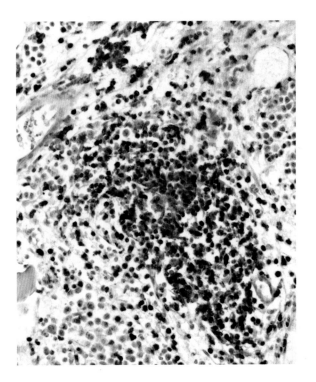

Figure 8-55

GERMINAL CENTER CELLS

Germinal center cells are seen on a bone marrow aspirate. Tingible body macrophages are also present (Wright stain).

Figure 8-56

BENIGN LYMPHOID AGGREGATE (CD3)

Immunoperoxidase staining for CD3 highlights the T cells in a benign lymphoid aggregate following myeloablative chemotherapy.

Table 8-4

COMPARISON OF BENIGN LYMPHOID AGGREGATES WITH OVERT NON-HODGKIN LYMPHOMA ON BONE MARROW SECTIONS[a]

Feature	Benign Lymphoid Aggregates	Non-Hodgkin Lymphoma
Number of aggregates	Usually only a few	Multiple, may be confluent
Location	Perivascular, adjacent to sinuses	Many patterns noted including paratrabecular or intrasinusoidal
Circumscription	Well circumscribed	Infiltrative margins
Cellular composition	Mature, small round lymphocytes typically predominate; occasional lymphoid aggregates have distinct germinal center[b] (Nuclear irregularity may be evident on H&E[c] sections)	Cytologic atypia may be present Variable cell size Nuclear irregularity may be prominent
Immunophenotype	T > B; T approximately = B B cells may be concentrated in center with T cells at periphery Plasma cells polyclonal Plasma cells may be highlighted by CD38/CD138[d]	Usually B cell predominance, except in rare T-NHL Light chain restriction may be detected in B-NHL Aberrant antigen coexpression on B cells such as CD5 or CD43
Genotype	Nonclonal	Clonal[e]

[a]Data from references 80, 81, 83, 84, and 91–94.
[b]Rare bone marrow infiltrates of marginal zone lymphoma may exhibit a germinal center.
[c]H&E = hematoxylin and eosin stain; NHL = non-Hodgkin lymphoma.
[d]CD138 also stains nonhematolymphoid cells (83).
[e]May get false negative results due to sampling (80,84)

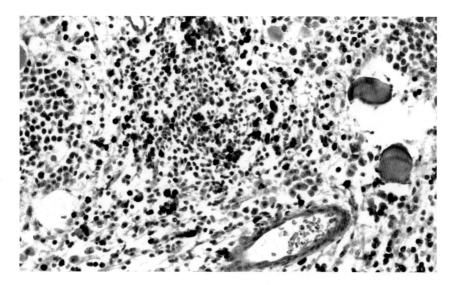

Figure 8-57

BENIGN LYMPHOID AGGREGATE (CD79a)

Benign lymphoid aggregate shows few admixed B cells in a bone marrow biopsy section following myeloablative chemotherapy.

Figure 8-58

BENIGN LYMPHOID AGGREGATE (CD20)

B cells within a benign lymphoid aggregate are highlighted by immunoperoxidase staining for CD20.

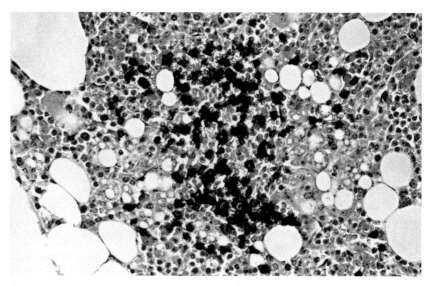

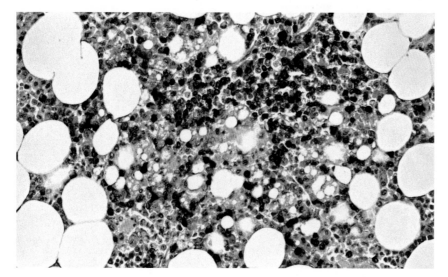

Figure 8-59

BENIGN LYMPHOID AGGREGATE (CD5)

A predominance of T cells in a benign lymphoid aggregate is highlighted by immunoperoxidase for CD5.

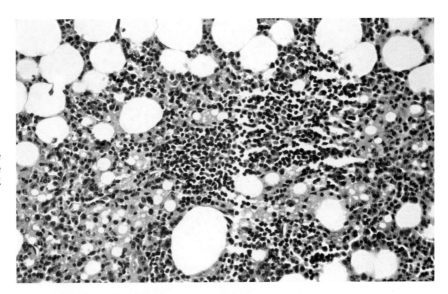

Figure 8-60

**LYMPHOID AGGREGATE
WITH LIPOGRANULOMA**

A benign lymphoid aggregate
with a lipogranuloma on a bone
marrow biopsy section (H&E
stain).

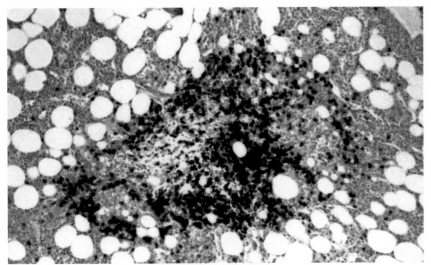

Figure 8-61

**BENIGN LYMPHID
AGGREGATE (CD20)**

B cells within a benign lymphoid aggregate are highlighted
by CD20 staining.

Figure 8-62

**BENIGN LYMPHOID
AGGREGATE (CD5)**

Abundant T cells within a
benign lymphoid aggregate
are highlighted by immunoperoxidase staining for CD5.

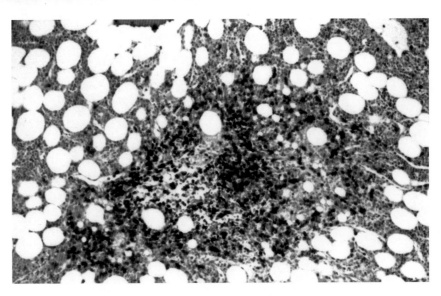

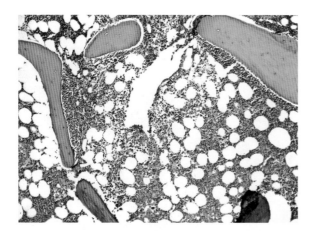

Figure 8-63

PARATRABECULAR INFILTRATE OF LYMPHOMA

Paratrabecular infiltrate in mantle cell lymphoma (H&E stain).

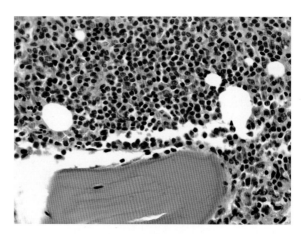

Figure 8-64

POORLY DELINEATED LYMPHOID INFILTRATE IN LYMPHOMA

Poorly delineated infiltrate of small lymphoid cells in a bone marrow involved by splenic marginal zone lymphoma (H&E stain).

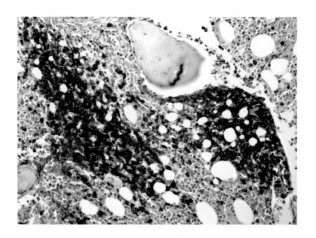

Figure 8-65

B-CELL LYMPHOMA (CD20)

CD20 highlights the B cells in the bone marrow involved by splenic marginal zone lymphoma.

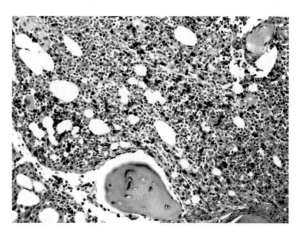

Figure 8-66

B-CELL LYMPHOMA (CD3)

CD3 highlights T cells in bone marrow involved by splenic marginal zone lymphoma. There are fewer T cells than seen in figure 8-64.

(fig. 8-63) (92,93). Intrasinusoidal collections of benign B cells, however, have been recently described in the bone marrow of patients with polyclonal B lymphocytosis (87). In addition, neoplastic lymphoid nodules tend to be poorly circumscribed (fig. 8-64) and show a clearcut B-cell predominance (figs. 8-65, 8-66).

The distinction between benign lymphoid aggregates and residual malignant B-cell lymphoma can be especially problematic after rituximab (anti-CD20) therapy (85). In these cases,

post-therapy T-cell aggregates can be multiple, poorly circumscribed, and even paratrabecular. Flow cytometric assessment for B-cell clonality may be helpful in resolving problematic cases as long as the lymphoid cells in question are well represented in the aspirate specimen. Alternative B-cell markers such as CD19 and CD79a must be used to assess for residual B-cell lymphoma following rituximab administration, because CD20 expression is masked by the binding of the anti-CD20 antibody.

Table 8-5

REACTIVE PLASMACYTOSIS IN BONE MARROW[a]

Feature	Comments
Associations	Cirrhosis
	Infections: HIV-1[b], other viral/bacterial infections
	Autoimmune/hypersensitivity: SLE, RA, drug reaction
	Solid tumors: carcinomas, Hodgkin lymphoma
	Leukemias: rare acute myelogenous leukemia
	Miscellaneous: following therapy, including myeloma therapy
Features	Plasmacytosis often occurs in conjunction with lymphoid aggregates and lipogranulomas
	Perivascular localization predominates
	May also see diffuse increase of individually dispersed plasma cells
	May see variety of morphologic features such as Mott cells, Russell bodies, flame cells, and binucleate forms
	Polyclonal by kappa/lambda assessment
	Positive for CD38, CD138, CD30, focal CD31
	Lack CD56, CD117

[a]Data from references 97, 99, 100, 102, and 106.
[b]HIV = human immunodeficiency virus; SLE = systemic lupus erythematosus; RA = rheumatoid arthritis.

POLYCLONAL PLASMACYTOSIS IN BONE MARROW

Systemic Illness

Plasma cells normally account for 1 to 4 percent of the cells in bone marrow biopsy sections (98). An increase in polyclonal plasma cells is a nonspecific finding associated with a variety of infections (especially HIV-1) and noninfectious systemic illnesses (especially autoimmune/hypersensitivity disorders and cirrhosis) (Table 8-5) (99,100,104). These benign plasma cells characteristically retain their normal perivascular distribution, mature nuclear and cytoplasmic features, and polyclonal kappa/lambda light chain expression (figs. 8-67–8-70). Reactive plasma cells, however, may be somewhat enlarged, may contain small nucleoli, and may be binucleated (1 to 5 percent) or, rarely, trinucleated (figs. 8-71–8-73). Secretory forms, including Russell bodies, Dutcher bodies, Mott cells, flame cells, and pseudo-Gaucher cells may also be seen (figs. 8-73, 8-74).

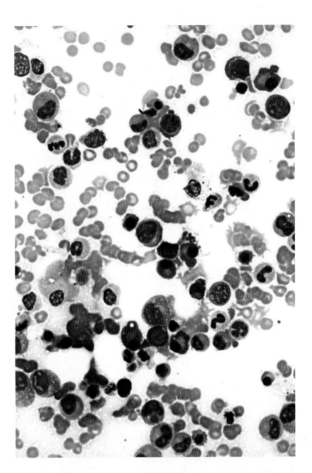

Figure 8-67

PLASMACYTOSIS

The increased plasma cells are increased on a bone marrow aspirate smear from a patient with thymoma and red blood cell aplasia (Wright stain).

Hematopoietic Failure

In addition to reactive plasmacytosis in systemic illnesses, bone marrow plasma cells may be relatively increased in the setting of profound hematopoietic failure, although absolute numbers may actually be normal in this situation. Rare patients with drug-induced hematopoietic failure may exhibit an absolute, not relative, predominance of plasma cells without substantial hematopoietic-associated hypocellularity (96). Likewise, case reports describe rare cases of significant reactive plasmacytosis in conjunction with cytokine-mediated recovery following therapy for myeloma, presenting a unique diagnostic challenge (101).

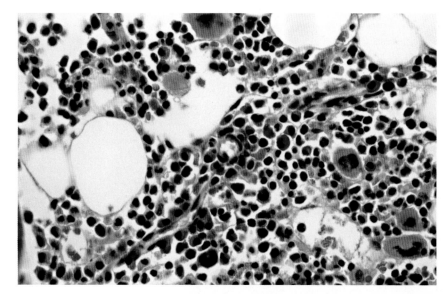

Figure 8-68

PERIVASCULAR PLASMA CELLS

A perivascular localization of benign plasma cells is evident on a core biopsy. Note the diagonal vessel (H&E stain).

Figure 8-69

PLASMA CELL HYPERPLASIA (CD138)

Plasma cell hyperplasia is highlighted on bone marrow biopsy section by an immunoperoxidase stain for CD138. Both perivascular and interstitial distribution are evident.

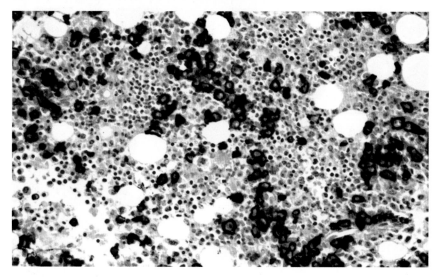

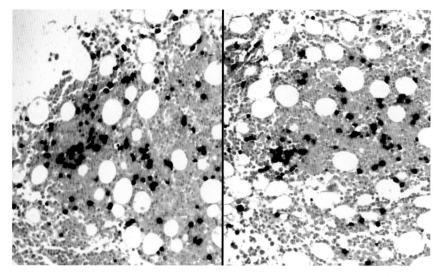

Figure 8-70

POLYCLONAL PLASMA CELLS (IN SITU HYBRIDIZATION)

Plasma cell hyperplasia with polyclonal plasma cells is evident by kappa (left) and lambda (right) in situ hybridization.

Figure 8-71

**ENLARGED REACTIVE
PLASMA CELL**

An enlarged reactive plasma
cell is evident in a bone marrow
aspirate smear (Wright stain).

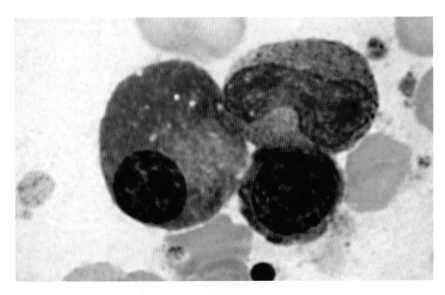

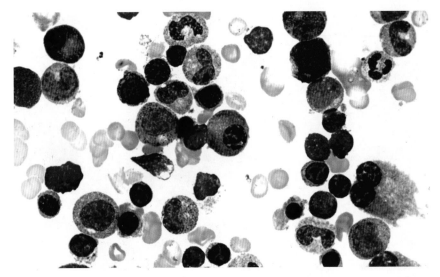

Figure 8-72

**BINUCLEATE REACTIVE
PLASMA CELL**

A binucleate plasma cell is
evident on a bone marrow aspirate
smear from a patient with plasma
cell hyperplasia (Wright stain).

Figure 8-73

**PLASMA CELLS WITH
SECRETORY VACUOLES**

A benign plasma cell with
"intranuclear" secretory vacuoles
(Dutcher body) (left) and a binucleate plasma cell with mild
nuclear immaturity (right) are
seen in two patients with benign
plasma cell hyperplasia (Wright
stain).

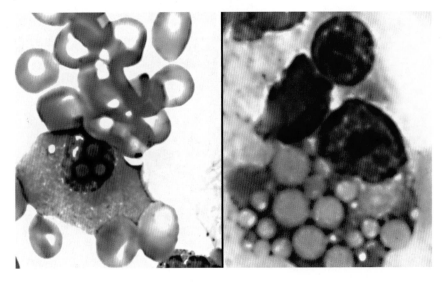

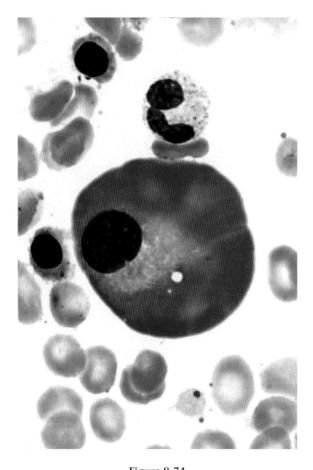

Figure 8-74

FLAMING PLASMA CELL

A flaming plasma cell is evident on a bone marrow aspirate smear in patient with plasma cell hyperplasia (Wright stain).

Monoclonal Gammopathy of Undetermined Significance

In patients with polyclonal plasmacytosis, serum protein studies often demonstrate polyclonal hypergammaglobulinemia. The detection of a monoclonal protein should prompt evaluation for a possible plasma cell dyscrasia. Many patients, usually elderly, have small, stable monoclonal plasma cell disorders termed monoclonal gammopathy of undetermined significance (MGUS) (103). Recent studies indicate that the risk of progression to overt myeloma in these patients is 1 percent/year (103). Unlike polyclonal plasmacytosis, the bone marrow plasma cells in patients with MGUS are typically, but

not always, monoclonal by standard immunoperoxidase light chain assessment. Like reactive plasmacytosis, however, the clonal plasma cells in MGUS are characteristically mature-appearing without cytologic atypia (105).

Differential Diagnosis of Non-Neoplastic Lymphoid and Plasma Cell Disorders

The differential diagnosis of non-neoplastic lymphoid and plasma cell disorders includes various clonal B-, T-, and plasma cell disorders. Although definitive distinction between benign and malignant disorders may hinge on molecular genetic analyses, often the integration of clinical, morphologic, and standard immunophenotypic information is all that is required. Patients with systemic disorders, either infectious or non-infectious, may exhibit a diffuse increase in T cells, discrete lymphoid aggregates, and polyclonal plasmacytosis, all reflecting an immune response to the underlying illness. Germinal center formation within lymphoid aggregates is especially likely in patients with autoimmune disorder/collagen vascular disease. In general, neoplastic lymphoid infiltrates in the bone marrow are more extensive, exhibit greater cytologic atypia, and exhibit distinctive infiltration patterns, all features not commonly associated with benign infiltrates.

Reactive plasmacytosis can be distinguished from monoclonal plasma cell disorders by standard immunophenotypic techniques. In addition to monotypic light chain expression, neoplastic plasma cells are characteristically CD56 positive, while normal plasma cells do not typically express this antigen (107–109). Loss of CD45 expression is also observed in about 90 percent of myelomas, while CD45 is expressed by reactive plasma cells. Reactive plasma cell infiltrates tend to maintain a normal perivascular location and do not form either sizeable nodules or sheets. The majority of benign plasma cells are morphologically mature without cytologic atypia. Monoclonal plasma cell disorders exhibit a broad biologic range, from indolent MGUS processes in which the bone marrow infiltration is minimal and plasma cells are cytologically unremarkable, to overt myeloma in which both the degree of cytologic atypia and the extent of bone marrow infiltration may be striking (fig. 8-75).

Figure 8-75

MULTIPLE MYELOMA

A markedly atypical plasma cell (left) and extensive bone marrow effacement highlighted with CD138 staining in a patient with multiple myeloma (right) (Wright, immunoperoxidase stain for CD138).

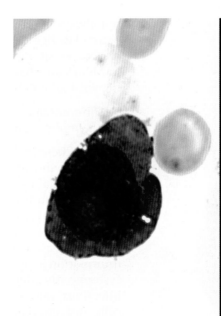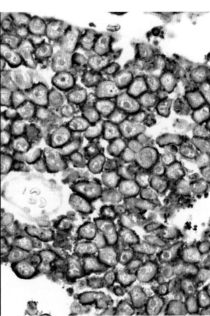

REFERENCES

Lymphocytes in Blood

1. Bigouret V, Hoffmann T, Arlettaz L, et al. Monoclonal T-cell expansions in asymptomatic individuals and in patients with large granular leukemia consist of cytotoxic effector T cells expressing the activating CD94:NKG2C/E and NKD2D killer cell receptors. Blood 2003;101:3198-204.

2. Comans-Bitter WM, de Groot R, van den Beemd R, et al. Immunophenotyping of blood lymphocytes in childhood. Reference values for lymphocyte subpopulations. J Pediatr 1997;130:388-93.

3. Delage R, Jacques L, Massinga-Loembe M, et al. Persistent polyclonal B-cell lymphocytosis: further evidence for a genetic disorder associated with B-cell abnormalities. Br J Haematol 2001;114:666-70.

4. Delage R, Roy J, Jacques L, Bernier V, Delage JM, Darveau A. Multiple bcl-2/Ig gene rearrangements in persistent polyclonal B-cell lymphocytosis. Br J Haematol 1997;97:589-95.

5. Denny T, Yogev R, Gelman R, et al. Lymphocyte subsets in healthy children during the first 5 years of life. JAMA 1992;267:1484-8.

6. Feugier P, De March AK, Lesesve JF, et al. Intravascular bone marrow accumulation in persistent polyclonal lymphocytosis: a misleading feature for B-cell neoplasm. Mod Pathol 2004;17:1087-96.

7. Foucar K. Reactive lymphoid proliferations in blood and bone marrow. In: Bone marrow pathology, 2nd ed. Chicago: ASCP Press; 2001:344-65.

8. Hewlett EL, Edwards KM. Clinical practice. Pertussis—not just for kids. N Engl J Med 2005;352:1215-22.

9. Himmelmann A, Gautschi O, Nawrath M, Bolliger U, Fehr J, Stahel RA. Persistent polyclonal B-cell lymphocytosis is an expansion of functional IgD+CD27+ memory B cells. Br J Haematol 2001;114:400-5.

10. Hodge G, Hodge S, Markus C, Lawrence A, Han P. A marked decrease in L-selectin expression by leucocytes in infants with Bordetella pertussis infection: leucocytosis explained? Respirology 2003;8:157-62.

11. Karandikar NJ, Hotchkiss EC, McKenna RW, Kroft SH. Transient stress lymphocytosis: an immunophenotypic characterization of the most common cause of newly identified adult lymphocytosis in a tertiary hospital. Am J Clin Pathol 2002;117:819-25.

12. Kotylo PK, Fineberg NS, Freeman KS, Redmond NL, Charland C. Reference ranges for lymphocyte subsets in pediatric patients. Am J Clin Pathol 1993;100:111-5.

13. Lamy T, Loughran TP Jr. Current concepts: large granular lymphocyte leukemia. Blood Rev 1999;13:230-40.

14. McCloskey TW, Cavaliere T, Bakshi S, et al. Immunophenotyping of T lymphocytes by three-color flow cytometry in healthy newborns, children, and adults. Clin Immunol Immunopathol 1997;84:46-55.

15. Miranda E, Loughran TJ. Chronic T-cell and NK-cell leukemias. In: Cheson BD, ed. Chronic lymphoid leukemias, 2nd ed: New York: Marcel Dekker; 2001:543-65.

16. Mossafa H, Malaure H, Maynadie M, et al. Persistent polyclonal B lymphocytosis with binucleated lymphocytes: a study of 25 cases. Br J Haematol 1999;104:486-93.

17. Ohga S, Nomura A, Takada H, Hara T. Immunological aspects of Epstein-Barr virus infection. Crit Rev Oncol Hematol 2002;44:203-15.

18. Peterson LC. Infectious mononucleosis. In: Kjeldsberg CR, ed. Practical diagnosis of hematologic disorders, 4th ed, vol 1. Chicago: ASCP Press; 2006:257-70.

19. Ventura KC, Hudnall SD. Hematologic differences in heterophile-positive and heterophile-negative infectious mononucleosis. Am J Hematol 2004;76:315-8.

20. Weisberger J, Cornfield D, Gorczyca W, Liu Z. Down-regulation of pan-T-cell antigens, particularly CD7, in acute infectious mononucleosis. Am J Clin Pathol 2003;120:49-55.

21. Wickramasinghe S. Abnormalities in leukocyte morphology and number. In: Wickramasinghe S, McCullough J, eds. Blood and bone marrow pathology. Edinburgh: Churchill Livingstone; 2003:299-320.

Normal Lymphocyte and Plasma Cell Parameters in Bone Marrow

22. Chilosi M, Adami F, Lestani M, et al. CD138/syndecan-1: a useful immunohistochemical marker of normal and neoplastic plasma cells on routine trephine bone marrow biopsies. Mod Pathol 1999;12:1101-6.

23. Clark P, Normansell DE. Phenotype analysis of lymphocyte subsets in normal human bone marrow. Am J Clin Pathol 1990;94:632-6.

24. Clark P, Normansell DE, Innes DJ, Hess CE. Lymphocyte subsets in normal bone marrow. Blood 1986;67:1600-6.

25. Costes V, Magen V, Legouffe E, et al. The Mi15 monoclonal antibody (anti-syndecan-1) is a reliable marker for quantifying plasma cells in paraffin-embedded bone marrow biopsy specimens. Hum Pathol 1999;30:1405-11.

26. Foucar K. Reactive lymphoid proliferations in blood and bone marrow. In: Bone marrow pathology, 2nd ed. Chicago: ASCP Press; 2001:344-65.

27. Girodon F, Favre B, Carli PM, et al. Minor dysplastic changes are frequently observed in the bone marrow aspirate in elderly patients without haematological disease. Clin Lab Haematol 2001;23:297-300.

28. Horny HP, Wehrmann M, Griesser H, Tiemann M, Bultmann B, Kaiserling E. Investigation of bone marrow lymphocyte subsets in normal, reactive, and neoplastic states using paraffin-embedded biopsy specimens. Am J Clin Pathol 1993;99:142-9.

29. Markey GM, Connolly N, Morris TC, Kettle P, Foster H. Plasma cell subtypes in bone marrow biopsies from patients without plasma cell dyscrasia. Br J Haematol 2001;114:958-9.

30. Martin P, Santon A, Bellas C. Neural cell adhesion molecule expression in plasma cells in bone marrow biopsies and aspirates allows discrimination between multiple myeloma, monoclonal gammopathy of uncertain significance and polyclonal plasmacytosis. Histopathology 2004;44:375-80.

31. O'Donnell LR, Alder SL, Balis UJ, Perkins SL, Kjeldsberg CR. Immunohistochemical reference ranges for B lymphocytes in bone marrow biopsy paraffin sections. Am J Clin Pathol 1995;104:517-23.

32. Rawstron AC, Owen RG, Davies FE, et al. Circulating plasma cells in multiple myeloma: characterization and correlation with disease stage. Br J Haematol 1997;97:46-55.

33. Rego E, Garcia A, Viana S, Falcao RP. Age-related changes of lymphocyte subsets in normal bone marrow biopsies. Cytometry 1998;34:22-9.

34. Rimsza L, Larson R, Winter S, et al. Benign hematogone-rich lymphoid proliferations can be distinguished from B-lineage acute lymphoblastic leukemia by integration of morphology, immunophenotype, adhesion molecule expression, and architectural features. Am J Clin Pathol 2000;114:66-75.

35. Rosse C, Kraemer MJ, Dillon TL, McFarland R, Smith NJ. Bone marrow cell populations of normal infants; the predominance of lymphocytes. J Lab Clin Med 1977;89:1225-40.

Constitutional Disorders with Abnormal Lymphocytes

36. Brunning RD. Morphologic alterations in nucleated blood and marrow cells in genetic disorders. Hum Pathol 1970;1:99-124.

37. Hansen HG, Graucob E. Hematologic cytology of storage diseases. New York: Springer-Verlag; 1985.

38. Muenzer J, Fisher A. Advances in the treatment of mucopolysaccharidosis type I. N Engl J Med 2004;350:1932-4.

39. Vellodi A. Lysosomal storage disorders. Br J Haematol 2005;128:413-31.

Increased Hematogones in Bone Marrow

40. Brady K, Atwater S, Lowell C. Flow cytometric detection of CD10 (cALLA) on peripheral blood B lymphocytes of neonates. Br J Haematol 1999;107:712-5.

41. Davis RE, Longacre TA, Cornbleet PJ. Hematogones in the bone marrow of adults. Immunophenotypic features, clinical settings, and differential diagnosis. Am J Clin Pathol 1994;102:202-11.

42. Dworzak MN, Fritsch G, Fleischer C, et al. Multiparameter phenotype mapping of normal and post-chemotherapy B lymphopoiesis in pediatric bone marrow. Leukemia 1997;11:1266-73.

43. Kallakury BV, Hartmann DP, Cossman J, Gootenberg JE, Bagg A. Posttherapy surveillance of B-cell precursor acute lymphoblastic leukemia. Value of polymerase chain reaction and limitations of flow cytometry. Am J Clin Pathol 1999;111:759-66.

44. Kroft SH. Role of flow cytometry in pediatric hematopathology. Am J Clin Pathol 2004;122 (Suppl):S19-32.

45. Kroft SH, Asplund SL, McKenna RW, Karandikar NJ. Haematogones in the peripheral blood of adults: a four-colour flow cytometry study of 102 patients. Br J Haematol 2004;126:209-12.

46. Leitenberg D, Rappeport JM, Smith BR. B-cell precursor bone marrow reconstitution after bone marrow transplantation. Am J Clin Pathol 1994;102:231-6.

47. Longacre TA, Foucar K, Crago S, et al. Hematogones: a multiparameter analysis of bone marrow precursor cells. Blood 1989;73:543-52.

48. Mandel M, Rechavi G, Neumann Y, et al. Bone marrow cell populations mimicking common acute lymphoblastic leukemia in infants with stage IV-S neuroblastoma. Acta Haematol 1991;86:86-9.

49. McKenna RW, Washington LT, Aquino DB, Picker LJ, Kroft SH. Immunophenotypic analysis of hematogones (B-lymphocyte precursors) in 662 consecutive bone marrow specimens by 4-color flow cytometry. Blood 2001;98:2498-507.

50. Rimsza L, Larson R, Winter S, et al. Benign hematogone-rich lymphoid proliferations can be distinguished from B-lineage acute lymphoblastic leukemia by integration of morphology, immunophenotype, adhesion molecule expression, and architectural features. Am J Clin Pathol 2000;114:66-75.

51. Rimsza LM, Douglas VK, Tighe P, et al. Benign B-cell precursors (hematogones) are the predominant lymphoid population in the bone marrow of preterm infants. Biol Neonate 2004;86:247-53.

52. Rimsza LM, Viswanatha DS, Winter SS, Leith CP, Frost JD, Foucar K. The presence of CD34+ cell clusters predicts impending relapse in pediatric ALL patients on maintenance chemotherapy. Am J Clin Pathol 1998;110:313-20.

53. Sandhaus LM, Chen TL, Ettinger LJ, Hirst-Allen A, Mehta K, Raskova J. Significance of increased proportion of CD10-positive cells in nonmalignant bone marrows of children. Am J Pediatr Hematol Oncol 1993;15:65-70.

54. Smedmyr B, Bengtsson M, Jakobsson A, Simonsson B, Oberg G, Totterman TH. Regeneration of CALLA (CD10+), TdT+ and double-positive cells in the bone marrow and blood after autologous bone marrow transplantation. Eur J Haematol 1991;46:146-51.

55. Tsao L, Colovai AI, Jiang JG, Bhagat G, Alobeid B. Characterizing CD43 expression in haematogones using multicolor flow cytometric analysis. Br J Haematol 2005;128:820-3.

56. van Lochem EG, Wiegers YM, van den Beemd R, Hahlen K, van Dongen JJ, Hooijkaas H. Regeneration pattern of precursor-B-cells in bone marrow of acute lymphoblastic leukemia patients depends on the type of preceding chemotherapy. Leukemia 2000;14:688-95.

57. van Wering ER, van der Linden-Schrever BE, Szczepanski T, et al. Regenerating normal B-cell precursors during and after treatment of acute lymphoblastic leukaemia: implications for monitoring of minimal residual disease. Br J Haematol 2000;110:139-46.

58. Vandersteenhoven AM, Williams JE, Borowitz MJ. Marrow B-cell precursors are increased in lymphomas or systemic diseases associated with B-cell dysfunction. Am J Clin Pathol 1993;100:60-6.

59. Vogel P, Erf LA, Rosenthal N. Hematological observations on bone marrow obtained by sternal puncture. Am J Clin Pathol 1937;7:436-47.

60. Weir EG, Cowan K, LeBeau P, Borowitz MJ. A limited antibody panel can distinguish B-precursor acute lymphoblastic leukemia from normal B precursors with four color flow cytometry: implications for residual disease detection. Leukemia 1999;13:558-67.

61. Wells DA, Sale GE, Shulman HM, et al. Multidimensional flow cytometry of marrow can differentiate leukemic from normal lymphoblasts and myeloblasts after chemotherapy and bone marrow transplantation. Am J Clin Pathol 1998;110:84-94.

62. Wolf E, Harms H, Winkler J, et al. Terminal deoxynucleotidyl transferase-positive cells in trephine biopsies following bone marrow or peripheral stem cell transplantation reflect vigorous B-cell generation. Histopathology 2005;46:442-50.

Diffuse Non-Neoplastic T-Cell Infiltrates in Bone Marrow

63. Barton AD. T-cell lymphocytosis associated with lymphocyte-rich thymoma. Cancer 1997;80:1409-17.

64. Caldwell CW, Poje E, Cooperstock M. Expansion of immature thymic precursor cells in peripheral blood after acute marrow suppression. Am J Clin Pathol 1991;95:824-7.

65. de Jong D, Richel DJ, Schenkeveld C, Boerrigter L, van 't Veer LJ. Oligoclonal peripheral T-cell lymphocytosis as a result of aberrant T-cell development in a cortical thymoma. Diagn Mol Pathol 1997;6:244-8.

66. Ehrlich GD, Han T, Bettigole R, et al. Human T-lymphotropic virus type I-associated benign transient immature T-cell lymphocytosis. Am J Hematol 1988;27:49-55.

67. Evans HL, Burks E, Viswanatha D, Larson RS. Utility of immunohistochemistry in bone marrow evaluation of T-lineage large granular lymphocyte leukemia. Hum Pathol 2000;31:1266-73.

68. Hoffacker V, Schultz A, Tiesinga JJ, et al. Thymomas alter the T-cell subset composition in the blood: a potential mechanism for thymoma-associated autoimmune disease. Blood 2000;96:3872-9.

69. Lassoued K, Oksenhendler E, Lambin JP, Cazals-Hatem D, Clauvel JP. Severe neutropenia associated with IgG2 subclass deficiency and bone marrow T-lymphocyte infiltration. Am J Hematol 1998;57:241-4.

70. Medeiros LJ, Bhagat SK, Naylor P, Fowler D, Jaffe ES, Stetler-Stevenson M. Malignant thymoma associated with T-cell lymphocytosis. A case report with immunophenotypic and gene rearrangement analysis. Arch Pathol Lab Med 1993;117:279-83.

71. Nakahara K, Utsunomiya A, Hanada S, et al. Transient appearance of CD3+CD8+ T lymphocytes with monoclonal gene rearrangement of T-cell receptor beta locus. Br J Haematol 1998;100:411-4.

72. Smith GP, Perkins SL, Segal GH, Kjeldsberg CR. T-cell lymphocytosis associated with invasive thymomas. Am J Clin Pathol 1994;102:447-53.

73. Smith P, Helbert M, Raftery M, Forster G, Cavenagh J. Paraproteins and monoclonal expansion of CD3+CD8+ CD56-CD57+ T lymphocytes in a patient with HIV infection. Br J Haematol 1999;105:85-7.

74. Viallard JF, Boiron JM, Parrens M, et al. Severe pancytopenia triggered by recombinant hepatitis B vaccine. Br J Haematol 2000;110:230-3.

Systemic Polyclonal Immunoblastic Proliferations Involving Bone Marrow

75. Koduri PR, Naides SJ. Transient blood plasmacytosis in parvovirus B19 infection: a report of two cases. Ann Hematol 1996;72:49-51.

76. Mongeon CA, Braziel RM, Leith CP, et al. Rapidly fatal multisystem polyclonal immunoblastic (IB) proliferations: a clinical, phenotypic and molecular analysis. Mod Pathol 1994;7:116A.

77. Peterson L, Marcelli A, Arthur D, et al. Systemic polyclonal immunoblastic proliferation: a distinct atypical lymphoproliferative disorder. Lab Invest 1998;78:138A.

78. Peterson LC, Kueck B, Arthur DC, Dedeker K, Brunning RD. Systemic polyclonal immunoblastic proliferations. Cancer 1988;61:1350-8.

79. Poje EJ, Soori GS, Weisenburger DD. Systemic polyclonal B-immunoblastic proliferation with marked peripheral blood and bone marrow plasmacytosis. Am J Clin Pathol 1992;98:222-6.

Benign Lymphoid Aggregates in Bone Marrow

80. Ben-Ezra J, Hazelgrove K, Ferreira-Gonzalez A, Garrett CT. Can polymerase chain reaction help distinguish benign from malignant lymphoid aggregates in bone marrow aspirates? Arch Pathol Lab Med 2000;124:511-5.

81. Bluth RF, Casey TT, McCurley TL. Differentiation of reactive from neoplastic small-cell lymphoid aggregates in paraffin-embedded marrow particle preparations using L-26 (CD20) and UCHL-1 (CD45RO) monoclonal antibodies. Am J Clin Pathol 1993;99:150-6.

82. Brunning RD, McKenna RW. Lesions simulating lymphoma and miscellaneous tumor-like lesions in the bone marrow. In: Brunning RD, McKenna RW, eds. Tumors of the bone marrow. AFIP Atlas of Tumor Pathology, 3rd Series, Fascicle 9. Washington, D.C.: American Registry of Pathology; 1994:409-37.

83. Chu P, Arber D, Weiss L. Expression of T/NK-cell and plasma cell antigens in nonhematopoietic epithelidoid neoplasms. Am J Clin Pathol 2003:64-70.

84. Coad JE, Olson DJ, Christensen DR, et al. Correlation of PCR-detected clonal gene rearrangements with bone marrow morphology in patients with B-lineage lymphomas. Am J Surg Pathol 1997;21:1047-56.

85. Douglas VK, Gordon LI, Goolsby CL, White CA, Peterson LC. Lymphoid aggregates in bone marrow mimic residual lymphoma following rituxan (rituximab) therapy for non-Hodgkin's lymphoma. Am J Clin Pathol 1999;112:844-53.

86. Farhi DC. Germinal centers in the bone marrow. Hematol Pathol 1989;3:133-6.

87. Feugier P, De March AK, Lesesve JF, et al. Intravascular bone marrow accumulation in persistent polyclonal lymphocytosis: a misleading feature for B-cell neoplasm. Mod Pathol 2004;17:1087-96.

88. Girodon F, Favre B, Carli PM, et al. Minor dysplastic changes are frequently observed in the bone marrow aspirate in elderly patients without haematological disease. Clin Lab Haematol 2001;23:297-300.

89. Karcher DS, Frost AR. The bone marrow in human immunodeficiency virus (HIV)-related disease. Morphology and clinical correlation. Am J Clin Pathol 1991;95:63-71.

90. Magalhaes SM, Filho FD, Vassallo J, Pinheiro MP, Metze K, Lorand-Metze I. Bone marrow lymphoid aggregates in myelodysplastic syndromes: incidence, immunomorphological characteristics and correlation with clinical features and survival. Leuk Res 2002;26:525-30; discussion, 531.

91. Rosenthal NS, Farhi DC. Bone marrow findings in connective tissue disease. Am J Clin Pathol 1989;92:650-4.

92. Salisbury JR, Deverell MH, Cookson MJ. Three-dimensional reconstruction of benign lymphoid aggregates in bone marrow trephines. J Pathol 1996;178:447-50.

93. Salisbury JR, Deverell MH, Seaton JM, Cookson MJ. Three-dimensional reconstruction of non-Hodgkin's lymphoma in bone marrow trephines. J Pathol 1997;181:451-4.

94. Thiele J, Zirbes TK, Kvasnicka HM, Fischer R. Focal lymphoid aggregates (nodules) in bone marrow biopsies: differentiation between benign hyperplasia and malignant lymphoma—a practical guideline. J Clin Pathol 1999;52:294-300.

95. Tsao L, Colovai AI, Jiang JG, Bhagat G, Alobeid B. Characterizing CD43 expression in haematogones using multicolor flow cytometric analysis. Br J Haematol 2005;128:820-3.

Polyclonal Plasmacytosis in Bone Marrow

96. Breier DV, Rendo P, Gonzalez J, Shilton G, Stivel M, Goldztein S. Massive plasmocytosis due to methimazole-induced bone marrow toxicity. Am J Hematol 2001;67:259-61.

97. Chilosi M, Adami F, Lestani M, et al. CD138/syndecan-1: a useful immunohistochemical marker of normal and neoplastic plasma cells on routine trephine bone marrow biopsies. Mod Pathol 1999;12:1101-6.

98. Costes V, Magen V, Legouffe E, et al. The Mi15 monoclonal antibody (anti-syndecan-1) is a reliable marker for quantifying plasma cells in paraffin-embedded bone marrow biopsy specimens. Hum Pathol 1999;30:1405-11.

99. Govender D, Harilal P, Dada M, Chetty R. CD31 (JC70) expression in plasma cells: an immunohistochemical analysis of reactive and neoplastic plasma cells. J Clin Pathol 1997;50:490-3.

100. Hyun BH, Kwa D, Gabaldon H, Ashton JK. Reactive plasmacytic lesions of the bone marrow. Am J Clin Pathol 1976;65:921-8.

101. Jego G, Avet-Loiseau H, Robillard N, et al. Reactive plasmacytoses in multiple myeloma during hematopoietic recovery with G- or GM-CSF. Leuk Res 2000;24:627-30.

102. Jego G, Robillard N, Puthier D, et al. Reactive plasmacytoses are expansions of plasmablasts retaining the capacity to differentiate into plasma cells. Blood 1999;94:701-12.

103. Kyle RA, Therneau TM, Rajkumar SV, et al. A long-term study of prognosis in monoclonal gammopathy of undetermined significance. N Engl J Med 2002;346:564-9.

104. Markey GM, Connolly N, Morris TC, Kettle P, Foster H. Plasma cell subtypes in bone marrow biopsies from patients without plasma cell dyscrasia. Br J Haematol 2001;114:958-9.

105. Milla F, Oriol A, Aguilar J, et al. Usefulness and reproducibility of cytomorphologic evaluations to differentiate myeloma from monoclonal gammopathies of unknown significance. Am J Clin Pathol 2001;115:127-35.

106. Rosenthal NS, Farhi DC. Reactive plasmacytosis and lymphocytosis in acute myeloid leukemia. Hematol Pathol 1994;8:43-51.

Differential Diagnosis

107. Lin P, Owens R, Tricot G, Wilson CS. Flow cytometric immunophenotypic analysis of 306 cases of multiple myeloma. Am J Clin Pathol 2004;121:482-8.

108. Martin P, Santon A, Bellas C. Neural cell adhesion molecule expression in plasma cells in bone marrow biopsies and aspirates allows discrimination between multiple myeloma, monoclonal gammopathy of uncertain significance and polyclonal plasmacytosis. Histopathology 2004;44:375-80.

109. Rawstron AC, Owen RG, Davies FE, et al. Circulating plasma cells in multiple myeloma: characterization and correlation with disease stage. Br J Haematol 1997;97:46-55.

9 DISORDERS OF BONE MARROW STROMA AND BONE

COMPONENTS OF BONE MARROW STROMA

Bone marrow stromal elements were initially recognized as the adherent cell layer in bone marrow culture systems; investigations using this cell culture model confirmed that bone marrow stromal cells were essential for the growth and support of hematopoietic elements (2–4,9). Subsequently, many fixed and migratory cell types have been shown to comprise the bone marrow stroma, including fixed fibroblasts, capillary and sinusoidal endothelial cells, macrophages/dendritic cells, adipose cells, endosteal cells, and adventitial reticular cells, migratory lymphocytes, and monocytes (see chapter 1 for more details) (8). As detailed in chapter 1, the bone marrow stroma provides the structural support for hematopoiesis, production of both stimulatory and inhibitory hematopoietic regulatory factors, and production of adhesion molecules essential for the microenvironmental specificity of stem/progenitor cell localization (1,3,7).

Macrophages and immune-accessory histiocytic cells, termed dendritic cells, are derived from hematopoietic progenitor cells. Adventitial reticular cells are located along the abluminal side of sinusoidal vessels; these cells have long thin cytoplasmic projections that encircle hematopoietic elements (8). Current evidence suggests that mesenchymal stem cells are a normal bone marrow constituent and give rise to mesenchymal bone marrow elements including fibroblasts, reticular cells, adipose cells, osteoblasts/osteocytes, and chrondroblasts/chondrocytes (2,5,6).

In addition to individual cell types, both blood vessels and bony trabeculae are constituents of the bone marrow structure. The bony trabeculae provide scaffolding support for hematopoiesis; the blood vessels are the conduits by which newly formed hematopoietic elements enter the systemic circulation and through which monocytes, dendritic cells, and lymphocytes migrate.

The stromal elements that are most readily apparent on bone marrow aspirate smears are macrophages, adipose cells, capillaries, and lymphocytes; other stromal constituents are typically inconspicuous (figs. 9-1, 9-2) (3). Although a role for mast cells in bone marrow stromal cell function has not been delineated, these cells are readily apparent in bone marrow aspirate particles and likely play a role in stromal cell activities (fig. 9-3). On bone marrow core biopsies, a variety of stromal and structural elements are evident, including bony trabeculae, blood vessels, adipose cells, macrophages, and lymphocytes (figs. 9-4, 9-5). In normal bone marrow specimens, the stroma is inconspicuous, but a variety of pathologic disorders can produce distinctive morphologic abnormalities of bone marrow stroma on aspirate and biopsy specimens (3). Similarly, pathologic vascular and bony disorders may also be evident on bone marrow core biopsy sections.

In this chapter, a spectrum of non-neoplastic bone marrow stromal disorders are discussed. Disorders of structural elements, including blood vessels and bony trabeculae, are presented (Table 9-1).

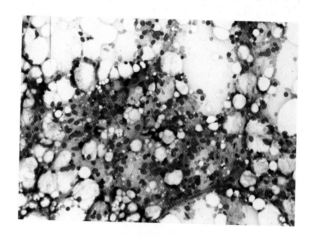

Figure 9-1

BONE MARROW ASPIRATE PARTICLES SHOWING STROMAL CELLS

Capillaries, histiocytes, and fat cells are seen (Wright stain).

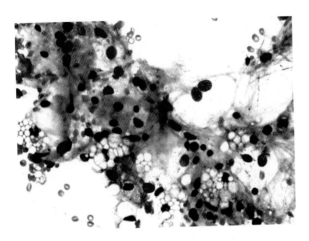

Figure 9-2

BONE MARROW ASPIRATE PARTICLE FOLLOWING CHEMOTHERAPY

The hematopoietic cells are markedly reduced, with a predominance of stromal elements (Wright stain).

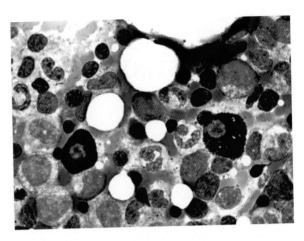

Figure 9-3

MAST CELLS IN BONE MARROW PARTICLE

Increased, dark-staining mast cells are evident (Wright stain).

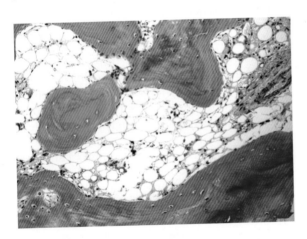

Figure 9-4

BONE MARROW STROMAL ELEMENTS

Stromal and structural elements are readily apparent in this profoundly hypocellular bone marrow core biopsy. A large caliber blood vessel, abundant fat cells, dispersed mononuclear lymphocytes and histiocytes, and bony trabeculae are seen (hematoxylin and eosin [H&E] stain). (Courtesy of Dr. C. Sever, Albuquerque, NM.)

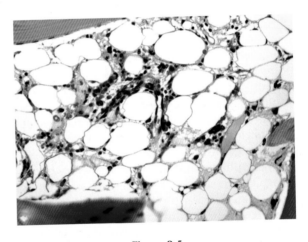

Figure 9-5

BONE MARROW STROMAL ELEMENTS

Intermediate magnification of a profoundly hypocellular bone marrow core biopsy shows small caliber blood vessels, fat cells, scattered lymphocytes and histiocytes, as well as bony trabeculae (H&E stain). (Courtesy of Dr. C. Sever, Albuquerque, NM.)

BONE MARROW STROMAL DISORDERS

Gelatinous Transformation of Bone Marrow

The presence of distinct foci of eosinophilic gelatinous extracellular material on bone marrow biopsy sections is an infrequent, although not rare, occurrence in a routine clinical setting, and varies with patient mix. This smooth stromal extracellular material is rich in hyaluronic acid. *Gelatinous transformation of the bone marrow* tends to be a focal, patchy process, as seen in bone marrow core biopsy sections, although in rare cases, extensive diffuse bone marrow involvement is evident (fig. 9-6). Bone marrow biopsy specimens that show gelatinous transformation also tend to exhibit hypocellularity and adipose cell atrophy in the areas of

Table 9-1	
NON-NEOPLASTIC STROMAL AND STRUCTURAL DISORDERS OF BONE MARROW	

Bone Marrow Stromal Disorders
Gelatinous transformation of bone marrow
Necrosis
Amyloid deposition
Fibrosis
Granulomatous and diffuse histiocytic disorders[a]
Iron disorders
Crystal deposition in bone marrow

Structural Disorders
Vascular abnormalities including neoangiogenesis
Acquired and constitutional bone abnormalities

[a]Infectious granulomatous disorders are detailed in chapter 10.

Table 9-2	
GELATINOUS TRANSFORMATION OF BONE MARROW[a,b]	
Morphologic features	Reduced cellularity Atrophy of adipose cells Accumulation of extracellular matrix material with a smooth, eosinophilic gelatinous appearance
Pathophysiology	Pathologic mechanisms unknown; key associations include: weight loss severe generalized illness cachexia anemia Eosinophilic gelatinous material is rich in hyaluronic acid (Alcian blue positive), which is not a typical constituent of normal bone marrow
Disease associations	Anorexia nervosa Acquired immunodeficiency syndrome (AIDS), alcoholism Malignant lymphomas Other solid tumors Infections Other severe acute illnesses or debilitating conditions

[a]Data from references 10–13.
[b]Other names for this bone marrow disorder include serous fat atrophy and starvation bone marrow.

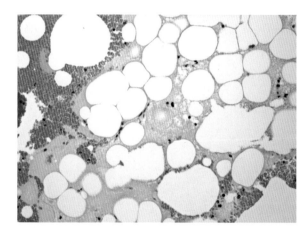

Figure 9-6

GELATINOUS TRANSFORMATION

Bone marrow core biopsy shows the smooth eosinophilic appearance of gelatinous transformation (H&E stain).

the gelatinous change (Table 9-2; figs. 9-7–9-9) (10–12). Although gelatinous transformation of the bone marrow may be appreciated on bone marrow aspirate smears in which hypocellular particles exhibit a smooth amorphous pinkish background substance, most cases are identified on core biopsy sections (figs. 9-6, 9-9, 9-10).

Gelatinous extracellular matrix material must be distinguished from both the granular stroma of fibrinoid necrosis and interstitial patches of amyloid deposition (see later sections of this chapter). Special stains are useful in distinguishing gelatinous transformation of the bone marrow (Alcian blue positive) from amyloid (Congo red positive and birefringent

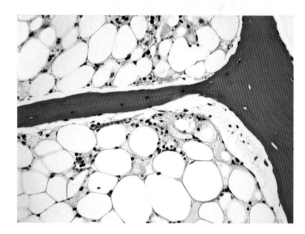

Figure 9-7

GELATINOUS TRANSFORMATION

Prominent gelatinous transformation results in patchy eosinophilic areas in this hypocellular bone marrow core biopsy from a patient with acquired immunodeficiency syndrome (AIDS) and osteopenia (H&E stain).

on polarization). Extensive aspiration artifact can also mimic gelatinous transformation of bone marrow (fig. 9-11).

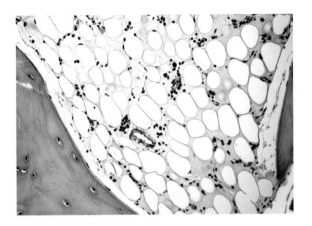

Figure 9-8

GELATINOUS TRANSFORMATION

Prominent dispersed gelatinous transformation of bone marrow is evidenced by eosinophilic areas within the stroma in a core biopsy from a patient with a markedly hypocellular bone marrow (H&E stain).

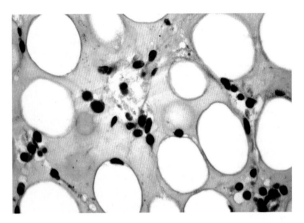

Figure 9-9

GELATINOUS TRANSFORMATION

The smooth eosinophilic to slightly basophilic appearance of gelatinous transformation of bone marrow is apparent at high magnification of a core biopsy section (H&E stain).

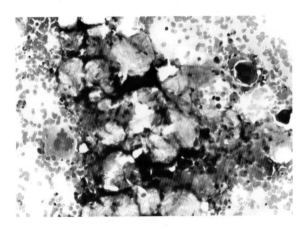

Figure 9-10

GELATINOUS TRANSFORMATION

Gelatinous transformation of bone marrow is apparent in this aspirate smear in which the particles have patchy, finely granular eosinophilic zones (Wright stain).

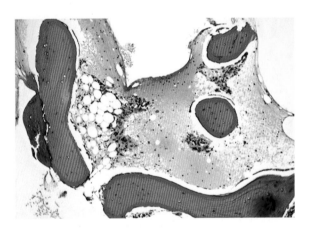

Figure 9-11

ASPIRATION ARTIFACT MIMICKING GELATINOUS TRANSFORMATION

On low magnification of a bone marrow core biopsy section, extensive aspiration artifact creates an appearance reminiscent of gelatinous transformation (H&E stain).

As delineated in Table 9-2, the pathophysiologic mechanisms responsible for this bone marrow stromal abnormality are unknown. Key "common denominators" linked to this relatively nonspecific bone marrow finding include weight loss, severe generalized illnesses of many types, cachexia, and anemia. Specific disease associations include anorexia nervosa, acquired immunodeficiency syndrome (AIDS), malignant lymphoma, and infections (11). Some authors postulate resolution of gelatinous transformation of the bone marrow, but sampling issues in follow-up bone marrow specimens must be taken into account, since gelatinous transformation of the bone marrow is typically a patchy process.

Bone Marrow Necrosis

Several types of necrosis have been delineated in bone marrow specimens. Most of the literature on bone marrow necrosis delineates cases of *ischemic coagulation necrosis* (19,25).

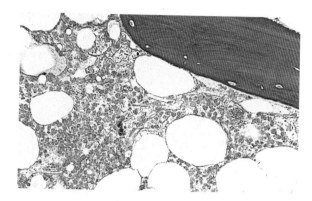

Figure 9-12

ISCHEMIC NECROSIS

Extensive ischemic necrosis is evident on this bone marrow biopsy section in which both bony trabeculae and the hematopoietic cavity show coagulation necrosis with ghosts of cell remnants but no discernible viable nuclei either within the hematopoietic area or within the lacunar spaces of the bony trabeculae (H&E stain).

This type of necrosis is evident in less than 5 percent of bone marrow specimens, and these aspirate specimens often have a "currant jelly" consistency, making smear preparations difficult to interpret. In general, however, there is extensive individual cell death with distorted smudgy nuclei and dissolution of cytoplasm. Ghost cell remnants are typically abundant (fig. 9-12). Adjacent bony trabeculae may be either viable or necrotic with osteocyte cell loss (figs. 9-12, 9-13). Bone marrow aspirate smears show numerous degenerate, distorted cells with prominent dissolution of the cytoplasm (fig. 9-14).

Many patients with ischemic coagulation necrosis present de novo with various underlying neoplastic and non-neoplastic disorders. Several diseases are associated with ischemic necrosis, including acute leukemias (especially acute lymphoblastic leukemia in children), lymphomas, acute chest syndrome in sickle cell anemia patients, severe infections, and antiphospholipid syndrome as well as other coagulopathies (16,17,19,20,22,23,25). Affected patients often have fever, severe bone pain, and pancytopenia (15,25). In cases such as acute chest syndrome complicating sickle cell anemia, normal hematopoietic elements are necrotic (fig. 9-15). The necrotic bone marrow is released into the circulation causing disseminated systemic fat embolization with multiorgan, especially pulmonary, complications (17,20).

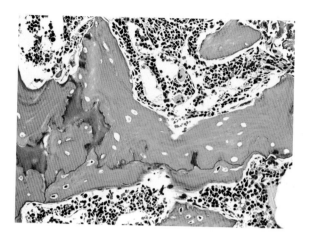

Figure 9-13

NECROTIC BONE TRABECULAE

Necrotic bony trabeculae are surrounded by a collar of new bone formation in a bone marrow core biopsy (H&E stain).

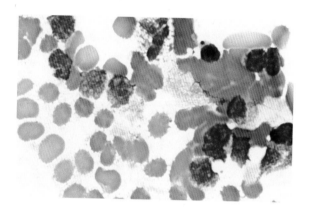

Figure 9-14

NECROTIC BONE MARROW CELLS

Necrotic cells on a bone marrow aspirate smear show degenerative changes, with poor delineation between nucleus and cytoplasm (Wright stain).

Various therapeutic regimens are another major cause of bone marrow necrosis. Potent multiagent chemotherapy is used to eradicate neoplastic infiltrates in bone marrow and other sites. Recent evidence suggests that chemotherapy for acute leukemia induces functional deregulation of bone marrow stromal cells and results in the increased production of inhibitory cytokines (18). Consequently, both hypocellularity and fibrinoid necrosis are predicted bone marrow findings following potent multiagent chemotherapy. *Fibrinoid necrosis* exhibits a granular appearance and is seen in conjunction

287

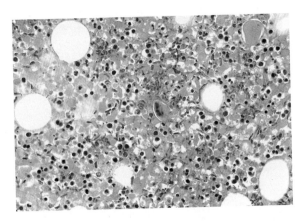

Figure 9-15

BONE MARROW NECROSIS

Extensive necrosis of normal bone marrow elements is evident in a patient with acute chest syndrome secondary to sickle/thalassemia (H&E stain).

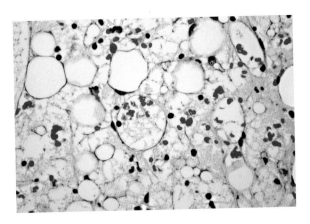

Figure 9-16

FIBRINOID NECROSIS

The eosinophilic granular appearance of fibrinoid necrosis is evident on this high-magnification photomicrograph of a bone marrow core biopsy section from a patient at day 15 of induction chemotherapy for acute leukemia (H&E stain).

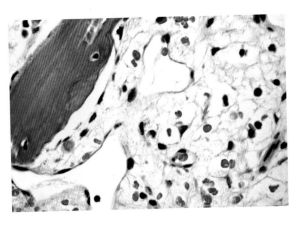

Figure 9-17

FIBRINOID NECROSIS

Acellular fibrillar appearance of the bone marrow stroma is evident in this bone marrow core biopsy section from a patient at day 8 of induction chemotherapy for acute leukemia (H&E stain).

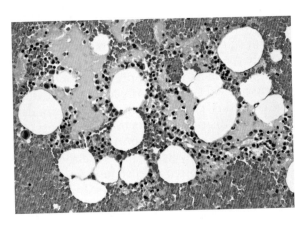

Figure 9-18

AMYLOID DEPOSITION

Bone marrow clot section shows multiple eosinophilic zones of amyloid deposition in a patient with primary amyloidosis.

with myeloablation and marked hypocellularity (fig. 9-16). Unlike coagulation necrosis, ghosts of individual dying cells are not a typical feature of fibrinoid necrosis, although it is possible that fibrinoid necrosis develops following coagulation necrosis. The finely granular abnormal bone marrow stroma has an eosinophilic, net-like appearance, and neither hematopoietic cells nor distinct adipose cells are conspicuous (figs. 9-16, 9-17). The differential diagnosis of fibrinoid necrosis includes aspiration artifact, gelatinous

transformation of bone marrow, and amyloid deposition (figs. 9-18, 9-19). The documentation of recent myeloablative chemotherapy is useful. With resolution, fibrinoid necrosis may appear more dense and homogeneous, sometimes even mimicking amyloid deposition (figs. 9-20–9-21).

In other situations, neoplastic bone marrow infiltrates undergo necrosis. In this situation, extensively necrotic tumor infiltrates are documented on initial, pretreatment bone marrow specimens. Rare reports describe idiosyncratic,

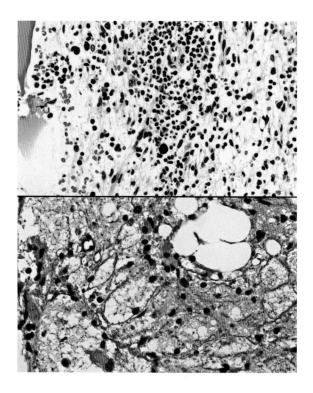

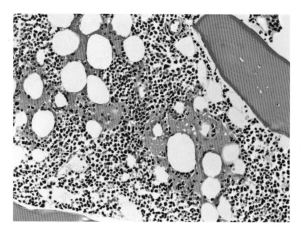

Figure 9-20

NECROTIC AMYLOID-LIKE MATERIAL

Distinct and discrete homogeneous eosinophilic foci, resembling amyloid, are seen in the bone marrow following induction chemotherapy in a child with acute lymphoblastic leukemia (H&E stain).

Figure 9-19

**FIBRINOID NECROSIS
AND ASPIRATION ARTIFACT**

Extensive aspiration artifact that mimics fibrinoid necrosis (bottom) is compared to resolving fibrinoid necrosis following potent multiagent chemotherapy (top) (H&E stain).

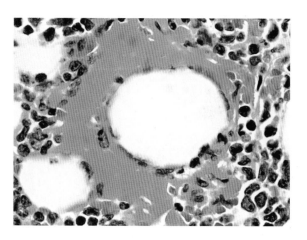

Figure 9-21

NECROTIC AMYLOID-LIKE MATERIAL

A bone marrow core biopsy section from a child receiving induction chemotherapy shows smudgy eosinophilic areas of stromal damage mimicking amyloid deposition (H&E stain).

massive ischemic necrosis following antineoplastic chemotherapy, other drug treatments, as well as following bone marrow transplantation (14,15,21,24,26). Late effects of bone marrow necrosis include bone marrow fibrosis, although restitution of hematopoiesis has also been documented (15,19).

Amyloid Deposition in Bone Marrow

Both non-neoplastic and neoplastic extramedullary *amyloid deposition disorders* are well known (28). Clonal disorders account for the majority of cases of amyloidosis involving bone marrow; only rare cases of secondary bone marrow amyloidosis have been described (29). The neoplastic disorders associated with bone marrow amyloidosis include primary systemic (AL) amyloidosis, overt multiple myeloma, and lymphoplasmacytic lymphomas/Waldenström macroglobulinemia (27).

Amyloid deposition in bone marrow has distinctive features on both aspirate smears and core biopsy sections. Although most frequently recognized on core biopsy sections, large amorphous, basophilic, cloud-like masses of amyloid may be evident within or adjacent to bone marrow particles on aspirate smears (fig. 9-22) (29). Aspirable amyloid collections may also be evident on clot sections (see fig. 9-18). These deposits correspond to the interstitial infiltrates of amyloid seen on

Figure 9-22

AMYLOID DEPOSITION

Amorphous, dark blue aggregates of amyloid are evident on this bone marrow aspirate smear from a patient with extensive amyloid replacement of bone marrow (Wright stain).

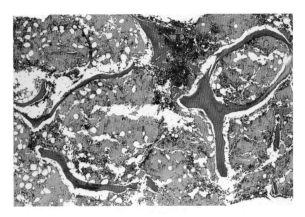

Figure 9-23

AMYLOID DEPOSITION

Low magnification of a bone marrow core biopsy section shows numerous confluent interstitial amyloid deposits throughout the medullary cavity. The osteopenia is striking (H&E stain).

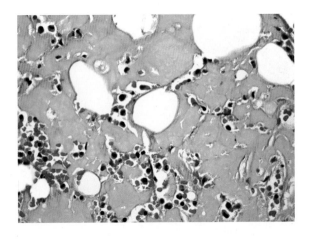

Figure 9-24

AMYLOID DEPOSITION

Bone marrow core biopsy section shows smudgy homogeneous eosinophilic confluent nodules in the interstitium of patient with primary amyloidosis (H&E stain).

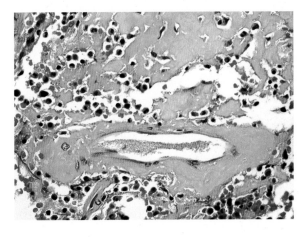

Figure 9-25

AMYLOID WITHIN INTERSTITIUM AND BLOOD VESSEL

Both interstitial and vessel wall infiltration by smudgy eosinophilic amyloid are evident on this bone marrow core biopsy section from a patient with primary amyloidosis (H&E stain).

core biopsy sections (figs. 9-23, 9-24). In addition to interstitial amyloid deposits, infiltration of the blood vessel wall may also be evident in bone marrow biopsy sections (fig. 9-25); there is a propensity for blood vessel wall involvement in amyloidosis (30). Indeed, amyloid deposits within the bone marrow of patients with systemic (AL) amyloidosis are often restricted to the vessel walls (fig. 9-26) (30).

In either interstitial or vessel wall sites, the amyloid deposition has a distinct smudgy, amorphous eosinophilic appearance on hematoxylin and eosin (H&E)-stained sections (see figs. 9-24, 9-25). Congo red stain is characteristically used to assess for amyloid deposition, which produces an apple-green birefringence with polarized light (fig. 9-26) (27,30). Although not generally required for diagnosis, the ultrastructural features of amyloid

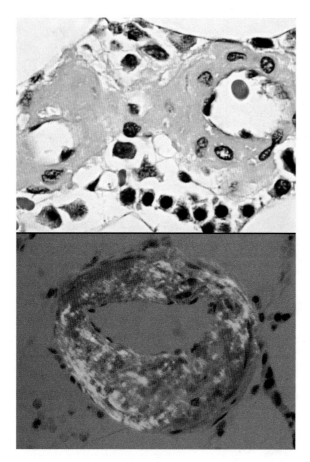

Figure 9-26

AMYLOID HIGHLIGHTED BY CONGO RED

This composite shows the H&E and polarized Congo red appearance of amyloid deposition within blood vessel walls in a bone marrow core biopsy section from a patient with amyloidosis (H&E, Congo red stains).

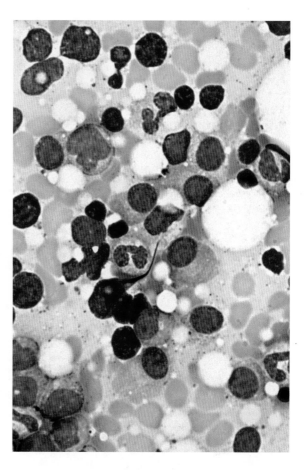

Figure 9-27

**INCREASED PLASMA CELLS IN PATIENT
WITH PRIMARY AMYLOIDOSIS**

Increased, cytologically mature-appearing plasma cells are evident on this bone marrow aspirate smear (Wright stain).

are very distinctive, and the β-pleated sheath configuration is virtually pathognomonic of amyloid (27). The assessment of plasma cells for clonality, morphologic dysplasia, and proportion within the bone marrow is essential in amyloid deposition disorders (figs. 9-27, 9-28).

The entities in the differential diagnosis of amyloid deposits in bone marrow include fibrinoid necrosis, gelatinous transformation of bone marrow, and, less likely, edema. Careful assessment of blood vessels is essential in these cases, since vessel wall abnormalities are unique to amyloidosis. In addition, clinical correlation and possible Congo red staining can resolve problematic cases.

Bone Marrow Fibrosis

Both reticulin and collagen fibers are produced by bone marrow stromal cells. These extracellular fiber types, although both within the collagen family, are distinguished by their biochemical properties and staining reactions.

Reticulin fibers are highlighted by silver stains, while collagen fibers are trichrome positive. Reticulin fibers are inconspicuous in normal bone marrow core biopsy sections; the silver stains highlight the delicate capillary/fiber meshwork produced by reticular cells of the normal bone marrow stroma (fig. 9-29) (42). Reticulin fibers are more numerous around larger caliber vessels and within lymphoid aggregates (fig. 9-30). They are also increased in association

Figure 9-28

PRIMARY AMYLOIDOSIS (IN SITU HYBRIDIZATION)

Kappa (left) and lambda (right) in situ hybridization reveal a monoclonal kappa population in the bone marrow core biopsy section of a patient with primary amyloidosis.

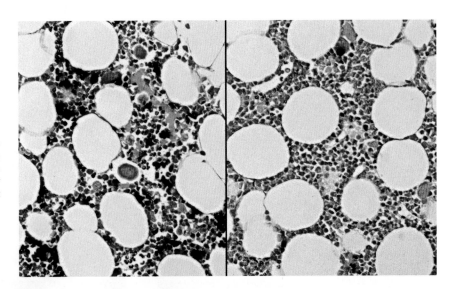

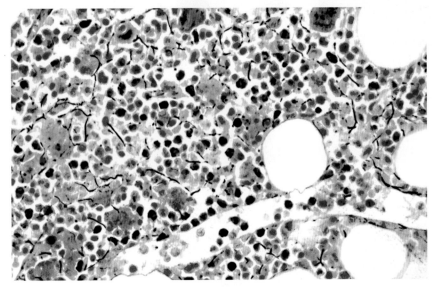

Figure 9-29

RETICULIN FIBERS

Delicate, lacy reticulin fibers support normal bone marrow hematopoietic cavity (reticulin stain).

Figure 9-30

RETICULIN FIBERS SURROUNDING BLOOD VESSEL

Increased reticulin fibers support blood vessels in a normal bone marrow core biopsy (reticulin stain).

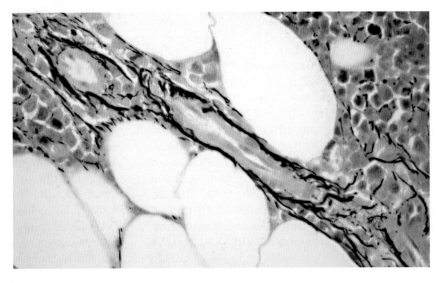

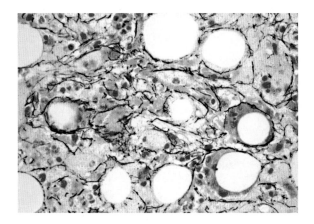

Figure 9-31

DIFFUSE INCREASE IN RETICULIN FIBERS

Diffuse increase in reticulin fibers is evident in this bone marrow core biopsy section (reticulin stain).

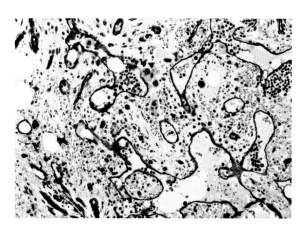

Figure 9-32

NEOANGIOGENESIS (CD34)

Prominent dilated sinuses with neoangiogenesis are evident at intermediate magnification in this bone marrow core biopsy section from a patient with advanced chronic idiopathic myelofibrosis (CD34 immunoperoxidase).

with numerous neoplastic bone marrow disorders (42). Reticulin fiber production and resorption in bone marrow is carefully regulated; the detection of significant reticulin fibrosis generally reflects an imbalance in these regulatory factors (fig. 9-31). Both systemic transforming growth factor-beta 1 (TGF-β1) and substance P have been linked to bone marrow reticulin fibrosis (34,36,39,40). In contrast, trichrome staining is typically absent in the stroma of normal bone marrow; the presence of trichrome-positive collagen fibers is instead indicative of a pathologic process.

Monocytes/macrophages as well as megakaryocytes play critical roles in the pathogenesis of *bone marrow fibrosis* (40). Monocyte/macrophage cytokine production is relevant to the balance of reticulin fiber production and resolution, while excessive intramedullary death of megakaryocytes and platelets is a pathologic process linked to reticulin and, eventually, collagen fibrosis. There is convincing evidence that bone marrow fibroblasts are nonclonal, even in those neoplastic disorders that characteristically exhibit bone marrow fibrosis (40). Neovascularization often accompanies bone marrow fibrosis (fig. 9-32).

Many non-neoplastic and neoplastic bone marrow disorders are associated with bone marrow fibrosis (Table 9-3). The extent of the reticulin and collagen fibrosis varies substantially based on the type of disorder and the disease duration in a given patient. The more extensive

Table 9-3
BONE MARROW DISORDERS WITH FIBROSIS[a]

Non-Neoplastic Disorders
Systemic infections including HIV-1[b] and granulomatous disorders
Collagen vascular disorders including SLE
Autoimmune myelofibrosis
Metabolic bone disorders including Paget disease, constitutional and acquired renal disorders
Following chemotherapy, radiation exposure, toxic insult
Following bone marrow necrosis
Osteopetrosis
Vitamin D deficiency
Pernicious anemia (occasional)
Gray platelet syndrome

Neoplastic Disorders
Chronic myeloproliferative disorders
Acute megakaryoblastic leukemia
Other myeloid neoplasms including systemic mast cell disease
Acute and chronic leukemias/lymphomas, notably hairy cell leukemia
Metastatic tumors including carcinomas and lymphomas
Myeloma (occasional)

[a]Data from references 31, 35–38, 41, and 42.
[b]HIV = human immunodeficiency virus; SLE = systemic lupus erythematosus.

the fibrosis, the more likely the bone marrow will be inaspirable.

Increased megakaryocyte/platelet turnover is a common cause of bone marrow fibrosis and is most notable in chronic myeloproliferative

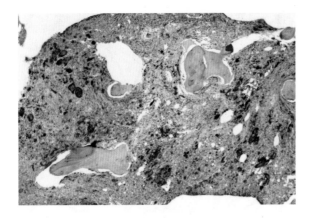

Figure 9-33

INCREASED MEGAKARYOCYTES (CD42b)

Immunoperoxidase staining for CD42b highlights clustered and strikingly increased megakaryocytes at low-power magnification in this bone marrow core biopsy from a patient with a chronic myeloproliferative disorder.

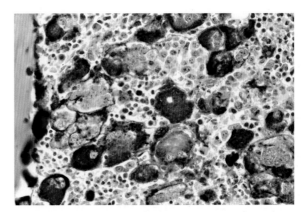

Figure 9-34

INCREASED MEGAKARYOCYTES (CD42b)

High-power magnification of a bone marrow core biopsy stained with CD42b reveals tremendously increased and clustered megakaryocytes in a patient with chronic myeloproliferative disorder and associated bone marrow fibrosis.

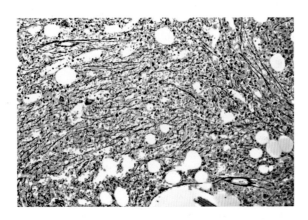

Figure 9-35

GRAY PLATELET SYNDROME

A diffuse increase in reticulin fibrosis is evident in this bone marrow core biopsy from a middle-aged patient with gray platelet syndrome (reticulin stain). (Courtesy of Dr. C. Sever, Albuquerque, NM.)

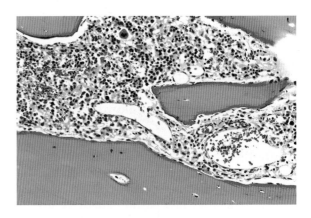

Figure 9-36

AUTOIMMUNE MYELOFIBROSIS

Intermediate magnification of a bone marrow core biopsy section from a patient with autoimmune myelofibrosis shows overall hypocellularity and dilated sinuses (H&E stain).

disorders, megakaryocytic leukemia, and even in rare constitutional disorders such as gray platelet syndrome (figs. 9-33–9-35) (35,41). Although infrequent in clinical practice, primary autoimmune myelofibrosis is a newly recognized non-neoplastic myelofibrotic disorder (31,38). Patients are anemic but lack the prominent teardrop erythrocytes and nucleated red blood cells that typify chronic myeloproliferative disorders. Other features of prototypic chronic myeloproliferative disorders such as

splenomegaly and a leukoerythroblastic blood picture are also absent in patients with primary autoimmune myelofibrosis. The bone marrow is characteristically hypercellular, with reticulin fibrosis, dilated sinuses, intrasinusoidal hematopoiesis, and increased megakaryocytes (figs. 9-36, 9-37). Although some serologic features of systemic lupus erythematosus are present, these patients do not fulfill the diagnostic criteria for a collagen vascular disease. A response to corticosteroid therapy has been documented.

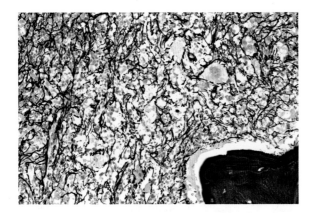

Figure 9-37

AUTOIMMUNE MYELOFIBROSIS

The reticulin stain in this bone marrow core biopsy section from a patient with autoimmune myelofibrosis reveals moderate to markedly diffuse reticulin fibrosis (reticulin stain).

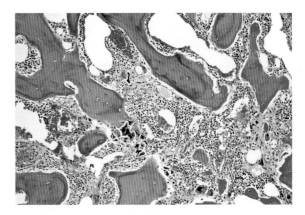

Figure 9-38

ADVANCED COLLAGEN FIBROSIS

Advanced and extensive collagen fibrosis in a bone marrow core biopsy section from a patient with end-stage chronic myelofibrosis (H&E stain).

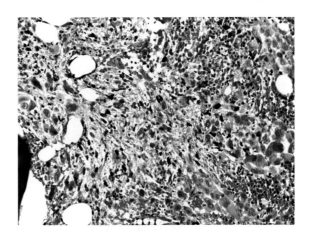

Figure 9-39

COLLAGEN FIBROSIS (TRICHROME)

The trichrome stain highlights collagen in a bone marrow core biopsy section from a patient with chronic myeloproliferative disorder.

The degree of bone marrow fibrosis should be estimated by the reticulin stain. Multiple technical factors must be taken into consideration when quantitation of reticulin fibrosis is attempted. Factors such as the thickness of the core biopsy section, fixation of the core biopsy, and staining methodologies all influence the number of fibers noted in a given area (33). Collagen fibrosis is less common than reticulin fibrosis, and this type of fibrosis may be a later event in pathologic processes (fig. 9-38). The trichrome stain can be used to assess collagen fibrosis, although special stains are not necessary to identify collagen, especially when extensive (fig. 9-39) (35). Since resorption of reticulin fibers is a physiologic process in bone marrow, resolution of reticulin fibrosis may occur following successful treatment of the underlying disorder (32); resolution of advanced collagen fibrosis is less common.

Granulomatous and Diffuse Histiocytic Disorders in Bone Marrow

Both fixed tissue macrophages/histiocytes and migratory monocytes are bone marrow stromal cells that have key regulatory activities. Macrophages/histiocytes and monocytes can be identified on both bone marrow aspirate smears and core biopsy sections. On aspirate smears, histiocytes are concentrated within bone marrow particles, while monocytes are typically sparse and admixed with other developing myeloid cells (fig. 9-40).

Aspirate Smears. Histiocytes may be abundant and even clustered on aspirate smears from patients with granulomatous infiltrates or diffuse histiocytic hyperplasias (fig. 9-41). They typically have abundant eosinophilic cytoplasm which may contain ingested cellular debris or iron (fig. 9-42). In infectious processes, organisms may be evident, while brisk ingestion of hematopoietic cells typifies the so-called hemophagocytic syndromes (figs. 9-43, 9-44). In hemophagocytic disorders, the physiologic cytokine balance is altered by many

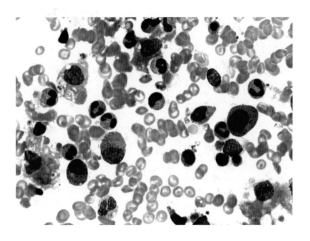

Figure 9-40

INCREASED HISTIOCYTES

Increased histiocytes are apparent in this bone marrow particle on aspirate smear (Wright stain).

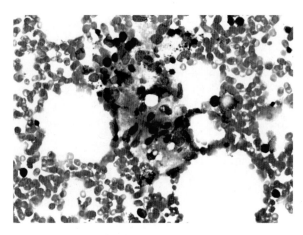

Figure 9-41

MICROGRANULOMA

The clumping of histiocytes that form the microgranuloma is apparent on the bone marrow aspirate smear from a child undergoing therapy for acute lymphoblastic leukemia (Wright stain).

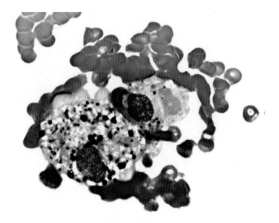

Figure 9-42

MACROPHAGE WITH INGESTED DEBRIS

On bone marrow aspirate smear, macrophages contain ingested debris (Wright stain).

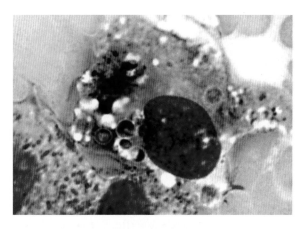

Figure 9-43

MACROPHAGE WITH INGESTED FUNGI

The macrophage contains ingested fungal organisms in a child with AIDS and secondary histoplasmosis (Wright stain). (Courtesy of P. Izadi, Los Angeles, CA.)

diverse underlying disease processes, resulting in unchecked histiocyte stimulation and avid phagocytosis (56).

Core Biopsy. Under physiologic conditions, monocytes and histiocytes are typically inconspicuous on bone marrow core biopsy sections, although they are evident on higher magnification, especially if histiocytes are diffusely increased or contain ingested material (fig. 9-45). Immunohistochemical stains such as CD68 highlight background stromal histiocytes (fig. 9-46).

Granulomas. *Granulomas,* cohesive collections of histiocytes, are better appreciated on bone marrow core biopsy sections than on aspirate smears. Bone marrow granulomas are segregated into different subtypes: epithelioid granulomas, caseating granulomas, ring-shaped granulomas, lipogranulomas, and rare foreign body type granulomas (Table 9-4) (49). All of these types are basically collections of epithelioid histiocytes (i.e., histiocytes with abundant eosinophilic cytoplasm) with various additional

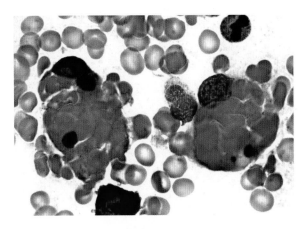

Figure 9-44

**INFECTION-ASSOCIATED
HEMOPHAGOCYTIC SYNDROME**

Increased histiocytes exhibiting tremendous erythrophagocytosis are evident on this bone marrow aspirate smear from a patient with infection-associated hemophagocytic syndrome (Wright stain). (Courtesy of Dr. C. Sever, Albuquerque, NM.)

Table 9-4
CAUSES OF EPITHELIOID GRANULOMAS IN BONE MARROW[a,b]

Systemic Infections	Neoplasms
Bacteria	Hodgkin lymphoma
Mycobacteria	Non-Hodgkin lymphomas
Brucellosis	Rare carcinomas
Tularemia	Rare myeloid neoplasms
Whipple disease (*Tropheryma whipplei*)	
Fungi	**Other Systemic Conditions**
Histoplasmosis	Rheumatologic and other
Cryptococcosis	autoimmune disorders
Coccidiomycosis	including SLE, sarcoidosis
Viruses	Idiosyncratic drug reactions
EBV[c]	—many agents described
CMV (may see ring forms)	BCG therapy
	Pneumoconiosis/silicosis
Hepatitis	
Rickettsia	
Q fever (ring forms typical)	
Ehrlichiosis	

[a]Data from references 47, 49, 57, 59, 62, and 64.
[b]See chapter 10 for a discussion of infectious granulomas.
[c]EBV = Epstein-Barr virus; CMV = cytomegalovirus; SLE = systemic lupus erythematosus; BCG = bacille Calmette-Guérin.

features such as central necrosis (caseating granuloma), central lipid vacuole or fibrin (ring granuloma), abundant foamy intracellular lipid-like material (lipogranuloma), or foreign

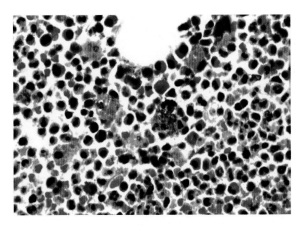

Figure 9-45

TINGIBLE BODY MACROPHAGES

High magnification of bone marrow core biopsy containing increased tingible body histiocytes (H&E stain).

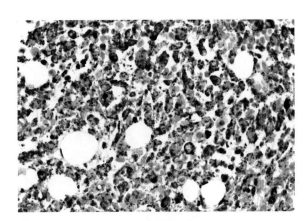

Figure 9-46

INCREASED HISTIOCYTES (CD68)

Immunoperoxidase staining for CD68 highlights a striking increase in interstitial histiocytes within this bone marrow core biopsy section from a patient with multiorgan histiocytosis following bone marrow transplantation.

material with multinucleated giant cells (foreign body granuloma) (figs. 9-47–9-50).

In some cases, the type of granuloma is a clue to the underlying pathologic process: caseating granulomas are much more characteristic of infectious processes, while lipogranulomas are essentially a normal finding in elderly patients. (Infectious disorders in bone marrow are discussed in detail in chapter 10). Other cell types that may be associated with bone marrow granulomas are plasma cells, lymphocytes, eosinophils, and neutrophils (fig. 9-51).

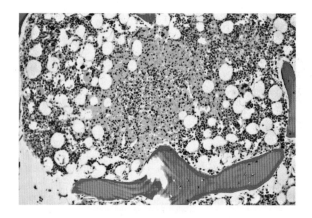

Figure 9-47

EPITHELIOID GRANULOMA

Low magnification shows an epithelioid granuloma on a bone marrow core biopsy from an AIDS patient with secondary mycobacterial infection (H&E stain).

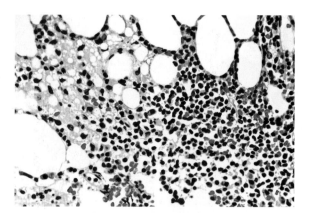

Figure 9-48

LIPOGRANULOMA

Bone marrow core biopsy with lipogranuloma contains foamy histiocytes adjacent to a lymphoid aggregate (H&E stain).

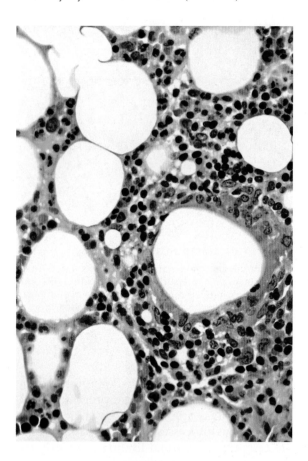

Figure 9-49

RING-SHAPED GRANULOMA

A ring-shaped granuloma with an empty central core is evident on this bone marrow core biopsy section from a patient with chronic renal failure (H&E stain).

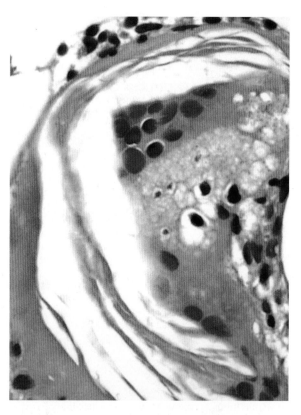

Figure 9-50

MULTINUCLEATED FOREIGN BODY GIANT CELL WITH KERATIN

A multinucleated foreign body giant cell reaction to keratinous material is evident in this sternal bone marrow clot section from a patient with a remote history of cardiac surgery (H&E stain). (Courtesy of Dr. B. Cabello-Inchausti, Plantation, FL.)

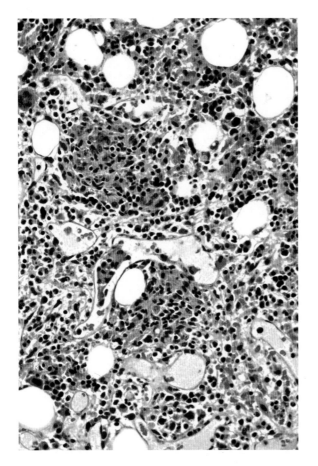

Figure 9-51

EPITHELIOID GRANULOMAS

Bone marrow core biopsy shows two epithelioid granulomas with admixed inflammatory cells (H&E stain).

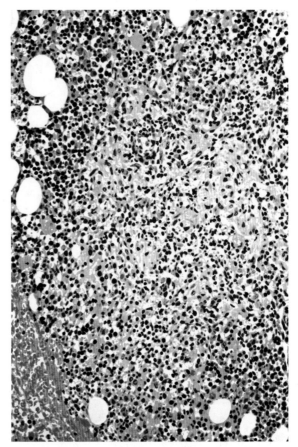

Figure 9-52

**LYMPHOMATOUS INFILTRATE
WITH ASSOCIATED GRANULOMAS**

An extensive lymphomatous infiltrate in this bone marrow biopsy section shows admixed epithelioid granulomas (H&E stain).

Epithelioid granulomas are identified in less than 5 percent of bone marrow specimens; they are more frequent in bone marrow specimens from immunocompromised or febrile patients (47). Epithelioid granulomas may be detected in bone marrow specimens from patients with a variety of disorders including systemic infections, neoplasms, immune disorders, environmental exposures, and idiosyncratic drug reactions (Table 9-4) (47,49,52,54,57). The most common infections inducing granulomas are mycobacteria and various fungal organisms (see chapter 10).

Bone marrow granulomas may also be apparent in either involved or uninvolved bone marrow in patients with Hodgkin and non-Hodgkin lymphomas (figs. 9-52, 9-53). In these cases the granulomas are not part of the neoplastic clone and instead are either recruited by lymphoma-associated factors or represent a host immune response directed against the neoplasm. In patients with primary myeloid neoplasms, it may be better to determine whether the associated histiocytic cells are clonal or reactive, but, if secondary infection can be excluded, there is no specific clinical need for this distinction.

Bone marrow granulomas are also seen with rheumatologic/collagen vascular disorders. Again, once secondary infections have been excluded, there is no specific clinical relevance to these granulomas. A variety of medications are linked to bone marrow granulomas, including the recently described association with amiodarone therapy (57).

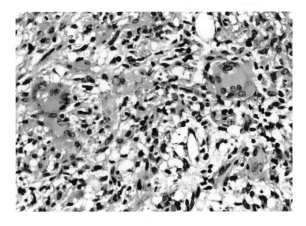

Figure 9-53

MARKED GRANULOMATOUS COMPONENT OF BONE MARROW LYMPHOMA

A marked granulomatous reaction, including Touton type giant cells, is evident in this high magnification photomicrograph of a bone marrow core biopsy section that was extensively effaced by non-Hodgkin lymphoma (H&E stain).

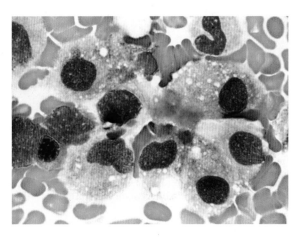

Figure 9-54

INCREASED BONE MARROW HISTIOCYTES

Markedly increased, cytologically bland histiocytes are evident in this bone marrow aspirate smear from a patient with infection-associated hemophagocytic syndrome (Wright stain). (Courtesy of Dr. C. Sever, Albuquerque, NM.)

Diffuse Increase in Histiocytes. A diffuse increase in non-neoplastic bone marrow histiocytes may reflect increased bone marrow cell turnover or a distinct pathologic process such as constitutional lysosomal storage diseases; infection-, constitutional-, or neoplasm-associated hemophagocytic syndromes; or rare idiosyncratic post-therapy benign histiocytic proliferations (figs. 9-54, 9-55) (58,63).

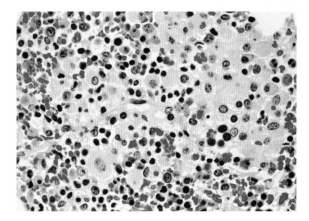

Figure 9-55

DIFFUSE INCREASE IN BONE MARROW HISTIOCYTES

This high magnification photomicrograph of a bone marrow core biopsy section shows a diffuse increase in cytologically bland histiocytes with abundant eosinophilic cytoplasm and small round nucleoli in this patient with striking bone marrow histiocytosis and infection-associated hemophagocytic syndrome (H&E stain). (Courtesy of Dr. C. Sever, Albuquerque, NM.)

Hemohagocytic Syndromes. Regardless of the underlying pathologic disorder, the hallmark of *hemophagocytic syndromes* is the avid ingestion of normal hematopoietic elements by histiocytes (figs. 9-56, 9-57) (43,53,60). These hemophagocytic histiocytes can be readily identified on either aspirate smears or core biopsy sections (figs. 9-57, 9-58). A constitutional immunodeficiency disorder, familial lymphohistiocytosis, is associated with a diffuse increase in bone marrow histiocytes and intermittent, possibly infection-associated, episodes of florid hemophagocytosis (figs. 9-59, 9-60) (58). Perforin gene mutations have been described in these patients (58).

Lysosomal Storage Diseases. The accumulation of abnormal breakdown products within histiocytes in patients with constitutional lysosomal storage disorders produces distinctive morphologic cells, such as Gaucher cells or Niemann-Pick histiocytes (see chapter 11 for details) (44,48,63). In Gaucher disease, the cytoplasm of the abundant histiocytes has a "crinkled tissue-paper" appearance, while numerous crisp cytoplasmic vacuoles characterize the histiocytes of Niemann-Pick disease (figs. 9-61–9-66). These storage cells are typically concentrated within bone marrow particles, but may be dispersed

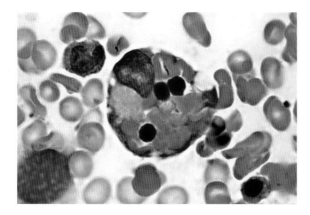

Figure 9-56

**INFECTION-ASSOCIATED
HEMOPHAGOCYTIC SYNDROME**

Striking hemophagocytosis with ingestion of erythrocytes as well as nucleated hematopoietic elements is evident on this bone marrow aspirate smear from a patient with infection-associated hemophagocytic syndrome. (Wright stain) (Courtesy of Dr. C. Sever, Albuquerque, NM.)

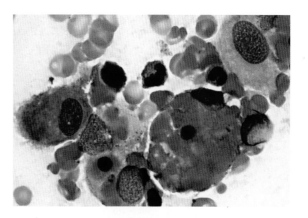

Figure 9-57

**INFECTION-ASSOCIATED
HEMOPHAGOCYTIC SYNDROME**

Abundant phagocytic and nonphagocytic histiocytes are evident in this bone marrow aspirate smear from a patient with infection-associated hemophagocytic syndrome (Wright stain). (Courtesy of Dr. C. Sever, Albuquerque, NM.)

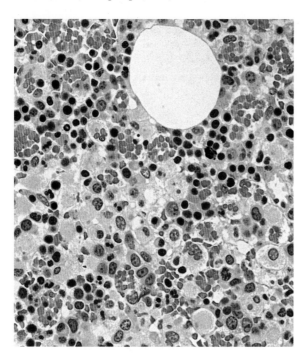

Figure 9-58

**INFECTION-ASSOCIATED
HEMOPHAGOCYTIC SYNDROME**

This intermediate magnification photomicrograph of a bone marrow core biopsy section from a patient with infection-associated hemophagocytic syndrome shows prominent erythrophagocytosis within the cytoplasm of histiocytes. A sack-like appearance is caused by ingested erythrocytes held closely together within the cytoplasm of the histiocytes (H&E stain). (Courtesy of Dr. C. Sever, Albuquerque, NM.)

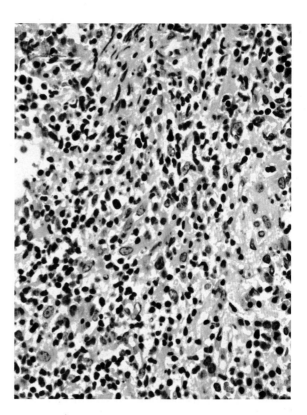

Figure 9-59

FAMILIAL LYMPHOHISTIOCYTOSIS

This bone marrow core biopsy section shows a striking increase in both histiocytes and lymphocytes in a child with familial lymphohistiocytosis (H&E stain). (Courtesy of Dr. J. Anastasi, Chicago, IL.)

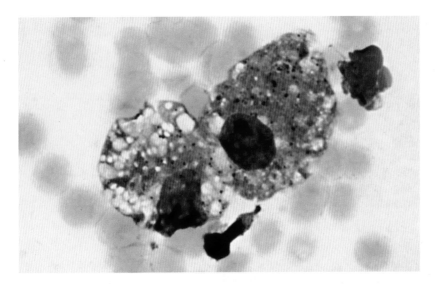

Figure 9-60

**FAMILIAL
LYMPHOHISTIOCYTOSIS**

Bone marrow aspirate smear
from a patient with familial lymphohistiocytosis shows increased, cytologically bland histiocytes with vacuolated, finely and coarsely granular
cytoplasm (Wright stain). (Courtesy
of Dr. J. Anastasi, Chicago, IL.)

Figure 9-61

GAUCHER DISEASE

Left: Gaucher cells have crinkly
cytoplasm, which is evident on a
bone marrow aspirate smear.
Right: Pseudo-Gaucher cells from
a patient with chronic myelogenous
leukemia (Wright stain). (Left image
courtesy of P. Izadi, Los Angeles,
CA.)

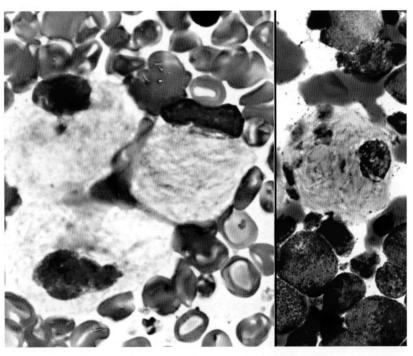

throughout aspirate smears (figs. 9-65, 9-66). A variant subtype of Neimann-Pick disease, so called sea blue histiocytosis, or ceroid histiocytosis, is characterized by an admixture of typical vacuolated, bubbly Niemann-Pick cells with dark blue histiocytes (fig. 9-67) (55,61). The bone marrow histiocytes, reticular cells, plasma cells, and osteoblasts of numerous other lysosomal storage diseases that are infrequent in clinical practice may contain abnormal cytoplasmic inclusions/vacuoles as well (46,50).

For all lysosomal storage diseases, definitive diagnosis is dependent upon the confirmation of the specific enzyme deficiency or other cellular defect (45,63).

Langerhans Cell Histiocytosis. Although uncommon, dendritic cell neoplasms such as *Langerhans cell histiocytosis* (LCH) occasionally manifest with prominent bone marrow infiltration. Although the cytologic features of LCH on aspirate smears are relatively nondescript, the distinct linear nuclear grooves on bone marrow

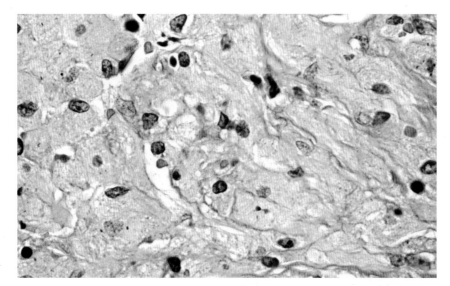

Figure 9-62

GAUCHER DISEASE

The Gaucher cells in a bone marrow core biopsy section have voluminous eosinophilic, crinkled cytoplasm and small, bland histiocyte nuclei (H&E stain).

Figure 9-63

NIEMANN-PICK DISEASE

Finely vacuolated Niemann-Pick type histiocytes are seen on a bone marrow aspirate smear from child with Niemann-Pick disease (Wright stain). (Courtesy of P. Izadi, Los Angeles, CA.)

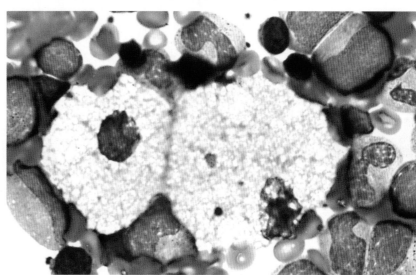

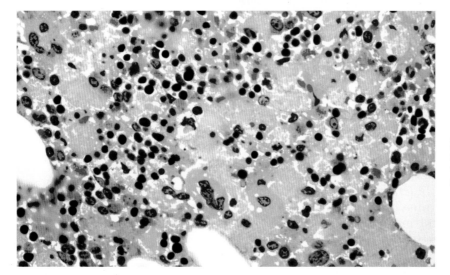

Figure 9-64

NIEMANN-PICK DISEASE

A prominent histiocytic infiltrate is evident on a bone marrow core biopsy from patient with Niemann-Pick disease (H&E stain).

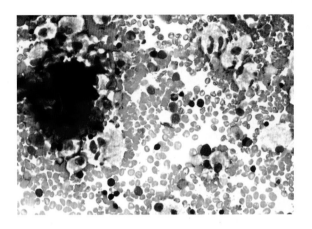

Figure 9-65

GAUCHER DISEASE

The bone marrow aspirate smear shows a marked increase in Gaucher type histiocytes, both within bone marrow particles and dispersed throughout the aspirate smear (Wright stain). (Courtesy of P. Izadi, Los Angeles, CA.)

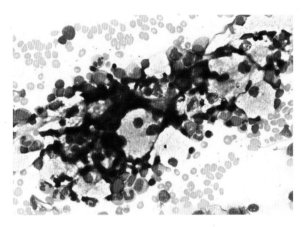

Figure 9-66

NIEMANN-PICK DISEASE

Abundant Niemann-Pick type histiocytes are evident in this bone marrow aspirate smear from a child with Niemann-Pick disease (Wright stain). (Courtesy of P. Izadi, Los Angeles, CA.)

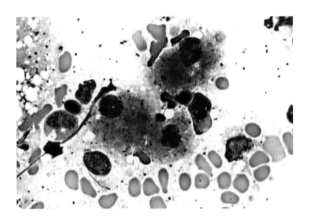

Figure 9-67

SEA BLUE HISTIOCYTES IN VARIANT NIEMANN-PICK DISEASE

An imprint smear shows deeply blue histiocytes, so-called sea blue histiocytes, in this patient with a variant of Niemann-Pick disease, termed either sea blue or ceroid histiocytosis (Wright stain).

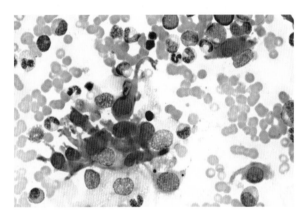

Figure 9-68

LANGERHANS CELL HISTIOCYTOSIS

Numerous stellate dendritic cells are present in this bone marrow aspirate in a child with extensive involvement by Langerhans cell histiocytosis (Wright stain). (Courtesy of Dr. S. Kroft, Milwaukee, WI.)

biopsy sections and CD1a expression by immunohistochemistry are useful in establishing the diagnosis (figs. 9-68–9-71).

Differential Diagnosis. The differential diagnosis of diffuse bone marrow histiocytic infiltrates is diverse and includes monocytic leukemias, histiocytic sarcomas, infections such as Whipple disease and mycobacterial infections, lymphomas (especially anaplastic large cell lymphomas), and histiocytic cell look-alikes (figs. 9-72–9-74) (51,54). Storage disease–type histiocytes can also be evident in bone marrow in high cell turnover conditions (see fig. 9-61).

Iron Disorders in Bone Marrow

Iron is an essential cellular nutrient and an essential component of hemoglobin. Although iron is also essential in enzymatic reduction/oxidation reactions, a primary role of iron is to provide a binding site for oxygen in the heme

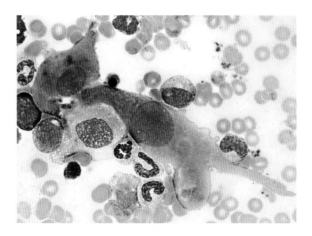

Figure 9-69

LANGERHANS CELL HISTIOCYTOSIS

The cytologic features of Langerhans cells are evident in a bone marrow aspirate smear from a child with extensive bone marrow involvement by Langerhans cell histiocytosis (Wright stain). (Courtesy of Dr. S. Kroft, Milwaukee, WI.)

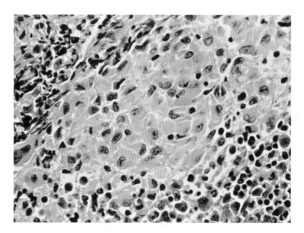

Figure 9-70

LANGERHANS CELL HISTIOCYTOSIS

Bone marrow core biopsy shows extensive involvement by Langerhans cell histiocytosis. These cells have large amounts of eosinophilic cytoplasm and irregular, two-folded nuclei with linear nuclear grooves. Note the eosinophilia (H&E stain). (Courtesy of Dr. S. Kroft, Milwaukee, WI.)

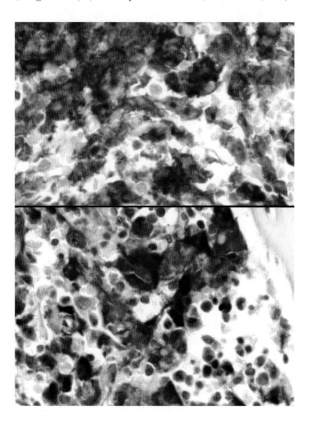

Figure 9-71

**LANGERHANS CELL HISTIOCYTOSIS
(CD1a, S-100 PROTEIN)**

CD1a (top) and S-100 protein (bottom) immunoperoxidase stains in bone marrow core biopsy specimens extensively involved by Langerhans cell histiocytosis.

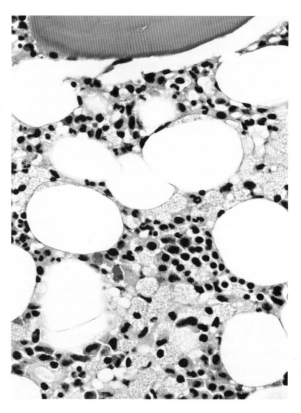

Figure 9-72

MYELOMA MIMICKING NIEMANN-PICK DISEASE

An interstitial infiltrate of distinctly vacuolated large cells mimics Niemann-Pick disease in a bone marrow core biopsy from patient with multiple myeloma (H&E stain).

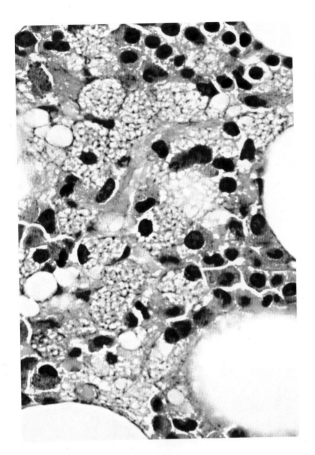

Figure 9-73

MYELOMA MIMICKING NIEMANN-PICK DISEASE

The numerous vacuolated neoplastic cells of a bone marrow biopsy involved by multiple myeloma mimic Niemann-Pick disease (H&E stain).

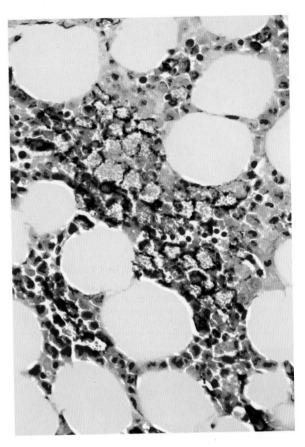

Figure 9-74

MYELOMA MIMICKING NIEMANN-PICK DISEASE (CD138)

Immunoperoxidase stain for CD138 highlights the vacuolated myeloma cells that mimic Niemann-Pick disease in this bone marrow core biopsy section.

component of hemoglobin (75). Increased amounts of iron can be toxic to cells, however, so iron homeostasis is a carefully regulated process beginning with iron absorption by intestinal epithelial cells, iron transport in plasma, and iron storage in hepatocytes and macrophages/histiocytes (68–70,72,75). At least two thirds of total host iron is contained within the erythrocytes and erythroid precursors (68).

Although there are many serologic tests and even a radiologic (magnetic resonance imaging) technique to assess storage iron, evaluation of bone marrow macrophages/histiocytes for iron content is a commonly used method to quantitate bone marrow storage iron (69,76). Abnormalities in the amount of storage iron in bone marrow macrophages are common

and include both decreased and increased iron stores based on assessing the bone marrow macrophages that are concentrated within particles (fig. 9-75). Usually, multiple particles are assessed using Prussian blue stains of bone marrow aspirate smears. For smears in which iron is virtually absent, it is essential to review the Prussian blue control for the adequacy of the stain. In cases of profound iron deficiency, both erythroid precursors and macrophages are virtually devoid of particulate blue iron. At the opposite end of the spectrum, specimens with increased storage iron exhibit strong, diffuse and granular blue positivity in the majority of macrophages (figs. 9-76, 9-77). In addition, brightly blue staining macrophage cytoplasmic fragments are commonly dispersed throughout

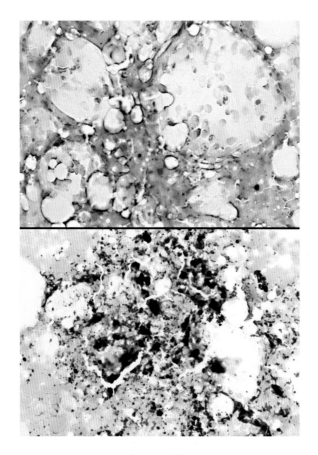

Figure 9-75

NORMAL AND INCREASED STORAGE IRON

Normal amounts of storage iron in an adult male (top) are compared to markedly increased storage iron in a chronically transfused patient (bottom) (Prussian blue stain).

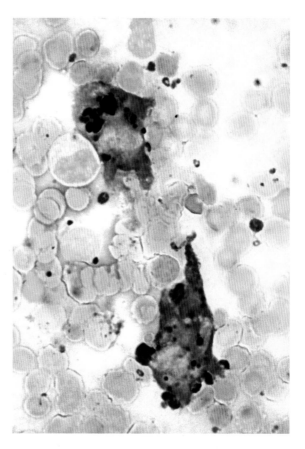

Figure 9-76

INCREASED MACROPHAGE IRON

Markedly positive iron staining of bone marrow macrophages. Prussian blue–positive cytoplasmic fragments of histiocytes are dispersed throughout the smear.

the smear (fig. 9-76). Because these fragments may overlay erythroid cells, it is important to distinguish them from actual erythroid iron.

Hemosiderin granules within bone marrow stromal macrophages may also be apparent on H&E-stained sections of bone marrow clot and core biopsy sections; however, due to loss of iron in processing, especially with decalcification, iron is assessed on bone marrow aspirate smears. Erythroid iron is simultaneously assessed. Normal erythroid precursors contain a few small iron granules within the cytoplasm. Excess erythroid iron is a common pathologic condition, and ringed sideroblasts may be evident (fig. 9-78). Increased storage iron with reduced erythroid iron is characteristic of anemia of chronic disease (see chapter 11).

Disorders associated with increased or decreased storage iron are listed on Table 9-5; iron deficiency is more commonly encountered in clinical practice than iron overload disorders. The most common cause of iron deficiency is decreased intake, often in conjunction with excess blood loss. This scenario is very typical for iron deficiency anemias that occur in reproductive-age females in which either heavy menses or pregnancy is a cause of the reduced iron stores when compensatory increased intake has not occurred (80). Likewise, chronic gastrointestinal tract bleeding is a frequent cause of reduced iron in males. Excess erythrocyte destruction can be linked to iron deficiency, especially if free hemoglobin is released into the plasma. Finally, therapeutic iron deficiency is the goal in

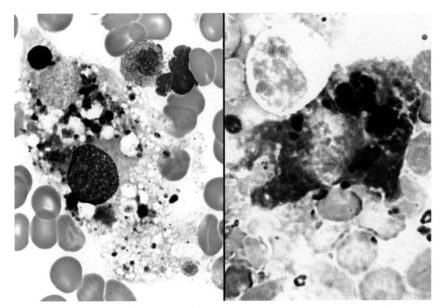

Figure 9-77

MACROPHAGE WITH INGESTED DEBRIS AND ABUNDANT IRON

The macrophages contain abundant hemosiderin as illustrated with Wright (left) and Prussian blue (right) staining. Prussian blue–positive cytoplasmic fragments of histiocytes are dispersed throughout the smear.

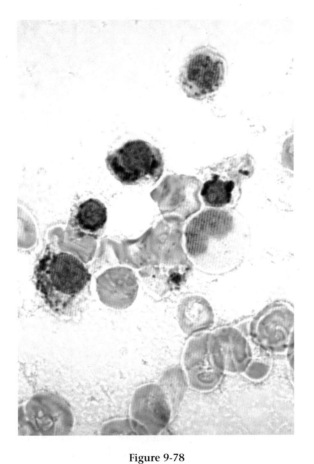

Figure 9-78

SIDEROBLASTIC ANEMIA

Numerous ringed sideroblasts are evident on this bone marrow aspirate smear from a patient with sideroblastic anemia (Prussian blue stain).

Table 9-5

CAUSES OF ABNORMAL AMOUNTS OF BONE MARROW STORAGE IRON[a]

Condition	Disorders/Comments
Decreased storage iron	Iron deficiency from inadequate intake or blood loss
	Selected chronic hemolytic anemias including PNH[b]
	Polycythemia vera
	Constitutional iron transport or metabolism disorders (parenchymal cell iron overload, but absent iron in bone marrow—rare)
Increased storage iron	Excess therapeutic/dietary intake such as chronic red blood cell transfusions, prolonged parenteral iron therapy, or prolonged ingestion of medicinal iron
	Iron-loading anemias such as thalassemias (secondary to chronic transfusions, often in conjunction with other iron regulatory defects)
	Chronic liver disease including alcoholic liver disease, viral hepatitis, and portacaval shunt
	Myelodysplastic syndromes
	Hereditary hemochromatosis (homozygous mutations in *HFE* gene—both juvenile and adult types described)
	Neonatal hemochromatosis
	Other hereditary iron overload disorders linked to mutations in other genes involved in iron transport or metabolism including ceruloplasmin (rare)

[a]Data from references 65, 66, 70–75, and 77–80.
[b]PNH = paroxysmal nocturnal hematuria.

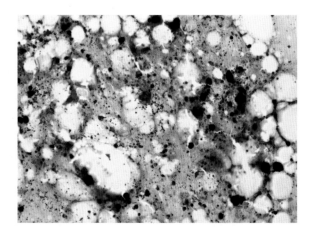

Figure 9-79

IRON OVERLOAD FROM CHRONIC TRANSFUSIONS

Massive iron overload secondary to chronic transfusions is highlighted by iron staining on this bone marrow aspirate smear (Prussian blue stain). (Courtesy of Dr.C. Sever, Albuquerque, NM.)

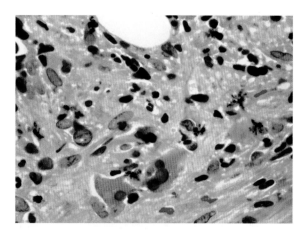

Figure 9-80

CRYSTALLINE FIXATIVE PRECIPITATE

A crystalline fixative precipitate is present on this bone marrow core biopsy specimen (H&E stain).

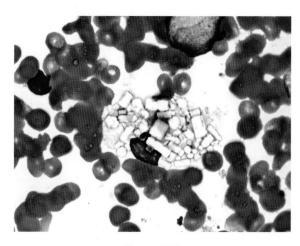

Figure 9-81

CYSTINOSIS

Cystinosis crystals in a bone marrow aspirate smear from a child with Fanconi renal disease (Wright stain).

patients with clonal disorders such as polycythemia vera which are linked to excess erythrocyte production (73).

Genetic disorders such as hemochromatosis and constitutional anemias are the most common causes of clinically significant iron overload conditions, which are associated with a wide range of multiorgan health problems (65,66,68,70,72,75,78,80). The genetic mechanisms for many types of adult and juvenile hemochromatosis have been delineated. Mutations in the *HFE* gene are linked to hereditary hemochromatosis type 1 (65,66,70–72,74,75). This disease trait occurs in about 1/200 to 400 Caucasians (66,67,74). Excess storage iron accumulation in many sites, including within bone marrow macrophages, is a feature of these genetic iron transport disorders. Iron overload secondary to chronic transfusion also results in dramatically increased storage iron (fig. 9-79).

Crystal Deposition in Bone Marrow

Although precipitated fixatives may be crystalline, pathologic crystals are only rarely encountered in bone marrow specimens (fig. 9-80). *Crystalline deposits* within the bone marrow stroma have been described in both constitutional and acquired disorders. Constitutional disorders with multiorgan crystal deposition include oxalosis and cystinosis; both of these rare autosomal

recessive metabolic disorders are characterized by chronic renal failure in addition to other multisystem abnormalities. Oxalosis is the consequence of alanine glyoxylate aminotransferase deficiency, while cystinosis results from the deficiency of a cystine carrier in the lysosomal membrane (fig. 9-81) (81,83,85,86). Bone marrow samples from patients with either oxalosis or cystinosis should exhibit the marked stromal and bone changes linked to renal osteodystrophy (see later in this chapter) (fig. 9-82).

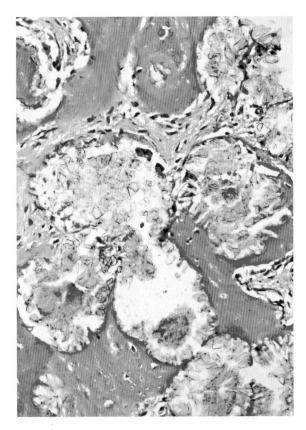

Figure 9-82

OXALOSIS

Extensive bone marrow involvement by oxalosis shows numerous crystals, foreign body reaction, and striking bony and stromal changes secondary to renal osteodystrophy (H&E stain).

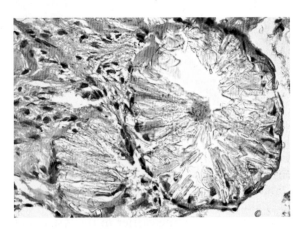

Figure 9-83

OXALOSIS

High magnification highlights the crystals with an associated foreign body giant cell reaction and stromal fibrosis (H&E stain).

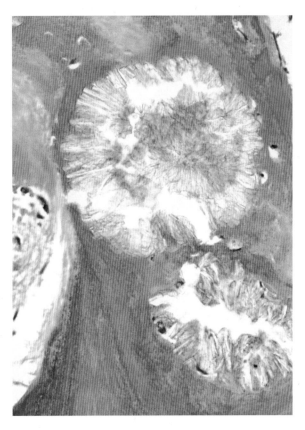

Figure 9-84

OXALOSIS

Oxalate crystal deposition within bony trabeculae in a patient with oxalosis (H&E stain).

The distinctive finding in these two metabolic disorders is the presence of crystals within the bone marrow stroma. In oxalosis, the crystals are very large and may be present within both stroma and bone matrix (figs. 9-83, 9-84) (82). The deposits cause a prominent foreign body giant cell reaction (fig. 9-85). In cystinosis, the crystals are less conspicuous at low-power magnification and are typically present within the macrophage cytoplasm (85). When identified on aspirate smears, oxalate crystals form long cords (fig. 9-86).

The acquired disorders linked to crystals in bone marrow stroma are also rare and include silica crystals in patients with pneumoconiosis and immunoglobulin crystals in patients with multiple myeloma (84,87). In myeloma patients the crystalline inclusions may be within neoplastic plasma cells as well as the stromal macrophages.

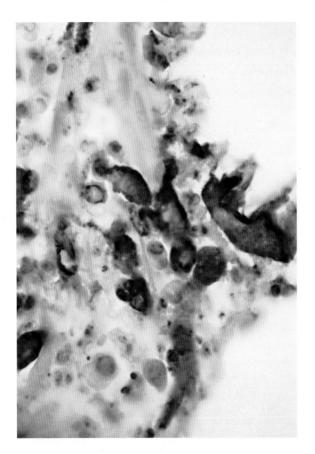

Figure 9-85

GRANULOMATOUS REACTION IN OXALOSIS (CD68)

Immunoperoxidase staining for CD68 highlights the extensive histiocytic reaction to oxalate crystal deposition within bone marrow in a patient with oxalosis.

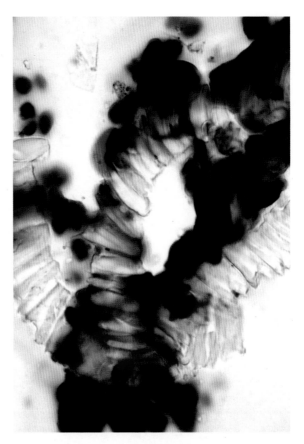

Figure 9-86

OXALOSIS CRYSTALS

Oxalosis crystals are evident on a bone marrow aspirate smear; string-like chords of stacked crystals are also seen (Wright stain).

STRUCTURAL DISORDERS OF BONE MARROW

Vascular Abnormalities Including Neoangiogenesis

Blood vessels should be routinely assessed on bone marrow core biopsy sections. Small caliber vessels are distributed in low numbers throughout the bone marrow parenchyma (fig. 9-87). The vascular abnormalities seen on bone marrow core biopsy sections are neoangiogenesis (increased capillary meshwork), intraluminal abnormal cells or substances, and abnormalities in blood vessel walls (Table 9-6).

Neoangiogenesis is common in various hematolymphoid neoplasms, but the capillary proliferation can be seen as part of bone marrow recovery following potent therapy for neoplasms or other

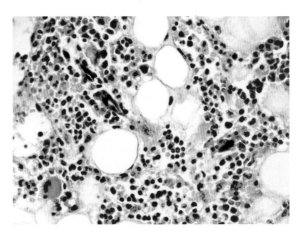

Figure 9-87

NORMAL VESSELS IN NORMAL BONE MARROW (CD34)

Immunoperoxidase stain for CD34 highlights the few blood vessels in a normal bone marrow core biopsy section.

311

Table 9-6

VASCULAR ABNORMALITIES IN BONE MARROW[a,b]

Abnormality	Comments
Increased capillary mesh-work as assessed by quantitative techniques	Neoangiogenesis is common in many hematolymphoid neoplasms in bone marrow including: Acute myeloid leukemia Myeloproliferative disorders Chronic myeloproliferative disorders Multiple myeloma Hairy cell leukemia Chronic lymphocytic leukemia Neoangiogenesis is also seen after therapy and toxic bone marrow insults
Abnormal cells or substances within vascular lumens	Emboli consisting of mucin or cholesterol described in rare bone marrow sections Intravascular thrombi noted in bone marrow of patients with thrombotic thrombocytopenic purpura Intravascular hematopoiesis, notably in chronic myeloproliferative disorders and autoimmune myelofibrosis Intravascular lymphoma rarely noted in bone marrow sections
Abnormal vessel wall	Amyloid deposits in bone marrow are most frequently restricted to vessel walls Giant cell arteritis detected rarely in bone marrow biopsy specimens

[a]Data from references 88, 90, and 92–97.
[b]Other rare abnormalities include localized angiomas, metastatic Kaposi sarcoma, and angiosarcomas.

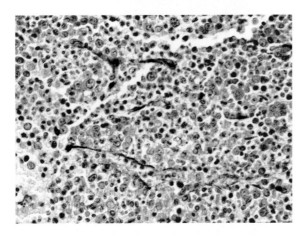

Figure 9-88

INCREASED VESSELS IN BONE MARROW (CD34)

Immunoperoxidase stain for CD34 highlights increased bone marrow vessels in a non-neoplastic condition.

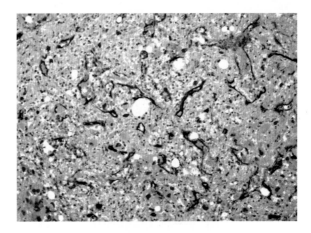

Figure 9-89

NEOANGIOGENESIS (CD34)

Marked neoangiogenesis is evident by CD34 staining for immunoperoxidase in this patient with chronic myelogenous leukemia in the accelerated phase.

toxic insults (figs. 9-88, 9-89) (88,92,93,96). Multiple factors play a role in driving neoangiogenesis, including vascular endothelial growth factor (VEGF) and syndecan 1 (89,96,98,100). Angiogenesis is assessed on core biopsy sections typically using immunohistochemical stains for CD34 to highlight capillaries. The number of these vessels per given area is compared to normal control specimens. This type of diffuse, generally tumor-related neoangiogenesis must be distinguished

from rare localized angiomas that involve bone marrow (fig. 9-89). Similarly, neoplastic vascular lesions such as Kaposi sarcoma and angiosarcoma rarely involve bone marrow (91).

Mucin and *cholesterol emboli* are occasionally noted within vessel lumens on bone marrow core biopsy sections, while *intravascular fibrin/platelet thrombi* may be noted in patients with coagulopathies such as thrombotic thrombocytopenic purpura (TTP) (fig. 9-90) (90,

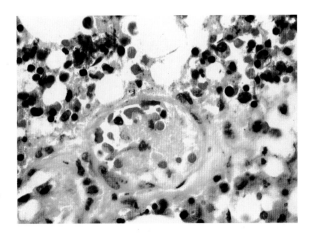

Figure 9-90

PLATELET THROMBI

A bone marrow core biopsy shows a vessel plugged with platelet thrombi in a patient with fatal thrombotic thrombocytopenic purpura (H&E stain).

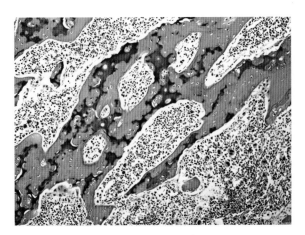

Figure 9-91

NORMAL BONE IN NEWBORN

Normal bone with incomplete ossification in a newborn (H&E stain).

94,95,97). As noted earlier in this chapter, smudgy, eosinophilic amyloid deposition within vessel walls is common in patients with primary systemic (AL) amyloidosis (99). This extracellular immunoglobulin deposition can be highlighted by apple-green birefringence on Congo red-stained sections.

Acquired and Constitutional Bone Abnormalities

Bony Trabeculae. The routine systematic evaluation of bony trabeculae is an important aspect of the examination of the bone marrow core biopsy. The detection of an abnormality of bony trabeculae may be a clue to an underlying metabolic disorder or evidence of a primary or metastatic neoplasm. The morphologic features of active bone production and remodeling are characteristic of bone marrow specimens from pediatric patients. Even in adults bone remodeling is ongoing to achieve mechanical support and to maintain appropriate calcium levels; however, this remodeling is not typically morphologically apparent in terms of conspicuous osteoclasts or osteoblasts in normal adult specimens (figs. 9-91–9-95) (102,111,115).

The systematic evaluation of bony trabeculae on core biopsy specimens includes an overall assessment of the size, thickness, shape, and contour of bony trabeculae, as well as a review of the cellular and matrix constituents of bony

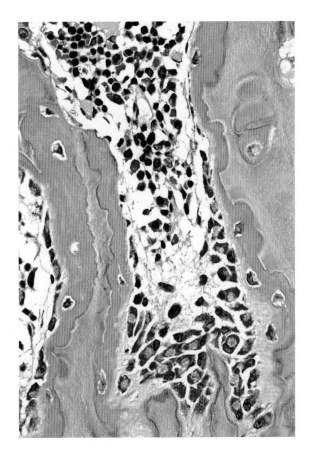

Figure 9-92

BONE REMODELING IN 9-MONTH-OLD

Prominent remodeling with osteoblast rimming, osteoid seams, and incomplete ossification in a bone marrow core biopsy specimen from 9-month-old baby (H&E stain).

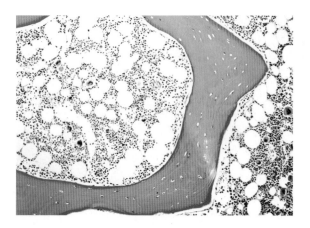

Figure 9-93

NORMAL BONY TRABECULAE IN 13-YEAR-OLD

Normal bone marrow trabeculae are lined by osteoblasts in a 13-year-old girl (H&E stain).

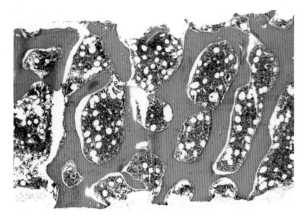

Figure 9-94

NORMAL BONY TRABECULAE IN 16-YEAR-OLD

Low magnification shows a normal bony trabecular configuration in a 16-year-old boy (H&E stain).

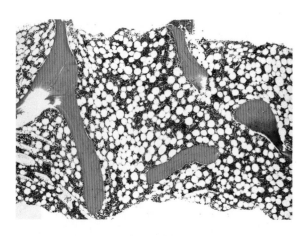

Figure 9-95

NORMAL BONY TRABECULAE IN 43-YEAR-OLD

Low magnification shows a normal bony trabecular configuration in a 43-year-old male (H&E stain).

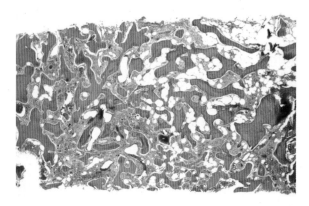

Figure 9-96

OSTEOSCLEROSIS

Thickened, anastomosing bony trabeculae in a patient with osteosclerosis (H&E stain).

trabeculae (Table 9-7). Because a generous core of intact bone marrow is necessary for optimal assessment of bone, both the length of the core biopsy and other factors must be considered, such as crush artifact and the presence of cortical bone and/or subcortical bone marrow immediately adjacent to the bony cortex. These regions of bone are not optimal for the evaluation of bony trabeculae. The relationship of individual bony trabeculae should be examined on low-power magnification. Some pathologic processes are associated with thickened, anastomosing bony trabeculae, resulting in much greater overall bone density than is evident in normal bone marrow (fig. 9-96).

The only cellular bony trabecular constituent that is typically apparent in bone marrow core biopsy specimens from healthy adults is the osteocyte, a mesenchymal cell derived from osteoblasts, which resides within lacunar spaces distributed throughout the mature mineralized bone (fig. 9-97). Dropout of osteocytes from lacunar spaces is a feature of necrotic bone (fig. 9-98).

Osteoblasts/Osteoclasts. In normal young patients and in patients with metabolic bone disorders, both osteoblasts and osteoclasts may

Table 9-7

EVALUATION OF BONY TRABECULAE[a]

Bony trabeculae	Anastomosing bone spicules provide structural support for hematopoietic (medullary) cavity
	Assess thickness, contours, spacing within medullary cavity
	A pattern of continuously connected, anastomosing bony trabeculae on routine microscopic assessment is pathologic
	Assess cell types associated with bony trabeculae
	Assess adjacent stroma for fibrosis or other abnormalities
Components of bony trabeculae	Components of mesenchymal stem cell origin: osteoblasts and osteocytes
	Components of hematopoietic origin: osteoclasts
	Mineralized bone predominates and contains osteocytes within lacunar spaces
	Osteoid (woven bone): consists of unmineralized newly formed bone matrix located along the periphery of mature bony trabeculae
	Osteoblasts (mononuclear cells) reside along periphery of bony trabeculae, produce osteoid, form a row of individual mononuclear cells along bony trabeculae in young patients
	Osteoclasts (multinucleated cells):
	located within scalloped indentations of bony trabeculae (Howship lacunae)
	resorb bone
	apparent in patchy distribution along bony trabeculae in specimens from pediatric patients
Stroma	Paratrabecular fibrosis is common in pathologic processes with prominent bone remodeling

[a]Data from references 102, 109, 111, 115, 116, and 118.

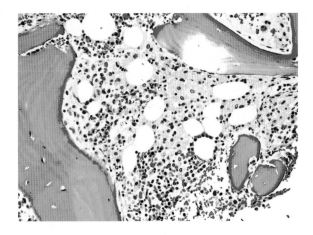

Figure 9-97

OSTEOCYTES WITHIN BONY TRABECULAE

Dark osteocyte nuclei are present within lacunar spaces in normal bony trabeculae from an adult (H&E stain).

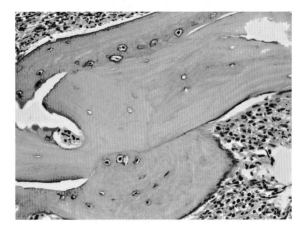

Figure 9-98

NECROTIC BONY TRABECULAE

Markedly thickened bony trabeculae with a central core of necrotic bone shows loss of osteocytes and a surrounding collar of viable new bone formation in a patient with resolving bone marrow necrosis (H&E stain).

be evident on bone marrow aspirate or core biopsy specimens (figs. 9-99, 9-100). Osteoblasts reside along the periphery of bony trabeculae and produce osteoid, so-called woven bone, which is unmineralized bone matrix (fig. 9-100). In conditions of active bone formation, osteoid seams may be apparent, with collars of new bone matrix surrounding mature, mineralized bone (fig. 9-101). Osteoblasts are mononuclear, mesenchymal stem cell–derived cells that line up individually along bony trabeculae (figs.

9-102, 9-103) (109). These cells are readily evident in bone marrow specimens from pediatric patients, but are inconspicuous in normal adult samples. In addition to the production of bone matrix, osteoblasts play a critical role in regulating osteoclast growth, maturation, and function (123). Recently, it has been determined that osteoblasts play a significant role in the regulation of hematopoiesis (see chapter 1).

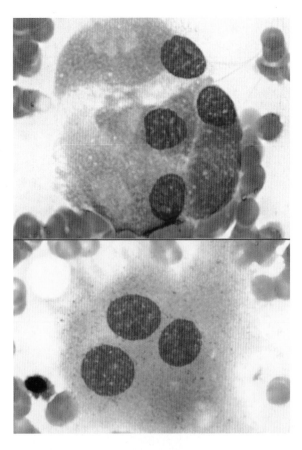

Figure 9-99

OSTEOBLASTS AND OSTEOCLAST

The cytologic features of osteoblasts (top) and an osteo-clast (bottom) are seen on bone marrow aspirate smears (Wright stain).

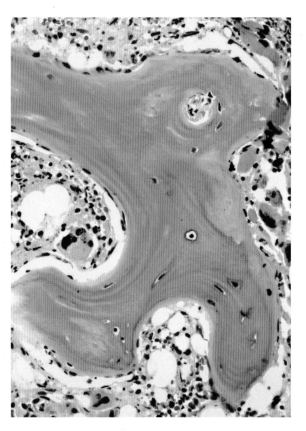

Figure 9-100

PROMINENT NEW BONE FORMATION

Prominent new bone formation with both increased osteoblasts and scattered osteoclasts in a bone marrow biopsy section from a patient with myeloproliferative disorder associated with marked bony changes (H&E stain). (Courtesy of Dr. C. Sever, Albuquerque, NM.)

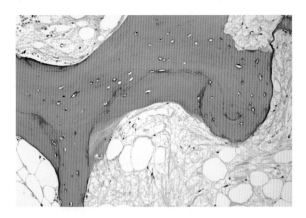

Figure 9-101

OSTEOID SEAM AND NEW BONE FORMATION

Intermediate magnification of a bone marrow core biopsy shows a prominent osteoid seam of new bone in widened bony trabeculae (H&E stain).

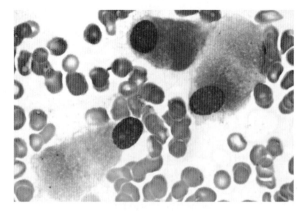

Figure 9-102

OSTEOBLASTS

Multiple osteoblasts with markedly eccentric nuclei are evident on a bone marrow aspirate smear (Wright stain).

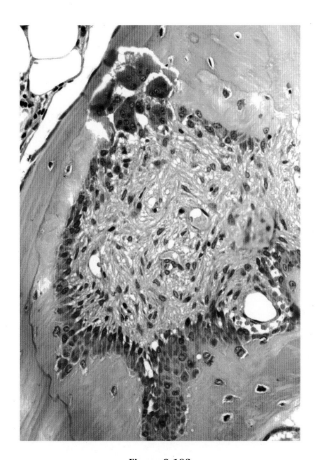

Figure 9-103

**RENAL OSTEODYSTROPHY
WITH OSTEOBLAST RIMMING**

A bone marrow core biopsy section from a patient with renal osteodystrophy shows marked osteoblast rimming of bony trabeculae, foci of increased osteoclasts within a lacunae, and prominent paratrabecular fibrosis (H&E stain).

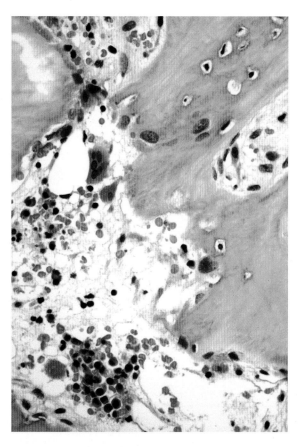

Figure 9-104

OSTEOCLASTS WITHIN LACUNAR SPACES

Osteoclasts within indented lacunar spaces are adjacent to bony trabeculae in a patient with Paget disease and prominent bony changes (H&E stain).

Multinucleated osteoclasts are monocyte/macrophage lineage–derived hematopoietic cells which reside in scalloped indentations (Howship lacunae) along the periphery of bony trabeculae (fig. 9-104) (116,123). In cell culture studies, fusion of myeloid dendritic cells resulted in osteoclasts in the presence of appropriate mediators (118). These cells resorb bone critical for bone remodeling. Similar to osteoblasts, osteoclasts are inconspicuous in bone marrow biopsy sections from normal adults.

Abnormal Bony Trabeculae. Any bone abnormality noted microscopically should be correlated with radiographic findings; findings such as *osteopenia* (thin bony trabeculae) or *osteosclerosis* (thickened bony trabeculae) may be sufficiently pronounced to be radiographically apparent. For cases with radiographic abnormalities, it is important for diagnostic decision making to determine whether the changes are localized or disseminated. In addition, laboratory testing, including measurement of calcium levels and various hormone assays, is often indicated in patients with bone abnormalities.

Osteopenia. The pathologic features of bony trabeculae are reviewed in Table 9-8. Pathologically thin, osteopenic bony trabeculae are more frequently noted in females, with an increasing incidence following menopause. Osteopenia may be seen in either male or female patients with chronic debilitating disorders (fig. 9-105). Defects in the homeostatic balance of bone production versus bone resorption have been

Table 9-8

PATHOLOGIC FEATURES OF BONY TRABECULAE[a,b]

Feature	Comments
Osteopenia	Thinned bony trabeculae Noted in osteoporosis as a generalized change, while patchy osteopenia may be evident in patients with chronic renal disorders Osteopenia may be patchy or generalized in myeloma patients, and lytic lesions are also typically present
Osteosclerosis	Increased bone remodeling with thickened bony trabeculae May be associated with anastomosing bony trabeculae, stromal fibrosis May be feature of metabolic bone disorder such as Paget disease or chronic renal failure-associated secondary hyperparathyroidism Also seen in many neoplastic processes such as chronic myeloproliferative disorders, systemic mast cell disease, myeloma variants, and metastatic carcinomas
Osteomalacia	Excess osteoid with defective mineralization Prominent osteomalacia linked to constitutional disorders or acquired disorders with reduced calcium or phosphorous (vitamin D deficiency, Fanconi syndrome, other renal disorders)
Osteopetrosis	Constitutional disorder linked to multiple genetic defects characterized by excess osteoblastic activity and stromal fibrosis Osteoclasts are abundant, but functionally defective Due to excessive bone formation and fibrosis, the hematopoietic cavity is severely attenuated

[a]Data from references 101, 108, 111, 112, 114, and 121–123.
[b]Patients with chronic renal disease or hyperparathyroidism exhibit a spectrum of pathologic features of bony trabeculae, which can vary over time.

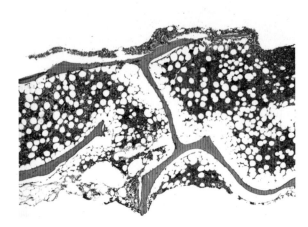

Figure 9-105

OSTEOPENIA

A bone marrow core biopsy shows striking osteopenia with an associated rim of fat cells (H&E stain).

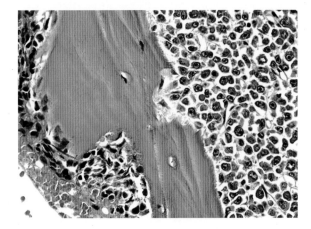

Figure 9-106

OSTEOLYTIC ACTIVITY IN MYELOMA

Osteolytic activity in multiple myeloma is evident on this high-power view of a bone marrow core biopsy section showing discrete foci of bone resorption (H&E stain).

postulated as a cause of osteopenia. Osteoporosis has also been described as a complication of various constitutional and acquired disorders or conditions, including Cushing disease, Marfan syndrome, Kostmann syndrome, and prolonged corticosteroid therapy (101,105,112). Several neoplastic disorders, most notably mul-tiple myeloma, are associated with marked bone resorption and osteolytic lesions (fig. 9-106) (108,122). The complex interaction of pathologic overstimulation of osteoclastic activity and inhibition of osteoblastic activity results in an imbalance favoring bone resorption in these patients (108,122).

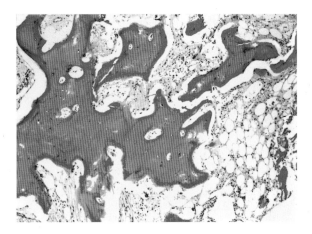

Figure 9-107

**BONY CHANGES IN CHRONIC
MYELOPROLIFERATIVE DISORDER**

Markedly thickened and scalloped bony trabeculae in a patient with chronic myeloproliferative disorder and associated bone marrow stromal fibrosis (H&E stain). (Courtesy of Dr. C. Sever, Albuquerque, NM.)

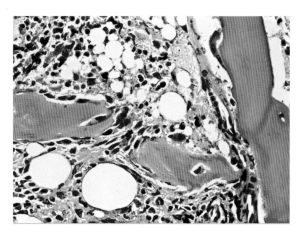

Figure 9-108

EXCESSIVE NEW BONE FORMATION

A bone marrow core biopsy section shows excessive new bone formation with osteoid and a marked increase in osteoblasts and osteoclasts (H&E stain). (Courtesy of Dr. C. Sever, Albuquerque, NM.)

Osteosclerosis. Thickened, osteosclerotic bony trabeculae can be a focal or diffuse abnormality; clinical and radiographic correlation, hematologic assessment, and laboratory testing must all be integrated to determine the etiology of cases of osteosclerosis (fig. 9-107). Thickened bony trabeculae with prominent scalloping and disorganized, mosaic cement lines is characteristic of Paget disease, a systemic metabolic bone disorder. Both osteoblasts and osteoclasts are markedly increased, and osteoclasts within the scalloped resorption bays may be enlarged and excessively multinucleated (fig. 9-108) (101,112,117).

Bone Abnormalities in Renal Disease. A wide range of bone abnormalities are associated with both constitutional and acquired renal function abnormalities. The nonspecific term *renal osteodystrophy* is often applied in bone marrow biopsy sections which demonstrate prominent bone remodeling and fibrosis (fig. 9-109).

In *osteomalacia*, defective mineralization causes wide osteoid seams to predominate. In some situations, there is such extensive osteoid formation that hematopoiesis is compromised (figs. 9-110, 9-111). Factors related to mineralization defects include hypophosphatemia, hypocalcemia, abnormal vitamin D metabolism, and aluminum toxicity. Many constitutional and acquired disorders are associated with calcium

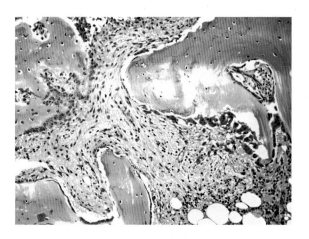

Figure 9-109

RENAL OSTEODYSTROPHY

The pathologic bone remodeling shows scalloping of bony trabeculae, and evidence of bone resorption and new bone formation in an adult with renal osteodystrophy (H&E stain). (Courtesy of Dr. S. Deodare, Toronto, Canada.)

and phosphorus abnormalities, while aluminum toxicity is linked to chronic dialysis and other therapies (120). Due to the key role of the kidney in phosphate homeostasis, both constitutional and acquired renal disorders are common causes of osteomalacia (103,104,107,113).

Chronic renal disease is one of the most common underlying disorders linked to many types of bony trabecular abnormalities including

319

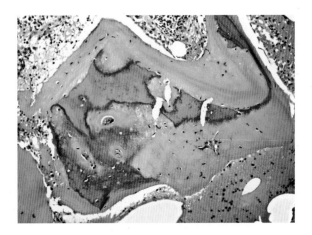

Figure 9-110

OSTEOMALACIA

Osteomalacia is highlighted by the extensive unmineralized bone matrix in this bone marrow core biopsy section (H&E stain).

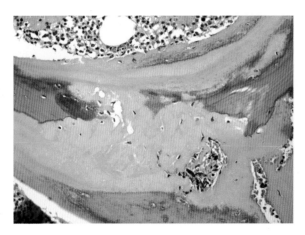

Figure 9-111

OSTEOMALACIA

Osteoid production without mineralization characterizes osteomalacia (H&E stain).

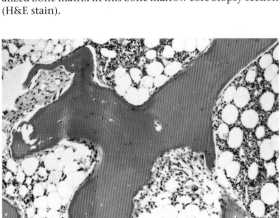

Figure 9-112

CHRONIC RENAL FAILURE

The striking bony changes in a patient with chronic renal failure include both thinning and thickening of bony trabeculae and active bone remodeling (H&E stain).

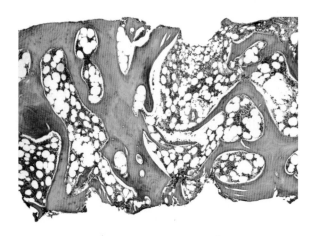

Figure 9-113

CHRONIC RENAL FAILURE

A bone marrow core biopsy shows the spectrum of thickened and thinned bony trabeculae typical of longstanding renal disease (H&E stain).

osteopenia, osteosclerosis, and osteomalacia (figs. 9-112, 9-113; see figs. 9-105 and 9-109). The development of secondary hyperparathyroidism in this patient population further exacerbates the metabolic bone disorder and, if sustained, produces osteitis fibrosa cystica (figs. 9-114, 9-115). The spectrum of bony trabeculae pathology in renal osteodystrophy varies based on disease duration, the development of secondary complications, and the type of treatment (103,113).

Osteopetrosis. A heterogeneous group of genetic disorders is linked to *osteopetrosis,* a phenomenon of excessive bone formation with defective osteoclast function, although osteoclasts are abundant (fig. 9-116) (106,119,123). Because osteoclasts are monocyte-derived, the hematopoietic defects are thought to be the cause of osteopetrotic disorders; bone marrow transplantation is the recommended therapy for these patients (119). Mutations in osteoclast

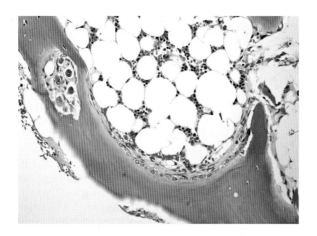

Figure 9-114

OSTEITIS FIBROSA CYSTICA

Osteitis fibrosa cystica is the result of secondary hyperparathyroidism due to chronic renal failure. Thick and thin bony trabeculae have increased osteoclastic and osteoblastic activity (H&E stain).

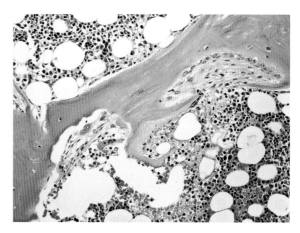

Figure 9-115

OSTEITIS FIBROSA CYSTICA

Cystic formation within bony trabeculae in a patient with osteitis fibrosa cystica secondary to the hyperparathyroidism associated with chronic renal disease (H&E stain).

ion channel protein genes, proton pump genes, and other gene defects have been identified in patients with osteopetrosis (110,119,123). Due to the extreme bone formation and the associated stromal fibrosis, the hematopoietic cavity is virtually effaced, resulting in severe hematologic compromise (fig. 9-116) (123).

EVALUATION OF STROMA

Pathologic disorders of bone marrow stroma and bone are common in clinical practice. Although some clues to these bone marrow stromal abnormalities can be derived from a review of bone marrow aspirate slides, the systematic evaluation of good quality bone marrow core biopsy sections is critical for the delineation of most stromal and all bone disorders. The detection of a morphologic abnormality of stroma and/or bone should prompt further assessment to identify the underlying cause of this abnormality. The critical role of bone marrow stromal cells in hematopoiesis is well recognized, and the impact of stromal defects on hematopoiesis is anticipated. Consequently, the diagnosis and

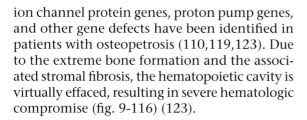

Figure 9-116

OSTEOPETROSIS

Remarkable osteoclast proliferation with jumbled bone formation and obliteration of the hematopoietic cavity is evident in this bone marrow core biopsy from a child with osteopetrosis (H&E stain). (Courtesy of Dr. C. Hanson, Rochester, MN.)

treatment of the underlying disorder producing the stromal or bone abnormality is essential.

REFERENCES

Components of Bone Marrow Stroma

1. Chan JY, Watt SM. Adhesion receptors on haematopoietic progenitor cells. Br J Haematol 2001;112:541-57.
2. Corre J, Planat-Benard V, Corberand JX, Penicaud L, Casteilla L, Laharrague P. Human bone marrow adipocytes support complete myeloid and lymphoid differentiation from human CD34 cells. Br J Haematol 2004;127:344-7.
3. Foucar K. Bone marrow in health and disease. Histopathology. 2002;41(Suppl 2):93-8.
4. Iwata M, Awaya N, Graf L, Kahl C, Torok-Storb B. Human marrow stromal cells activate monocytes to secrete osteopontin, which down-regulates Notch1 gene expression in CD34+ cells. Blood 2004;103:4496-502.
5. Kawada H, Fujita J, Kinjo K, et al. Nonhematopoietic mesenchymal stem cells can be mobilized and differentiate into cardiomyocytes after myocardial infarction. Blood 2004;104:3581-7.
6. Lakshmipathy U, Verfaillie C. Stem cell plasticity. Blood Rev 2005;19:29-38.
7. Nilsson SK, Johnston HM, Coverdale JA. Spatial localization of transplanted hemopoietic stem cells: inferences for the localization of stem cell niches. Blood 2001;97:2293-9.
8. Vega F, Medeiros LJ, Lang WH, Mansoor A, Bueso-Ramos C, Jones D. The stromal composition of malignant lymphoid aggregates in bone marrow: variations in architecture and phenotype in different B-cell tumours. Br J Haematol 2002;117:569-76.
9. Wynn RF, Hart CA, Corradi-Perini C, et al. A small proportion of mesenchymal stem cells strongly expresses functionally active CXCR4 receptor capable of promoting migration to bone marrow. Blood 2004;104:2643-5.

Gelatinous Transformation of Bone Marrow

10. Abella E, Feliu E, Granada I, et al. Bone marrow changes in anorexia nervosa are correlated with the amount of weight loss and not with other clinical findings. Am J Clin Pathol 2002;118:582-8.
11. Bohm J. Gelatinous transformation of the bone marrow: the spectrum of underlying diseases. Am J Surg Pathol 2000;24:56-65.
12. Fraser JR, Laurent TC, Laurent UB. Hyaluronan: its nature, distribution, functions and turnover. J Intern Med 1997;242:27-33.
13. Seaman JP, Kjeldsberg CR, Linker A. Gelatinous transformation of the bone marrow. Hum Pathol 1978;9:685-92.

Bone Marrow Necrosis

14. Aboulafia DM, Demirer T. Fatal bone marrow necrosis following fludarabine administration in a patient with indolent lymphoma. Leuk Lymphoma 1995;19:181-4.
15. Aydogdu I, Erkurt MA, Ozhan O, et al. Reversible bone marrow necrosis in a patient due to overdosage of diclofenac sodium. Am J Hematol 2006;81:298.
16. Bulvik S, Aronson I, Ress S, Jacobs P. Extensive bone marrow necrosis associated with antiphospholipid antibodies. Am J Med 1995;98:572-4.
17. Castro O, Brambilla DJ, Thorington B, et al. The acute chest syndrome in sickle cell disease: incidence and risk factors. The Cooperative Study of Sickle Cell Disease. Blood 1994;84:643-9.
18. Corazza F, Hermans C, Ferster A, Fondu P, Demulder A, Sariban E. Bone marrow stroma damage induced by chemotherapy for acute lymphoblastic leukemia in children. Pediatr Res 2004;55:152-8.
19. Diebold J, Molina T, Camilleri-Broet S, et al. Bone marrow manifestations of infections and systemic diseases observed in bone marrow trephine biopsy review. Histopathology 2000;37:199-211.
20. Liem RI, O'Gorman MR, Brown DL. Effect of red cell exchange transfusion on plasma levels of inflammatory mediators in sickle cell patients with acute chest syndrome. Am J Hematol 2004;76:19-25.
21. Limentani SA, Pretell JO, Potter D, et al. Bone marrow necrosis in two patients with acute promyelocytic leukemia during treatment with all-trans retinoic acid. Am J Hematol 1994;47:50-55.
22. Lowenthal EA, Wells A, Emanuel PD, Player R, Prchal JT. Sickle cell acute chest syndrome associated with parvovirus B19 infection: case series and review. Am J Hematol 1996;51:207-13.
23. Medoff BD, Shepard JA, Smith RN, Kratz A. Case records of the Massachusetts General Hospital. Case 17-2005. A 22-year-old woman with back and leg pain and respiratory failure. N Engl J Med 2005;352:2425-34.
24. Mori A, Hashino S, Imamura M, et al. Bone marrow infarction due to acute graft-versus-host disease in an acute lymphoblastic leukemia patient after unrelated bone marrow transplantation. Bone Marrow Transplant 1998;21:615-7.
25. Paydas S, Ergin M, Baslamisli F, et al. Bone marrow necrosis: clinicopathologic analysis of 20 cases and review of the literature. Am J Hematol 2002;70:300-5.

26. Seki Y, Koike T, Yano M, et al. Bone marrow necrosis with dyspnea in a patient with malignant lymphoma and plasma levels of thrombomodulin, tumor necrosis factor-alpha, and D-dimer. Am J Hematol 2002;70:250-3.

Amyloid Deposition in Bone Marrow

27. Guidelines Working Group of UK Myeloma Forum; British Committee for Standards in Haematology, British Society for Haematology. Guidelines on the diagnosis and management of AL amyloidosis. Br J Haematol 2004;125:681-700.

28. Kaplan B, Martin BM, Livneh A, Pras M, Gallo GR. Biochemical subtyping of amyloid in formalin-fixed tissue samples confirms and supplements immunohistologic data. Am J Clin Pathol 2004;121:794-800.

29. Leung KF, Ma ES. Amyloid deposits in the bone marrow. Br J Haematol 2003;121:679.

30. Swan N, Skinner M, O'Hara CJ. Bone marrow core biopsy specimens in AL (primary) amyloidosis. A morphologic and immunohistochemical study of 100 cases. Am J Clin Pathol 2003;120:610-6.

Bone Marrow Fibrosis

31. Bass RD, Pullarkat V, Feinstein DI, Kaul A, Winberg CD, Brynes RK. Pathology of autoimmune myelofibrosis. Am J Clin Pathol 2001;116:211-6.

32. Beham-Schmid C, Apfelbeck U, Sill H, et al. Treatment of chronic myelogenous leukemia with the tyrosine kinase inhibitor STI571 results in marked regression of bone marrow fibrosis. Blood 2002;99:381-3.

33. Buesche G, Georgii A, Kreipe HH. Diagnosis and quantification of bone marrow fibrosis are significantly biased by the pre-staining processing of bone marrow biopsies. Histopathology 2006;48:133-48.

34. Chagraoui H, Komura E, Tulliez M, Giraudier S, Vainchenker W, Wendling E. Prominent role of TGF-beta 1 in thrombopoietin-induced myelofibrosis in mice. Blood 2002;100:3495-503.

35. Foucar K. Miscellaneous disorders of bone marrow, including stromal and bone abnormalities. Bone marrow pathology, 2nd ed. Chicago: ASCP Press; 2001:546-84.

36. Foucar K. Bone marrow stroma in health and disease. Histopathology 2002;41(Suppl 2):93-98.

37. Gruner BA, DeNapoli TS, Elshihabi S, et al. Anemia and hepatosplenomegaly as presenting features in a child with rickets and secondary myelofibrosis. J Pediatr Hematol Oncol 2003;25:813-5.

38. Pullarkat V, Bass RD, Gong JZ, Feinstein DI, Brynes RK. Primary autoimmune myelofibrosis: definition of a distinct clinicopathologic syndrome. Am J Hematol 2003;72:8-12.

39. Rameshwar P, Chang VT, Thacker UF, Gascon P. Systemic transforming growth factor-beta in patients with bone marrow fibrosis—pathophysiological implications. Am J Hematol 1998; 59:133-42.

40. Rameshwar P, Joshi DD, Yadav P, et al. Mimicry between neurokinin-1 and fibronectin may explain the transport and stability of increased substance P immunoreactivity in patients with bone marrow fibrosis. Blood 2001;97:3025-31.

41. Reilly JT. Idiopathic myelofibrosis: pathogenesis, natural history and management. Blood Rev 1997;11:233-42.

42. Vega F, Medeiros LJ, Lang WH, Monsoor A, Bueso-Ramos C, Jones D. The stromal composition of malignant lymphoid aggregates in bone marrow: variations in architecture and phenotype in different B-cell tumours. Br J Haematol 2002;117:569-76.

Granulomatous and Diffuse Histiocytic Disorders in Bone Marrow

43. Allory Y, Challine D, Haioun C, et al. Bone marrow involvement in lymphomas with hemophagocytic syndrome at presentation: a clinicopathologic study of 11 patients in a Western institution. Am J Surg Pathol 2001;25:865-74.

44. Boot RG, Verhoek M, de Fost M, et al. Marked elevation of the chemokine CCL18/PARC in Gaucher disease: a novel surrogate marker for assessing therapeutic intervention. Blood 2004;103:33-9.

45. Boven LA, van Meurs M, Boot RG, et al. Gaucher cells demonstrate a distinct macrophage phenotype and resemble alternatively activated macrophages. Am J Clin Pathol 2004;122:359-69.

46. Brunning RD. Morphologic alterations in nucleated blood and marrow cells in genetic disorders. Hum Pathol 1970;1:99-124.

47. Eid A, Carion W, Nystrom JS. Differential diagnoses of bone marrow granuloma. West J Med 1996;164:510-5.

48. Foucar K. Histiocytic disorders involving bone marrow. In: Bone marrow pathology, 2nd ed. Chicago: ASCP Press; 2001:520-41.

49. Foucar K. Miscellaneous disorders of bone marrow, including stromal and bone abnormalities. In: Bone marrow pathology, 2nd ed. Chicago: ASCP Press; 2001:546-84.

50. Hansen HG, Graucob E. Hematologic cytology of storage diseases: New York: Springer-Verlag; 1985.

51. Hornick JL, Jaffe ES, Fletcher CD. Extranodal histiocytic sarcoma: clinicopathologic analysis of 14 cases of a rare epithelioid malignancy. Am J Surg Pathol 2004;28:1133-44.

52. Hussong J, Peterson LR, Warren JR, Peterson LC. Detecting disseminated Mycobacterium avium complex infections in HIV-positive patients. The usefulness of bone marrow trephine biopsy specimens, aspirate cultures, and blood cultures. Am J Clin Pathol 1998;110:806-9.

53. Janka G, Imashuku S, Elinder G, Schneider M, Henter JI. Infection- and malignancy-associated hemophagocytic syndromes. Secondary hemophagocytic lymphohistiocytosis. Hematol Oncol Clin North Am 1998;12:435-44.

54. Krober SM, Kaiserling E, Horny HP, Weber A. Primary diagnosis of Whipple's disease in bone marrow. Hum Pathol 2004;35:522-5.

55. Landas S, Foucar K, Sando GN, Ellefson R, Hamilton HE. Adult Niemann-Pick disease masquerading as sea blue histiocyte syndrome: report of a case confirmed by lipid analysis and enzyme assays. Am J Hematol 1985;20:391-400.

56. Mazodier K, Marin V, Novick D, et al. Severe imbalance of IL-18/IL-18BP in patients with secondary hemophagocytic syndrome. Blood 2005;106:3483-9.

57. Mukhopadhyay S, Mukhopadhyay S, Abraham NZ Jr, Jones LA, Howard L, Gajra A. Unexplained bone marrow granulomas: is amiodarone the culprit? A report of 2 cases. Am J Hematol 2004;75:110-2.

58. Onciu M. Histiocytic proliferations in childhood. Am J Clin Pathol 2004;122(Suppl):S128-36.

59. Pelstring RJ, Kim CK, Lower EE, Swerdlow SH. Marrow granulomas in coal workers' pneumoconiosis. A histologic study with elemental analysis. Am J Clin Pathol 1988;89:553-6.

60. Risdall RJ, McKenna RW, Nesbit ME, et al. Virus-associated hemophagocytic syndrome: a benign histiocytic proliferation distinct from malignant histiocytosis. Cancer 1979;44:993-1002.

61. Silverstein MN, Ellefson RD, Ahern EJ. The syndrome of the sea-blue histiocyte. N Engl J Med 1970;282:1-4.

62. Srigley JR, Vellend H, Palmer N, et al. Q-fever. The liver and bone marrow pathology. Am J Surg Pathol 1985;9:752-8.

63. Vellodi A. Lysosomal storage disorders. Br J Haematol 2005;128:413-31.

64. Young JF, Goulian M. Bone marrow fibrin ring granulomas and cytomegalovirus infection. Am J Clin Pathol 1993;99:65-8.

Iron Disorders in Bone Marrow

65. Adams PC, Reboussin DM, Barton JC, et al. Hemochromatosis and iron-overload screening in a racially diverse population. N Engl J Med 2005;352:1769-78.

66. Ajioka RS, Kushner JP. Hereditary hemochromatosis. Semin Hematol 2002;39:235-41.

67. Andersen RV, Tybjaerg-Hansen A, Appleyard M, Birgens H, Nordestgaard BG. Hemochromatosis mutations in the general population: iron overload progression rate. Blood 2004;103:2914-9.

68. Andrews NC. A genetic view of iron homeostasis. Semin Hematol 2002;39:227-34.

69. Brittenham GM, Badman DG; National Institute of Diabetes and Digestive and Kidney Diseases (NIDDK) Workshop. Noninvasive measurement of iron: report of an NIDDK workshop. Blood 2003;101:15-9.

70. Camaschella C. Understanding iron homeostasis through genetic analysis of hemochromatosis and related disorders. Blood 2005;106:3710-7.

71. De Gobbi M, Roetto A, Piperno A, et al. Natural history of juvenile haemochromatosis. Br J Haematol 2002;117:973-9.

72. Donovan A, Andrews NC. The molecular regulation of iron metabolism. Hematol J 2004;5:373-80.

73. Foucar K. Miscellaneous disorders of bone marrow, including stromal and bone abnormalities. In: Bone marrow pathology, 2nd ed. Chicago: ASCP Press; 2001:546-84.

74. Franchini M. Hereditary iron overload: update on pathophysiology, diagnosis, and treatment. Am J Hematol 2006;81:202-9.

75. Heeney MM, Andrews NC. Iron homeostasis and inherited iron overload disorders: an overview. Hematol Oncol Clin North Am 2004;18:1379-403, ix.

76. Jensen PD. Evaluation of iron overload. Br J Haematol 2004;124:697-711.

77. Nittis T, Gitlin JD. The copper-iron connection: hereditary aceruloplasminemia. Semin Hematol 2002;39:282-9.

78. Ponka P. Rare causes of hereditary iron overload. Semin Hematol 2002;39:249-62.

79. Roetto A, Daraio F, Porporato P, et al. Screening hepcidin for mutations in juvenile hemochromatosis: identification of a new mutation (C70R). Blood 2004;103:2407-9.

80. Whitfield JB, Treloar S, Zhu G, Powell LW, Martin NG. Relative importance of female-specific and non-female-specific effects on variation in iron stores between women. Br J Haematol 2003;120:860-6.

Crystal Deposition in Bone Marrow

81. Cochat P. Primary hyperoxaluria type 1. Kidney Int 1999;55:2533-47.

82. Gherardi G, Poggi A, Sisca S, Calderaro V, Bonucci E. Bone oxalosis and renal osteodystrophy. Arch Pathol Lab Med 1980;104:105-11.

83. Halil O, Farringdon K. Oxalosis: an unusual cause of leucoerythroblastic anaemia. Br J Haematol 2003;122:2.

84. Pelstring RJ, Kim CK, Lower EE, Swerdlow SH. Marrow granulomas in coal workers' pneumoconiosis. A histologic study with elemental analysis. Am J Clin Pathol 1988;89:553-6.

85. Quinn JP, Royston D, Murphy PT. Bone marrow findings in hereditary cystinosis with renal failure. Am J Hematol 2004;76:79.

86. Shotelersuk V, Larson D, Anikster Y, et al. CTNS mutations in an American-based population of cystinosis patients. Am J Hum Genet 1998;63:1352-62.

87. Yamamoto T, Hishida A, Honda N, Ito I, Shirasawa H, Nagase M. Crystal-storing histiocytosis and crystalline tissue deposition in multiple myeloma. Arch Pathol Lab Med 1991;115:351-4.

Vascular Abnormalities Including Neoangiogenesis

88. Aguayo A, Kantarjian H, Manshouri T, et al. Angiogenesis in acute and chronic leukemias and myelodysplastic syndromes. Blood 2000;96:2240-5.

89. Bussolati B, Ahmed A, Pemberton H, et al. Bifunctional role for VEGF-induced heme oxygenase-1 in vivo: induction of angiogenesis and inhibition of leukocytic infiltration. Blood 2004;103:761-6.

90. Cahalin PA, Pawade J. Giant cell arteritis detected by bone marrow trephine. Br J Haematol 2002;118:687.

91. Foucar K. Miscellaneous disorders of bone marrow, including stromal and bone abnormalities. In: Bone marrow pathology, 2nd ed. Chicago: ASCP Press; 2001:546-84.

92. Mangi MH, Newland AC. Angiogenesis and angiogenic mediators in haematological malignancies. Br J Haematol 2000;111:43-51.

93. Munshi NC, Wilson C. Increased bone marrow microvessel density in newly diagnosed multiple myeloma carries a poor prognosis. Semin Oncol 2001;28:565-9.

94. Nabhan C, Kwaan HC. Current concepts in the diagnosis and management of thrombotic thrombocytopenic purpura. Hematol Oncol Clin North Am 2003;17:177-99.

95. Nosanchuk J, Terzian J, Posso M. Circulating mucopolysaccharide (mucin) in two adults with metastatic adenocarcinoma. Detection in peripheral blood smear and at autopsy. Arch Pathol Lab Med 1987;111:545-8.

96. Parikh AA, Ellis LM. The vascular endothelial growth factor family and its receptors. Hematol Oncol Clin North Am 2004;18:951-71, vii.

97. Pierce JR Jr, Wren MV, Cousar JB Jr. Cholesterol embolism: diagnosis antemortem by bone marrow biopsy. Ann Intern Med 1978;89:937-8.

98. Rollin S, Lemieux C, Maliba R, et al. VEGF-mediated endothelial P-selectin translocation: role of VEGF receptors and endogenous PAF synthesis. Blood 2004;103:3789-97.

99. Swan N, Skinner M, O'Hara CJ. Bone marrow core biopsy specimens in AL (primary) amyloidosis. A morphologic and immunohistochemical study of 100 cases. Am J Clin Pathol 2003;120:610-6.

100. Yuan K, Hong TM, Chen JJ, Tsai WH, Lin MT. Syndecan-1 up-regulated by ephrinB2/EphB4 plays dual roles in inflammatory angiogenesis. Blood 2004;104:1025-33.

Acquired and Constitutional Bone Abnormalities

101. Bain BJ. Diseases of bone. In: Bain BJ, Clark DM, Lampert IA, eds. Bone marrow pathology, 2nd ed. Oxford: Blackwell Science; 1996:307-14.

102. Bain BJ. The normal bone marrow. In: Bain BJ, Clark DM, Lampert IA, eds. Bone marrow pathology, 2nd ed. Oxford: Blackwell Science; 1996:1-50.

103. Ballanti P, Coen G, Mazzaferro S, et al. Histomorphometric assessment of bone turnover in uraemic patients: comparison between activation frequency and bone formation rate. Histopathology 2001;38:571-83.

104. Baum M. The Fanconi syndrome of cystinosis: insights into the pathophysiology. Pediatr Nephrol 1998;12:492-7.

105. Bishop NJ, Williams DM, Compston JC, Stirling DM, Prentice A. Osteoporosis in severe congenital neutropenia treated with granulocyte colony-stimulating factor. Br J Haematol 1995;89:927-8.

106. Chen CJ, Chao TY, Chu DM, Janckila AJ, Cheng SN. Osteoblast and osteoclast activity in a malignant infantile osteopetrosis patient following bone marrow transplantation. J Pediatr Hematol Oncol 2004;26:5-8.

107. Clarke BL, Wynne AG, Wilson DM, Fitzpatrick LA. Osteomalacia associated with adult Fanconi's syndrome: clinical and diagnostic features. Clin Endocrinol (Oxf) 1995;43:479-90.

108. Colucci S, Brunetti G, Rizzi R, et al. T cells support osteoclastogenesis in an in vitro model derived from human multiple myeloma bone disease: the role of the OPG/TRAIL interaction. Blood 2004;104:3722-30.

109. Corre J, Planat-Benard V, Corberand JX, Penicaud L, Casteilla L, Laharrague P. Human bone marrow adipocytes support complete myeloid and lymphoid differentiation from human CD34 cells. Br J Haematol 2004;127:344-7.

110. Dai XM, Ryan GR, Hapel AJ, et al. Targeted disruption of the mouse colony-stimulating factor 1 receptor gene results in osteopetrosis, mononuclear phagocyte deficiency, increased primitive progenitor cell frequencies, and reproductive defects. Blood 2002;99:111-20.

111. Foucar K. Miscellaneous disorders of bone marrow, including stromal and bone abnormalities. In: Bone marrow pathology, 2nd ed. Chicago: ASCP Press; 2001:546-84.

112. Gruber HE, Stauffer ME, Thompson ER, Baylink DJ. Diagnosis of bone disease by core biopsies. Semin Hematol 1981;18:258-78.

113. Hruska KA, Teitelbaum SL. Renal osteodystrophy. N Engl J Med 1995;333:166-74.

114. Lacy MQ, Gertz MA, Hanson CA, Inwards DJ, Kyle RA. Multiple myeloma associated with diffuse osteosclerotic bone lesions: a clinical entity distinct from osteosclerotic myeloma (POEMS syndrome). Am J Hematol 1997;56:288-93.

115. Manolagas SC, Jilka RL. Bone marrow, cytokines, and bone remodeling. Emerging insights into the pathophysiology of osteoporosis. N Engl J Med 1995;332:305-11.

116. Massey HM, Flanagan AM. Human osteoclasts derive from CD14-positive monocytes. Br J Haematol 1999;106:167-70.

117. Murrin RJ, Harrison P. Abnormal osteoclasts and bone marrow fibrosis in Paget's disease of the bone. Br J Haematol 2004;124:3.

118. Rivollier A, Mazzorana M, Tebib J, et al. Immature dendritic cell transdifferentiation into osteoclasts: a novel pathway sustained by the rheumatoid arthritis microenvironment. Blood 2004;104:4029-37.

119. Schulz AS, Classen CF, Mihatsch WA, et al. HLA-haploidentical blood progenitor cell transplantation in osteopetrosis. Blood 2002;99:3458-60.

120. Spivak JL. The blood in systemic disorders. Lancet 2000;355:1707-12.

121. Terpos E, Politou M, Rahemtulla A. New insights into the pathophysiology and management of bone disease in multiple myeloma. Br J Haematol 2003;123:758-69.

122. Tian E, Zhan F, Walker R, et al. The role of the Wnt-signaling antagonist DKK1 in the development of osteolytic lesions in multiple myeloma. N Engl J Med 2003;349:2483-94.

123. Tolar J, Teitelbaum SL, Orchard PJ. Osteopetrosis. N Engl J Med 2004;351:2839-49.

BONE MARROW FEATURES OF SYSTEMIC INFECTIONS

GENERAL CONCEPTS

This chapter describes the bone marrow morphology associated with a variety of infectious disorders. For many systemic infections, the bone marrow findings are nonspecific but compatible with a reactive process. Even when nonspecific, the morphologic evaluation of the bone marrow in conjunction with the clinical history serves to further direct workup, including the need for special stains, cultures, serologies, or molecular studies (see chapter 2).

Ideally, bone marrow aspirates for cultures should be drawn at the time of the initial bone marrow procedure for any patient suspected of having an infection. Fresh bone marrow without anticoagulant, placed immediately into blood culture bottles and/or viral transport media, is preferred. For nonaspirable bone marrows, a fresh biopsy may be disaggregated to supply cells for cultures; transportation of intact biopsies requires media containing no antibiotics. When cultures are desired after the initial procedure, specimens held in heparin are preferred over other anticoagulants due to their less significant effects on microbial suppression (6). Unstained aspirate smears and touch preparations of all bone marrows should be saved in the event that special stains, such as fluorescent auramine-rhodamine, become necessary.

Two examples of nonspecific bone marrow manifestations of systemic infection are granulomas and hemophagocytic syndrome. These are discussed in detail in separate sections of this chapter. Some infectious diseases are associated with specific findings: the identification of organisms in smear or biopsy preparations or the occurrence of specific cellular changes elicited by an organism that are pathognomonic of infection, such as the viral inclusions in endothelial cells infected by cytomegalovirus (CMV).

While the focal point of this chapter is to discuss bone marrow morphology, the peripheral blood may be more informative for some infections. Organisms may be visualized on Wright-stained peripheral smears for a number of diseases including malaria, ehrlichiosis, babesiosis, trypanosomiasis, meningococcemia, plague, relapsing fever due to *Borrelia* organisms (7), candidiasis (1,2,4), disseminated histoplasmosis (3), and fungemia or bacteremia associated with immunosuppression (figs. 10-1, 10-2) (5,8). Therefore, both nonspecific and specific peripheral blood findings are included for each of the entities discussed.

A series of dynamic alterations occur in the peripheral blood and bone marrow of patients with systemic infections, resulting in evolution and change during the course of the disease. This must be considered when comparing patient results to those described in the literature for a disease process. As susceptibility to a systemic infection also increases in individuals who are immunosuppressed, the medical history becomes important in the interpretation of findings. Chemotherapy, tissue transplantation, idiosyncratic drug reactions, or underlying disease (i.e., autoimmune disorders, acquired immunodeficiency syndrome [AIDS]) create additional morphologic alterations in the

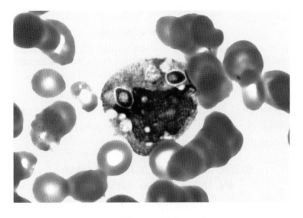

Figure 10-1

***CANDIDA* INFECTION**

A peripheral blood smear shows the yeast forms of *Candida* in a monocyte (Wright stain).

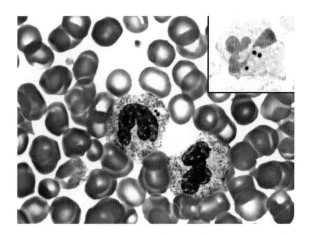

Figure 10-2

GRAM-POSITIVE BACTERIA

A circulating neutrophil contains gram-positive bacteria (diplococci) in patient with sepsis (Wright stain; insert, Gram stain).

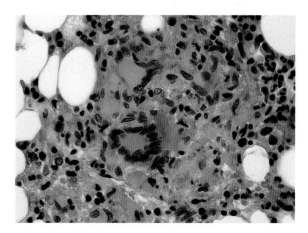

Figure 10-4

GRANULOMAS WITH MULTINUCLEATED GIANT CELLS

Epithelioid granulomas with multinucleated giant cells are present in a bone marrow biopsy section from a patient with tuberculosis (hematoxylin and eosin [H&E] stain).

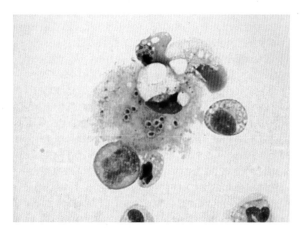

Figure 10-3

FUNGAL ORGANISMS

Fungal organisms are present within the macrophage cytoplasm on a bone marrow aspirate smear from a female with fever and pancytopenia (Wright stain).

peripheral blood and bone marrow that may mask or detract from those associated with a secondary infection.

BONE MARROW GRANULOMAS IN INFECTIOUS DISEASES

A *granuloma* is an inflammatory reaction to a systemic infection, neoplasm, drug, or noninfectious condition that is often chronic in nature. Information on granulomatous infiltrates relating to noninfectious processes is discussed in chapter

9. Granulomas are observed in 1 to 2 percent of bone marrows and are more frequently seen in patients with fever of unknown origin (10). They are a valuable histologic clue to the presence of an opportunistic infection; approximately one third of granulomas in large studies are related to an infectious etiology. This number increases substantially (up to 80 percent) in certain patient populations (those with AIDS, transplant recipients) that are exposed to specific disease entities, particularly in endemic areas (45).

Performing step sections on trephine biopsies of bone marrow and recognizing unusual patterns of macrophage (histiocyte) proliferation improves the yield for identifying granulomas. A review of aspirate smears for organisms is an important adjunct to the evaluation of trephine biopsy sections when granulomas are identified. Bacterial and fungal organisms are often easier to visualize on routine Wright-Giemsa- or Giemsa-stained slides than in hematoxylin and eosin (H&E)-stained sections (fig. 10-3).

Epithelioid granulomas are one of the most frequent forms of granuloma found in bone marrow. They appear as relatively well-circumscribed nodules composed of epithelioid histiocytes with variably admixed and surrounding lymphocytes, plasma cells, eosinophils, and neutrophils. Multinucleated giant cells, created by the fusion of monocytes and macrophages, may be present (fig. 10-4) (29).

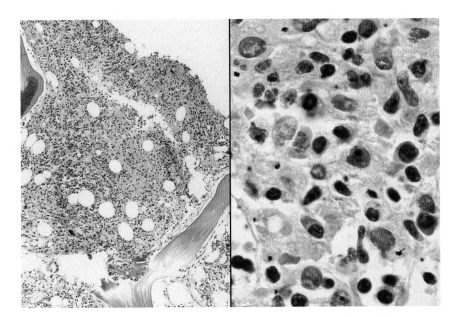

Figure 10-5

GRANULOMAS IN HUMAN IMMUNODEFICIENCY VIRUS (HIV) INFECTION

Poorly delineated lympho-histiocytic aggregates in a bone marrow biopsy from an HIV-positive female who presented with fever and pancytopenia (H&E stain).

Figure 10-6

RING GRANULOMA IN Q FEVER

Ring granulomas are composed of epithelioid histiocytes and neutrophils radially arranged around a central clear space composed of fat. Although not pronounced in this bone marrow biopsy, surrounding eosinophilic fibrinoid material is often present (H&E stain).

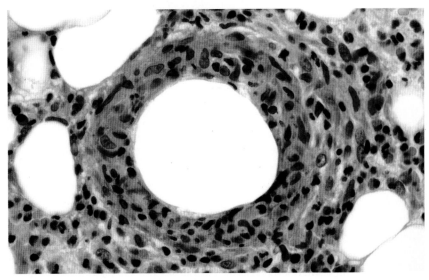

Organisms that typically elicit granuloma formation in normal individuals may not do so in immunocompromised patients. In AIDS patients, granulomas often manifest as either poorly defined aggregates of epithelioid histiocytes or vague lymphohistiocytic aggregates (fig. 10-5) (30). In the post-transplantation setting, nonspecific collections of epithelioid histiocytes are frequent and are often negative for microorganisms by special stains, even when culture positive. The appearance of histiocytic infiltrates may vary for a given infection. For example, three types of macrophage proliferations have been described in patients with disseminated histoplasmosis: epithelioid granulomas, diffuse macrophage proliferations, and loose aggregates of macrophages (13).

Infectious causes of granulomas are listed in Table 10-1, along with the peripheral blood and bone marrow findings that may be seen in response to the designated organisms. Certain granulomas have configurations that aid in the differential diagnosis, although none is sufficiently specific for reliable identification (12). Doughnut-ring granulomas are found in prolonged and severe Q fever infection (fig. 10-6) but may also be seen in rare cases of *Mycobacterium avium* complex infection, brucellosis, leishmaniasis, typhoid fever, Lyme disease,

Table 10-1

SYSTEMIC INFECTIONS ASSOCIATED WITH BONE MARROW GRANULOMAS[a]

Disease/Organism	Peripheral Blood Findings	Additional Bone Marrow Findings[b]	References
Bacterial			
Brucellosis	Pancytopenia, thromobocyto-penia (idiopathic thrombocy-topenia purpura), microangio-pathic hemolytic anemia	Hypo-, normo-, or hypercellular marrow; possible hemophagocytosis, increased histiocytes, eosinophils, or plasma cells	9, 21, 34, 50
Typhoid fever (*Salmonella typhi*)	Thrombocytopenia, anemia, rare leukopenia	Myeloid hyperplasia, possible increased lymphocytes and/or monocytes, hemopha-gocytosis, Leishman-Donovan (LD) bodies	28, 39, 46
Q fever[c]	Pancytopenia	Small ring granulomas, increase in fat, depressed myeloid series, angiitis, necrosis, hemophagocytosis	18, 41, 44
Leishmaniasis (Kala-azar)	Pancytopenia, dysplasia of any lineage, cryoglobulinemia (rare)	Atypia of any lineage, hemophagocytosis, reticulin fibrosis, amastigotes in Giemsa-stained smears	32, 36, 38, 43, 49
Mycobacterium avium complex	Anemia (often severe)	Erythroid hypoplasia, failure of erythroid mat-uration, aplastic anemia, lymphohistiocytic lesions, clusters of epithelioid histiocytes, pseudo-Gaucher cells	14, 16, 17, 47
Mycobacterium tuberculosis	Normochromic normocytic anemia, thrombocytopenia, lymphopenia, monocytopenia, pancytopenia, neutrophilia, lymphocytosis and/or monocytosis	Erythroid hypoplasia, +/- granulomas with central necrosis, patchy marrow necrosis, Langerhans type giant cells, hemophagocy-tosis, pseudo-Gaucher cells	14, 22, 30, 35, 40
Ehrlichia	See text		
Fungal			
Cryptococcus	Lymphopenia, other cytopenias, microangiopathic hemolytic anemia (DIC[d], rare)	Hemophagocytosis, number of findings related to underlying disorder (AIDS, immunosuppression)	31, 33, 48
Histoplasma	See text		
Viral			
Hepatitis	Cytopenias (possibly immune mediated)	Slightly hypocellular marrow, increased lymph-ocytes and/or plasma cells, aplastic anemia	15a, 26, 27
Epstein-Barr Virus[e]	See text		
Cytomegalovirus[f]	See text		

[a]These findings are based on reports in the literature and are not all inclusive.
[b]Rare reports of bone marrow granulomas in: Lyme disease (24), Legionnaires disease (20), Rocky Mountain spotted fever (12), tularemia, candidiasis (19), coccidioidomycosis (11), paracoccidiomycosis, *Saccharomyces cerevisiae*, and Whipple disease (23). Clusters of foamy histiocytes are seen in: *Mycobacterium leprae* (37,42).
[c]Q fever is rare in the United States.
[d]DIC = disseminated intravascular coagulation; AIDS = acquired immunodeficiency syndrome.
[e]Epstein-Barr virus is best evaluated by in situ hybridization. LMP is frequently negative.
[f]Cytomegalovirus in situ hybridization may be falsely positive in biopsy sections.

and infections caused by hepatitis A virus, Ep-stein-Barr virus (EBV), and CMV (10,15,25). A prominent cause of central necrosis (caseation) in granulomas is *Mycobacterium tuberculosis*, but a number of fungal infections also show this finding. Increased monocytes or histiocytes in the absence of granuloma formation are seen in a variety of bacterial infections, particularly tuberculosis, subacute bacterial endocarditis, and syphilis. The spirochetes of syphilis may cause widespread interstitial inflammation and invasion of vessel walls.

The etiology of bone marrow granulomas can be discovered in a majority of cases by correlating the patient's clinical history with the morphol-ogy, and the results of immunohistochemical,

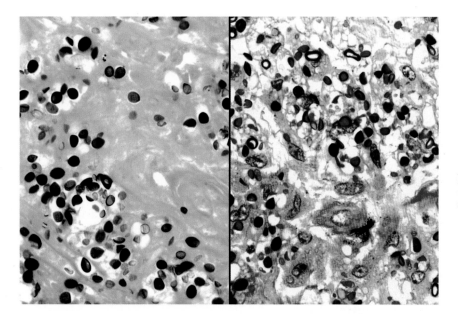

Figure 10-7

**SPECIAL STAINS
FOR FUNGUS**

Histoplasmosis is highlighted by Gomori methenamine silver (GMS)-diastase (left) and periodic acid–Schiff (PAS) (right) stains.

microbiologic, and serologic techniques. This includes a detailed review of the drug history as a potential cause of granuloma formation. Special stains for microorganisms detect a higher percentage of fungal organisms than bacterial organisms in biopsy sections, including *Mycobacterium* sp (fig. 10-7). Both acid-fast bacillus (AFB), or auramine rhodamine, and fungal stains should be applied to all biopsies that contain granulomas from immunosuppressed patients, as more than one type of organism may be present (i.e., mixed infection), particularly in the setting of human immunodeficiency virus (HIV) infection. The most commonly encountered fungal organism in nonimmunosuppressed patients is *Candida albicans*. Typhoid fever is one of the few diseases for which bone marrow cultures yield a higher rate of positivity than peripheral blood cultures.

FUNGAL INFECTIONS ASSOCIATED WITH IMMUNOSUPPRESSION

Patients undergoing chemotherapy, bone marrow transplantation, or solid organ transplantation have a high risk for developing fungal infections due to periods of profound neutropenia. The type of infection is influenced by the medical condition of the patient, geographic location, and type of antifungal prophylaxis used in the treatment facility or community. *Aspergillus* species and *Candida* are the most common invasive fungal organisms identified, although any fungus may cause disease in a patient with significant neutropenia (53,57). Among recipients of solid organ transplants, *Candida* infections dominate in patients receiving liver, kidney, or pancreas transplants, while *Aspergillus* is more frequent in patients with lung or heart transplants (56). Cryptococcosis, fusariosis, zygomycosis, and phaeohypomycosis have been reported in transplant recipients as well (51,55).

Drugs that cause immunosuppression, particularly when used for long-term therapy, increase the risk of infection by *Cryptococcus*, invasive *Aspergillus*, and *Zygomycetes* (52). Infliximab (Remicade), a powerful immune-modulating drug, has been associated with military tuberculosis, invasive histoplasmosis, and cryptococcosis (54,58,59).

HUMAN IMMUNODEFICIENCY VIRUS INFECTION

AIDS was first described as a new disease entity in 1981 following the unexplained occurrence of *Pneumocystis carinii* pneumonia and Kaposi sarcoma in previously healthy homosexual men (63). HIV, an RNA lentivirus, was isolated from a patient with lymphadenopathy in 1983 and identified as the etiologic agent of AIDS, transmissible by sexual contact, blood products, intrauterine exposure, or through breast milk. Currently, approximately 40 million people worldwide have this viral infection (60).

HIV infects host cells by binding to the cell surface protein CD4 in conjunction with a chemokine coreceptor, usually CXCR4 or CCR5, depending on the viral strain. The initial cells infected are bone marrow–derived dendritic cells in mucus membranes and skin. These dendritic cells migrate to lymphoid organs and deliver virus to CD4-positive T cells, allowing initial viral replication to occur in regional lymph nodes (termed the HIV window for testing). Viral replication in the lymphoid tissues reaches a critical point when sufficient cell destruction causes a release of virus into circulation, usually 3 to 6 weeks after initial infection.

This viremia is coupled with symptoms in approximately 50 to 70 percent of patients, and is entitled the "acute HIV syndrome." Symptoms persist from one to several weeks and are similar to those of other acute viral infections, ranging from sore throat, fever, muscle aches, lymphadenopathy, and nausea and vomiting, to rashes and neurologic complications. Accompanying peripheral blood changes may be indistinguishable from those of infectious mononucleosis or an infectious mononucleosis-like syndrome (66). Transient neutropenia, thrombocytopenia, or more rarely, pancytopenia may occur (61). The symptoms gradually subside and peripheral blood findings normalize as the patient develops an immune response to the virus.

A long period of clinical latency ensues during which the death of productively infected cells occurs through multiple cellular and humoral immune mechanisms. In untreated patients, enhanced apoptosis of uninfected CD4-positive T cells takes place as well as the destruction of infected cells (68). Loss of CD4-positive T cells is masked initially by an increase in CD8-positive T cells. By the time clinical symptoms become apparent, this steady state is unbalanced toward an exponential increase in viral burden. With a progressive decline in immunologic function, patients with AIDS develop a variety of illnesses, including opportunistic infections, malignancies, and degenerative diseases. In pediatric patients, pulmonary disorders, growth failure, and a progressive decline in neurologic function and neurodevelopment are particularly prominent.

Historically, 80 percent of AIDS patients have died of secondary infections, most often bacterial in nature. This is changing in industrial countries due to improved prophylaxis and the introduction of highly active antiretroviral therapy (HAART) in 1996 (64,67). Zidovudine (AZT) continues to be the first line of therapy, with HAART reserved for worsening infection as defined by specific criteria (60). Drug-induced cytopenias and pancytopenia are problematic side effects of zidovudine therapy in contrast to their less frequent occurrence with the newer drugs. In addition to a decline in deaths due to opportunistic infections, the incidence of many HIV-related malignant neoplasms, such as Kaposi sarcoma and lymphomas other than Burkitt lymphoma/leukemia, has also dropped (62,65). HAART and newer therapeutic agents improve the immune status, quality of life, and overall survival of HIV-infected individuals.

Peripheral Blood and Bone Marrow Findings in Patients with AIDS

The peripheral blood and bone marrow findings in AIDS patients have been well-described since the 1980s (Tables 10-2, 10-3). One of the first clinical signs of HIV infection, often appearing during the period of clinical latency, is HIV-associated thrombocytopenia. The primary mechanism for thrombocytopenia in early stage infection is peripheral platelet destruction mediated by either antiplatelet antibodies or platelet-bound immune complexes, similar to immune thrombocytopenia (ITP) but involving different antigenic targets (79,84,92). Megakaryocytes are directly infected by the virus and, in later stages of infection, production defects dominate (91,94). HIV-infected persons with thrombocytopenia are usually asymptomatic, even when platelet counts are extremely low. The thrombocytopenia frequently responds to antiretroviral therapy, particularly zidovudine.

Additional cytopenias are commonly seen on peripheral blood evaluation by the time an AIDS-defining diagnosis occurs, with an inverse correlation found between the HIV-1 plasma viral load and hematologic values (94). In many patients, reconstitution of all blood cell lineages occurs after months of HAART therapy due to the amelioration of stem cell activity, restoration of stromal cell function, and normalization of the production of cytokines and chemokines (76). Anemia may remain a significant problem, however, and is an independent risk factor for decreased survival in the post-HAART era (87,89).

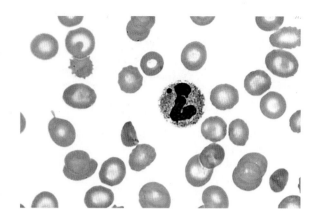

Figure 10-8

**NUCLEAR INCLUSION BODY
IN NEUTROPHIL CYTOPLASM**

A Howell-Jolly body-like nuclear inclusion is present in a peripheral blood neutrophil from a patient with HIV infection. This single round inclusion body represents an "apoptotic" nuclear fragment that is seen most commonly in patients on retroviral therapy (Wright stain). (Courtesy of Dr. P. Ward, Duluth, MN.)

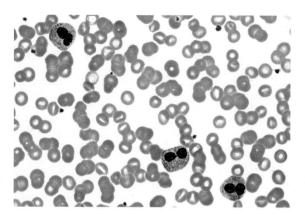

Figure 10-9

**NEUTROPHIL ATYPIA IN HUMAN
IMMUNODEFICIENCY VIRUS INFECTION**

Pelger-Hüet type neutrophils are one form of peripheral blood cell atypia present in patients with HIV infection (Wright stain). (Courtesy of Dr. S. Kroft, Milwaukee, WI.)

The cause of the anemia is typically multifactorial, as HIV acts through antibody-mediated or direct mechanisms to decrease erythroid production; concurrent infections, neoplasms, or therapeutic agents play secondary roles (71,74). Macrocytosis is usually associated with zidovudine therapy, but may also be seen in untreated patients, with one possible cause being decreased vitamin B$_{12}$ absorption. Moore et al. (88) documented schistocytes in one fourth of peripheral blood films from hospitalized AIDS patients; however, only 7 percent of these patients had symptoms of a thrombotic microangiopathic process (fever, anemia, thrombocytopenia, renal or neurologic dysfunction, and fever).

Neutropenia is less common and severe since HAART, particularly with the concurrent use of cytokine therapy. Neutropenia most often relates to failure of myeloid production and is the result of the HIV infection itself or is an adverse effect following treatment with antiretroviral agents or antibiotics. A distinctive finding in a subset of patients with AIDS is the presence of deeply basophilic Howell-Jolly body–like inclusions in neutrophils, which likely represent "apoptotic" nuclear fragments similar to those seen in red blood cells (RBCs) (fig. 10-8) (72,95). Similar neutrophil fragments may be observed after treatment with immunosuppressive or chemotherapeutic drugs, such as mycophenolate mofetil (77). Progressive lymphopenia is observed in over 90 percent of AIDS patients as a result of CD4-positive T-cell loss.

Dysplastic features, detailed in Table 10-2, are usually mild and correlate with the degree of anemia and thrombocytopenia. These changes are not as widespread as observed in an overt myelodysplastic syndrome, however, concurrent therapeutic agents may accentuate the effects (fig. 10-9) (78). AIDS patients do not have an increased incidence of myelodysplastic syndromes.

Since the introduction of HAART therapy, fewer bone marrow evaluations are being performed for single lineage cytopenias and more are being done for fever of unknown origin and pancytopenia (97,99). Nevertheless, similar morphologic features are still observed. The bone marrow evaluation provides the most information in symptomatic patients who have a CD4 count under 50/µL and hematocrit less than 25 percent or CD4 less than 21/µL, fever, and cytopenias (80,85). Even in these individuals, the procedure is often one of last resort after peripheral blood cultures, serologies, urine antigen evaluation for histoplasmosis, and radiographic studies are noncontributory (81).

Early bone marrow examinations may be beneficial in extremely ill patients in whom the immediate identification of an organism by special stains would prompt aggressive treatment,

Table 10-2

PERIPHERAL BLOOD FINDINGS IN ADVANCED HUMAN IMMUNODEFICIENCY VIRUS
(HIV) INFECTION AND ACQUIRED IMMUNODEFICIENCY SYNDROME (AIDS)[a]

Cytopenia	Peripheral Blood Findings	Comments
Anemia	Usually normochromic normocytic Nonspecific anisopoikilocytosis Mild to moderate schistocytes (micro-angiopathic hemolytic anemia) Rouleaux formation secondary to hypergammaglobulinemia MCV[b] may be increased, especially in patients receiving zidovudine[c] Absence of polychromasia (reticulocytopenia)	Often correlates with disease severity and is multifactorial in etiology including: anemia of chronic disease decreased production (drug or viral effect) iron deficiency other nutritional deficiencies (folate, vitamin B_{12} deficiency) infection (particularly parvovirus) bleeding
Lymphopenia (majority)	Possibly variant (reactive) forms including cells with lobulated nuclei	Loss of CD4+ T cells; flow cytometry will show decreased CD4:CD8 T-cell ratio
Neutropenia	Often atypical features: hypogranularity, pseudo-Pelger-Hüet nuclei, bizarre nuclear shapes, circulating giant metamyelocytes, Howell-Jolly body-like inclusions Toxic changes: left shift, toxic granulation, Döhle bodies Cytoplasmic vacuolation	Decreased production (drug or viral effect) Infrequent antibody-mediated destruction Toxic changes if intercurrent infection or receiving G-CSF therapy. Cytoplasmic vacuolation associated with sepsis
Thrombocytopenia	Often mild to moderate	ITP-like disorder in early disease Production defect in advanced disease

[a]Data from references 69, 71, 72, 75, 88, 92, 95, and 96.
[b]MCV = mean corpuscular volume; G-CSF = granulocyte colony-stimulating factor; ITP = immune thrombocytopenic purpura.
[c]Used as a marker for drug compliance in patients receiving zidovudine.

or for those in whom a neoplastic or primary hematologic process is strongly suspected (70). Keiser et al. (80) found that bone marrow evaluation provided a unique infectious diagnosis in only 10 percent of patients analyzed. The yield for diagnosing mycobacterial or fungal infections by bone marrow versus peripheral blood cultures is similar. Bone marrows with granulomas are four times more likely to have positive cultures, while histologically identifiable organisms are seen in fewer than one third of culture-positive bone marrows (83).

Bone marrows are frequently hypercellular except late in the course of disease (see features listed in Table 10-3). When the HIV status of a patient is unknown, the bone marrow morphology may suggest a myelodysplastic syndrome, a myeloproliferative disorder, a low-grade lymphoma, or a plasma cell dyscrasia. Insufficient erythropoiesis may relate to an inadequate erythropoietin response; the administration of erythropoietin is usually beneficial in increasing erythroid production and decreasing transfusion requirements. Dysplastic changes may

involve all three hematopoietic cell lines (98). A compilation of the bone marrow findings, particularly bare megakaryocytic nuclei, plasmacytosis, gelatinous transformation, and giant metamyelocytes should prompt recognition of HIV-1 infection (figs. 10-10, 10-11) (73,78,93). Reticulin fibrosis is also common (90).

Opportunistic Infections Associated with AIDS

The CD4-positive T-cell count and HIV viral load are important laboratory parameters for predicting an increased risk of developing specific opportunistic infections. HIV-infected persons who develop opportunistic infections in the post-HAART era are often unaware of their HIV status, do not have available therapy (most people infected throughout the world), are nonadherent or intolerant to antiretroviral therapy, or develop drug resistance. The most common opportunistic organisms seen in the bone marrow in the absence of HAART therapy are *Mycobacterium avium* complex (fig. 10-12), *Mycobacterium tuberculosis, Cryptococcus neoformans,* and *Histoplasma capsulatum* (102,109).

Table 10-3

BONE MARROW ABNORMALITIES IN ADVANCED HUMAN IMMUNODEFICIENCY VIRUS (HIV) INFECTION AND ACQUIRED IMMUNODEFICIENCY SYNDROME (AIDS)[a,b]

Common Abnormalities (>30% of Bone Marrows)[c] with Possible Associated Findings	
Hypercellularity	Architectural disorganization with poorly formed erythroid islands, hyperplasias of any or all lineages; less frequent - intravascular hematopoiesis and abnormally localized megakaryocytes (adjacent to bony trabeculae)
Dyserythropoiesis	Megaloblastic maturation, multinucleation with rare bizarre immature forms, nuclear irregularity, internuclear chromatin bridge formation, delayed hemoglobinization, irregular cytoplasmic clearing, basophilic stippling, left-shifted maturation
Dysgranulopoiesis	*Giant metamyelocytes, detached nuclear fragments,* delayed nuclear maturation, hyposegmentation, nucleoli in myelocytes, persistent cytoplasmic basophilia, hypogranularity, increased large primary granules, left-shifted maturation
Abnormal mega-karyocytes	Clusters, *bare megakaryocytic nuclei,* small size, hypolobation, nuclear fragmentation with multiple discrete nuclei
Plasmacytosis	Polyclonal, interstitial and perivascular
Gelatinous transformation	Associated with weight loss; possible necrosis
Reticulin fibrosis	May be induced by infection or neoplasm
Iron store alterations	Increased with decreased erythroid iron (anemia of chronic disease), increased with normal erythroid iron (ringed sideroblasts uncommon), or decreased with decreased erythroid iron (iron deficiency)
Less Common Abnormalities (<30% of Bone Marrows) with Possible Associated Findings	
Hypocellularity	Affected by increased viral load, intercurrent infection, treatment regimen
Red cell aplasia	Seen with parvovirus B19 infection, other infections (CMV, MAC)[d], zidovudine therapy
Lymphoid aggregates	*Frequently large and poorly circumscribed with polymorphous composition* including mixed T cells and B cells, +/- histiocytes, plasma cells, and eosinophils; occasionally well-circumscribed with predominance of small lymphocytes
Increased histiocytes	Interstitial or aggregates, hemophagocytosis may be evident
Increased eosinophils	Mixed eosinophilic and basophilic granulation in precursors
Granulomas	May see in absence of identified secondary infection
Neoplasms	High grade B-cell lymphomas, classic Hodgkin lymphoma, Kaposi sarcoma (rare in marrow)

[a]Data from references 73, 75, 78, 86, 93, and 98.
[b]Compilation of findings most helpful in suggesting a diagnosis of HIV infection are in italics.
[c]Pediatric populations show less overt cellular dysplasia or stromal changes.
[d]CMV = cytomegalovirus; MAC = *Mycobacterium avium* complex.

Mycobacteria are seen less frequently than fungal organisms since the advent of HAART (113). *M. avium* complex organisms are usually present in large numbers within bone marrow macrophages but occasionally are difficult to find in routine biopsy sections, especially in the absence of a significant inflammatory infiltrate. They present as a negative image on Wright-Giemsa–stained aspirate smears and may be mistaken as indicative of a storage disease (fig. 10-13). *M. tuberculosis* elicits a granulomatous response, with or without caseous necrosis.

Stains for mycobacteria are less sensitive than blood or bone marrow cultures or polymerase chain reaction (PCR) evaluation of bone marrow specimens (100,101,107). The single best stain for the detection of mycobacteria is a fluorescent auramine rhodamine stain, although its sensitivity is limited to only 40 to 50 percent (106). The less sensitive AFB stain is more commonly performed due to its widespread availability (fig. 10-14).

H. capsulatum is the most common fungus found in the bone marrow of AIDS patients. Intracellular (within neutrophils or monocytes) or extracellular yeast forms of *H. capsulatum* are observed also in the blood films of up to 40 percent of infected patients (fig. 10-15) (104). Similar dissemination occurs in children under 2 years of age in endemic

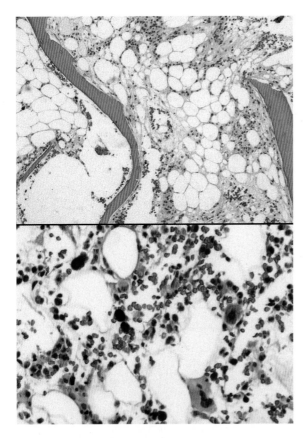

Figure 10-10

ACQUIRED IMMUNODEFICIENCY SYNDROME (AIDS)

Top: Marked bone marrow hypocellularity with areas of gelatinous transformation in an adult male with advanced AIDS. Bony trabeculae are osteopenic (H&E stain).

Bottom: Multiple bare megakaryocytic nuclei in a bone marrow biopsy from an HIV-positive female (H&E stain).

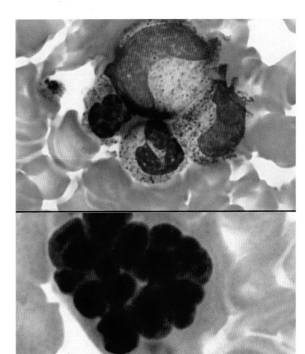

Figure 10-11

ACQUIRED IMMUNODEFICIENCY SYNDROME (AIDS)

Bone marrow aspirate smear from an AIDS patient with an unknown medication history. The cellular atypia consists of giant metamyelocytes (top) and marked erythroid multi-nucleation (bottom) (Wright stain). (Courtesy of P. Izadi, Los Angeles, CA.)

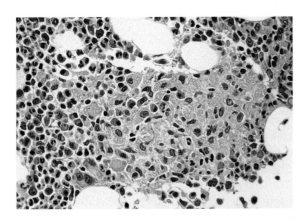

Figure 10-12

GRANULOMA WITH *MYCOBACTERIUM AVIUM* COMPLEX

AIDS patient with bone marrow granulomas containing *Mycobacterium avium* complex (H&E stain).

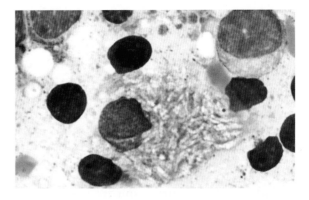

Figure 10-13

***MYCOBACTERIUM AVIUM* COMPLEX**

Negative images of presumable intracellular rod-like organisms are within macrophages on Wright-stained aspirate smears from the same patient as in figure 10-12.

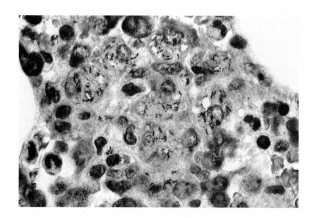

Figure 10-14

MYCOBACTERIUM AVIUM COMPLEX

An acid-fast bacteria stain in bone marrow highlights *Mycobacterium avium* complex in an AIDS patient with histiocytic infiltrates.

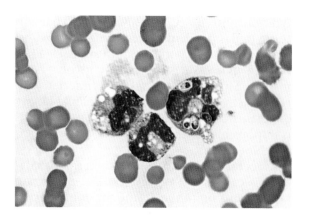

Figure 10-15

HISTOPLASMOSIS CAPSULATUM

Peripheral blood monocytes contain *Histoplasmosis capsulatum* organisms. The organisms have a crescent or ring shape and many are surrounded by a halo (Wright stain).

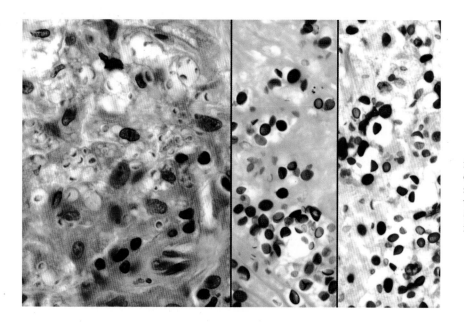

Figure 10-16

HISTOPLASMOSIS CAPSULATUM

Extensive granulomatous infiltration with *Histoplasma* organisms is seen on an H&E-stained section (left) with better visualization after GMS-diastase (middle) and PAS (right) staining.

areas. The bone marrows of immunosuppressed individuals with histoplasmosis commonly have irregular lymphohistiocytic aggregates or diffuse sheets of macrophages rather than the more common epithelioid granulomas seen in immunocompetent individuals. Organisms are often obvious in H&E-stained sections, although they are better seen on Gomori methenamine silver (GMS) and periodic acid–Schiff (PAS)–stained sections or in Wright-Giemsa–stained aspirate smears (fig. 10-16). Stains are most often positive in patients with markedly elevated low density lipoprotein (LDH) levels (105). Infrequently, a reactive hemophagocytic syndrome is associated with disseminated histoplasmosis (103).

Additional fungi that infect AIDS patients are similar to those that infect other patients with T-cell depletion: *Candida albicans, Pneumocystis jiroveci* (formerly *Pneumocystis carinii*), *Cryptococcus neoformans,* and *Penicillium marneffei.* These organisms, in addition to rarer species such as *Rhodotorula glutinis* and *Hansenula anomala,* have been described in peripheral blood smears of AIDS patients (108,111,112). They are typically surrounded by well-delineated halos in the cytoplasm of leukocytes (artifact). *P. marneferii* is endemic in parts of Southeast Asia (111), while *P. jiroveci* does not usually involve bone marrow. Monocytes/macrophages infected with HIV function poorly in the intracellular killing of organisms, while dysfunction of neutrophils is responsible for the increased severity of candidal infections.

Visceral leishmaniasis, also termed kala-azar, is caused by the intracellular protozoan *Leishmania infantum* found in countries of the Mediterranean basin and the Middle East. Approximately 50 to 75 percent of new cases occurring in Europe occur in HIV-positive patients (110). The patients often do not have the normal clinical presentation of fever, malaise, anorexia, weight loss, and hepatosplenomegaly, making the diagnosis more challenging. Visceral leishmaniasis is also caused by *Leishmania donovani* (India and Africa) and *Leishmania chagasi* (North and South America).

HIV-infected patients with parvovirus B19 have unusual bone marrow manifestations (described further later). Dysregulation of B-cell activation and the inability of the cells to respond to antigen are two of the mechanisms responsible for the increase in certain bacterial infections seen among those with advanced HIV disease. Continually improved therapy has resulted in persons with AIDS being infected by previously unrecognized or seldom identified pathogens, such as *Enterocytozoon*, *Cyclospora*, and oxacillin-resistant *Staphylococcus aureus* (113).

Herpesvirus 8–Associated Multicentric Castleman Disease

Herpesvirus 8 (HHV8) is the causative agent of Kaposi sarcoma but is also associated with atypical lymphoproliferative disorders and hematologic malignancies (e.g., primary effusion lymphoma) in patients with HIV infection. The etiology of these disorders is likely related to the ability of HHV8-specific genes to cause cell transformation in vitro and in vivo (115).

Multicentric Castleman disease (MCD) develops in patients with HIV infection and is induced by HHV8-infected B cells. Such patients have the typical symptoms of MCD: fever, generalized lymphadenopathy, hepatosplenomegaly, and hematologic abnormalities. The clinical outcome is often poor with a high risk of lymphoma development (116).

Peripheral blood and bone marrow findings in patients with HIV-associated MCD overlap with the reactive/dysplastic changes normally seen with HIV infection, including anemia, thrombocytopenia, normal or reduced leukocytes, bone marrow hypercellularity with architectural disorganization, trilineage atypia, mild eosinophilic hyperplasia, plasmacytosis, and reticulin fibrosis (114). The features that are more specific to MCD are plasmablasts/immunoblasts that are immunoreactive for HHV8-latent nuclear antigen in the interstitium and within mantle zones of lymphoid follicles. In a small number of cases, small lymphoid aggregates with hyalinized/depleted germinal centers are present (114).

INFECTIOUS MONONUCLEOSIS (EPSTEIN-BARR VIRUS)

Epstein-Barr virus (EBV) is a DNA virus that infects much of the world population; the most common pattern of disease is a clinically silent infection of infancy or childhood (119,134). When primary infection occurs later, during adolescent or early adulthood (10 to 30 years of age), EBV frequently causes heterophil antibody-positive *infectious mononucleosis*, a typically benign, self-limited disorder. In a small number of individuals, infectious mononucleosis may be severe or fatal, particularly when EBV-associated *hemophagocytic syndrome* develops (118,142,146). These individuals are often immunocompromised because of an inherited immunodeficiency disorder, such as X-linked lymphoproliferative syndrome, immunosuppressive therapy, or AIDS (121,132). EBV also plays a role in the development of post-transplant lymphoproliferative disorders and certain malignancies, including Burkitt lymphoma, Hodgkin lymphoma, diffuse large B-cell lymphoma, natural killer cell lymphoproliferative disorders, leiomyosarcoma, and nasopharyngeal carcinoma (125,136,145).

EBV infectious mononucleosis was first described in the early 1900s when patients with markedly atypical lymphocytes were mistakenly reported as having spontaneous remissions of acute leukemia (123). It was not until 1920 that Sprunt and Evans (141) described infectious mononucleosis as a clinical entity and differentiated the appearance of the reactive

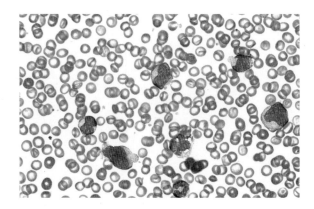

Figure 10-17

EPSTEIN-BARR VIRUS (EBV) INFECTION

The peripheral blood shows variant lymphocytes in a patient with EBV infectious mononucleosis (Wright stain).

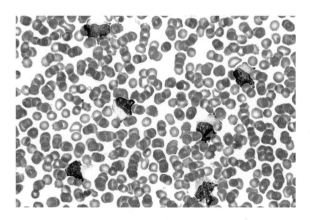

Figure 10-19

DOWNEY TYPE II LYMPHOCYTES

Downey type II cells are abundant in this peripheral blood smear from an adolescent male with EBV infectious mononucleosis. The cells are intermediate in size, with a moderately condensed nuclear chromatin pattern and inconspicuous nucleoli. The relatively abundant pale gray-blue cytoplasm shows radial or peripheral basophilia and spreads with an amoeboid appearance that indents adjacent erythrocytes. The cytoplasm may contain a few small azurophilic granules, which is better visualized at higher power (Wright stain).

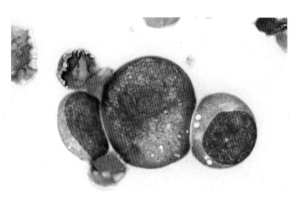

Figure 10-18

DOWNEY TYPE III LYMPHOCYTE

A Downey type III lymphocyte is seen between two other lymphocytes in the peripheral blood of a 16-year-old girl with EBV infectious mononucleosis. Downey type III cells are large immunoblasts with abundant, deeply basophilic cytoplasm. Nuclei are often round-oval, with fine to moderately coarse chromatin, distinct parachromatin, and visible nucleoli (Wright stain).

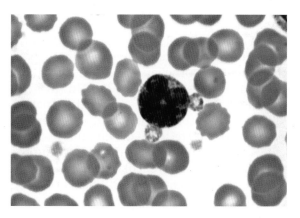

Figure 10-20

DOWNEY TYPE I LYMPHOCYTE

The smaller Downey type I cell is most often seen in children with primary EBV infection. The nucleus is usually indented or lobated, and contains condensed chromatin and inconspicuous nucleoli. The less abundant cytoplasm is basophilic or foamy in appearance and infrequently contains azurophilic granules (Wright stain).

lymphocytes from the more uniform lymphoblasts characteristic of acute leukemia (fig. 10-17). A few years later, Downey and McKinlay (120) provided a detailed morphologic description of the atypical lymphocytes seen in infectious mononucleosis, referred to as Downey type I, II, and III lymphocytes. These are illustrated in figures 10-18–10-20, although differentiation between the lymphocyte types is not required in clinical practice. Nevertheless, recognition that Downey types II and III lymphocytes are commonly seen in infectious mononucleosis, while Downey type I lymphocytes are more customarily seen in other reactive conditions or in young children with EBV infection, may help in the peripheral blood interpretation.

Table 10-4

PERIPHERAL BLOOD FINDINGS IN INFECTIOUS MONONUCLEOSIS[a]

Minimal morphologic criteria for diagnosis (present in >90% of cases)
 Lymphocytes and monocytes comprise >50% of the leukocytes
 >10% reactive lymphocytes per 100 white blood cells
 Marked lymphocyte heterogeneity

Additional findings
 Mild thrombocytopenia common (1/3 cases)
 Mild to moderate neutropenia (relatively rare)
 Plasma cells or plasmacytoid lymphocytes infrequent
 Spherocytes and polychromasia secondary to autoimmune hemolytic anemia (0.5-3% of cases)[b]
 Red blood cell clumping due to cold agglutinin[c]

[a]Data from references 117, 122, 127, 128, and 130.
[b]Autoimmune hemolytic anemia due to red blood cell autoantibodies (primarily anti-i).
[c]Immunoglobulin (Ig)M cold agglutinin is seen in 70 to 80% of patients; only a subset manifests as red blood cell clumping on the blood film.

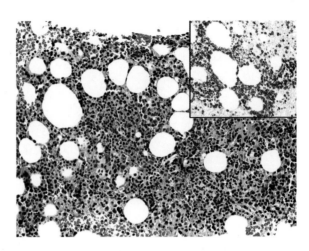

Figure 10-21

LYMPHOCYTOSIS IN EPSTEIN-BARR VIRUS INFECTION

A bone marrow clot section from a patient with infectious mononucleosis shows lymphocytosis with increased CD3-positive T cells (insert) (H&E, immunoperoxidase stain for CD3).

EBV infects B cells in the oropharynx, with subsequent dissemination of virus throughout the reticuloendothelial system, causing polyclonal activation of B cells (126). This incites a prominent cytotoxic/suppressor T cell and natural killer (NK) cell response that eventually curbs viral proliferation and restrains the immune response (135,147). It is the T cells that constitute the atypical lymphocytes circulating in the peripheral blood of patients with EBV infection.

Patients with infectious mononucleosis typically present with a mild to moderate leukocytosis (10,000 to 20,000/µL), pharyngitis, splenomegaly (about 50 percent of cases), lymphadenopathy (over 90 percent cases, usually cervical), mild hepatitis, and malaise (134). Lymphocytosis is detectable approximately 1 week after initiation of symptoms, peaking at 2 to 3 weeks and persisting for up to 8 weeks. Peripheral blood memory B cells remain latently infected for the lifetime of the individual, with the possibility of reactivation during periods of immunosuppression (140).

Additional peripheral blood findings associated with infectious mononucleosis are listed in Table 10-4. The heterophil antibody (monospot) test is confirmative; however, heterophil antibodies lag behind peripheral blood smear changes and a negative result does not

exclude the diagnosis. In clinically suspicious cases, testing should be repeated 1 to 2 weeks later or specific serologic tests for EBV should be obtained. The differential diagnosis includes infectious mononucleosis type syndromes (described later). Primary EBV infection in young children is heterophil negative in approximately half of the cases and neutropenia may be the only cytopenia present (138). Rarely, autoimmune hemolytic anemia may be the main initial manifestation of EBV infection. Antibody responses may result in the appearance of rheumatoid factor or the production of antinuclear, antiplatelet, and rarely, antineutrophil antibodies (124,139,144).

A bone marrow evaluation is not indicated for the diagnosis of infectious mononucleosis, and similar to lymph node or tonsillar biopsies in these patients, can lead to unnecessary additional testing and inappropriate concern for a neoplastic disorder. Most commonly, nonspecific reactive changes are found, including lymphocytosis, plasmacytosis, subtle granuloma formation (small, non-necrotizing), and infrequently, histiocytosis (fig. 10-21) (131). Scattered immunoblasts are present and may resemble Hodgkin and Reed-Sternberg cells (fig. 10-22). Immunoblasts are immunoreactive for latent membrane protein (LMP) or positive

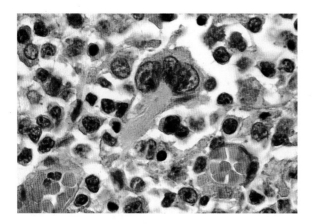

Figure 10-22

IMMUNOBLAST IN EPSTEIN-BARR VIRUS INFECTION

A bone marrow biopsy from a teenaged girl with infectious mononucleosis shows cells resembling Reed-Sternberg cells (H&E stain).

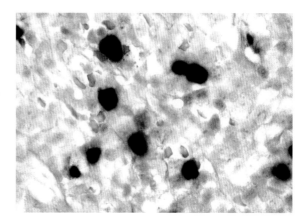

Figure 10-23

EPSTEIN-BARR VIRUS INFECTION

Cells are positive by in situ hybridization for EBV RNA (EBER).

by in situ hybridization studies for EBV RNA (EBER) (fig. 10-23).

The degree of the bone marrow abnormalities relates to the severity of the EBV infection and whether or not an individual is immunocompromised. Expanded populations of atypical immunoblasts are common in immunodeficient individuals (fig. 10-24). These individuals may also develop a hematologic picture that mimics a myelodysplastic/chronic myeloproliferative disorder, with bone marrow hypercellularity, sustained left-shifted neutrophilia, and a histiocytosis that disrupts the normal bone marrow architecture (these features may be seen with CMV and parvovirus infections as well). Patients with antibodies to circulating RBCs or platelets have associated lineage hyperplasias as the bone marrow attempts to compensate for the peripheral cell loss. Rarely, transient bone marrow suppression, aplasia, or amegakaryocytosis develop (129,137). Patients with fatal EBV infection have bone marrow findings that simulate the histopathologic findings observed in other organs including a polymorphous lymphoid infiltrate, histiocytosis, necrosis, lymphoid depletion, and/or hemophagocytosis (133,146). EBV is the most common agent identified in systemic hemophagocytic syndromes, with the exuberant T-cell cytokine reaction being responsible for the fatal outcome (143).

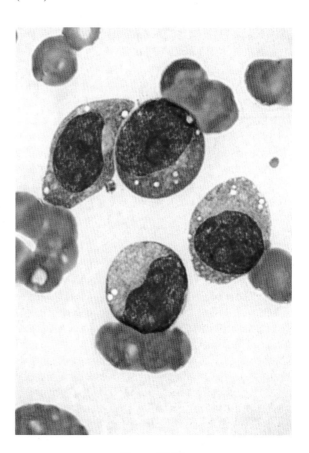

Figure 10-24

EPSTEIN-BARR VIRUS INFECTION

A bone marrow aspirate smear from a child with AIDS and secondary EBV infection shows a prominent population of immunoblasts, representing the T-cell response to EBV infection (Wright stain). (Courtesy of P. Izadi, Los Angeles, CA.)

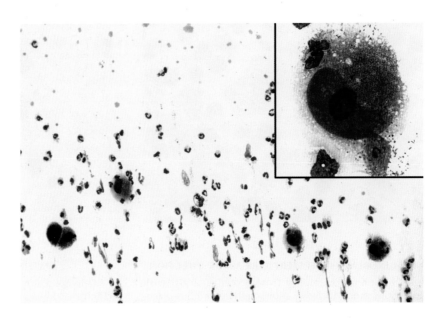

Figure 10-25

CYTOMEGALOVIRUS

Cytomegalovirus-infected endothelial cells are concentrated at the feathered edge of this peripheral blood smear. The cells are large, have abundant basophilic cytoplasm, and have an eccentric nucleus that is flattened on the inner side (insert) (Wright stain). (Courtesy of Dr. S. Kroft, Milwaukee, WI.)

INFECTIOUS MONONUCLEOSIS TYPE SYNDROMES

Peripheral blood and bone marrow findings that are indistinguishable from those of EBV infection are most frequently seen in association with CMV infection, but may also be observed with the acute HIV syndrome, as well as infections caused by hepatitis viruses, HHV6, and *Toxoplasma* (148,174,175). The bone marrow may appear aplastic due to the suppression of hematopoiesis (170).

Cytomegalovirus

The second most common cause of an infectious mononucleosis type syndrome, after EBV, is *CMV infection* (159,177). This usually occurs in adults 20 to 30 years of age but is also seen in older adults (155). Unlike EBV infectious mononucleosis, CMV-infected patients rarely have pharyngitis or tonsillitis, and the lymphadenopathy and splenomegaly are less severe. Laboratory abnormalities are similar, with the possibility of cold agglutinins, rheumatoid factor, mixed cryoglobulinemia, antinuclear antibodies, and anticomplementary activity. Immunocompromised solid organ transplant recipients or patients who have undergone chemotherapy may develop life-threatening infections, usually from reactivation of latent CMV infection (162,168a).

The peripheral blood smear shows a relative lymphocytosis with more than 50 percent lymphocytes, including 10 percent or more

variant forms. Increases of large granular lymphocytes and NK cells are common (153,157). Thrombocytopenia and hemolytic anemia occur regularly in children with congenital CMV disease but are less frequent in healthy adults with CMV mononucleosis (154). Rarely, circulating CMV-infected endothelial cells may be found concentrated at the lateral edges of the blood film or in buffy coat preparations from immunosuppressed patients with severe active infection (160). These cells are indicative of endothelial damage and are pathognomonic for CMV infection (fig. 10-25) (152,168).

Bone marrow specimens from patients infected with CMV may be similar to those from EBV-infected patients, with lymphoid aggregates, granulomatous infiltrates, myeloid and megakaryocytic suppression, and less commonly, trilineage hypoplasia (figs. 10-26, 10-27) (149,163,172,173). CMV may cause delayed or failed engraftment in stem cell transplant recipients. While CD14-positive monocytes are the major viral reservoir during latent infection, multiple cell types are infected during active infection, particularly in immunosuppressed patients, including endothelial cells, neutrophils, and lymphocytes (150).

The detection of viral inclusions in biopsy sections, particularly "owl-eye" inclusions, confirmed by immunohistochemistry or in situ hybridization, is diagnostic for CMV infection (fig. 10-28) (165,167). As nuclear inclusions are

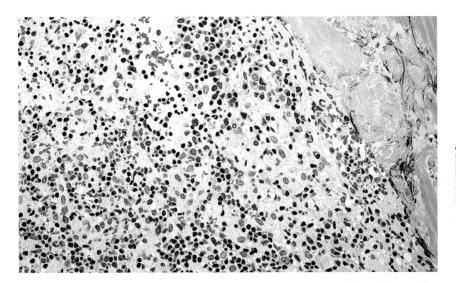

Figure 10-26

CYTOMEGALOVIRUS

Bone marrow biopsy from a patient with acute cytomegalovirus infection shows a granulomatous infiltrate with increased lymphocytes and decreased megakaryocytes (H&E stain).

Figure 10-27

CYTOMEGALOVIRUS

The majority of lymphocytes in the cytomegalovirus-infected bone marrow are CD3-positive T cells (left), with a mixture of CD4-positive (middle) and CD8-positive (right) cells (immunoperoxidase stains for CD3, CD4, CD8).

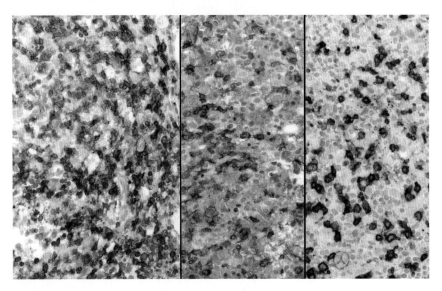

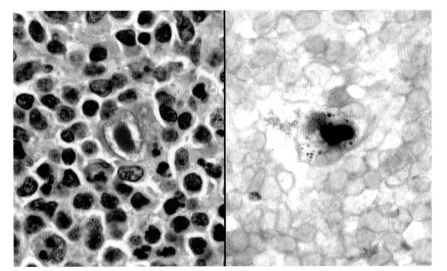

Figure 10-28

CYTOMEGALOVIRUS

A cytomegalic cell with a nuclear inclusion (or so-called owl-eye cell) in a biopsy section from a cytomegalovirus-infected individual. Cowdry owl-eye inclusion bodies are present within mesenchymal cells (e.g., endothelial cells, fibrocytes) and sometimes inflammatory cells (left; H&E stain). In situ hybridization for cytomegalovirus is positive (right).

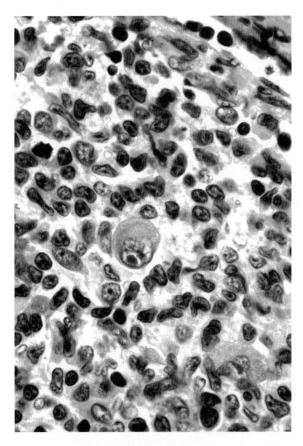

Figure 10-29

CYTOMEGALOVIRUS

A cell infected with cytomegalovirus resembles a Reed-Sternberg cell (H&E stain).

found in only 20 to 37 percent of cases (150, 169), the diagnosis often depends on other findings (168a). Virally infected cells may resemble Hodgkin and Reed-Sternberg cells and may be CD15 positive, raising the possibility of Hodgkin lymphoma (fig. 10-29) (171). Uncommonly, fibrin ring granulomas, a florid hemophagocytic syndrome, or secondary immune thrombocytopenic purpura occur (151,156,166,178). Sustained atypical monocytoses that resemble a myelodysplastic syndrome or myeloproliferative disorder, such as juvenile myelomonocytic leukemia, have been reported (158,176).

T-cell receptor (TCR)-gamma gene rearrangements have been described in rare cases of prolonged CMV mononucleosis or during infection in postsplenectomy patients, and are considered to be a part of the immune response to CMV infec-

tion (153,164). The CMV pp65 antigenemia assay is more specific for the diagnosis of both primary and reactivated CMV infection in immunocompromised patients than antibody titers (161).

PARVOVIRUS INFECTION

Humans are the only known host for *parvovirus B19 infection*. The clinical manifestations of infection depend on the age, and hematologic and immunologic status of the host. Pregnant women with primary infection have a 5 to 10 percent risk of an abnormal outcome, manifested by fetal or congenital anemia, spontaneous abortion, or hydrops fetalis (186,200). In this regard, B19 infection should be excluded in any child suspected of having congenital anemia (e.g., Diamond-Blackfan anemia) (188). The most common expression of infection is erythema infectiosum in children (Fifth disease), and arthralgias and arthritis in adults (60 percent of females and 30 percent of males) (187). A small subset of children with recent-onset arthritis also have evidence of B19 infection (196). For the majority of immunocompetent children and adults, parvovirus B19 is a self-limited infection that results in life-long immunity.

The transmission of this small DNA virus occurs via respiratory secretions, blood products, or from mother to fetus (181,187). The virus binds to blood group P antigen receptors on erythroid precursors, megakaryocytes, endothelial cells, and fetal myocytes. Viral entry into cells requires activated B1 integrin coreceptors, present only on erythroid progenitors, making erythroid progenitors the sole site of viral replication (203). In bone marrow specimens, the virus induces cell cycle arrest and is directly cytotoxic to the erythroid cells (183,199). The viral proteins appear to have toxic effects on other cell populations, such as megakaryocytes and myeloid precursors (191,202).

The majority of parvovirus B19-infected individuals have a transient arrest of erythropoiesis that results in a hemoglobin drop of approximately 1 g/dL; recovery of erythropoiesis occurs in 10 to 19 days (187). Some patients develop transient aplastic crisis (pure red cell aplasia) or transient erythroblastopenia of childhood (201). Transient aplastic crisis is most commonly seen in patients with an underlying hemolytic disorder, such as hereditary spherocytosis, thalassemia, autoimmune hemolytic anemia, malaria, or RBC enzyme deficiencies (e.g., pyruvate kinase deficiency) (184). Those with decreased RBC production, as in iron deficiency anemia, may also rarely experience this phenomenon. For patients with chronic hemolytic anemia, the abrupt cessation of erythropoiesis in the face of a markedly shortened RBC lifespan leads to a rapid and potentially life-threatening fall in the hemoglobin level. Supportive care and RBC transfusions usually result in recovery in approximately 2 weeks.

Pure red cell aplasia develops in immunocompromised individuals with persistent parvovirus B19 infection who fail to produce neutralizing antibodies that effectively eradicate the virus (195). This is most commonly reported in immunosuppressed patients such as those with AIDS, congenital immunodeficiency syndromes, lymphoproliferative disorders, myeloid disorders, and rheumatologic disorders managed with steroid therapy, as well as transplant recipients (179,180,184). These patients often present with hypoproliferative anemia (chronic anemia of uncertain etiology). Parvovirus B19 infection has also been associated with rare cases of hemophagocytic syndrome among children and adults, and with aplastic anemia (198). A possible connection with chronic neutropenia of infancy and childhood is less clear (182,197).

Specific treatment, such as intravenous immunoglobulin, may be necessary for patients with underlying hematologic disorders who do not respond to supportive care (184). In immunosuppressed patients, temporary cessation of the immunosuppressive agent or intravenous immunoglobulin therapy is indicated.

Peripheral blood smears from patients with parvovirus B19 infection demonstrate normochromic normocytic anemia with reticulocytopenia that is resistant to erythropoietin therapy. Careful review of the RBC morphology may uncover an underlying hematologic disorder, such as hereditary spherocytosis (fig. 10-30) or sickle cell anemia. White blood cell (WBC) and platelet counts are normal or show varying degrees of lymphopenia, neutropenia, thrombocytopenia, or plasmacytosis, which occur 6 to 10 days after the initial infection (191,193). The thrombocytopenia is either immune-mediated or the result of bone marrow suppression (189,190).

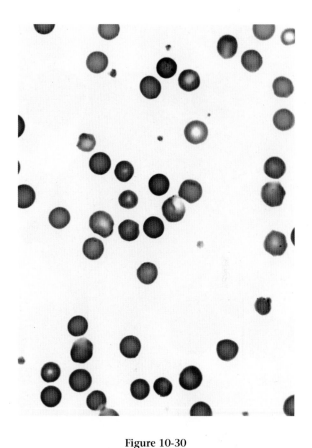

Figure 10-30

PARVOVIRUS B19 INFECTION

A peripheral blood smear from a patient with hereditary spherocytosis shows an absence of reticulocytes due to parvovirus B19 infection (Wright stain).

Giant proerythroblasts, alternatively referred to as lantern cells, are the hallmark of parvovirus B19 infection, but their presence or absence alone is not diagnostic (192). Viral inclusions are often easier to detect in biopsy sections rather than in stained bone marrow aspirate smears; smear interpretation is improved after formalin fixation for 15 minutes (194). Generally, the scattered giant proerythroblasts are large and have fine megaloblastoid chromatin (fig. 10-31) (192). Infected proerythroblasts lose their normal tinctorial quality and show nuclear swelling with dissolution of the nucleus. Little maturation occurs beyond the proerythroblast stage due to the viral cytopathic effects (figs. 10-32, 10-33).

Viral-associated suppression of the myeloid or megakaryocytic lineages may be seen and rare cases of severe bone marrow necrosis have been reported (187,202). Intranuclear viral inclusions

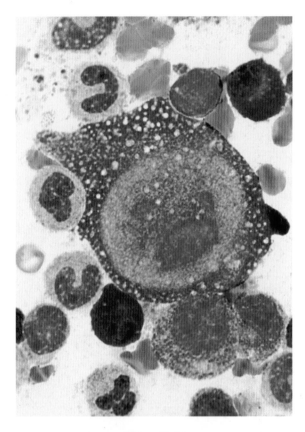

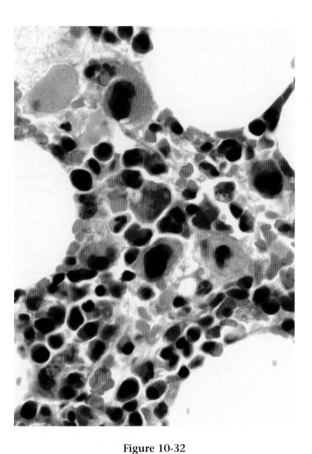

Figure 10-31

PARVOVIRUS B19 INFECTION

A giant proerythroblast in the bone marrow aspirate smear from a patient with parvovirus B19 infection. These cells are large (25 to 32 μm in diameter) and show cytopathic viral effects with large nuclear inclusions, occasional "dog-ear" cytoplasmic projections, and vacuolation (Wright stain).

Figure 10-32

PARVOVIRUS B19 INFECTION

Atypical megakaryocytes are in the bone marrow core biopsy from a patient with marked anemia, decreased erythropoiesis, and parvovirus B19 infection (H&E stain).

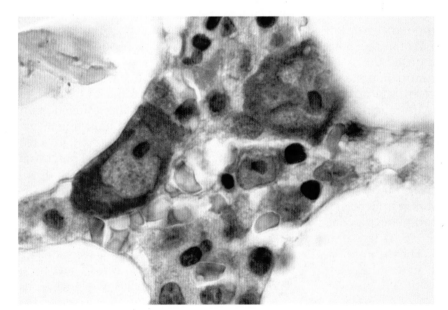

Figure 10-33

PARVOVIRUS B19 INFECTION

Hemoglobin A immunoperoxidase stain highlights a few proerythroblasts while other stages of erythroid maturation are markedly reduced in a bone marrow biopsy from a patient with parvovirus B19 infection. Hemoglobin A may not stain the earliest erythroid precursors.

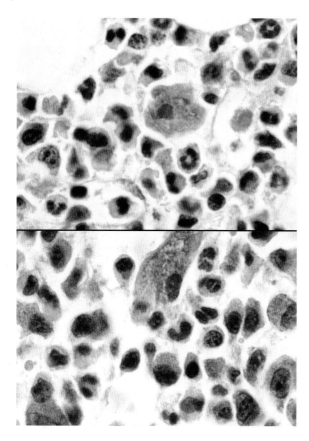

Figure 10-34

**PARVOVIRUS B19
NUCLEAR INCLUSIONS**

A hypercellular bone marrow biopsy section from a patient with AIDS shows proerythroblasts with eosinophilic nuclear inclusion bodies, which in some cells compress the chromatin against the nuclear membrane (H&E stain).

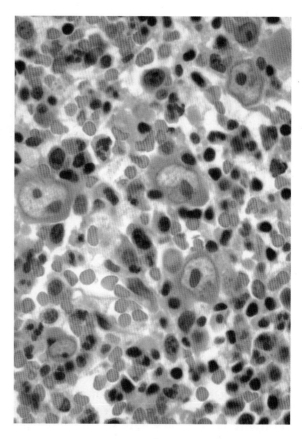

Figure 10-35

PARVOVIRUS B19 IN IMMUNOSUPPRESSED PATIENT

A bone marrow core biopsy from an immunosuppressed patient with giant proerythroblasts that contain prominent eosinophilic nuclear inclusion bodies. Increased maturing erythroid precursors are present in the background (H&E stain).

are most prominent in severe infections, particularly of immunocompromised hosts (fig. 10-34) (185). Immunocompromised individuals, in contrast to others with parvovirus B19 infection, may have a hypercellular bone marrow with an erythroid hyperplasia showing maturation (fig 10-35). Viral tolerance allows for the development of infected erythroid cells past the pronormoblast stage in these individuals (185). Asynchronous hemoglobinization occurs in the more mature erythroid precursors.

The diagnosis of acute or chronic parvovirus B19 infection may be made by immunohistochemistry or in situ hybridization for parvovirus B19 DNA on tissue sections (fig. 10-36). Serologic assays for parvovirus B19-specific immunoglobulin (Ig)M and IgG may be negative in infected

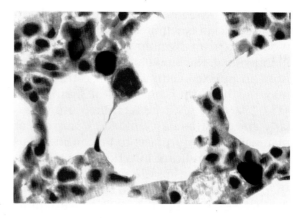

Figure 10-36

IN SITU HYBRIDIZATION FOR PARVOVIRUS B19

An immunohistochemical stain for parvovirus B19 highlights infected cells in this bone marrow biopsy section.

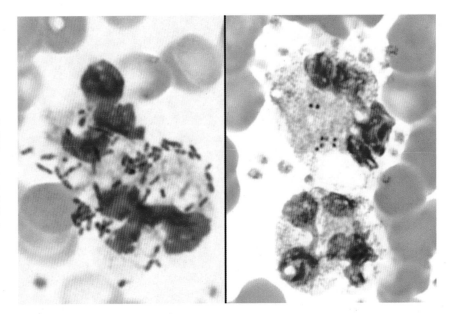

Figure 10-37

BACTERIA IN NEUTROPHILS

Left: Intracellular bacteria (rods) are seen in circulating neutrophils in a 2-year-old child with sepsis.

Right: Cocci are within neutrophils of an adult with sepsis.

The collections of bacteria appear uniform in shape (Wright stain). (Courtesy of Dr. P. Ward, Duluth, MN.)

individuals who are immunosuppressed. IgM antibodies frequently appear only after the disappearance of the viremia. Therefore, PCR analysis of DNA in serum is recommended due to its greater sensitivity and specificity. PCR positivity lasts 2 to 5 months and indicates either active or recent infection (198).

BACTERIAL INFECTIONS

Sepsis

The identification of bacteria in leukocytes in routine blood smears is often unexpected and typically correlates with overwhelming sepsis and a grave prognosis. Immediate notification of the clinician is required. When this finding is observed in an asymptomatic or less severely ill individual, the blood may have been drawn from an infected central venous catheter and may not have the same clinical significance (227). Bacteria must be identified intracellularly and must be differentiated from cellular material or other artifacts to be considered as evidence of significant infection.

Bacterial organisms are usually uniform in shape, present in groups, and tend to lie within distinct vacuoles (fig. 10-37) (221). Neutrophils have features of activation, including toxic granulation, Döhle bodies, and vacuolation (see chapter 5). Staphylococcal organisms (especially *Staphylococcus aureus*) and *Neisseria meningitidis*

are the most commonly detected organisms in blood smears (212,225,230). For organisms with a more unusual appearance, a Gram stain of the peripheral smear helps to confirm the presence of bacteria and differentiate between gram-negative and gram-positive organisms for treatment purposes (214).

Bordetella Pertussis

Bordetella pertussis, a small, gram-negative coccobacillus, is the etiologic agent of *whooping cough*, or "violent cough," and one of the few bacterial organisms that causes lymphocytosis. Whooping cough is primarily a disease of infants and children who have not been immunized, with 60 percent of cases occurring in children less than 5 years of age. However, immunization boosters have not been routinely given beyond childhood in the United States and an increased incidence of disease is being reported in adolescents and adults, who are a major source of infection for unimmunized or partially immunized children (less than 3 doses of pertussis-containing vaccine) (218,223). Symptoms are generally most severe in infants; fatal cases in infants account for more than 90 percent of deaths from pertussis (218). Infants may present with apnea and cyanosis in the absence of cough, making the clinical diagnosis more difficult. The illness can be severe and protracted in adults, with a mean duration of symptoms of 5 to 7 weeks (204).

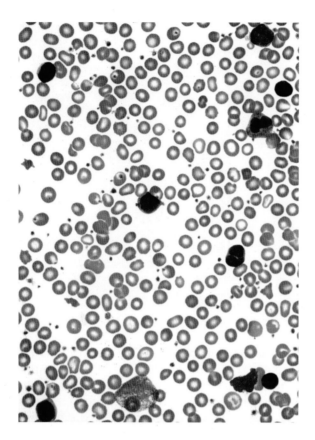

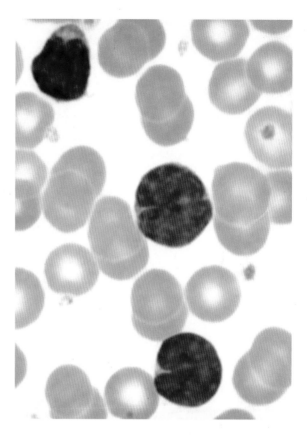

Figure 10-38

BORDETELLA PERTUSSIS INFECTION

A peripheral blood smear from a child with *Bordetella pertussis* infection shows a predominance of small mature-appearing lymphocytes (Wright stain).

Figure 10-39

BORDETELLA PERTUSSIS INFECTION

At high power, occasional lymphocytes with cleaved nuclei are seen. More convoluted nuclei were also present (Wright stain).

The characteristic hematologic feature of pertussis is a leukocytosis with lymphocyte predominance (229). In infants, the total WBC count may exceed 50,000/μL, with increased neutrophils, monocytes, or platelets in addition to the lymphocytosis (222). The leukocytosis can be responsible for infant death due to the formation of cellular aggregates that cause pulmonary hypertension (215). Regardless of age, the WBC count is typically elevated during the time of early respiratory symptoms but by the time many patients seek medical care, particularly adults, only one third display significant leukocytosis or lymphocytosis (217). Previously immunized adults or partially immunized children have a less severe leukocyte reaction (204).

Evaluation of the lymphocyte morphology is an important clue to the diagnosis, especially in infants with atypical clinical findings. Lymphocytes appear uniformly mature, with condensed chromatin and scant cytoplasm (fig. 10-38). The majority are T cells that frequently exhibit cleaved or convoluted nuclei (12 to 56 percent of lymphocytes) (fig. 10-39) (222). Occasional immunoblasts and plasma cells are seen. Lymphocytes have markedly reduced L-selectin expression, perhaps induced by pertussis toxin. This prevents the homing of the T cells to tissues and increases their number in circulation (219,220).

In classic cases, the clinical diagnosis is usually straightforward. A definitive diagnosis in other cases requires the growth of the organism in culture or detection with DNA molecular biology techniques or direct fluorescein-labeled immunofluorescent antibody stains (209). Respiratory secretions and pernasal nasopharyngeal swabs are optimal specimens (215).

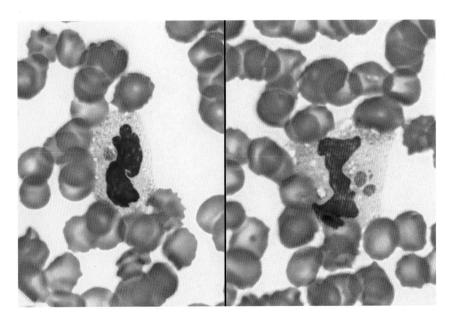

Figure 10-40

EHRLICHIOSIS

Circulating neutrophils contain morulae of *Anaplasma phago-cytophilia*, which are of similar but less intense coloration than the nucleus. The morulae (Latin for mulberry) are arranged in spherical groups with irregular edges (Wright stain). (Courtesy of Dr. P. Nguyen, Rochester, MN.)

Ehrlichiosis

Ehrlichia are obligate intracellular gram-negative bacteria belonging to the recently reorganized family Anaplasmataceae (228). Three species produce disease in humans: *E. chaffeensis,* which causes human monocytic ehrlichiosis (HME); *Anaplasma phagocytophilia*, which causes human granulocytotropic anaplasmosis (HGA, formally termed human granulocytic ehrlichiosis), and *E. ewingii*, which causes rare granulocytic disease, with increased frequency in transplant patients (226a). The geographic distribution of *E. chaffeensis* and *A. phagocytophilia* reflect regions of the United States where their hard-tick vectors reside (210a). HME is concentrated in the south-central, southeastern, and mid-Atlantic states, while HGA is common in the northeastern states, northwest Wisconsin, eastern Minnesota, and Pacific northwest states. Although the clinical symptoms are similar, HME more often results in serious disease with hospitalization required for approximately 50 percent of patients and a mortality rate of 2 to 3 percent (224,228). Patients with HME can develop a septic shock-like syndrome, especially if immunosuppressed (210a). The mortality rate for patients with HGA is lower, at 0.5 to 1.0 percent.

The distinctive laboratory findings at disease presentation include mild to moderate thrombocytopenia (70 to 90 percent of cases), mild to moderate leukopenia (consisting of lymphopenia and/or neutropenia), and elevation of serum hepatic transaminase levels (205). Granulocytes may have toxic changes and lymphocytes include large cells with basophilic cytoplasm (216). Anemia may develop and a rebound lymphocytosis occurs during recovery (207).

The identification of morulae in either circulating monocytes (HME) or granulocytes (HGA) is diagnostic in the appropriate clinical setting. Morulae are cytoplasmic membrane-bound vacuoles with irregular edges that contain hundreds to thousands of clustered gram-negative bacteria (fig. 10-40). Infected cells typically contain only 1 or 2 morulae, although as many as 15 may be seen in immunosuppressed individuals. Finding morulae requires patience and skill. They are present in less than 0.2 percent of circulating WBCs in HME infection; examination of buffy coats facilitates detection (216). The percentage of peripheral blood films with detectable morulae varies greatly in the literature (3 to 80 percent), with a higher number seen with HGA infection (50 to 80 percent) and in immunosuppressed individuals (216).

When *Ehrlichia* organisms are not seen in peripheral blood smears, the bone marrow becomes the most extensively studied tissue. The histopathologic bone marrow findings are inconsistent, and are likely to change during the course of the disease. Normocellular or hypercellular bone marrows are most frequently

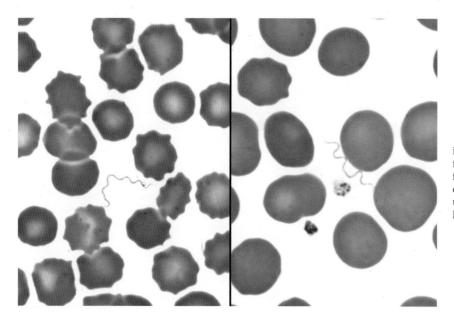

Figure 10-41

BORRELIA

Spirochetes (*Borrelia*) are seen in the peripheral blood smears from patients with relapsing fever. Spirochetes are extracellular organisms that vary from 8 to 30 um in length and have 3 to 10 helical coils (Wright stain).

described, with myeloid and/or megakaryocytic hyperplasia (210,224). Granulomas, aggregates of foamy histiocytes, increased plasma cells, and erythrophagocytosis are present in a smaller proportion of cases. HGA organisms preferentially infect more mature rather than immature granulocytic cells in bone marrow (206).

The majority of patients infected with *Ehrlichia* organisms are seronegative during the first few weeks of acute infection (60 to 97 percent) (226). Thus, therapeutic decisions must be based on clinical suspicion, the peripheral blood findings, and PCR analysis (sensitivity of 60 to 85 percent, high degree of false positive results). Human ehrlichiosis became a nationally reportable disease to the Centers for Disease Control (CDC) in 1999. The organisms are susceptible to tetracyclines and their derivatives, particularly doxycycline.

Borrelia (Relapsing Fever)

Spirochetes of the genus *Borrelia* are responsible for causing relapsing fever, a relatively rare disease seen primarily in the western regions of the United States and Canada (211). The disease is usually tick transmitted and may involve at least 15 different species of *Borrelia*. The spirochetes identified in the peripheral blood film are pathognomonic for infection and are commonly discovered incidentally when the diagnosis is not suspected clinically (fig. 10-41). Spirochetes are present in the blood during febrile episodes,

which start approximately 1 week after infection, last 3 days on average, and recur with subsequent relapses (213). When the diagnosis is suspected, acridine-orange staining of buffy coat preparations optimizes evaluation (208).

PROTOZOA INFECTIONS

Malaria (*Plasmodium* Species)

Malarial infections in humans are caused by four species of *Plasmodium*, spread by the female *Anopheles* mosquito: *P. falciparum, P. vivax, P. ovale* and *P. malariae*. Infections are seen throughout the United States, with 1,528 cases reported in 2005 (263). They occur primarily in persons returning from endemic areas of the world, such as tropical regions of sub-Saharan Africa, Southeast Asia, the Middle East, and Latin America. The diagnosis of malaria is based on the identification of parasites in circulating RBCs; the morphologic features help to distinguish the plasmodia type (Table 10-5). In acutely ill patients, at least three negative smears in 48 hours are normally required to exclude infection.

Individuals with malaria develop cyclical chills and rigors followed by high fevers that correspond temporally to RBC lysis as organisms (schizonts) mature. Additional clinical findings include headache, fatigue, arthralgias, myalgias, abdominal pain, hepatosplenomegaly, and thrombocytopenia (up to 80 percent of patients). Thrombocytopenia is caused by

Table 10-5

MORPHOLOGIC DIFFERENCES BETWEEN MALARIAL PARASITES IN PERIPHERAL BLOOD SMEARS[a]

	Infected Erythrocytes		Parasite Stages Circulating In Blood	Parasites Chromatin Dot	Pigment	Specific Features
	Size	Schüffner Stippling[b]				
Plasmodium falciparum	Normal	−	Rings, often multiple, +/− gametocytes	Often double	Black, in gametocytes	Thin delicate rings Crescent-/cigar-/banana-shaped gametocytes
Plasmodium vivax	Enlarged	+	All	Single	Gold/brown	Thicker rings Ameboid trophozoites Increased merozoites per cell (12-24) in random configuration
Plasmodium ovale	Enlarged[c]	+	All	Single	Dark brown	Round, compact trophozoites 8-12 trophozoites per cell in rosette configuration
Plasmodium malariae	Normal	−	All, few rings	Inverted	Dark brown, coarse	Round, compact trophozoites 8-12 trophozoites per cell in rosette configuration

[a]Data from reference 234.
[b]Schüffner stippling is the presence of numerous small pink granules in the cytoplasm of infected erythrocytes, except for those with early ring forms. Identification is highly dependent on stain quality.
[c]Erythrocytes infected with *P. ovale* are often oval (>20%) or fimbriated (irregular projections of the cell margins).

platelet phagocytosis induced by the platelet binding of malarial antigens and antiparasite antibodies, along with the splenic pooling of platelets (249). In addition to direct RBC lysis, anemia occurs through phagocytosis of both parasitized and nonparasitized erythrocytes, and by T-cell cytokine-mediated suppression of erythropoiesis (231,236,257). Dyserythropoiesis and ineffective erythropoiesis may be seen in the bone marrow (266), along with macrophage hyperplasia, plasmacytosis, and increased eosinophils (265). The microvasculature of the bone marrow may be obstructed by parasitized RBCs in severe *P. falciparum* infection.

A severe *malarial anemia syndrome* is found in endemic areas with moderate to high malarial transmission rates. It occurs primarily in younger children (1 to 3 years of age) and is a leading cause of death in this age group (261). Extravascular removal of nonparasitized RBCs, in conjunction with inadequate bone marrow erythropoiesis, accounts for the significant anemia, even among those with relatively low parasite burdens (241).

The morphologic assessment of malaria requires an initial evaluation for *P. falciparum*. This organism is responsible for the greatest number of malarial complications and deaths in non-immune individuals. As *P. falciparum* invades erythrocytes of all stages, high parasite loads are seen in fulminate infections (more than 20 percent of RBCs). The organism is frequently drug resistant and unlike other plasmodia, induces specialized receptors on infected RBCs that adhere to the microvasculature, producing microvascular disease and secondary organ dysfunction (235). While a detailed description of the parasite's life cycle is beyond the scope of this section, *P. falciparum* is primarily seen as small, sometimes multiple ring forms (early trophozoites) within erythrocytes on blood films (fig. 10-42). More mature asexual forms are absent due to their sequestration in the peripheral vasculature. Sexual forms (gametocytes) may develop from trophozoites, usually after treatment, and are distinguished by their distinctive crescent/banana/sausage shape (fig. 10-43).

P. vivax and *P. ovale* infections produce a similar clinical disease. These organisms have the ability to live in more temperate regions of the world compared to *P. falciparum*. Dormant hypnozoite liver stages permit parasite survival during colder periods of the year; active forms may arise months to years later (242). The dormant liver phase requires specialized treatment to eradicate the organisms. These plasmodia preferentially

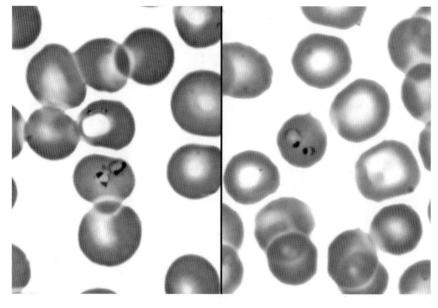

Figure 10-42

PLASMODIUM FALCIPARUM

Plasmodium falciparum (malaria) is seen in normal-sized peripheral blood erythrocytes. Infected erythrocytes may contain more than one ring form (multiple organisms), as illustrated here. The ring forms are small (less than 2 μm) and delicate, with 1 to 2 deep red chromatin masses. More mature forms (late trophozoites and schizonts) are usually absent (Wright stain).

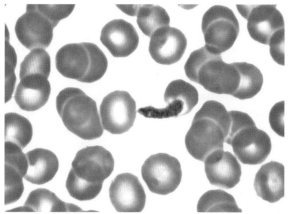

Figure 10-43

PLASMODIUM FALCIPARUM GAMETOCYTE

Infection with *Plasmodium falciparum* is frequently associated with a high level of parasitemia (over 5 percent of red blood cells infected) and exclusively ring forms. An exception is the presence of occasional large gametocytes, which are diagnostic for *P. falciparum*. As shown here, a gametocyte has a banana or crescent/sausage shape (Wright stain).

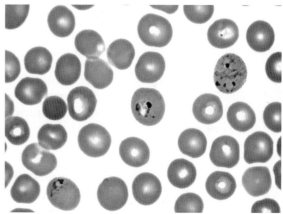

Figure 10-44

PLASMODIUM VIVAX

A peripheral blood smear from a 20-year-old female who recently traveled to India and developed spiking fevers upon return to the United States. Enlarged erythrocytes contain single ring forms with a single red chromatin mass and blue cytoplasm. One erythrocyte (upper right) contains a maturing *Plasmodium vivax* trophozoite with a complex ameboid form, which is less round or compact than that seen in *P. ovale* or *P. malariae* infections (Wright stain).

invade reticulocytes through reticulocyte-binding proteins; this is reflected in the larger than normal size of the parasitized RBCs in the circulation (fig. 10-44). The favored invasion of reticulocytes limits parasitemia (usually less than 1 percent of RBCs infected) and multiple stages of the organism circulate due to the lack of peripheral sequestration (fig. 10-45). Duffy antigen is the receptor used by *P. vivax* to invade

erythrocytes; its absence in black populations protects against *P. vivax* infection (258).

P. malariae invades old erythrocytes, rarely produces acute illness in normal hosts, and may persist for years in infected individuals. The parasitemia is usually minimal and symptoms are typically mild except in rare children with glomerulonephritis (260).

Figure 10-45

PLASMODIUM VIVAX

Mature schizonts occupy nearly the entire erythrocyte in this young woman with *Plasmodium vivax* infection. Schizonts contain 12 to 24 merozoites, which are formed from cytoplasmic and chromatin divisions. The merozoites are randomly arranged in the cells, each distinguishable by its chromatin mass. Central yellow/black pigment may be seen with maturation. Merozoites are released into circulation and infect other erythrocytes when red blood cells lyse (Wright stain).

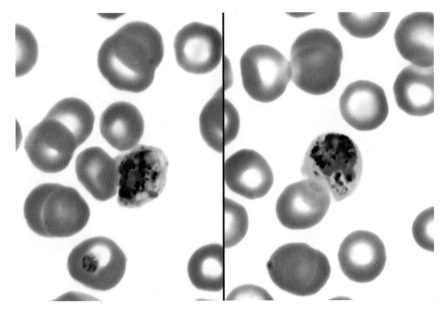

The automated hematology analyzer is being used to screen for the possibility of malaria in peripheral blood (244,248). Testing is based on the presence of hemozoin-containing pigment produced by plasmodia within neutrophils and monocytes. PCR is gaining greater acceptance as a sensitive and specific method for detecting *Plasmodium* species in blood (250a).

Babesiosis

Babesia, an intraerythrocytic protozoan transmitted by ticks, is commonly confused with malaria organisms. *Babesia microti* is endemic along the northeast coast of the United States (253). Several as yet unnamed *Babesia* organisms (WA$_1$, CA$_1$, and MO$_1$) are found in the upper midwest and North Pacific states (238,246,247). Transmission of these organisms also occurs perinatally and by blood transfusion (245,255). *Babesia* organisms typically cause a mild malaria-like syndrome that may be severe in patients who are elderly, immunocompromised, or splenectomized. Exchange transfusions may be required for those with severe disease. Hemolytic anemia and thrombocytopenia are common.

Babesia merozoites resemble the ring forms of plasmodia, particularly *P. falciparum,* but are smaller and often have a central clear vacuole and no evidence of hemozoin pigment, Schüffner stippling, or schizont or gametocyte forms (fig. 10-46). *Babesia* merozoites invade mature erythrocytes and eventually lyse the cells. Para-sitemia commonly involves 1 to 20 percent of erythrocytes. In splenectomized individuals, it may be as high as 85 percent of RBCs (254). The degree of parasitemia may not correlate with the severity of the symptoms.

An infrequent but diagnostic finding is the coalescence of four mature merozoites within an erythrocyte, such that the four chromatin masses form a "Maltese cross." Organisms with three chromatin dots are also unique to *Babesia* organisms as plasmodia have one or two chromatin masses. *Babesia* organisms, unlike plasmodia, may be seen extracellularly. Infection is usually confirmed by the indirect immunofluorescence antibody test (IFAT). Serologic and PCR-based diagnostic tests are available in reference laboratories.

Trypanosomiasis

Two species of trypanosomes are pathogenic in humans: *Trypanosoma cruzi*, the causative agent of American trypanosomiasis (or Chagas disease) and *T. brucei* complex, responsible for African sleeping sickness (or African trypanosomiasis). *T. cruzi* organisms are transmitted to humans by the reduviid bug (kissing bug). Acute Chagas disease should be considered in any individual who has had a recent transfusion in an endemic area (predominantly South and Central America), infants born to *T. cruzi*-infected mothers, or recent residents from an endemic area (239,251,252).

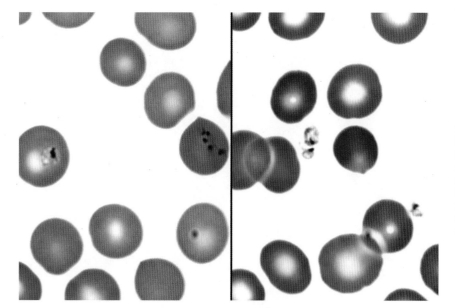

Figure 10-46

BABESIA MICROTI

Intracellular and extracellular ring forms of *Babesia* are present in this peripheral blood film from a 57-year-old man. Multiple rings with four chromatin dots are seen in the erythrocytes (left). Unlike malaria, extraerythrocytic rings with round, ovoid, or pear shapes are also present (right) (Wright stain).

Figure 10-47

TRYPANOSOMIASIS

A peripheral blood smear with extracellular trypomastigotes of *Trypanosomiasis brucei gambiense*. Trypomastigotes typically range from 20 to 30 µm in size and have a C-shape with a central nucleus. A single flagellum originates at one end, near the kinetoplast, and runs along the body of the parasite, extending beyond as a free, thread-like structure. This is enveloped by an undulating membrane (Wright stain).

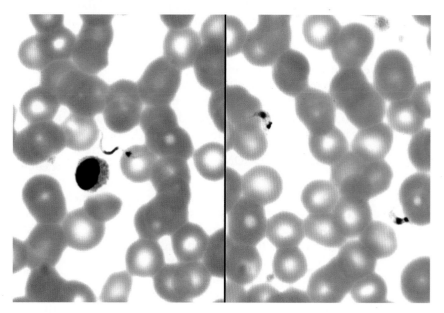

African trypanosomiasis is transmitted primarily by tsetse flies, which reside solely in Africa. *T. brucei* complex includes two morphologically similar trypanosomes that infect humans: *T. brucei gambiense* (rural West Africa) and *T. brucei rhodesiense* (game reserves of East Africa) (237,250). *T. brucei gambiense* infections may be accompanied by a normochromic normocytic anemia, often with brisk reticulocytosis, due to immune-mediated hemolysis (263). Moderate leukocytosis and mild thrombocytopenia may also be observed (262).

In acutely infected patients, the diagnosis can be made by identifying trypomastigotes in peripheral blood or buffy coat specimens (243,259). The trypomastigote forms of *T. cruzi* and *T. brucei* are best characterized by the presence of a single flagellum originating near a kinetoplast (fig. 10-47). *T. cruzi* has a larger kinetoplast than *T. brucei* but is otherwise morphologically similar. *T. brucei* organisms multiply in the blood stream and cause a higher parasitemia than *T. cruzi*. Additional specimens, such as lymph nodes, bone marrow aspirates, and pericardial or cerebrospinal

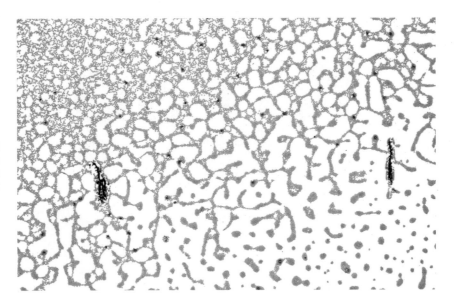

Figure 10-48

FILARIASIS

Two microfilariae are present at the feathered edge of this peripheral blood smear from a patient infected by *Loa loa* (Wright stain).

fluid, may be required to make the diagnosis in immunocompromised individuals. Methods for the PCR detection of trypanosome DNA are also available (232).

Effective treatment options are limited for patients with trypanosomiasis, but with the recent publication of *T. brucei* and *T. cruzi* genome sequences, the development of targeted drugs and vaccines is expected (233,240,256).

HELMINTH INFECTIONS

Filariasis

Filariae are tissue dwelling roundworms (nematodes) with a complex life cycle that includes the transmission of larval forms to humans through mosquito or fly bites (271). Mature worms of three species pathogenic to humans produce circulating microfilariae that are observable in the peripheral blood: *Wuchereria bancrofti* (tropics and subtropics), *Brugia malayi* (South Asia), and *Loa loa* (Central and West Africa) (269). The first two parasites cause lymphadenitis, lymphatic obstruction, and, more rarely, elephantiasis (267). *L. Loa* infection produces eosinophilia and transient subcutaneous swellings (Calabar swellings). Although the number of circulating microfilariae is often low, the diagnosis is most easily accomplished by the identification of these organisms in peripheral blood. Fingerstick specimens provide a greater yield of microfilariae than peripheral venipunctures, while midnight blood draws are necessary to collect the nocturnally

circulating *W. bancrofti* and *B. malayi*. When smears are negative for organisms, a concentration method should be used (268).

Microfilariae are large ribbon-like structures (175 to 300 µm in length) that are best seen along the lateral edges of smears (fig. 10-48) (270). Pathogenic microfilariae can be differentiated from nonpathogenic forms by the presence of an outer sheath that extends beyond the ends of the organisms. This sheath may be difficult to detect in Giemsa-stained smears, except as a negative image, and speciation then relies on the placement of nuclei in the tail (268). The tip of the tail contains a continuous column of nuclei in *L. loa*; two isolated nuclei in *B. malayi*; and no nuclei in *W. bancrofti* (fig. 10-49).

EMERGING INFECTIONS

This section focuses on two infections that have recently appeared and result in significant morbidity and mortality in humans.

Hantavirus Pulmonary Syndrome

Hantavirus pulmonary syndrome (HPS), also termed *hantavirus cardiopulmonary syndrome*, is one of the most lethal of acute human viral infections. The causal agent of HPS, discovered in 1993 during an outbreak in the southwestern United States, is Sin Nombre virus (SNV) (277). The deer mouse (*Peromyscus maniculatus*) is the primary reservoir of this previously unknown hantavirus, seen throughout North and South America. As of 2002, HPS has been confirmed

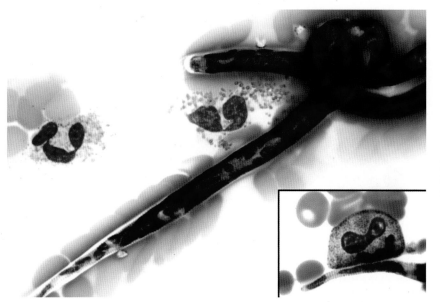

Figure 10-49

FILARIASIS

Two high-power views of *Loa loa* tails (sheathed microfilaria) show nuclei extending to the tips of the tails (Wright stain).

in 31 states in the United States, with a case fatality rate of 33 to 60 percent (279).

Human SNV infection occurs via the inhalation of contaminated aerosols of rodent urine, feces, or saliva (283). An initial viral prodrome with nonspecific clinical symptoms lasts for 2 to 10 days. The antiviral immune response adversely affects endothelial cells of the pulmonary microvasculature, spleen, and lymph nodes. Clinical deterioration is abrupt, with lung capillary leakage, pulmonary edema, and cardiogenic shock (273,286). In fatal cases, cardiogenic shock causes death within 3 days after the onset of respiratory symptoms. As intensive care management with possible utilization of extracorporeal membrane oxygenation (ECMO) constitutes the primary treatment for this infectious disease, prompt identification of the infection is critical to the prevention of rapidly fulminant disease (275).

The complete blood count (CBC) and peripheral blood smear findings are important screening tools for presumptive HPS (278,281). Lymphocytes are usually normal or decreased in number, although this may vary. Thrombocytopenia is an early and consistent abnormality, while elevation of the hematocrit indicates capillary leakage and hemoconcentration. These hematologic findings lack specificity individually, but together with a mildly to moderately left-shifted granulocytosis, absence of significant toxic granulation, and increase in immunoblasts/plasma cells, impart a high index of

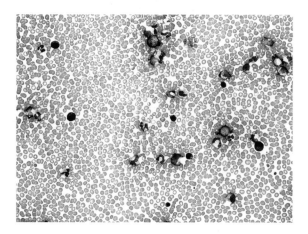

Figure 10-50

HANTAVIRUS PULMONARY SYNDROME

A peripheral blood smear from an older woman with fatal hantavirus pulmonary syndrome. A scanning view shows hemoconcentration, a granulocytic left shift, immunoblasts, and circulating normoblasts (Wright stain).

suspicion for SNV infection (figs. 10-50–10-52) (281). The identification of at least four of the five criteria listed in Table 10-6, in the presence of radiographic diffuse pulmonary infiltrates, provides a sensitivity of 96 percent and specificity of 99 percent for HPS. However, confirmation of SNV infection should be made using a more definitive test, such as an IgM-detecting enzyme-linked immunosorbent assay or reverse transcriptase (RT)-PCR (280).

357

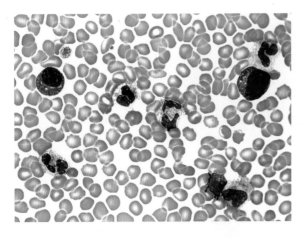

Figure 10-51

HANTAVIRUS PULMONARY SYNDROME

Higher magnification of figure 10-50 shows that the neutrophilic cells do not have significant toxic changes. Two large immunoblasts have deeply basophilic cytoplasm. The immunoblasts (T cell and B cell) are often more numerous along the feathered and lateral edges of the smear (Wright stain).

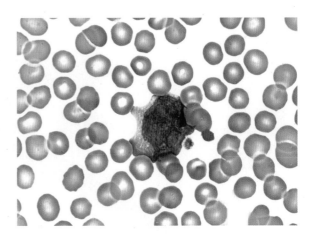

Figure 10-52

HANTAVIRUS PULMONARY SYNDROME

Immunoblasts are large cells (15 to 25 μm) with moderately abundant, often deeply basophilic cytoplasm. They have a large reticular nucleus that contains variably prominent nucleoli. Circulating plasmacytoid cells have the same clinical significance as immunoblasts in hantavirus pulmonary syndrome (Wright stain).

Table 10-6

FIVE CRITERIA PREDICTIVE OF HANTAVIRUS CARDIOPULMONARY SYNDROME[a,b]

Criteria	Interpretation
Increased hematocrit	Yes = >50% for males, >48% for females
Left shift of granulocytes	Yes = myelocytes present
Absence of moderate or severe toxic changes in granulocytes	Yes = absence of toxic granulation or minimal change in a minority of neutrophils No = prominent toxic granulation and Döhle bodies with variable vacuolization in the majority of neutrophils
Thrombocytopenia	Yes = platelet count <150,000/μL
Increased immunoblasts or plasma cells	Yes = >10% of total lymphocyte count

[a]Data from reference 281.
[b]Cases fulfilling four of five criteria have a positive predictive value of approximately 83% and a negative predictive value of 99.8% in high prevalence areas. The positive predictive value is lower in areas of low Sin Nombre virus (SNV) prevalence. Requires serologic confirmation. All cases fulfilling five of five criteria have positive confirmed serology to date.

Evaluation of serial platelet counts helps in the differential diagnosis of HPS as these patients show a more significant platelet decline (more than 20,000/μL per 12-hour period) than observed with other infections of possible consideration (plaque, tularemia, brucellosis, or Rocky Mountain spotted fever). In the prodromal phase, the blood findings may be subtle, and if at least four of the five criteria listed in Table 10-6 are not met in a patient exposed to SNV, a repeat CBC with morphologic review every 4 hours generally clarifies the diagnosis.

Severe Acute Respiratory Syndrome

A new disease, *severe acute respiratory syndrome* (SARS), first presented in November 2002 in China, spread to Hong Kong in February 2003, and was followed by a global outbreak that ended in July 2003 (282,285). A novel coronavirus (SARS-CoV) was discovered to be responsible for the disease which resulted in 774 deaths (276,288). Morbidity and mortality from infection was greater with increasing age; no deaths occurred among patients in the 0 to 24 year age range.

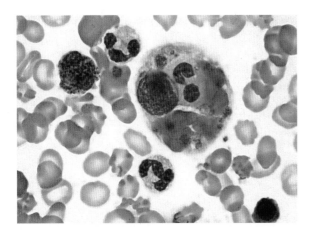

Figure 10-53

HEMOPHAGOCYTIC SYNDROME

A bone marrow aspirate smear shows a macrophage ingesting red blood cells, neutrophils, and platelets in a patient with an infection-associated hemophagocytic syndrome (Wright stain).

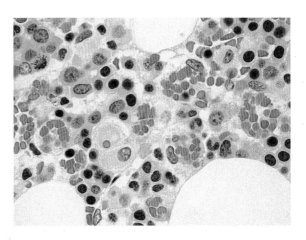

Figure 10-54

HEMOPHAGOCYTIC SYNDROME

Macrophages filled with red blood cells are prominent in the bone marrow biopsy section from the same patient as in figure 10-53 (H&E stain).

The symptoms are nonspecific: high fever, lower respiratory tract symptoms, and malaise (272). Greater than 50 percent of patients have initial neutrophilia (over 4,000/μL) with a subsequent drop in WBC counts due to a marked decreased in CD4- and CD8-positive T cells and NK cells (274,284). A moderate lymphopenia occurs in 70 to 98 percent of patients during the course of the disease (274,282,287). A unique finding for a viral infection is the absence of reactive-appearing lymphocytes.

INFECTION-ASSOCIATED HEMOPHAGOCYTIC SYNDROME

Hemophagocytic syndrome (HPS) may occur as a primary/familial disorder or as a secondary/reactive disorder due to a variety of infections, neoplasms, or collagen vascular disease (also see chapter 9) (289,293,302). Children and adults with secondary HPS develop an acute illness with fever, hepatosplenomegaly, cytopenias effecting two or more lineages, hypertriglyceridemia, and hypofibrinogenemia (291). Anemia is the most common cytopenia observed (80 percent) with approximately half of the patients having leukopenia or thrombocytopenia.

The bone marrow is commonly hypercellular with a striking histocytic proliferation. The histocytes show evidence of active phagocytosis of cells in the erythroid and granulocytic lineages,

and less frequently, platelets (fig. 10-53) (292). The hemophagocytosis is usually evident in both the bone marrow aspirate smears and biopsy sections (fig. 10-54). This may be accompanied by myeloid hyperplasia with possible disruption of maturation, an interstitial T-cell infiltrate, and erythroid hypoplasia. While the hemophagocytosis is usually obvious, determining the underlying condition that causes the HPS (infectious versus neoplastic) is problematic. Individuals with an underlying neoplasm may have similar bone marrow findings to those with an infectious process, even in the absence of bone marrow involvement by the neoplasm.

Infection-associated HPS is generally of viral etiology, particularly EBV, but also occurs secondary to a variety of bacterial and parasitic infections (see Table 10-1) (289,291,294,296–298,301). EBV-associated HPS includes two distinct disease entities: 1) patients with *X-linked lymphoproliferative* (XLP) *disorder* and 2) sporadic cases with *hemophagocytic lymphohistiocytosis* (HLH). Both are caused by an abnormal T-cell immune response to EBV-infected cells. Patients with XLP tend to be young boys with mutations of the *SAP/SH2D1A* gene that encodes a signaling activation molecule–associated protein (SAP) (300). A nonfunctioning SAP protein leads to abnormal T-cell activation and enhanced Th1 cytokine production in response to EBV-infected B cells. Other gene mutations, such as for the X-linked inhibitor of apoptosis, *XIAP*, are being discovered (296a). Patients with HLH do not have an underlying genetic abnormality or gender bias; EBV directly infects T cells and NK cells rather than B cells as in XLP. EBV latent membrane protein (LMP-1) mediates signaling in infected T cells, reduces *SAP* gene expression, and upregulates Th1 cytokines, causing T-cell

activation through a mechanism similar to that seen with XLP (290).

The XLP patients who survive infectious mononucleosis develop dysgammaglobulinemia and lymphomas (299). Rare presentations of XLP have been reported in adults, and in association with aplastic anemia or lymphocytic vasculitis (295).

REFERENCES

General Concepts

1. Berrouane Y, Bisiau H, Le Baron F, Cattoen C, Duthilleul P, Dei Cas E. Candida albicans blastoconidia in peripheral blood smears from non-neutropenic surgical patients. J Clin Pathol 1998;51:537-8.
2. Chao TY, Kuo CC, Hseuh EJ, Yang YF, Wang CC. Diagnosis of fungemia in bone marrow transplantation patients by examination of peripheral blood smears. Bone Marrow Transplant 1994;14:647-9.
3. Mesa H, Pambuccian S, Ferrieri P, et al. A case of systemic histoplasmosis diagnosed in a peripheral blood smear. Br J Haematol 2004;127:241.
4. Monihan JM, Jewell TW, Weir GT. Candida parapsilosis diagnosed by peripheral blood smear. Arch Pathol Lab Med 1986;110:1180-1.
5. Supparatpinyo K, Sirisanthana T. Disseminated Penicillium marneffei infection diagnosed on examination of a peripheral blood smear of a patient with human immunodeficiency virus infection. Clin Infect Dis 1994;18:246-7.
6. Weijmer MC, Debets-Ossenkopp YJ, Van De Vondervoort FJ, ter Wee PM. Superior antimicrobial activity of trisodium citrate over heparin for catheter locking. Nephrol Dial Transplant 2002;17:2189-95.
7. Yagupsky P, Moses S. Neonatal Borrelia species infection (relapsing fever). Am J Dis Child 1985;139:74-6.
8. Yao JD, Arkin CF, Doweiko JP, Hammer SM. Disseminated cryptococcosis diagnosed on peripheral blood smear in a patient with acquired immunodeficiency syndrome. Am J Med 1990;89:100-2.

Bone Marrow Granulomas in Infectious Diseases

9. al-Eissa YA, Assuhaimi SA, al-Fawaz IM, Higgy KE, al-Nasser MN, al-Mobaireek KF. Pancytopenia in children with brucellosis: clinical

manifestations and bone marrow findings. Acta Haematol 1993;89:132-6.
10. Bhargava V, Farhi DC. Bone marrow granulomas: clinicopathologic findings in 72 cases and review of the literature. Hematol Pathol 1988;2:43-50.
11. Blair JE, Smilack JD, Caples SM. Coccidioidomycosis in patients with hematologic malignancies. Arch Intern Med 2005;165:113-7.
12. Bodem CR, Hamory BH, Taylor HM, Kleopfer L. Granulomatous bone marrow disease. A review of the literature and clinicopathologic analysis of 58 cases. Medicine (Baltimore). 1983;62:372-83.
13. Davies SF, McKenna RW, Sarosi GA. Trephine biopsy of the bone marrow in disseminated histoplasmosis. Am J Med 1979;67:617-22.
14. Dunn P, Kuo MC, Sun CF. Pseudo-Gaucher cells in mycobacterial infection: a report of two cases. J Clin Pathol 2005;58:1113-4.
15. Eid A, Carion W, Nystrom JS. Differential diagnoses of bone marrow granuloma. West J Med 1996;164:510-5.
15a. Fernandez AB. An unusual case of autoimmune hemolytic anemia in treatment naive hepatitis C virus infection. Hematology 2006;11:385-7.
16. Fox BC, Ross DD, Huang AB, Gabrielson EW, Furth PA. Mycobacterial disease associated with aplastic anaemia. J Infect 1989;19:157-65.
17. Gascon P, Sathe SS, Rameshwar P. Impaired erythropoiesis in the acquired immunodeficiency syndrome with disseminated Mycobacterium avium complex. Am J Med 1993;94:41-8.
18. Hufnagel M, Niemeyer C, Zimmerhackl LB, Tuchelmann T, Sauter S, Brandis M. Hemophagocytosis: a complication of acute Q fever in a child. Clin Infect Dis 1995;21:1029-31.
19. Jagadha V, Andavolu RH, Huang CT. Granulomatous inflammation in the acquired immune deficiency syndrome. Am J Clin Pathol 1985;84:598-602.

20. Johnson BE, Lynch SR, Park CH. Myelosuppression in Legionnaires' disease. Arch Intern Med 1982;142:1377-8.
21. Karakukcu M, Patiroglu T, Ozdemir MA, Gunes T, Gumus H, Karakukcu C. Pancytopenia, a rare hematologic manifestation of brucellosis in children. J Pediatr Hematol Oncol 2004;26:803-6.
22. Ko YC, Lee CT, Cheng YF, et al. Hypercalcaemia and haemophagocytic syndrome: rare concurrent presentations of disseminated tuberculosis in a dialysis patient. Int J Clin Pract 2004;58:723-5.
23. Krober SM, Kaiserling E, Horny HP, Weber A. Primary diagnosis of Whipple's disease in bone marrow. Hum Pathol 2004;35:522-5.
24. Kvasnicka HM, Thiele J, Ahmadi T. Bone marrow manifestation of Lyme disease (Lyme Borreliosis). Br J Haematol 2003;120:723.
25. Lobdell DH. 'Ring' granulomas in cytomegalovirus hepatitis. Arch Pathol Lab Med 1987;111:881-2.
26. Lu J, Basu A, Melenhorst JJ, Young NS, Brown KE. Analysis of T-cell repertoire in hepatitis-associated aplastic anemia. Blood 2004;103:4588-93.
27. Mahrous S, Abdel-Monem A, Mangoud A, et al. Haematologial manifestations in HCV infected patients at Sharkia Governerate, Egypt. J Egypt Soc Parasitol 2004;34:417-28.
28. Mert A, Tabak F, Ozaras R, Ozturk R, Aki H, Aktuglu Y. Typhoid fever as a rare cause of hepatic, splenic, and bone marrow granulomas. Intern Med 2004;43:436-9.
29. Most J, Spotl L, Mayr G, Gasser A, Sarti A, Dierich MP. Formation of multinucleated giant cells in vitro is dependent on the stage of monocyte to macrophage maturation. Blood 1997;89:662-71.
30. Nichols L, Florentine B, Lewis W, Sattler F, Rarick MU, Brynes RK. Bone marrow examination for the diagnosis of mycobacterial and fungal infections in the acquired immunodeficiency syndrome. Arch Pathol Lab Med 1991;115:1125-32.
31. Numata K, Tsutsumi H, Wakai S, Tachi N, Chiba S. A child case of haemophagocytic syndrome associated with cryptococcal meningoencephalitis. J Infect 1998;36:118-9.
32. Ozyurek E, Ozcay F, Yilmaz B, et al. Hemophagocytic lymphohistiocytosis associated with visceral leishmaniasis: a case report. Pediatr Hematol Oncol 2005;22:409-14.
33. Pantanowitz L, Omar T, Sonnendecker H, Karstaedt AS. Bone marrow cryptococcal infection in the acquired immunodeficiency syndrome. J Infect 2000;41:92-4.
34. Pappas G, Kitsanou M, Christou L, Tsianos E. Immune thrombocytopenia attributed to brucellosis and other mechanisms of Brucella-induced thrombocytopenia. Am J Hematol 2004;75:139-41.
35. Paydas S, Ergin M, Baslamisli F, et al. Bone marrow necrosis: clinicopathologic analysis of 20 cases and review of the literature. Am J Hematol 2002;70:300-5.
36. Rocha Filho FD, Ferreira FV, Mendes Fde O, et al. Bone marrow fibrosis (pseudo-myelofibrosis) in human kala-azar. Rev Soc Bras Med Trop 2000;33:363-6.
37. Sen R, Sehgal PK, Dixit V, et al. Lipid-laden macrophages in bone marrow of leprosy patients. Lepr Rev 1991;62:374-80.
38. Sheikha A. Dyserythropoiesis in 105 patients with visceral leishmaniasis. Lab Hematol 2004;10:206-11.
39. Shin BM, Paik IK, Cho HI. Bone marrow pathology of culture proven typhoid fever. J Korean Med Sci 1994;9:57-63.
40. Singh KJ, Ahluwalia G, Sharma SK, Saxena R, Chaudhary VP, Anat M. Significance of haematological manifestations in patients with tuberculosis. J Assoc Physicians India 2001;49:788, 790-4.
41. Srigley JR, Vellend H, Palmer N, et al. Q-fever. The liver and bone marrow pathology. Am J Surg Pathol 1985;9:752-8.
42. Suster S, Cabello-Inchausti B, Robinson MJ. Nongranulomatous involvement of the bone marrow in lepromatous leprosy. Am J Clin Pathol 1989;92:797-801.
43. Tanoli ZM, Rai ME, Gandapur AS. Clinical presentation and management of visceral leishmaniasis. J Ayub Med Coll Abbottabad 2005;17:51-3.
44. Travis LB, Travis WD, Li CY, Pierre RV. Q fever. A clinicopathologic study of five cases. Arch Pathol Lab Med 1986;110:1017-20.
45. Vilalta-Castel E, Valdes-Sanchez MD, Guerra-Vales JM, et al. Significance of granulomas in bone marrow: a study of 40 cases. Eur J Haematol 1988;41:12-6.
46. Wain J, Pham VB, Ha V, et al. Quantitation of bacteria in bone marrow from patients with typhoid fever: relationship between counts and clinical features. J Clin Microbiol 2001;39:1571-6.
47. Wiley EL, Perry A, Nightingale SD, Lawrence J. Detection of Mycobacterium avium-intracellulare complex in bone marrow specimens of patients with acquired immunodeficiency syndrome. Am J Clin Pathol 1994;101:446-51.
48. Wong KF, Ma SK, Chan JK, Lam KW. Acquired immunodeficiency syndrome presenting as marrow cryptococcosis. Am J Hematol 1993;42:392-4.
49. Yarali N, Fisgin T, Duru F, Kara A. Myelodysplastic features in visceral leishmaniasis. Am J Hematol 2002;71:191-5.
50. Yildirmak Y, Palanduz A, Telhan L, Arapoglu M, Kayaalp N. Bone marrow hypoplasia during Brucella infection. J Pediatr Hematol Oncol 2003;25:63-4.

Fungal Infections Associated with Immunosuppression

51. Baddley JW, Stroud TP, Salzman D, Pappas PG. Invasive mold infections in allogeneic bone marrow transplant recipients. Clin Infect Dis 2001;32:1319-24.

52. Kontoyiannis DP, Wessel VC, Bodey GP, Rolston KV. Zygomycosis in the 1990s in a tertiary-care cancer center. Clin Infect Dis 2000;30:851-6.

53. Marr KA, Patterson T, Denning D. Aspergillosis. Pathogenesis, clinical manifestations, and therapy. Infect Dis Clin North Am 2002;16:875-94, vi.

54. Myers A, Clark J, Foster H. Tuberculosis and treatment with infliximab. N Engl J Med 2002;346:623-6.

55. Procop GW, Roberts GD. Emerging fungal diseases: the importance of the host. Clin Lab Med 2004;24:691-719, vi-vii.

56. Singh N, Husain S. Aspergillus infections after lung transplantation: clinical differences in type of transplant and implications for management. J Heart Lung Transplant 2003;22:258-66.

57. Walsh TJ, Groll A, Hiemenz J, Fleming R, Roilides E, Anaissie E. Infections due to emerging and uncommon medically important fungal pathogens. Clin Microbiol Infect 2004;10(Suppl 1):48-66.

58. Warris A, Bjorneklett A, Gaustad P. Invasive pulmonary aspergillosis associated with infliximab therapy. N Engl J Med 2001;344:1099-100.

59. Wood KL, Hage CA, Knox KS, et al. Histoplasmosis after treatment with anti-tumor necrosis factor-alpha therapy. Am J Respir Crit Care Med 2003;167:1279-82.

AIDS

60. AIDS epidemic update 2006. Available at: www.unaids.org/enHIV_data/2006GlobalReport.

61. Bain BJ. The haematological features of HIV infection. Br J Haematol 1997;99:1-8.

62. Eltom MA, Jemal A, Mbulaiteye SM, Devesa SS, Biggar RJ. Trends in Kaposi's sarcoma and non-Hodgkin's lymphoma incidence in the United States from 1973 through 1998. J Natl Cancer Inst 2002;94:1204-10.

63. Gottlieb MS, Schroff R, Schanker HM, et al. Pneumocystis carinii pneumonia and mucosal candidiasis in previously healthy homosexual men: evidence of a new acquired cellular immunodeficiency. N Engl J Med 1981;305:1425-31.

64. Krentz HB, Kliewer G, Gill MJ. Changing mortality rates and causes of death for HIV-infected individuals living in Southern Alberta, Canada from 1984 to 2003. HIV Med 2005;6:99-106.

65. Mbulaiteye SM, Parkin DM, Rabkin CS. Epidemiology of AIDS-related malignancies an international perspective. Hematol Oncol Clin North Am 2003;17:673-96, v.

66. Steeper TA, Horwitz CA, Hanson M, et al. Heterophil-negative mononucleosis-like illnesses with atypical lymphocytosis in patients undergoing seroconversions to the human immunodeficiency virus. Am J Clin Pathol 1988;90:169-74.

67. Yeni PG, Hammer SM, Carpenter CC, et al. Antiretroviral treatment for adult HIV infection in 2002: updated recommendations of the International AIDS Society-USA Panel. JAMA 2002;288:222-35.

68. Yue FY, Kovacs CM, Dimayuga RC, et al. Preferential apoptosis of HIV-1-specific CD4+ T cells. J Immunol 2005;174:2196-204.

Peripheral Blood and Bone Marrow Findings in Patients with AIDS

69. Adetifa IM, Temiye EO, Akinsulie AO, Ezeaka VC, Iroha EO. Haematological abnormalities associated with paediatric HIV/AIDS in Lagos. Ann Trop Paediatr 2006;26:121-5.

70. Akpek G, Lee SM, Gagnon DR, Cooley TP, Wright DG. Bone marrow aspiration, biopsy, and culture in the evaluation of HIV-infected patients for invasive mycobacteria and histoplasma infections. Am J Hematol 2001;67:100-6.

71. Bain BJ. The haematological features of HIV infection. Br J Haematol 1997;99:1-8.

72. Godwin JH. Howell-Jolly body-like inclusions. Am J Clin Pathol 1994;102:389-90.

73. Gordon S, Lee S. Naked megakaryocyte nuclei in bone marrows of patients with acquired immunodeficiency syndrome: a somewhat specific finding. Mod Pathol 1994;7:166-8.

74. Harbol AW, Liesveld JL, Simpson-Haidaris PJ, Abboud CN. Mechanisms of cytopenia in human immunodeficiency virus infection. Blood Rev 1994;8:241-51.

75. Harris CE, Biggs JC, Concannon AJ, Dodds AJ. Peripheral blood and bone marrow findings in patients with acquired immune deficiency syndrome. Pathology 1990;22:206-11.

76. Isgro A, Aiuti A, Leti W, et al. Immunodysregulation of HIV disease at bone marrow level. Autoimmun Rev 2005;4:486-90.

77. Kahwash E, Gewirtz AS. Howell-Jolly body-like inclusions in neutrophils. Arch Pathol Lab Med 2003;127:1389-90.

78. Karcher DS, Frost AR. The bone marrow in human immunodeficiency virus (HIV)-related disease. Morphology and clinical correlation. Am J Clin Pathol 1991;95:63-71.

79. Karpatkin S, Nardi M, Green D. Platelet and coagulation defects associated with HIV-1-infection. Thromb Haemost 2002;88:389-401.

80. Keiser P, Rademacher S, Smith JW. Utility of bone marrow culture and biopsy in the diagnosis of disseminated infections in AIDS. Am J Hematol 1997;56:1-4.

81. Ker CC, Hung CC, Huang SY, et al. Comparison of bone marrow studies with blood culture for etiological diagnosis of disseminated mycobacterial and fungal infection in patients with acquired immunodeficiency syndrome. J Microbiol Immunol Infect 2002;35:89-93.

82. Khandekar MM, Deshmukh SD, Holla VV, et al. Profile of bone marrow examination in HIV/AIDS patients to detect opportunistic infections, especially tuberculosis. Indian J Pathol Microbiol 2005;48:7-12.

83. Kilby JM, Marques MB, Jaye DL, Tabereaux PB, Reddy VB, Waites KB. The yield of bone marrow biopsy and culture compared with blood culture in the evaluation of HIV-infected patients for mycobacterial and fungal infections. Am J Med 1998;104:123-8.

84. Koefoed K, Ditzel HJ. Identification of talin head domain as an immunodominant epitope of the antiplatelet antibody response in patients with HIV-1-associated thrombocytopenia. Blood 2004;104:4054-62.

85. Llewelyn MJ, Noursedeghi M, Dogan A, Edwards SG, Miller RF. Diagnostic utility of bone marrow sampling in HIV-infected patients since the advent of highly active antiretroviral therapy. Int J STD AIDS 2005;16:686-90.

86. Marche C, Tabbara W, Michon C, Clair B, Bricaire F, Matthiessen L. Bone marrow findings in HIV infection: a pathological study. Prog AIDS Pathol 1990;2:51-60.

87. Mocroft A, Kirk O, Barton SE, et al. Anaemia is an independent predictive marker for clinical prognosis in HIV-infected patients from across Europe. EuroSIDA study group. AIDS 1999;13:943-50.

88. Moore RD. Schistocytosis and a thrombotic microangiopathy-like syndrome in hospitalized HIV-infected patients. Am J Hematol 1999;60:116-20.

89. Moore RD. Anemia and human immunodeficiency virus disease in the era of highly active antiretroviral therapy. Semin Hematol 2000;37(Suppl 6):18-23.

90. O'Malley DP, Sen J, Juliar BE, Orazi A. Evaluation of stroma in human immunodeficiency virus/acquired immunodeficiency syndrome-affected bone marrows and correlation with CD4 counts. Arch Pathol Lab Med 2005;129:1137-40.

91. Sato T, Sekine H, Kakuda H, Miura N, Sunohara M, Fuse A. HIV infection of megakaryocytic cell lines. Leuk Lymphoma 2000;36:397-404.

92. Scaradavou A. HIV-related thrombocytopenia. Blood Rev 2002;16:73-6.

93. Schneider DR, Picker LJ. Myelodysplasia in the acquired immune deficiency syndrome. Am J Clin Pathol 1985;84:144-52.

94. Servais J, Nkoghe D, Schmit JC, et al. HIV-associated hematologic disorders are correlated with plasma viral load and improve under highly active antiretroviral therapy. J Acquir Immune Defic Syndr 2001;28:221-5.

95. Slagel DD, Lager DJ, Dick FR. Howell-Jolly body-like inclusions in the neutrophils of patients with acquired immunodeficiency syndrome. Am J Clin Pathol 1994;101:429-31.

96. Sloand E. Hematologic complications of HIV infection. AIDS Rev 2005;7:187-96.

97. Tanaka PY, Hadad DJ, Barletti SC, de Souza SA, Calore EE. Bone marrow biopsy in the diagnosis of infectious and non-infectious causes in patients with advanced HIV infection. J Infect 2007'54:362-6.

98. Tripathi AK, Misra R, Kalra P, Gupta N, Ahmad R. Bone marrow abnormalities in HIV disease. J Assoc Physicians India 2005;53:705-10.

99. Zhao X, Sun NC, Witt MD, Keller M, Niihara Y. Changing pattern of AIDS: a bone marrow study. Am J Clin Pathol 2004;121:393-401.

Opportunistic Infections Associated with AIDS

100. Escobedo-Jaimes L, Cicero-Sabido R, Criales-Cortez JL, et al. Evaluation of the polymerase chain reaction in the diagnosis of miliary tuberculosis in bone marrow smear. Int J Tuberc Lung Dis 2003;7:580-6.

101. Hussong J, Peterson LR, Warren JR, Peterson LC. Detecting disseminated Mycobacterium avium complex infections in HIV-positive patients. The usefulness of bone marrow trephine biopsy specimens, aspirate cultures, and blood cultures. Am J Clin Pathol 1998;110:806-9.

102. Keiser P, Rademacher S, Smith JW. Utility of bone marrow culture and biopsy in the diagnosis of disseminated infections in AIDS. Am J Hematol 1997;56:1-4.

103. Koduri PR, Chundi V, DeMarais P, Mizock BA, Patel AR, Weinstein RA. Reactive hemophagocytic syndrome: a new presentation of disseminated histoplasmosis in patients with AIDS. Clin Infect Dis 1995;21:1463-5.

104. Kurtin PJ, McKinsey DS, Gupta MR, Driks M. Histoplasmosis in patients with acquired immunodeficiency syndrome. Hematologic and bone marrow manifestations. Am J Clin Pathol 1990;93:367-72.

105. Luther JM, Lakey DL, Larson RS, et al. Utility of bone marrow biopsy for rapid diagnosis of febrile illnesses in patients with human immunodeficiency virus infection. South Med J 2000;93:692-7.

106. Marques MB, Waites KB, Jaye DL, Kilby JM, Reddy VV. Histologic examination of bone marrow core biopsy specimens has limited value in the diagnosis of mycobacterial and fungal infections in patients with the acquired immunodeficiency syndrome. Ann Diagn Pathol 2000;4:1-6.

107. Mert A, Bilir M, Tabak F, et al. Miliary tuberculosis: clinical manifestations, diagnosis and outcome in 38 adults. Respirology 2001;6:217-24.

108. Monihan JM, Jewell TW, Weir GT. Candida parapsilosis diagnosed by peripheral blood smear. Arch Pathol Lab Med 1986;110:1180-1.

109. Nichols L, Florentine B, Lewis W, Sattler F, Rarick MU, Brynes RK. Bone marrow examination for the diagnosis of mycobacterial and fungal infections in the acquired immunodeficiency syndrome. Arch Pathol Lab Med 1991;115:1125-32.

110. Pasquau F, Ena J, Sanchez R, et al. Leishmaniasis as an opportunistic infection in HIV-infected patients: determinants of relapse and mortality in a collaborative study of 228 episodes in a Mediterreanean region. Eur J Clin Microbiol Infect Dis 2005;24:411-8.

111. Supparatpinyo K, Sirisanthana T. Disseminated Penicillium marneffei infection diagnosed on examination of a peripheral blood smear of a patient with human immunodeficiency virus infection. Clin Infect Dis 1994;18:246-7.

112. Yao JD, Arkin CF, Doweiko JP, Hammer SM. Disseminated cryptococcosis diagnosed on peripheral blood smear in a patient with acquired immunodeficiency syndrome. Am J Med 1990;89:100-2.

113. Zhao X, Sun NC, Witt MD, Keller M, Niihara Y. Changing pattern of AIDS: a bone marrow study. Am J Clin Pathol 2004;121:393-401.

HHV8-Associated Multicentric Castleman Disease

114. Bacon CM, Miller RF, Noursadeghi M, McNamara C, Du MQ, Dogan A. Pathology of bone marrow in human herpes virus-8 (HHV8)-associated multicentric Castleman disease. Br J Haematol 2004;127:585-91.

115. Malnati MS, Dagna L, Ponzoni M, Lusso P. Human herpesvirus 8 (HHV-8/KSHV) and hematologic malignancies. Rev Clin Exp Hematol 2003;7:375-405.

116. Oksenhendler E, Boulanger E, Galicier L, et al. High incidence of Kaposi sarcoma-associated herpesvirus-related non-Hodgkin lymphoma in patients with HIV infection and multicentric Castleman disease. Blood 2002;99:2331-6.

Infectious Mononucleosis (Epstein-Barr Virus)

117. Carter RL. Platelet levels in infectious mononucleosis. Blood 1965;25:817-21.

118. Chuang HC, Lay JD, Hsieh WC, et al. Epstein-Barr virus LMP1 inhibits the expression of SAP gene and upregulates Th1 cytokines in the pathogenesis of hemophagocytic syndrome. Blood 2005;106:3090-6.

119. Cohen JI. Epstein-Barr virus infection. N Engl J Med 2000;343:481-92.

120. Downey H, McKinlay C. Acute lymphadenosis compared with acute lymphatic leukemia. Arch Intern Med 1923;32:82-112.

121. Engel P, Eck MJ, Terhorst C. The SAP and SLAM families in immune responses and X-linked lymphoproliferative disease. Nat Rev Immunol 2003;3:813-21.

122. Eriksson KF, Holmberg L, Bergstrand CG. Infectious mononucleosis and agranulocytosis. Scand J Infect Dis 1979;11:307-9.

123. Hall A. A case resembling acute lymphatic leukaemia, ending in complete recovery. Proc R Soc Med 1915;8:15-9.

124. Hermann J, Demel U, Stunzner D, Daghofer E, Tilz G, Graninger W. Clinical interpretation of antineutrophil cytoplasmic antibodies: parvovirus B19 infection as a pitfall. Ann Rheum Dis 2005;64:641-3.

125. Herrmann K, Niedobitek G. Epstein-Barr virus-associated carcinomas: facts and fiction. J Pathol 2003;199:140-5.

126. Hochberg D, Souza T, Catalina M, Sullivan JL, Luzuriaga K, Thorley-Lawson DA. Acute infection with Epstein-Barr virus targets and overwhelms the peripheral memory B-cell compartment with resting, latently infected cells. J Virol 2004;78:5194-204.

127. Horwitz CA, Henle W, Henle G, Schapiro R, Borken S, Bundtzen R. Infectious mononucleosis in patients aged 40 to 72 years: report of 27 cases, including 3 without heterophil-antibody responses. Medicine (Baltimore) 1983;62:256-62.

128. Horwitz CA, Moulds J, Henle W, et al. Cold agglutinins in infectious mononucleosis and heterophil-antibody-negative mononucleosis-like syndromes. Blood 1977;50:195-202.

129. Iishi Y, Kosaka M, Mizuguchi T, et al. Suppression of hematopoiesis by activated T-cells in infectious mononucleosis associated with pancytopenia. Int J Hematol 1991;54:65-73.

130. Karzon DT. Infectious mononucleosis. Adv Pediatr 1976;22:231-65.

131. Krause JR, Kaplan SS. Bone marrow findings in infectious mononucleosis and mononucleosis-like diseases in the older adult. Scand J Haematol 1982;28:15-22.

132. Latour S, Veillette A. Molecular and immunological basis of X-linked lymphoproliferative disease. Immunol Rev 2003;192:212-24.

133. Lukes R, Cox F. Clinical and morphologic findings in 30 fatal cases of infectious mononucleosis. Am J Pathol 1958;34:586.

134. Macsween KF, Crawford DH. Epstein-Barr virus—recent advances. Lancet Infect Dis 2003;3:131-40.

135. Precopio ML, Sullivan JL, Willard C, Somasundaran M, Luzurlaga K. Differential kinetics and specificity of EBV-specific CD4+ and CD8+ T cells during primary infection. J Immunol 2003;170:2590-8.

136. Rezk SA, Weiss LM. Epstein-Barr virus-associated lymphoproliferative disorders. Hum Pathol 2007;38:1293-304.

137. Rosenfeld SJ, Young NS. Viruses and bone marrow failure. Blood Rev 1991;5:71-7.

138. Schmitz H, Volz D, Krainick-Riechert C, Scherer M. Acute Epstein-Barr virus infections in children. Med Microbiol Immunol (Berl) 1972;158:58-63.

139. Sevilla J, del Carmen Escudero M, Jimenez R, et al. Severe systemic autoimmune disease associated with Epstein-Barr virus infection. J Pediatr Hematol Oncol 2004;26:831-3.

140. Souza TA, Stollar BD, Sullivan JL, Luzuriaga K, Thorley-Lawson DA. Peripheral B cells latently infected with Epstein-Barr virus display molecular hallmarks of classical antigen-selected memory B cells. Proc Natl Acad Sci U S A 2005;102:18093-8.

141. Sprunt T, Evans F. Mononuclear leukocytosis in reaction to acute infections ("infectious mononucleosis"). John Hopkins Hosp Bull 1920;31:410.

142. Sumegi J, Huang D, Lanyi A, et al. Correlation of mutations of the SH2D1A gene and Epstein-Barr virus infection with clinical phenotype and outcome in X-linked lymphoproliferative disease. Blood 2000;96:3118-25.

143. Takada H, Takahata Y, Nomura A, Ohga S, Mizuno Y, Hara T. Increased serum levels of interferon-gamma-inducible protein 10 and monokine induced by gamma interferon in patients with haemophagocytic lymphohistiocytosis. Clin Exp Immunol 2003;133:448-53.

144. Tanaka M, Kamijo T, Koike K, et al. Specific autoantibodies to platelet glycoproteins in Epstein-Barr virus-associated immune thrombocytopenia. Int J Hematol 2003;78:168-70.

145. Thorley-Lawson DA, Gross A. Persistence of the Epstein-Barr virus and the origins of associated lymphomas. N Engl J Med 2004;350:1328-37.

146. Wick MJ, Woronzoff-Dashkoff KP, McGlennen RC. The molecular characterization of fatal infectious mononucleosis. Am J Clin Pathol 2002;117:582-8.

147. Williams H, McAulay K, Macsween KF, et al. The immune response to primary EBV infection: a role for natural killer cells. Br J Haematol 2005;129:266-74.

Infectious Mononucleosis Type Syndromes

148. Akashi K, Eizuru Y, Sumiyoshi Y, et al. Brief report: severe infectious mononucleosis-like syndrome and primary human herpesvirus 6 infection in an adult. N Engl J Med 1993;329:168-71.

149. Crapnell K, Zanjani E, Chaudhuri A, Ascensao JL, St Jear S, Maciejewski JP. In vitro infection of megakaryocytes and their precursors by human cytomegalovirus. Blood 2000;95:487-93.

150. Emery VC. Investigation of CMV disease in immunocompromised patients. J Clin Pathol 2001;54:84-8.

151. Fisgin T, Yarali N, Duru F, Kara A. CMV-induced immune thrombocytopenia and excessive hematogones mimicking an acute B-precursor lymphoblastic leukemia. Leuk Res 2003;27:193-6.

152. Grefte A, van der Giessen M, van Son W, The TH. Circulating cytomegalovirus (CMV)-infected endothelial cells in patients with an active CMV infection. J Infect Dis 1993;167:270-7.

153. Han XY, Lin P, Amin HM, et al. Postsplenectomy cytomegaloviral mononucleosis: marked lymphocytosis, TCRgamma gene rearrangements, and impaired IgM response. Am J Clin Pathol 2005;123:612-7.

154. Harris AI, Meyer RJ, Brody EA. Cytomegalovirus-induced thrombocytopenia and hemolysis in an adult [letter]. Ann Intern Med 1975;83:670-1.

155. Horwitz CA, Henle W, Henle G, et al. Clinical and laboratory evaluation of cytomegalovirus-induced mononucleosis in previously healthy individuals. Report of 82 cases. Medicine (Baltimore) 1986;65:124-34.

156. Janka G, Imashuku S, Elinder G, et al. Infection- and malignancy-associated hemophagocytic syndromes. Secondary hemophagocytic lymphohistiocytosis. Hematol Oncol Clin North Am 1998;12:435-44.

157. Kano Y, Shiohara T. Current understanding of cytomegalovirus infection in immunocompetent individuals. J Dermatol Sci 2000;22:196-204.

158. Kirby MA, Weitzman S, Freedman MH. Juvenile chronic myelogenous leukemia: differentiation from infantile cytomegalovirus infection. Am J Pediatr Hematol Oncol 1990;12:292-6.

159. Klemola E, Kaariainen L, von Essen R, Haltia K, Koivuniemi A, von Bonsdorff CH. Further studies on cytomegalovirus mononucleosis in previously healthy individuals. Acta Med Scand 1967;182:311-22.

160. Kroft SH. Infectious diseases manifested in the peripheral blood. Clin Lab Med 2002;22:253-77.

161. Lesprit P, Scieux C, Lemann M, Carbonelle E, Modai J, Molina JM. Use of the cytomegalovirus (CMV) antigenemia assay for the rapid diagnosis of primary CMV infection in hospitalized adults. Clin Infect Dis 1998;26:646-50.

162. Ljungman P. Risk assessment in haaematopoitic stem cell transplantation: viral status. Best Pract Res Clin Haematol 2007;20:209-17.

163. Magalhaes SM, Duarte FB, Vassallo J, Costa SC, Lorand-Metze I. Multiple lymphoid nodules in bone marrow biopsy in immunocompetent patient with cytomegalovirus infection: an immunohistochemical analysis. Rev Soc Bras Med Trop 2001;34:365-8.

164. Mathew P, Hudnall SD, Elghetany MT, Payne DA. T-gamma gene rearrangement and CMV mononucleosis. Am J Hematol 2001;66:64-6.

165. Mattes FM, McLaughlin JE, Emery VC, Clark DA, Griffiths PD. Histopathological detection of owl's eye inclusions is still specific for cytomegalovirus in the era of human herpesviruses 6 and 7. J Clin Pathol 2000;53:612-4.

166. Mizutani K, Azuma E, Komada Y, et al. An infantile case of cytomegalovirus induced idiopathic thrombocytopenic purpura with predominant proliferation of CD10 positive lymphoblast in bone marrow. Acta Paediatr Jpn 1995;37:71-4.

167. Penchansky L, Krause JR. Identification of cytomegalovirus in bone marrow biopsy. South Med J 1979;72:500-1.

168. Pooley RJ, Peterson L, Finn WG, Kroft SH. Cytomegalovirus-infected cells in routinely prepared peripheral blood films in immunosuppressed patients. Am J Clin Pathol. 1999;112:108-12.

168a. Proceedings from the 5th International Cytomegalovirus Conference. Stockholm, Sweden, May 21-24, 1995. Scand J Infect Dis Suppl 1995;99:1-120.

169. Rasing LA, De Weger RA, Verdonck LF, et al. The value of immunohistochemistry and in situ hybridization in detecting cytomegalovirus in bone marrow transplant recipients. APMIS 1990;98:479-88.

170. Rosenfeld SJ, Young NS. Viruses and bone marrow failure. Blood Rev 1991;5:71-7.

171. Rushin JM, Riordan GP, Heaton RB, Sharpe RW, Cotelingam JD, Jaffe ES. Cytomegalovirus-infected cells express Leu-M1 antigen. A potential source of diagnostic error. Am J Pathol 1990;136:989-95.

172. Sindre H, Tjoonnfjord GE, Rollag H, et al. Human cytomegalovirus suppression of and latency in early hematopoietic progenitor cells. Blood 1996;88:4526-33.

173. Sing GK, Ruscetti FW. Preferential suppression of myelopoiesis in normal human bone marrow cells after in vitro challenge with human cytomegalovirus. Blood 1990;75:1965-73.

174. Steeper TA, Horwitz CA, Hanson M, et al. Heterophil-negative mononucleosis-like illnesses with atypical lymphocytosis in patients undergoing seroconversions to the human immunodeficiency virus. Am J Clin Pathol 1988;90:169-74.

175. Thami GP, Kanwar AJ, Goyal A. Heterophil negative infectious mononucleosis like syndrome due to hepatitis B virus. J Assoc Physicians India 2000;48:921-2.

176. Toyoda H, Ido M, Hori H, et al. A case of juvenile myelomonocytic leukemia with concomitant cytomegalovirus infection. J Pediatr Hematol Oncol 2004;26:606-8.

177. Wreghitt TG, Teare EL, Sule O, Devi R, Rice P. Cytomegalovirus infection in immunocompetent patients. Clin Infect Dis 2003;37:1603-6.

178. Young JF, Goulian M. Bone marrow fibrin ring granulomas and cytomegalovirus infection. Am J Clin Pathol 1993;99:65-8.

Parvovirus Infection

179. Abkowitz J, Brown K, Wood RW, Kovach NL, Green SW, Young NS. Clinical relevance of parvovirus B19 as a cause of anemia in patients with human immunodeficiency virus infection. J Infect Dis 1997;176:269-73.

180. Bertoni E, Rosati A, Zanazzi M, et al. Aplastic anemia due to B19 parvovirus infection in cadaveric renal transplant recipients: an underestimated infectious disease in the immunocompromised host. J Nephrol 1997;10:152-6.

181. Brown KE, Young NS, Alving BM, Barbosa LH. Parvovirus B19: implications for transfusion medicine. Summary of a workshop. Transfusion 2001;41:130-5.

182. Bux J, Behrens G, Jaeger G, Welte K. Diagnosis and clinical course of autoimmune neutropenia in infancy: analysis of 240 cases. Blood 1998;91:181-6.

183. Chisaka H, Morita E, Yaegashi N, Sugamura K. Parvovirus B19 and the pathogenesis of anaemia. Rev Med Virol 2003;13:347-59.

184. Corcoran A, Doyle S. Advances in the biology, diagnosis and host-pathogen interactions of parvovirus B19. J Med Microbiol 2004;53:459-75.

185. Crook T, Rogers BB, McFarland R, et al. Unusual bone marrow manifestations of parvovirus B19 infection in immunocompromised patients. Hum Pathol 2000;31:161-8.

186. Eis-Hubinger AM, Dieck D, Schild R, Hansmann M, Schneweis KE. Parvovirus B19 infection in pregnancy. Intervirology 1998;41:178-84.

187. Heegaard ED, Brown KE. Human parvovirus B19. Clin Microbiol Rev 2002;15:485-505.

188. Heegaard ED, Hasle H, Skibsted L, Bock J, Brown KE. Congenital anemia caused by parvovirus B19 infection. Pediatr Infect Dis J 2000;19:1216-8.

189. Heegaard ED, Rosthoj S, Petersen BL, Nielsen S, Karup Pedersen F, Hornsleth A. Role of parvovirus B19 infection in childhood idiopathic thrombocytopenic purpura. Acta Paediatr 1999;88:614-7.

190. Inoue S, Kinra NK, Mukkamala SR, Gordon R. Parvovirus B-19 infection: aplastic crisis, erythema infectiosum and idiopathic thrombocytopenic purpura. Pediatr Infect Dis J 1991;10:251-3.

191. Kaplan C, Morinet F, Cartron J. Virus-induced autoimmune thrombocytopenia and neutropenia. Semin Hematol 1992;29:34-44.

192. Koduri PR. Novel cytomorphology of the giant proerythroblasts of parvovirus B19 infection. Am J Hematol 1998;58:95-9.

193. Koduri PR, Naides SJ. Transient blood plasmacytosis in parvovirus B19 infection: a report of two cases. Ann Hematol 1996;72:49-51.

194. Krause JR, Penchansky L, Knisely AS. Morphological diagnosis of parvovirus B19 infection. A cytopathic effect easily recognized in air-dried, formalin-fixed bone marrow smears stained with hematoxylin-eosin or Wright-Giemsa. Arch Pathol Lab Med 1992;116:178-80.

195. Kurtzman GJ, Ozawa K, Cohen B, Hanson G, Oseas R, Young NS. Chronic bone marrow failure due to persistent B19 parvovirus infection. N Engl J Med 1987;317:287-94.

196. Lehmann HW, Knoll A, Kuster RM, Modrow S. Frequent infection with a viral pathogen, parvovirus B19, in rheumatic diseases of childhood. Arthritis Rheum 2003;48:1631-8.

197. McClain K, Estrov Z, Chen H, Mahoney DH Jr. Chronic neutropenia of childhood: frequent association with parvovirus infection and correlations with bone marrow culture studies. Br J Haematol 1993;85:57-62.

198. Mishra B, Malhotra P, Ratho RK, Singh MP, Varma S, Varma N. Human parvovirus B19 in patients with aplastic anemia. Am J Hematol 2005;79:166-7.

199. Morita E, Nakashima A, Asao H, Sato H, Sugamura K. Human parvovirus B19 nonstructural protein (NS1) induces cell cycle arrest at G(1) phase. J Virol 2003;77:2915-21.

200. Nunoue T, Kusuhara K, Hara T. Human fetal infection with parvovirus B19: maternal infection time in gestation, viral persistence and fetal prognosis. Pediatr Infect Dis J 2002;21:1133-6.

201. Prassouli A, Papadakis V, Tsakris A, et al. Classic transient erythroblastopenia of childhood with human parvovirus B19 genome detection in the blood and bone marrow. J Pediatr Hematol Oncol 2005;27:333-6.

202. Srivastava A, Bruno E, Briddell R, et al. Parvovirus B19-induced perturbation of human megakaryocytopoiesis in vitro. Blood 1990;76:1997-2004.

203. Weigel-Kelley KA, Yoder MC, Srivastava A. Alpha5beta1 integrin as a cellular coreceptor for human parvovirus B19: requirement of functional activation of beta1 integrin for viral entry. Blood 2003;102:3927-33.

Bacterial Infections

204. Aoyama T, Takeuchi Y, Goto A, Iwai H, Murase Y, Iwata T. Pertussis in adults. Am J Dis Child 1992;146:163-6.

205. Bakken JS, Aguero-Rosenfeld ME, Tilden RL, et al. Serial measurements of hematologic counts during the active phase of human granulocytic ehrlichiosis. Clin Infect Dis 2001;32:862-70.

206. Bayard-McNeeley M, Bansal A, Chowdhury I, et al. In vivo and in vitro studies on Anaplasma phagocytophilum infection of the myeloid cells of a patient with chronic myelogenous leukaemia and human granulocytic ehrlichiosis. J Clin Pathol 2004;57:499-503.

207. Caldwell CW, Everett ED, McDonald G, Yesus YW, Roland WE. Lymphocytosis of gamma/delta T cells in human ehrlichiosis. Am J Clin Pathol 1995;103:761-6.

208. Chatel G, Gulletta M, Matteelli A, et al. Short report: Diagnosis of tick-borne relapsing fever by the quantitative buffy coat fluorescence method. Am J Trop Med Hyg 1999;60:738-9.

209. Dragsted DM, Dohn B, Madsen J, Jemsen JS. Comparison of culture and PCR for detection of Bordetella pertussis and Bordetella parapertussis under routine laboratory conditions. J Med Microbiol 2004;53:749-54.

210. Dumler JS, Dawson JE, Walker DH. Human ehrlichiosis: hematopathology and immunohistologic detection of Ehrlichia chaffeensis. Hum Pathol 1993;24:391-6.

210a. Dumler JS, Madigan JE, Pusterla N, Bakken JS. Ehrlichioses in humans: epidemiology, clinical presentation, diagnosis, and treatment. Clin Infect Dis 2007;45(Suppl 1):S45-51.

211. Dworkin MS, Schwan TG, Anderson DE Jr. Tick-borne relapsing fever in North America. Med Clin North Am 2002;86:417-33, viii-ix.

212. Falkinburg L, West E, Yazbak F. Phagocytosis of staphylococci seen in peripheral blood smear. JAMA 1992;182:869.

213. Felsenfeld O. Borreliae, human relapsing fever, and parasite-vector-host relationships. Bacteriol Rev 1965;29:46-74.

214. Fife A, Hill D, Barton C, Burden P. Gram negative septicaemia diagnosed on peripheral blood smear appearances. J Clin Pathol 1994;47:82-4.

215. Frydenberg A, Starr M. Pertussis. Presentation, investigation and management. Aust Fam Physician 2004;33:317-9.

216. Hamilton KS, Standaert SM, Kinney MC. Characteristic peripheral blood findings in human ehrlichiosis. Mod Pathol 2004;17:512-7.

217. Heininger U, Klich K, Stehr K, Cherry JD. Clinical findings in Bordetella pertussis infections: results of a prospective multicenter surveillance study. Pediatrics 1997;100:E10.

218. Hewlett EL, Edwards KM. Clinical practice. Pertussis—not just for kids. N Engl J Med 2005;352:1215-22.

219. Hodge G, Hodge S, Markus C, Lawrence A, Han P. A marked decrease in L-selectin expression by leucocytes in infants with Bordetella pertussis infection: leucocytosis explained? Respirology 2003;8:157-62.

220. Hudnall SD, Molina CP. Marked increase in L-selectin-negative T cells in neonatal pertussis. The lymphocytosis explained? Am J Clin Pathol 2000;114:35-40.

221. Kroft SH. Infectious diseases manifested in the peripheral blood. Clin Lab Med 2002;22:253-77.

222. Kubic VL, Kubic PT, Brunning RD. The morphologic and immunophenotypic assessment of the lymphocytosis accompanying Bordetella pertussis infection. Am J Clin Pathol 1991;95:809-15.

223. Munoz FM. Pertussis in infants, children, and adolescents: diagnosis, treatment, and prevention. Semin Pediatr Infect Dis 2006;17:14-9.

224. Paddock CD, Childs JE. Ehrlichia chaffeensis: a prototypical emerging pathogen. Clin Microbiol Rev 2003;16:37-64.

225. Selby DM, Gautier G, Luban NL, Campos M. Overwhelming neonatal septicemia diagnosed upon examination of peripheral blood smears. Clin Pediatr (Phila) 1990;29:706-9.

226. Stone JH, Dierberg K, Aram G, Dumler DS. Human monocytic ehrlichiosis. JAMA 2004;292:2263-70.

226a. Thomas LD, Hongo I, Bloch KC, Tang YW, Dummer S. Human ehrlichiosis in transplant recipients. Am J Transplant 2007;7:1641-7.

227. Torlakovic E, Hibbs JR, Miller JS, Litz CE. Intracellular bacteria in blood smears in patients with central venous catheters. Arch Intern Med 1995;155:1547-50.

228. Walker DH, Dumler JS. Human monocytic and granulocytic ehrlichioses. Discovery and diagnosis of emerging tick-borne infections and the critical role of the pathologist. Arch Pathol Lab Med 1997;121:785-91.

229. Ward PC. The lymphoid leukocytoses. Postgrad Med 1980;67:217-23.

230. Young EJ, Cardella TA. Meningococcemia diagnosed by peripheral blood smear. JAMA 1988;260:992.

Protozoa Infections

231. Ayi K, Turrini F, Piga A, Arese P. Enhanced phagocytosis of ring-parasitized mutant erythrocytes: a common mechanism that may explain protection against falciparum malaria in sickle trait and beta-thalassemia trait. Blood 2004;104:3364-71.

232. Becker S, Franco JR, Simarro PP, Stich A, Abel PM, Steverding D. Real-time PCR for detection of Trypanosoma brucei in human blood samples. Diagn Microbiol Infect Dis 2004;50:193-9.

233. Berriman M, Ghedin E, Hertz-Fowler C, et al. The genome of the African trypanosome Trypanosoma brucei. Science 2005;309:416-22.

234. CAP Hematology and Clinical Microscopy Resource Committee. Microorganisms. In: Glassy EF, ed. Color atlas of hematology. Northfield, IL: College of American Pathologists; 1998:274-5.

235. Chakravorty SJ, Craig A. The role of ICAM-1 in Plasmodium falciparum cytoadherence. Eur J Cell Biol 2005;84:15-27.

236. Chang KH, Stevenson MM. Malarial anaemia: mechanisms and implications of insufficient erythropoiesis during blood-stage malaria. Int J Parasitol 2004;34:1501-16.

237. Chretien JP, Smoak BL. African trypanosomiasis: changing epidemiology and consequences. Curr Infect Dis Rep 2005;7:54-60.

238. Conrad PA, Kjemtrup AM, Carreno RA, et al. Description of Babesia duncani n.sp. (Apicomplexa: Babesiidae) from humans and its differentiation from other piroplasms. Int J Parasitol 2006;36:779-89.

239. Di Pentima MC, Hwang LY, Skeeter CM, Edwards MS. Prevalence of antibody to Trypanosoma cruzi in pregnant Hispanic women in Houston. Clin Infect Dis 1999;28:1281-5.

240. El-Sayed NM, Myler PJ, Bartholomeu DC, et al. The genome sequence of Trypanosoma cruzi, etiologic agent of Chagas disease. Science 2005;309:409-15.

241. Evans KJ, Hansen DS, van Rooijen N, Buckingham LA, Schofield L. Severe malarial anemia of low parasite burden in rodent models results from accelerated clearance of uninfected erythrocytes. Blood 2006;107:1192-9.

242. Fairhurst R, Wellems T. Plasmodium species (malaria). In: Mandell G, Bennett J, Dolin R, eds. Principles and practice of infectious diseases, 6th ed. New York: Churchill Livingstone; 2005:3121-44.

243. Feilij H, Muller L, Gonzalez Cappa SM. Direct micromethod for diagnosis of acute and congenital Chagas' disease. J Clin Microbiol 1983;18:327-30.

244. Fourcade C, Casbas MJ, Belaouni H, Gonzalez JJ, Garcia PJ, Pepio MA. Automated detection of malaria by means of the haematology analyser Coulter GEN.S. Clin Lab Haematol 2004;26:367-72.

245. Fox LM, Wingerter S, Ahmed A, et al. Neonatal babesiosis: case report and review of the literature. Pediatr Infect Dis J 2006;25:169-73.

246. Herwaldt BL, de Bruyn G, Pieniazek NJ, et al. Babesia divergens-like infection, Washington State. Emerg Infect Dis 2004;10:622-9.

247. Herwaldt BL, Springs FE, Roberts PP, et al. Babesiosis in Wisconsin: a potentially fatal disease. Am J Trop Med Hyg 1995;53:146-51.

248. Huh J. Jung J, Yoon H, Chung W. Pseudoeosinophilia associated with malaria infection determined in the Sysmex XE-2100 hematology analyzer. Ann Hematol 2005;84;400-2.

249. Jaff MS, McKenna D, McCann SR. Platelet phagocytosis: a probable mechanism of thrombocytopenia in Plasmodium falciparum infection. J Clin Pathol 1985;38:1318-9.

250. Jelinek T, Bisoffi Z, Bonazzi L, et al. Cluster of African trypanosomiasis in travelers to Tanzanian national parks. Emerg Infect Dis 2002;8:634-5.

250a. Johnston S, Pieniazek NJ, Xayavong MV, Slemenda SB, Wilkins PP, da Silva AJ. PCR as a confirmatory technique for laboratory diagnosis of malaria. J Clin Microbiol 2006;44:1087-9.

251. Kirchhoff LV. American trypanosomiasis (Chagas' disease)—a tropical disease now in the United States. N Engl J Med 1993;329:639-44.

252. Kirchhoff LV, Paredes P, Lomeli-Guerrero A, et al. Transfusion-associated Chagas disease (American trypanosomiasis) in Mexico: implications for transfusion medicine in the United States. Transfusion 2006;46:298-304.

253. Krause PJ, McKay K, Gadbaw J, et al. Increasing health burden of human babesiosis in endemic sites. Am J Trop Med Hyg 2003;68:431-6.

254. Kroft SH. Infectious diseases manifested in the peripheral blood. Clin Lab Med 2002;22:253-77.

255. Leiby DA, Chung AP, Gill JE, et al. Demonstrable parasitemia among Connecticut blood donors with antibodies to Babesia microti. Transfusion 2005;45:1804-10.

256. Luscher A, de Koning HP, Maser P. Chemotherapeutic strategies against Trypanosoma brucei: drug targets vs. drug targeting. Curr Pharm Des 2007;13:555-67.

257. McDevitt MA, Xie J, Gordeuk V, Bucala R. The anemia of malaria infection: role of inflammatory cytokines. Curr Hematol Rep 2004;3:97-106.

258. Mu J, Joy DA, Duan J, et al. Host switch leads to emergence of Plasmodium vivax malaria in humans. Mol Biol Evol 2005;22:1686-93.

259. Murray M, Murray PK, McIntyre WI. An improved parasitological technique for the diagnosis of African trypanosomiasis. Trans R Soc Trop Med Hyg 1977;71:325-6.

260. Olowu WA, Adelusola KA. Pediatric acute renal failure in southwestern Nigeria. Kidney Int 2004;66:1541-8.

261. Reyburn H, Mbatia R, Drakeley C, et al. Association of transmission intensity and age with clinical manifestations and case fatality of severe Plasmodium falciparum malaria. JAMA 2005;293:1461-70.

262. Robins-Browne RM, Schneider J, Metz J. Thrombocytopenia in trypanosomiasis. Am J Trop Med Hyg 1975;24:226-31.

263. Thwing J, Skarbinski J, Newman RD, et al; Centers for Disease Control and Prevention. Malaria surveillance—United States, 2005. MMWR Surveill Summ 2007;56:23-40.

264. Wery M, Mulumba PM, Lambert PH, Kazyumba L. Hematologic manifestations, diagnosis, and immunopathology of African trypanosomiasis. Semin Hematol 1982;19:83-92.

265. Wickramasinghe SN, Abdalla SH. Blood and bone marrow changes in malaria. Baillieres Best Pract Res Clin Haematol 2000;13:277-99.

266. Wickramasinghe SN, Looareesuwan S, Nagachinta B, White NJ. Dyserythropoiesis and ineffective erythropoiesis in Plasmodium vivax malaria. Br J Haematol 1989;72:91-9.

Helminth Infections

267. Addiss DG, Dimock KA, Eberhard ML, Lammie PJ. Clinical, parasitologic, and immunologic observations of patients with hydrocele and elephantiasis in an area with endemic lymphatic filariasis. J Infect Dis 1995;171:755-8.

268. Eberhard ML, Lammie PJ. Laboratory diagnosis of filariasis. Clin Lab Med 1991;11:977-1010.

269. Figueredo-Silva J, Noroes J, Cedenho A, Dreyer G. The histopathology of bancroftian filariasis revisited: the role of the adult worm in the lymphatic-vessel disease. Ann Trop Med Parasitol 2002;96:531-41.

270. Kroft SH. Infectious diseases manifested in the peripheral blood. Clin Lab Med 2002;22:253-77.

271. Melrose WD. Lymphatic filariasis: new insights into an old disease. Int J Parasitol 2002;32:947-60.

Emerging Infections

272. Booth CM, Matukas LM, Tomlinson GA, et al. Clinical features and short-term outcomes of 144 patients with SARS in the greater Toronto area. JAMA 2003;289:2801-9.

273. Chang B, Crowley M, Campen M, Koster F. Hantavirus cardiopulmonary syndrome. Semin Respir Crit Care Med 2007;28:193-200.

274. Chng WJ, Lai HC, Earnest A, Kuperan P. Haematological parameters in severe acute respiratory syndrome. Clin Lab Haematol 2005;27:15-20.

275. Crowley MR, Katz RW, Kessler R, et al. Successful treatment of adults with severe hantavirus pulmonary syndrome with extracorporeal membrane oxygenation. Crit Care Med 1998;26:409-14.

276. Drosten C, Gunther S, Preiser W, et al. Identification of a novel coronavirus in patients with severe acute respiratory syndrome. N Engl J Med 2003;348:1967-76.

277. Duchin JS, Koster FT, Peters CJ, et al. Hantavirus pulmonary syndrome: a clinical description of 17 patients with a newly recognized disease. The Hantavirus Study Group. N Engl J Med 1994;330:949-55.

278. Foucar K. Constitutional and reactive myeloid disorders. Bone marrow pathology, 2nd ed. Chicago: ASCP Press; 2001:146-72.

279. Graziano KL, Tempest B. Hantavirus pulmonary syndrome: a zebra worth knowing. Am Fam Physician 2002;66:1015-20.

280. Hjelle B, Jenison S, Torrez-Martinez N, et al. Rapid and specific detection of Sin Nombre virus antibodies in patients with hantavirus pulmonary syndrome by a strip immunoblot assay suitable for field diagnosis. J Clin Microbiol 1997;35:600-8.

281. Koster F, Foucar K, Hjelle B, et al. Rapid presumptive diagnosis of hantavirus cardiopulmonary syndrome by peripheral blood smear review. Am J Clin Pathol 2001;116:665-72.

282. Lee N, Hui D, Wu A, et al. A major outbreak of severe acute respiratory syndrome in Hong Kong. N Engl J Med 2003;348:1986-94.

283. Mills JN, Corneli A, Young JC, Garnson LE, Khan AS, Ksiazek TG. Hantavirus pulmonary syndrome—United States: updated recommendations for risk reduction. Centers for Disease Control and Prevention. MMWR Recomm Rep 2002;51:1-12.

284. The involvement of natural killer cells in the pathogenesis of severe acute respiratory syndrome. Am J Clin Pathol 2004;121:507-11.

285. Peiris JS, Guan Y, Yuen KY. Severe acute respiratory syndrome. Nat Med 2004;10:S88-97.

286. Ramos MM, Overturf GD, Crowley MR, Rosenberg RB, Hjelle B. Infection with Sin Nombre hantavirus: clinical presentation and outcome in children and adolescents. Pediatrics 2001;108:E27.

287. Wong RS, Wu A, To KF, et al. Haematological manifestations in patients with severe acute respiratory syndrome: retrospective analysis. BMJ 2003;326:1358-62.

288. Zhong NS, Zheng BJ, Li YM, et al. Epidemiology and cause of severe acute respiratory syndrome (SARS) in Guangdong, People's Republic of China, in February, 2003. Lancet 2003;362:1353-8.

Infection-Associated Hemophagocytic Syndrome

289. Chen CJ, Huang YC, Jaing TH, et al. Hemophagocytic syndrome: a review of 18 pediatric cases. J Microbiol Immunol Infect 2004;37:157-63.

290. Chuang HC, Lay JD, Hsieh WC, et al. Epstein-Barr virus LMP1 inhibits the expression of SAP gene and upregulates Th1 cytokines in the pathogenesis of hemophagocytic syndrome. Blood 2005;106:3090-6.

291. Fisman DN. Hemophagocytic syndromes and infection. Emerg Infect Dis 2000;6:601-8.

292. Florena AM, Iannitto E, Quintini G, Franco V. Bone marrow biopsy in hemophagocytic syndrome. Virchows Arch 2002;441:335-44.

293. Henter JI, Arico M, Elinder G, Imashuku S, Janka G. Familial hemophagocytic lymphohistiocytosis. Primary hemophagocytic lymphohistiocytosis. Hematol Oncol Clin North Am 1998;12:417-33.

294. Imashuku S, Hibi S, Ohara T, et al. Effective control of Epstein-Barr virus-related hemophagocytic lymphohistiocytosis with immunochemotherapy. Histiocyte Society. Blood 1999;93:1869-74.

295. Kanegane H, Ito Y, Ohshima K, et al. X-linked lymphoproliferative syndrome presenting with systemic lymphocytic vasculitis. Am J Hematol 2005;78:130-3.

296. Mizukane R, Kadota Ji J, Yamaguchi T, et al. An elderly patient with hemophagocytic syndrome due to severe mycoplasma pneumonia with marked hypercytokinemia. Respiration 2002;69:87-91.

296a. Rigaud S, Fondaneche MC, Lambert N, et al. XIAP deficiency in humans causes and X-linked lymphoproliferative syndrome. Nature 2006;444:110-4.

297. Risdall RJ, Brunning RD, Hernandez JI, Gordon DH. Bacteria-associated hemophagocytic syndrome. Cancer 1984;54:2968-72.

298. Risdall RJ, McKenna RW, Nesbit ME, et al. Virus-associated hemophagocytic syndrome: a benign histiocytic proliferation distinct from malignant histiocytosis. Cancer 1979;44:993-1002.

299. Seemayer TA, Gross TG, Egeler RM, et al. X-linked lymphoproliferative disease: twenty-five years after the discovery. Pediatr Res 1995;38:471-8.

300. Sumegi J, Seemayer TA, Huang D, et al. A spectrum of mutations in SH2D1A that causes X-linked lymphoproliferative disease and other Epstein-Barr virus-associated illnesses. Leuk Lymphoma 2002;43:1189-201.

301. Takagi M, Unno A, Maruyama T, Kaneko K, Obinata K. Human herpesvirus-6 (HHV-6)-associated hemophagocytic syndrome. Pediatr Hematol Oncol 1996;13:451-6.

302. Woda BA, Sullivan JL. Reactive histiocytic disorders. Am J Clin Pathol 1993;99:459-63.

11 NONINFECTIOUS SYSTEMIC DISEASES AND MISCELLANEOUS BONE MARROW CONDITIONS

ANEMIA OF CHRONIC DISEASE

Although the complex pathophysiologic mechanisms are not entirely resolved, *anemia of chronic disease* is generally defined by a constellation of clinical, morphologic, and laboratory parameters (Table 11-1). Patients typically develop mild to moderate normocytic normochromic anemia several months following the onset of a chronic inflammatory disorder, chronic infection, or neoplastic disorder. A common feature of these diverse disorders is a sustained immune reaction, which is linked to both disruption of iron homeostasis and impaired erythropoieses (1–3,5,8,11). Iron resorption declines and iron is shunted into storage cells, producing the paradoxical bone marrow picture of reduced sideroblastic iron in conjunction with increased macrophage storage iron that typifies anemia of chronic disease (fig. 11-1). Recent publications suggest a major role of hepcidin overproduction as the key mediator of anemia of chronic disease, influencing not only iron homeostasis, but also erythroid progenitor cell proliferation and survival (1–3,8). Because

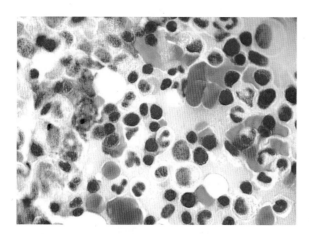

Figure 11-1

INCREASED STORAGE IRON

Storage iron is increased but erythroid iron is absent in this bone marrow aspirate smear (Prussian blue stain).

Table 11-1

FEATURES OF ANEMIA OF CHRONIC DISEASE[a]

Clinical
Development of anemia 1-2 months after onset of a variety of types of chronic diseases including: chronic inflammatory disorders, chronic infections, neoplasms, end organ failure disorders such as chronic liver disease, and chronic rejection after solid organ transplantation

Blood
Usually normocytic normochromic anemia with normal mean corpuscular volume, mean corpuscular hemoglobin concentration, and red cell distribution width
Inappropriately low reticulocyte count

Iron Studies
Decreased serum/plasma iron
Decreased transferrin (total iron-binding capacity)
Decreased transferrin saturation
Normal to increased ferritin
Normal to slightly increased serum transferrin receptor levels
Increased hepcidin levels in plasma and urine

Bone Marrow
Normal or mildly reduced numbers of erythroid precursors
Decreased sideroblasts (iron-containing erythroid precursor cells)
Increased storage iron within macrophages/histiocytes

Pathophysiologic Mechanisms
Cross regulation between immune function and iron homeostasis results in mildly decreased erythrocyte survival time, inadequate bone marrow response to anemia due to blunted erythropoietin response, apoptosis of erythroid precursors, and increased retention of iron within macrophages
Many cytokines and other immunoregulatory factors implicated in this complex pathophysiologic disorder including IL1[a], IL6, IL10, TNF-α, IFN-γ, TGF-β, and a newly recognized hepatic antimicrobial peptide, hepcidin, an acute phase reactant in infections and other inflammatory processes which also downregulates iron absorption and upregulates iron uptake by storage cells
Key role for hepcidin as chief mediator of ACD supported by recent literature in that hepcidin not only influences iron homeostasis but also inhibits erythroid progenitor cell proliferation and survival

[a]Data from references 1–12.

[b]IL = interleukin; TNF-α = tumor necrosis factor alpha; IFN-γ = interferon gamma; TGF-β = tumor growth factor beta; ACD = anemia of chronic disease.

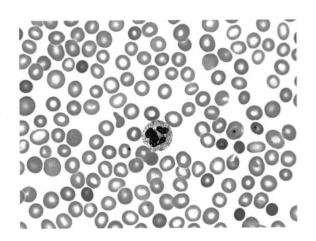

Figure 11-2

**AUTOIMMUNE HEMOLYTIC ANEMIA AND
IDIOPATHIC THROMBOCYTOPENIA PURPURA (ITP)**

Postsplenectomy persistence of autoimmune hemolytic anemia and ITP in a patient with systemic lupus erythematosus and associated Evan syndrome.

of the overlap in laboratory parameters, most emphasis is placed on distinguishing anemia of chronic disease from iron deficiency anemia (see chapter 4) (11,12).

Anemia of chronic disease is the predominant hematologic abnormality in patients with systemic noninfectious disorders. In addition to anemia of chronic disease, other blood and bone marrow findings may be evident in association with collagen vascular disorders, congenital and acquired immunodeficiency disorders, other constitutional disorders, chronic renal failure, and chronic alcoholism. Distinctive hematologic abnormalities are also linked to pregnancy, toxic exposures, and unique post-therapy changes.

COLLAGEN VASCULAR (RHEUMATOLOGIC) DISORDERS

Collagen vascular (rheumatologic) disorders are the prototypic systemic illnesses associated with anemia of chronic disease. This disease association is not unexpected, since the cytokine-mediated immune aberrations responsible for collagen vascular disorders are directly linked to the abnormalities in iron homeostasis that produce the anemia of chronic disease. These patients can also have concurrent treatable vitamin deficiency–associated anemia such as salicylate-induced folate deficiency, pernicious

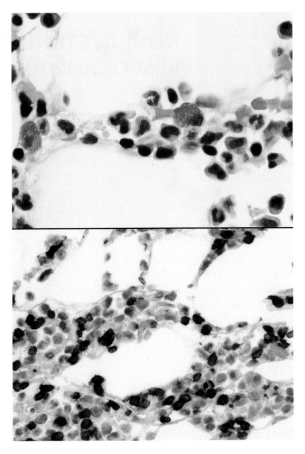

Figure 11-3

**RHEUMATOID ARTHRITIS WITH
DIFFUSE INCREASE IN T CELLS**

This bone marrow core biopsy shows a hypocellular bone marrow from a patient with rheumatoid arthritis in which a prominent diffuse increase in T cells was identified by immunohistochemical staining (hematoxylin and eosin [H&E] stain, top; immunoperoxidase stain for CD3, bottom).

anemia due to vitamin B_{12} deficiency, autoimmune hemolytic anemia, and T-cell–mediated pure red cell aplasia (fig. 11-2) (13,25).

Other immune-mediated cytopenias are also common in patients with collagen vascular disorders (19,26). Neutropenia, and less often red cell aplasia, are prevalent in patients with rheumatoid arthritis and have been linked to T-cell large granular lymphocytic leukemias/proliferations (figs. 11-3, 11-4) (26). In contrast, the neutropenia noted in patients with systemic lupus erythematosus (SLE) has been linked to either immune-mediated peripheral destruction of neutrophils or bone marrow apoptotic mechanisms (fig. 11-5) (17).

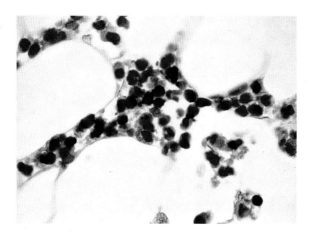

Figure 11-4

INCREASED CYTOTOXIC SUPPRESSOR T CELLS IN RHEUMATOID ARTHRITIS–ASSOCIATED RED CELL APLASIA

A diffuse increase in cytotoxic suppressor T cells is highlighted by T-cell restricted intracellular antigen (TIA)-1 positivity in this bone marrow core biopsy from a patient with rheumatoid arthritis and associated red cell aplasia (immunoperoxidase stain for TIA-1).

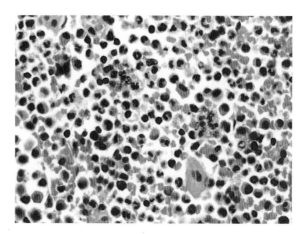

Figure 11-5

INCREASED HISTIOCYTES CONTAINING INGESTED NEUTROPHILS

This bone marrow core biopsy shows histiocytes containing large numbers of ingested and partially degenerated neutrophils (H&E stain).

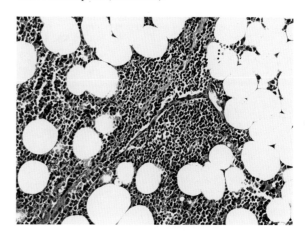

Figure 11-6

LYMPHOID AGGREGATE IN COLLAGEN VASCULAR DISEASE

Bone marrow core biopsy from a patient with collagen vascular disease shows an associated lymphoid aggregate (H&E stain).

Coagulopathies are very common in this patient population, notably the antiphospholipid syndrome, thrombotic thrombocytopenic purpura, and other thrombotic disorders, which are especially prevalent in patients with SLE (15,16,23,25). Factors that play a role in SLE-associated thrombotic events include abnormal platelet activation, antiphospholipid antibody persistence and subtype, and endothelial cell apoptosis (15,16, 23). Although collagen vascular disorders such as SLE typically manifest in adolescence and adulthood, the neonatal lupus syndrome is a well-recognized complication in infants born to mothers with anti-Ro autoantibodies (14,27). In addition to antibody-mediated cytopenias, these neonates may have complete congenital heart block and cutaneous rash (14).

The bone marrow findings in patients with collagen vascular disorders are variable (24). In addition to the anemia of chronic disease, both polyclonal plasmacytosis and lymphoid aggregates are common findings. These lymphoid aggregates may contain hyperplastic germinal centers (figs. 11-6, 11-7). In addition to evaluating these lymphoid aggregates, the bone marrow should be assessed for abnormal diffuse lymphocytic infiltrates, especially increases in cytotoxic, suppressor CD3-positive, CD8-positive, and T-cell restricted intracellular antigen (TIA)-1–posi-

tive T cells (see figs. 11-3, 11-4). These abnormal T-cell infiltrates may reflect a clonal or nonclonal large granular lymphocytic infiltration.

Other less common bone marrow findings in patients with collagen vascular disorders include single or multilineage aplasia, myelofibrosis with megakaryocytic hyperplasia mimicking a chronic myeloproliferative disease, hemophagocytosis usually secondary to infection, and infiltration by malignant lymphoma (figs. 11-8,

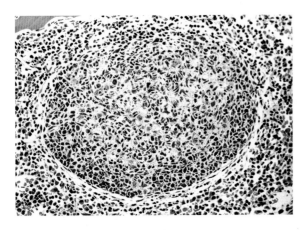

Figure 11-7

LYMPHOID AGGREGATE WITH GERMINAL CENTER IN COLLAGEN VASCULAR DISEASE

Lymphoid aggregate contains a germinal center in a bone marrow core biopsy from a patient with collagen vascular disease (H&E stain).

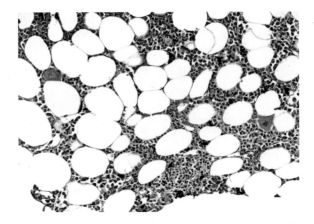

Figure 11-8

COLLAGEN VASCULAR DISEASE WITH RED CELL APLASIA

Hemoglobin A immunohistochemical stain highlights only rare residual erythroblasts in a patient with collagen vascular disease–associated pure red cell aplasia.

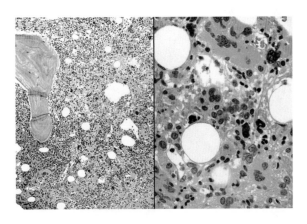

Figure 11-9

MYELOPROLIFERATIVE-LIKE PATTERN IN SEVERE RHEUMATOID ARTHRITIS

Composite low- and high-magnification view reveals a chronic myeloproliferative disorder-like picture with increased cellularity, dilated sinuses, and increased mega-karyocytes in a patient with severe rheumatoid arthritis (H&E stain). (Courtesy of Dr. C. Sever, Albuquerque, NM.)

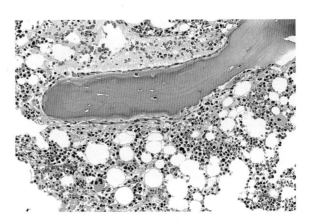

Figure 11-10

BONE REMODELING IN SYSTEMIC LUPUS ERYTHEMATOSUS IN A PATIENT WITH HYPERCALCEMIA

Bone marrow core biopsy shows prominent bony remodeling in a 32-year-old woman with systemic lupus erythematosus and hypercalcemia. (Courtesy of Dr. C. Sever, Albuquerque, NM.)

11-9) (18,24). Both Hodgkin and non-Hodgkin lymphomas (most cases) have been described in patients with collagen vascular disorders (18,20). Methotrexate therapy, commonly used to treat rheumatoid arthritis, is associated with subsequent malignant lymphoma, and pathogenic roles for either Epstein-Barr (EBV) virus or *p53* mutations have been postulated (18).

Bony abnormalities, ranging from osteopenia to osteosclerosis, are evident on bone marrow core biopsy sections from patients with collagen vascular disorders. Osteopenia may be the consequence of corticosteroid therapy, while osteomalacia or osteosclerosis may result from secondary chronic renal failure in this patient population (see chapter 9 for additional illustrations) (fig. 11-10) (24). In addition to these overt morphologic aberrations,

Table 11-2

CONSTITUTIONAL IMMUNODEFICIENCY DISORDERS[a]

Category	Exemplary Type(s)	Gene Loci Mutations/ Pathogenetic Features	Hematologic Manifestations
Combined lymphocyte defects	X-linked severe combined immun-odeficiency	Xq13.1 gene locus; defect in IL2-R[b] and receptors for other cytokines due to mutations in shared protein; autosomal recessive forms also described	Abnormalities linked to secondary infections; increased incidence of EBV-associated NHL
	DiGeorge syndrome	22q11.2 and other loci; embryonic defect in thymic and other organ development of pharyngeal pouch derivatives	Abnormalities linked to secondary infections; cases of EBV-associated LPD noted; rare cases of aplastic anemia
Antibody deficiencies	X-linked agamma-globulinemia	*XLA*, Xq22 gene loci; defect of B-cell specific tyrosine kinase	Abnormalities linked to secondary infections; increased incidence of leukemias and lymphomas
	Common variable immunodeficiency disorder	Neither genetic loci nor pathogenesis clearcut; heterogeneous defects; late onset of B- and T-cell functional and regulatory defects; T-cell and dendritic cell defects postulated	Increased incidence in abnormal multiorgan lymphoid infiltrates and overt lymphomas; propensity for bacterial infections
Other distinctive syndromes	Wiskott-Aldrich syndrome	Xp11.3 (*WASP*) gene locus; *WASP* gene involved in cytoskeleton	Thrombocytopenia with small plate-lets; increased hypolobulated mega-karyocytes in bone marrow; marked increase in leukemias, NHL, and HL
	Ataxia telangiectasia	11q22-q23, *ATM* gene locus, DNA repair defect in *ATM* gene results in progres-sive neurodegeneration	Marked increased in leukemia, HL, NHL, and other solid tumors
	Familial hemophago-cytic lymphohistio-cytosis	Several types, 2 gene loci reported: 9q21.3-22 and 10q21-22; perforin gene (10q22) defect results in impaired nat-ural killer and cytotoxic T-cell activity Other gene mutations described	Pancytopenia; extensive histiocytic in-filtration of bone marrow with hemo-phagocytosis initiated by infection Eventual bone marrow hypoplasia or aplasia
Phagocyte disorders	Chediak-Higashi syndrome	1q42-q44, *CHS* gene locus; defect in CHS gene results in faulty lysosome assembly leading to giant granules	Distinctive enlarged granules in all granulated cells; patients often develop hemophagocytic syndrome and/or fatal EBV-related LPD
	Chronic granulo-matous disease	Mutations in genes that encode the various units of the superoxide-generating phagocyte NADPH oxidase system	Bone marrow usually shows reactive features; not a major site of histiocytic/ granulomatous infiltration

[a]Data from references 28, 29, 32–35, 37–45, 47, and 48.

[b]IL = interleukin; EBV = Epstein-Barr virus; HL = Hodgkin lymphoma; NHL = non-Hodgkin lymphoma; LPD = lymphop-roliferative disorders; NADPH = nicotinamide adenine dinucleotide phosphate.

abnormalities in bone marrow progenitor cell reserves and bone marrow stromal cell func-tion have been noted in patients with collagen vascular disorders, notably those with SLE and rheumatoid arthritis (21,22).

CONSTITUTIONAL AND ACQUIRED IMMUNODEFICIENCY DISORDERS

A comprehensive review of constitutional im-munodeficiency disorders is beyond the scope of this Fascicle. Instead, only hematologic and bone marrow features are reviewed, while categories and exemplary types of constitutional immunodefi-ciency disorders are highlighted in Table 11-2,

along with information regarding gene loci mutations and pathogenetic features.

The hematologic manifestations of patients with constitutional immunodeficiency disor-ders are generally fairly nonspecific, reflecting the predictable sequelae of recurrent infec-tions (Table 11-2). Small platelets and reduced megakaryocyte lobulation are characteristic of the Wiskott-Aldrich syndrome (fig. 11-11) (29). Patients with Chediak-Higashi syndrome have dramatic pathologic findings such as the pres-ence of enlarged cytoplasmic granules, which are readily apparent in all types of granulated cells including large granular lymphocytes (figs.

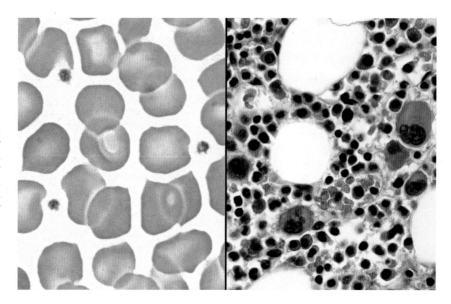

Figure 11-11

WISKOTT-ALDRICH SYNDROME

The peripheral blood (left) and bone marrow core biopsy (right) smears from a patient with Wiskott-Aldrich syndrome show minute platelets in blood and increased small, hypolobulated megakaryocytes in bone marrow (Wright, H&E stains).

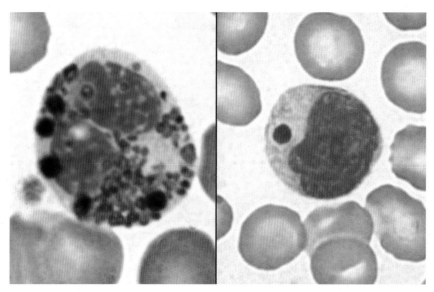

Figure 11-12

CHEDIAK-HIGASHI SYNDROME

The morphologic features of an eosinophil (left) and lymphocyte (right) are seen in a peripheral blood smear from a child with Chediak-Higashi syndrome (Wright stain). (Courtesy of P. Izadi, Los Angeles, CA.)

11-12–11-15) (43). The bone marrow in these patients may also show histiocytic hyperplasia with hemophagocytosis; EBV-associated lymphoproliferative disorders are also common (31,39,46). Secondary neoplasms, often EBV-associated, may develop in patients with many other types of constitutional immunodeficiency disorders, and the bone marrow may be a site of involvement in these cases (Table 11-2).

Bone marrow histiocytic hyperplasia with hemophagocytic syndrome can be the consequence of severe secondary infections in patients with many other types of constitutional immunodeficiency disorders, although this finding is particularly prevalent in patients with Chediak-Higashi syndrome or in those with familial hemophagocytic lymphohistiocytosis. The latter is a natural killer/cytotoxic T-cell disorder associated with perforin gene mutations (figs. 11-16–11-18) (34,38,40). Pancytopenia is common during florid hemophagocytic episodes.

Acquired immunodeficiency syndrome (AIDS) is the prototypic acquired immunodeficiency disorder, although patients undergoing transplantation or receiving sustained chemotherapy also manifest many of the long-term sequelae of chronic

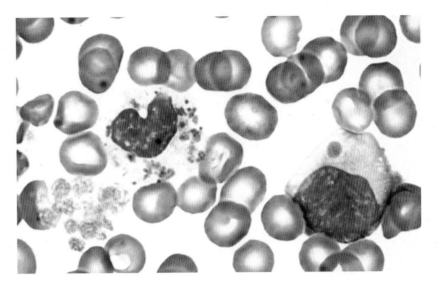

Figure 11-13

CHEDIAK-HIGASHI SYNDROME

Abnormal granulation occurs within neutrophils, lymphocytes, and platelets (Wright stain). (Courtesy of Dr. R. Brynes, Los Angeles, CA.)

Figure 11-14

CHEDIAK-HIGASHI SYNDROME

Hypercellular bone marrow with abnormal granulation in all stages of granulocytic maturation, including eosinophils and eosinophil precursors, in a patient with Chediak-Higashi syndrome (Wright-Giemsa stain.) (Courtesy of Dr. R. Brynes, Los Angeles, CA.)

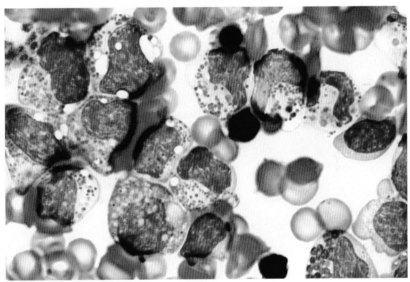

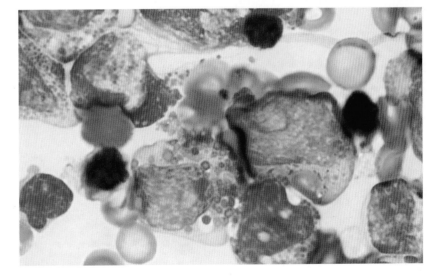

Figure 11-15

CHEDIAK-HIGASHI SYNDROME

Huge abnormal cytoplasmic granules in promyelocytes in conjunction with abnormal granulation in maturing granulocytic and eosinophilic elements in a patient with Chediak-Higashi syndrome (Wright-Giemsa stain). (Courtesy of Dr. R. Brynes, Los Angeles, CA.)

Figure 11-16

INFECTION-ASSOCIATED HEMOPHAGOCYTIC SYNDROME

An increase in histiocytes, some of which show marked erythrophagocytosis, is evident in this bone marrow aspirate smear from a patient with infection-associated hemophagocytic syndrome and underlying immunodeficiency (Wright stain). (Courtesy of Dr. C. Sever, Albuquerque, NM.)

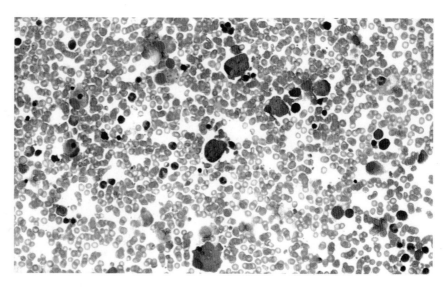

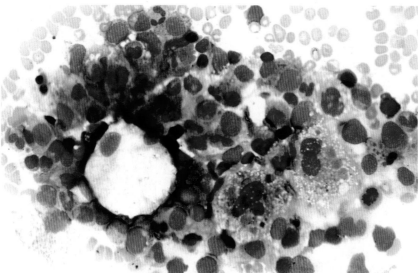

Figure 11-17

FAMILIAL HEMOPHAGOCYTIC LYMPHOHISTIOCYTOSIS

Increased and abnormal histiocytes are seen in a bone marrow aspirate from a patient with familial hemophagocytic lymphohistiocytosis (Wright stain). (Courtesy of P. Izadi, Los Angeles, CA.)

Figure 11-18

FAMILIAL HEMOPHAGOCYTIC LYMPHOHISTIOCYTOSIS

Both hemophagocytic histiocytes and nonphagocytic histiocytes are evident in this bone marrow aspirate smear from a patient with familial hemophagocytic lymphohistiocytosis (Wright stain). (Courtesy of P. Izadi, Los Angeles, CA.)

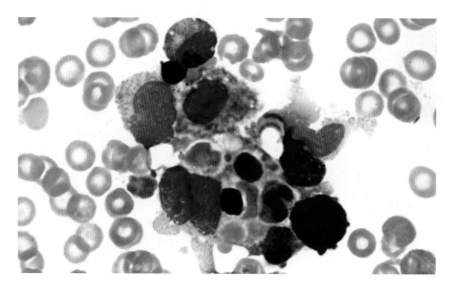

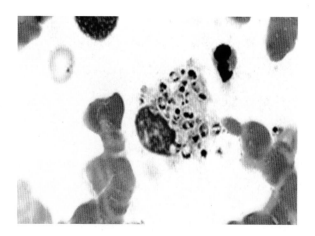

Figure 11-19

MACROPHAGE CONTAINING HISTOPLASMA

The macrophage has ingested *Histoplasma* organisms in this bone marrow aspirate from a patient with acquired immunodeficiency syndrome (AIDS) and secondary histoplasmosis (Wright stain).

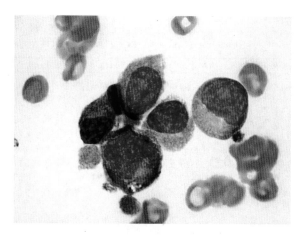

Figure 11-20

SECONDARY EPSTEIN-BARR VIRUS INFECTION

A spectrum of activated lymphocytes is seen in a bone marrow aspirate from a child with human immunodeficiency virus (HIV) and secondary Epstein-Barr virus infection (Wright-Giemsa stain). (Courtesy of P. Izadi, Los Angeles, CA.)

immunodeficiency. The blood and bone marrow features of AIDS and other infectious disorders are detailed in chapter 10. Briefly, numerous blood and bone marrow abnormalities are noted in AIDS patients, including such nonspecific findings as variably severe blood cytopenias, gelatinous transformation of bone marrow, plasmacytosis, mild reticulin fibrosis of bone marrow, and variably atypical lymphoid aggregates in core biopsies. Secondary bone marrow infections are also common in AIDS and other chronically immunosuppressed patients (see chapter 10) (figs. 11-19, 11-20).

Similar to constitutional immunodeficiency disorders, *infection-associated hemophagocytic syndrome* may be evident in the bone marrow of patients with acquired immunodeficiency. The development of secondary neoplasms, often EBV-related, is a major clinical problem in this patient population, and bone marrow is often a site of involvement by these secondary neoplasms (fig. 11-21) (30,36).

LYSOSOMAL STORAGE DISEASES AND OTHER CONSTITUTIONAL DISORDERS

A diffuse or patchy increase in morphologically distinctive histiocytes within bone marrow characterizes some lipidoses, autosomal recessive lysosomal enzyme deficiency disorders. These lipidoses include *Gaucher disease, Niemann-Pick*

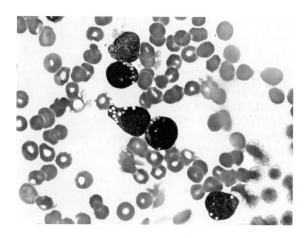

Figure 11-21

BURKITT LEUKEMIA/LYMPHOMA

Bone marrow effacement by Burkitt leukemia/lymphoma is seen in an immunocompromised patient (Wright stain).

disease, and a variant of Niemann-Pick disease termed *sea blue histiocyte syndrome* (Table 11-3) (49,50,53,56). (See chapter 9 for discussion and additional illustrations.)

The distinctive morphologic features in these disorders result from the accumulation within histiocytes of a substrate protein due to the enzyme deficiency. The unique morphologic features of storage disease type histiocytes, such as Gaucher, Niemann-Pick, and sea blue

Table 11-3

HEMATOLOGIC AND BONE MARROW FEATURES OF SELECTED LYSOSOMAL STORAGE DISEASES[a]

Disorder (category)	Blood Features	Bone Marrow Features	Comments
Gaucher disease (lipidosis)	Cytopenias linked to splenomegaly and bone marrow infiltration	Diffuse increase in histiocytes with crinkled cytoplasm	Multiple genetic types Acid β-glucosidase deficiency (accumulation of glucosylceramide [glucocerebroside])
Niemann-Pick disease (lipidosis)	Cytopenias linked to splenomegaly and bone marrow infiltration	Diffuse increase in prominently vacuolated histiocytes	Acid sphingomyelinase enzyme defect (accumulation of sphingomyelin)
Sea blue histiocytosis (lipidosis)		Diffuse increase in both vacuolated and sea blue histiocytes	Variant of Niemann-Pick disease
Mucopolysaccharidosis (Hurler disease)	Granulated, vacuolated lymphocytes	Granules or inclusions in reticular cells, plasma cells, and osteoblasts	α-L-iduronidase enzyme defect (disorder of glycosaminoglycan [mucopolysaccharide] degradation)
Sialidosis (mucolipidosis)	Granulated, vacuolated lymphocytes	Foamy histiocytes	α-neuraminidase enzyme defect (disorder of glycoprotein degradation)

[a]Data from references 49–56.

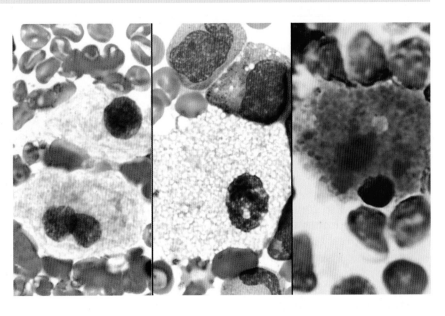

Figure 11-22

STORAGE DISEASE TYPE HISTIOCYTES

Gaucher cells (left), a Niemann-Pick cell (center), and a sea blue histocyte (right) are seen (Wright stain).

histiocytes, are best appreciated on bone marrow aspirate smears, although the morphologic features of bone marrow core biopsy sections are also reasonably distinctive (figs. 11-22, 11-23). The extent of bone marrow replacement is best assessed on core biopsy sections (fig. 11-23).

Gaucher histiocytes are characterized by small, round to oval nuclei and voluminous amounts of eosinophilic cytoplasm with distinct crinkled, striated cytoplasm. Niemann-Pick cells exhibit a similar low nuclear to cytoplasmic ratio, while the voluminous cytoplasm is uniformly finely vacuolated. Sea blue histiocyte

syndrome has, in addition to Niemann-Pick cells, histiocytes with deeply basophilic cytoplasm as seen by Wright-Giemsa staining (fig. 11-22) (53). Hybrid morphologic forms may also be evident, with partial blue cytoplasm and diffuse vacuolization.

Histiocytes morphologically indistinguishable from those of Gaucher, Niemann-Pick, and sea blue histiocytes may be present in bone marrow specimens of patients with high cell turnover conditions or hyperlipidemic disorders (50). Consequently, the presence of distinctive storage disease type histiocytes in bone marrow

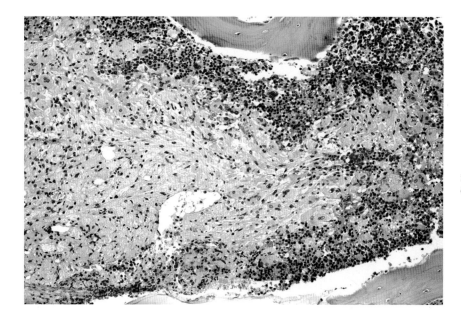

Figure 11-23

GAUCHER DISEASE

Extensive bone marrow efface-ment in a child with Gaucher disease (H&E stain).

Figure 11-24

SIALIDOSIS

Peripheral blood lymphocytes show large abnormal granules in conjunction with vacuoles in an infant with sialidosis (Wright stain).

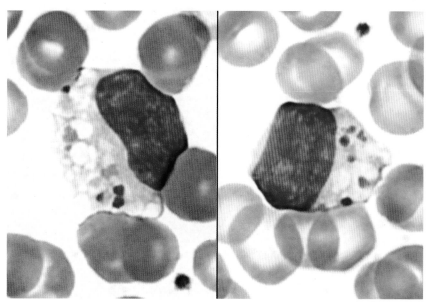

is insufficient for a definitive diagnosis of a lysosomal storage disease. Instead, definitive diagnosis requires assay of enzyme levels or some other type of genotypic confirmation (55,56). Recombinant enzyme replacement therapy is available for patients with some storage disorders, notably recombinant glucocerebrosidase for Gaucher disease (54,56).

A variety of other types of lysosomal storage diseases, including *mucolipidoses* and *mucopoly-saccharidoses*, may also manifest with hemato-

logic and bone marrow abnormalities (Table 11-3). Common blood findings in these rare disorders include lymphocytes with distinct vacuoles and granules, often surrounded by halos (fig. 11-24) (49,51). In some lysosomal storage diseases, the neutrophils or eosinophils may show intense granulation (49,51). Distinctive bone marrow cells in patients with mucolipidoses and mucopolysaccharidoses include morphologically abnormal histiocytes, reticular cells, plasma cells, and osteoblasts (51). These

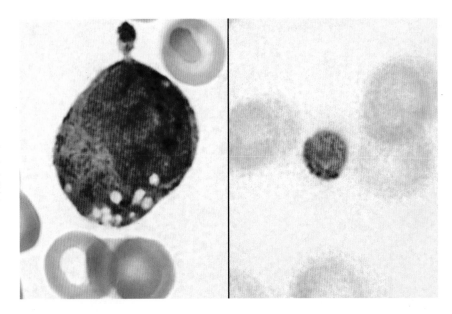

Figure 11-25

PEARSON SYNDROME

Vacuolated myeloid precursors are associated with ringed sideroblasts in an infant with Pearson syndrome (Wright stain). (Courtesy of Dr. L. Contis, Pittsburgh, PA.)

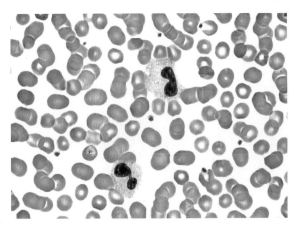

Figure 11-26

FAMILIAL PELGER-HÜET ANOMALY

Peripheral blood smear from patient with familial Pelger-Hüet anomaly shows hyposegmentation (Wright stain). (Courtesy of Dr. S. Kroft, Milwaukee, WI.)

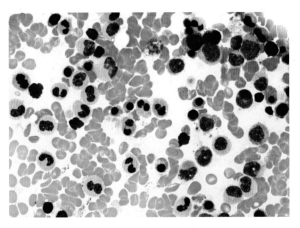

Figure 11-27

FAMILIAL PELGER-HÜET ANOMALY

Bone marrow aspirate smear from a patient with familial Pelger-Hüet anomaly shows hyposegmentation of neutrophils (Wright stain). (Courtesy of Dr. S. Kroft, Milwaukee, WI.)

abnormalities often consist of granules, vacuoles, or other cytoplasmic inclusions.

Other rare constitutional disorders, such as *Pearson syndrome,* can manifest with multilineage cytopenias and distinct bone marrow abnormalities (52). This mitochondrial defect disorder is characterized by vacuolated myeloid and erythroid precursors and ringed sideroblasts (fig. 11-25). Distinctive blood and bone marrow findings have also been described in patients with the familial *Pelger-Hüet anomaly,* characterized by

distinctive neutrophil hyposegmentation in both blood and bone marrow, while all other features of neutrophils are normal (figs. 11-26, 11-27).

Myelokathexis is another rare constitutional disorder with unique blood and bone marrow findings, largely localized to the myeloid lineage. Despite bone marrow hypercellularity, the nuclei of the granulocytic cells show distinctive segmentation abnormalities in conjunction with neutropenia (see chapter 5) (figs. 11-28, 11-29). The bone marrow features of constitutional

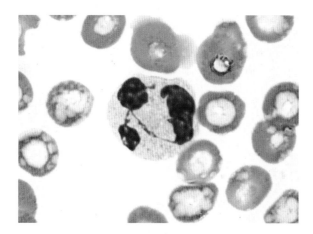

Figure 11-28

MYELOKATHEXIS

The peripheral blood smear from a child with myelo-kathexis and profound neutropenia shows abnormal neutrophil segmentation (Wright-Giemsa stain). (Courtesy of Dr. S. Kroft, Milwaukee, WI.)

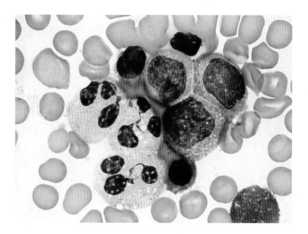

Figure 11-29

MYELOKATHEXIS

Bone marrow aspirate smear from a patient with myelokathexis shows prominent myeloid hyperplasia in conjunction with striking segmentation abnormalities of maturing neutrophils (Wright-Giemsa stain.) (Courtesy of Dr. S. Kroft, Milwaukee, WI.)

primary hematologic disorders such as *Diamond-Blackfan anemia* (constitutional red cell aplasia), *Fanconi anemia* (constitutional aplastic anemia), *Kostmann syndrome* (constitutional agranulocytosis), and *thrombocytopenia with absent radii* (a constitutional amegakaryocytosis) are reviewed in the lineage-specific chapters of this book as well as in chapter 7.

CHRONIC RENAL FAILURE

Anemia is the most frequent hematologic abnormality in patients with *chronic renal failure,* although coagulopathies, largely due to platelet function defects, are also prevalent in this population (63). Reduced erythropoietin production due to the renal failure is the dominant factor producing anemia in these patients, but many other cofactors contribute to the severity of the anemia, especially in patients on chronic dialysis. These include chronic blood loss, shortened red blood cell (RBC) survival time, and erythrocyte and bone marrow toxins introduced through dialysis (61,63). Despite these significant cofactors, a dramatic response to recombinant human erythropoietin is characteristic in chronic renal failure patients (58). The development of antierythropoietin antibodies, however, is a recently recognized cause of dramatic normocytic normochromic anemia with absent reticulocytes in this patient population (figs. 11-30, 11-31) (57,59).

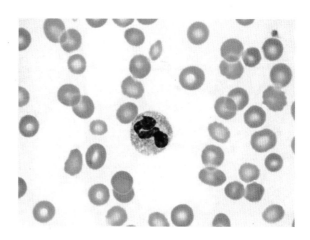

Figure 11-30

RED CELL APLASIA SECONDARY TO ANTIERYTHROPOIETIN ANTIBODIES

Profound normocytic normochromic anemia with absent polychromasia is seen in a peripheral blood smear from a patient with renal failure on erythropoietin therapy who developed antierythropoietin antibodies (Wright stain). (Courtesy of Dr. Q. Y. Zhang, Albuquerque, NM.)

At the opposite end of the spectrum, renal transplant patients, patients with certain types of glomerulonephritis, and patients with some renal tumors develop erythrocytosis secondary to physiologically inappropriate erythropoietin production (63). In these conditions, erythrocyte counts are elevated, resulting in

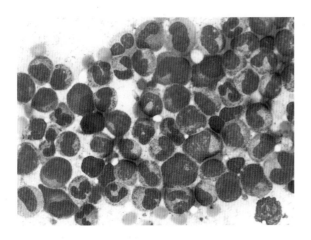

Figure 11-31

RED CELL APLASIA SECONDARY TO ANTIERYTHROPOIETIN ANTIBODIES

Bone marrow aspirate smear shows abundant granulocytic cells, but virtually absent erythroid elements, in a patient with chronic renal failure on erythropoietin who developed antierythropoietin antibodies (Wright stain). (Courtesy of Dr. Q. Y. Zhang, Albuquerque, NM.)

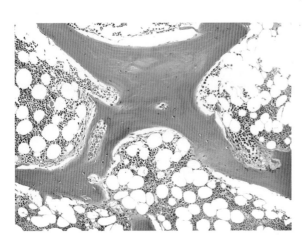

Figure 11-32

OSTEITIS FIBROSA CYSTICA

Bone marrow core biopsy section shows prominent bony changes compatible with osteitis fibrosa cystica in a patient with secondary hyperparathyroidism from chronic renal failure (H&E stain).

increased levels of hemoglobin and an elevated hematocrit. Other lineages are generally unremarkable (see chapter 4 for a discussion of erythrocytosis).

A bone marrow examination is not generally required in the management of patients with chronic renal failure. However, bone marrow

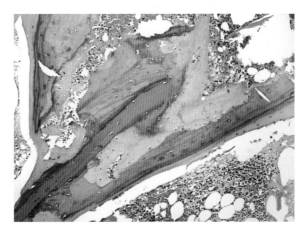

Figure 11-33

OSTEOMALACIA

Wide osteoid seams of unmineralized bone are evident in this bone marrow core biopsy from patient with Fanconi renal disease and osteomalacia (H&E stain).

examination may be necessary in patients with refractory, unexplained cytopenias or other medical problems. Bony trabecular abnormalities are the most striking pathologic finding in this patient population (see chapter 9 for additional illustrations). A variety of underlying conditions are responsible for these bony trabecular abnormalities. One of these is secondary hyperparathyroidism-related osteitis fibrosa cystica, which induces myelofibrosis and increased bone remodeling (fig. 11-32). Similarly, striking osteomalacia with defective mineralization of osteoid is caused by hypophosphatemia, hypocalcemia, and abnormal vitamin D metabolism, all common events in advanced chronic renal disease (fig. 11-33) (60,62). Aluminum deposition from dialysis is a major factor linked to osteomalacia in chronic dialysis patients (62). Mixed features of osteosclerosis, osteomalacia, and even osteopenia are common, and the features of bony trabeculae can change over time in these patients (fig. 11-34).

CHRONIC ALCOHOLISM

Hematologic abnormalities are very common in patients with *chronic alcoholism*: anemia and coagulopathies predominate (65,66,70). The causes of anemia include the anemia of chronic disease, direct toxic effects of alcohol on the bone marrow, various nutritional deficiencies, RBC survival defects, and hemodilution (figs. 11-35–11-37)

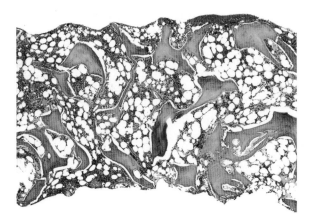

Figure 11-34

CHRONIC RENAL FAILURE

Bone marrow core biopsy from a patient with chronic renal failure illustrates the mixed features of bone pathology secondary to various pathologic processes linked to the duration of the renal failure (H&E stain).

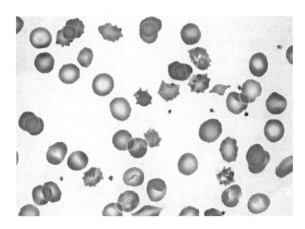

Figure 11-35

ALCOHOLIC LIVER DISEASE AND RENAL FAILURE

A peripheral blood smear from a patient with alcoholic liver disease and renal failure shows severe anemia, acanthocytes, burr cells, and fragments (Wright stain).

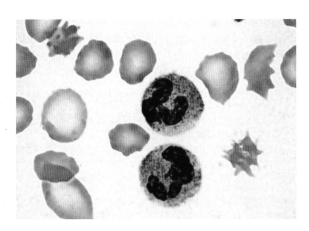

Figure 11-36

ALCOHOLIC LIVER DISEASE AND RENAL FAILURE

Acanthocytes in the blood of a patient with alcoholic liver disease and renal failure (Wright stain).

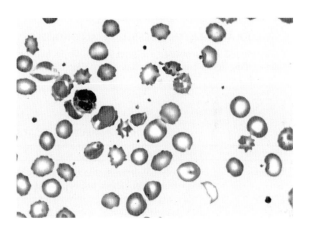

Figure 11-37

ALCOHOLIC LIVER DISEASE AND SEPSIS

A peripheral blood smear from a patient with alcoholic liver disease and sepsis shows severe anemia, macrocytosis, acanthocytes, target cells, and scattered hypochromic erythrocytes (Wright stain).

(65). The predominant mechanism causing the anemia can vary over time. Impaired synthesis of coagulation factors and, frequently, thrombocytopenia contribute to the coagulopathy that is common in alcoholic patients (70).

Although bone marrow examination is generally not required to assess mild to moderate anemia in patients with chronic alcoholism, bone marrow examination may be required to evaluate for infection, unexplained multilineage cytopenias or severe cytopenias, or other abnormalities (67). Storage iron may be markedly

increased or absent depending upon the dominant disease process and the degree of chronic blood loss or inadequate intake in an individual patient. Florid megaloblastic hematopoiesis typifies folate (most common) or vitamin B_{12} deficiencies, while ringed sideroblasts are abundant in rare patients with alcohol-induced sideroblastic anemia (see chapter 4 for illustrations) (66). Other chronic alcoholism-related abnormalities include vacuolated erythroid precursors, a morphologic manifestation of alcohol toxicity, and rare cases of profound bone marrow multilineage hypoplasia secondary to alcohol toxicity (fig. 11-38) (64,67–69).

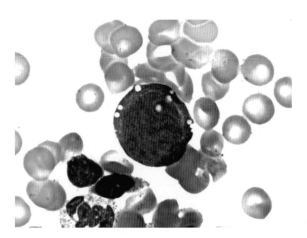

Figure 11-38

VACUOLATED ERYTHROBLASTS IN ALCOHOLISM

Vacuolated erythroblasts are seen in the bone marrow aspirate smear from a patient with alcoholism (Wright stain).

PREGNANCY-ASSOCIATED BONE MARROW DISORDERS

Hematologic aberrations are common in pregnancy. Physiologic processes include an underlying hypercoagulable state, which results from both the increased clotting factors and decreased anticoagulant levels that are present throughout gestation, and third-trimester events such as dilutional anemia and benign gestational thrombocytopenia (Table 11-4) (74,76,78,79). Clinically significant pathologic hematologic conditions are nutritional deficiency–associated anemia, various pathologic coagulopathies and thrombotic microangiopathies, immune-mediated thrombocytopenic purpura, and even overt hematolymphoid neoplasms (Table 11-4; fig. 11-39).

For many of these conditions, hematologic/laboratory assessment is all that is necessary; bone marrow examination is not typically required for most pregnancy-associated hematologic disorders. The levels of fetal stores of iron, folate, and vitamin B$_{12}$ (cobalamin) may be reduced in gravid patients with dietary deficiencies. Com-

Table 11-4

PREGNANCY-ASSOCIATED HEMATOLOGIC DISORDERS[a]

Disorder	Comments
Anemia	Dilutional anemia in 3rd trimester is physiologic Nutritional deficiency, especially iron deficiency, common in pregnancy Folate and vitamin B$_{12}$ deficiencies also noted in pregnancy; can affect fetus, newborn Rare constitutional or acquired red cell aplasias may complicate pregnancy (see chapter 4)
Coagulopathy	Hypercoagulable state physiologic during pregnancy; linked to increased thrombotic risk Additional pathologic disorders can complicate pregnancy including hereditary disorders, antiphospholipid syndrome, DIC[b] (many initiating factors), and HUS/TTP-like thrombotic microangiopathic disorders with RBC fragmentation and thrombocytopenia which occur either throughout pregnancy (e.g., hereditary disorders, antiphospholipid syndrome) or in the peripartum period (e.g., HUS/TTP)
Thrombocyto-penia	Benign, physiologic, gestational thrombocytopenia occurs late in pregnancy in 5-10% of pregnant females; no complications for mother or fetus Many other causes of clinically significant thrombocytopenia may occur throughout pregnancy, including ITP, other immune-related disorders such as SLE, and various coagulopathy-associated thrombocytopenias including DIC, HUS/TTP, amniotic fluid embolus, acute fatty liver of pregnancy
ITP	Bone marrow examination may be required to establish diagnosis of ITP in gravid patients (see chapter 6)
Aplastic anemia	Bone marrow examination necessary in patients with significant pancytopenia; incidence of aplastic anemia not likely increased above age-related background rates (see chapter 7)
Neoplasms	Bone marrow examination required for various leukemias and lymphomas that may occur in pregnant patients similar to the age-related incidence of these disorders; treatment decision making problematic due to concerns about fetal toxicities

[a]Data from references 71–84.

[b]DIC = disseminated intravascular coagulation; HUS = hemolytic uremic syndrome; TTP = thrombotic thrombocytopenic purpura; RBC = red blood cell; SLE = systemic lupus erythematosus; ITP = immune thrombocytopenic purpura.

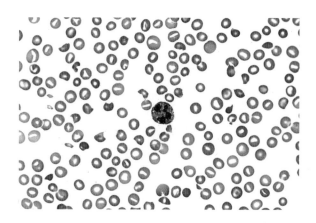

Figure 11-39

MICROANGIOPATHIC HEMOLYTIC ANEMIA

The peripheral blood smear shows the typical features of microangiopathic hemolytic anemia which include severe anemia and thrombocytopenia in conjunction with polychromasia, microspherocytes, and fragmented erythrocytes (Wright stain).

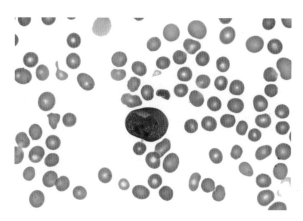

Figure 11-40

MEGALOBLASTIC ANEMIA IN INFANT

A peripheral blood smear from a 6-month-old infant with a mean corpuscular volume (MCV) of 92 and circulating erythroblasts with a megaloblastic chromatin configuration linked to vitamin B_{12} deficiency. The mother is vegan (Wright stain). (Courtesy of Dr. X. Yao, Burbank, CA.)

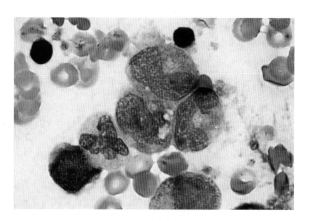

Figure 11-41

MEGALOBLASTIC ANEMIA IN INFANT

Bone marrow aspirate smear from a 6-month-old infant shows marked megaloblastic changes in the granulocytic lineage due to early onset vitamin B_{12} deficiency linked to dietary restrictions of mother (vegan mother) (Wright stain). (Courtesy of Dr. X. Yao, Burbank, CA.)

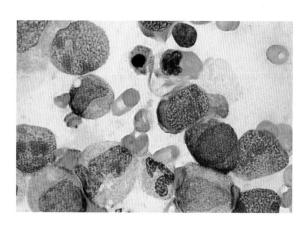

Figure 11-42

MEGALOBLASTIC ANEMIA IN INFANT

A bone marrow aspirate smear shows striking megaloblastic changes of erythroid and granulocytic cells in a 7-month-old infant with vitamin B_{12} deficiency secondary to maternal dietary restrictions (vegan mother) (Wright stain). (Courtesy of Dr. C. Kjeldsberg, Salt Lake City, UT.)

plications in the neonate and young infant may develop if stores and subsequent dietary levels are insufficient to support the rapid growth of the infant (see chapter 4) (figs. 11-40–11-42).

Bone marrow examination may be necessary in gravid patients with suspected immune thrombocytopenic purpura, aplastic anemia, or hematolymphoid neoplasms. The incidence rates in pregnancy for these three entities paral-

lel the rates of age-matched populations (83). Therapy for neoplasms that manifest during pregnancy is particularly challenging due to the risk of fetal complications.

HEAVY METAL TOXICITIES

Arsenic toxicity produces dramatic abnormalities in blood and bone marrow, which may be misinterpreted as either myelodysplasia or megaloblastic

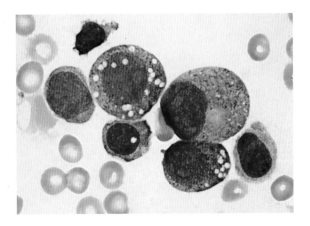

Figure 11-43
COPPER DEFICIENCY

Vacuolated myeloid precursors in a bone marrow aspirate from a 1-year-old boy on total parenteral nutrition who developed profound copper deficiency as well as red cell aplasia (Wright stain).

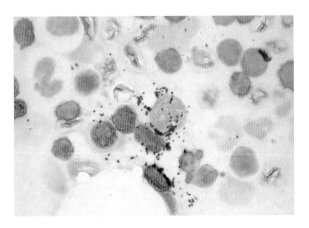

Figure 11-45
COPPER DEFICIENCY

Ringed sideroblasts are evident in this bone marrow aspirate smear from a patient who developed zinc-induced copper deficiency following ingestion of large doses of zinc as a health supplement (Prussian blue stain).

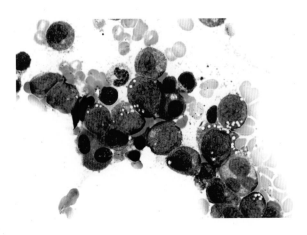

Figure 11-44
COPPER DEFICIENCY

Copper deficiency in an adult female manifests as vacuolization of erythroid and granulocytic precursors (Wright stain).

anemia (86,87). Since arsenic is now once again being used as a therapeutic agent, it is important to recognize hematologic aberrations linked to this agent (85,89). Although neurologic and gastrointestinal symptoms generally predominate, peripheral blood manifestations of arsenic toxicity include anemia, macrocytosis, coarse basophilic stippling, and circulating multinucleated normoblasts. The bone marrow is typically markedly hypercellular, with erythroid hyperplasia, striking megaloblastic changes in myeloid and erythroid lineages, and bizarre dyserythropoiesis with striking karyorrhexis (86,87). Myeloblasts are not typically increased, and levels of both folate and vitamin B_{12} are normal.

Excessive zinc therapy or supplementation can induce *copper deficiency*, which is linked to pancytopenia with paradoxical erythroid hyperplasia in the bone marrow, although the myeloid lineage may be suppressed (88,90,91). Bone marrow changes in copper deficiency include vacuolization of myeloid and erythroid precursors, megaloblastic changes, and variable numbers of ringed sideroblasts. The blood changes include neutropenia and variable microcytosis (figs. 11-43–11-45) (91).

UNIQUE POST-THERAPY EFFECTS IN BONE MARROW

Potent multiagent chemotherapy produces dramatic changes in non-neoplastic bone marrow, including a marked reduction in all lineages as a nonspecific consequence of cytotoxic therapy in a site of physiological high cell proliferation. Cell ablation is characterized by individual cell death, which progresses to widespread cell dropout. The extent of multilineage bone marrow suppression depends on the myelotoxicity of the chemotherapy regimen; the degree of bone marrow suppression is generally assessed by sequential

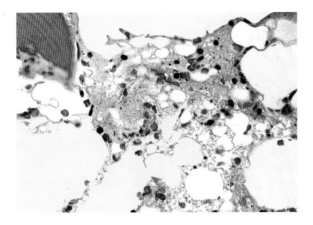

Figure 11-46

INDUCTION CHEMOTHERAPY DAMAGE

Bone marrow core biopsy section shows extensive fibrinoid necrosis and virtual absence of hematopoietic elements in a patient on induction therapy for acute leukemia (H&E stain).

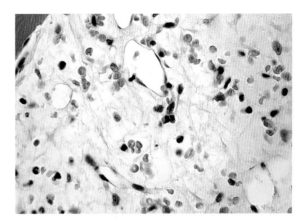

Figure 11-47

INDUCTION CHEMOTHERAPY DAMAGE

Bone marrow core biopsy from patient on day 8 of induction therapy for acute leukemia shows virtual absence of hematopoietic elements and damaged bone marrow stroma (H&E stain).

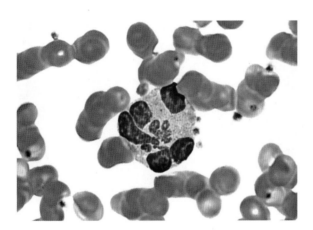

Figure 11-48

CHEMOTHERAPY DAMAGE

The peripheral blood shows a giant hypersegmented neutrophil in a patient recovering from potent chemotherapy (Wright stain).

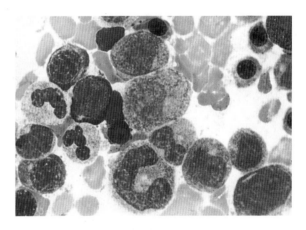

Figure 11-49

CHEMOTHERAPY DAMAGE

Megaloblastic changes in granulocytic elements are evident in this bone marrow aspirate smear following chemotherapy for acute leukemia (Wright stain).

blood counts. For patients undergoing induction chemotherapy for acute leukemia, sequential assessment of bone marrow during the first month of therapy is used to determine the rapidity and extent of eradication of the neoplastic clone. In this patient population, complete myeloablation is the goal (figs. 11-46, 11-47). Atypical features of regenerating hematopoietic cells may be evident during bone marrow recovery, including nuclear lobulation of erythroid cells and other erythroid abnormalities (figs. 11-48, 11-49). In patients un-

dergoing therapy for extramedullary neoplasms, bone marrow examination is not generally required unless cytopenias are prolonged or other possible pathologic processes, such as secondary infection or tumor dissemination to bone marrow, are suspected.

Idiosyncratic drug reactions or toxic exposures can result in prolonged aplasia in rare patients (figs. 11-50–11-53) (94,96). Dysplastic features, most striking in erythroid elements but also affecting other lineages, can occur in patients

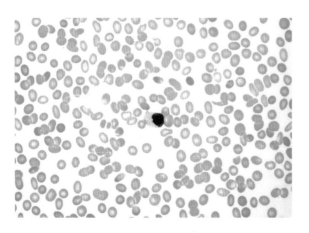

Figure 11-50

METHOTREXATE-INDUCED AGRANULOCYTOSIS

The peripheral blood shows profound neutropenia (Wright stain). (Courtesy of Dr. C. Sever, Albuquerque, NM.)

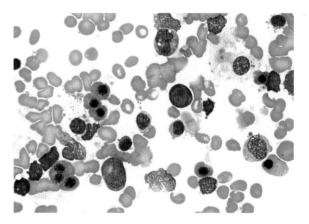

Figure 11-51

METHOTREXATE-INDUCED AGRANULOCYTOSIS

Profound granulocytic hypoplasia and increased histiocytes in the bone marrow of a patient who developed methotrexate-induced agranulocytosis (Wright stain). (Courtesy of Dr. C. Sever, Albuquerque, NM.)

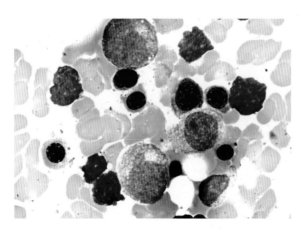

Figure 11-52

METOCLOPRAMIDE-INDUCED AGRANULOCYTOSIS

A bone marrow aspirate from patient with metoclopramide-induced agranulocytosis shows only occasional immature granulocytic cells (Wright stain). (Courtesy of Dr. C. Sever, Albuquerque, NM.)

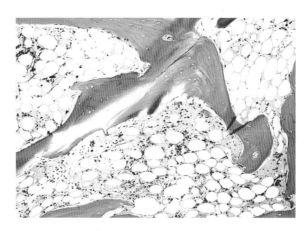

Figure 11-53

METHOTREXATE-INDUCED APLASTIC ANEMIA

A bone marrow core biopsy section from a patient who developed methotrexate-induced aplastic anemia shows profound hematopoietic aplasia (H&E stain.) (Courtesy of Dr. C. Sever, Albuquerque, NM.)

receiving antineoplastic chemotherapy or other medications such as methotrexate or valproic acid (figs. 11-54–11-56) (92,95,99). These erythroid changes include karyorrhexis, megaloblastic changes, and nuclear lobulation. Medication-associated sideroblastic anemia is also encountered in clinical practice (fig. 11-57). One distinctive medication-associated bone marrow abnormality is the defect in mitoses that can be seen in patients on colchicine (figs. 11-58, 11-59).

Recombinant cytokines, such as granulocyte–colony-stimulating factor (G-CSF), granulocyte/monocyte–colony-stimulating factor (GM-CSF), erythropoietin, and even thrombopoietin, may be given to accelerate bone marrow regeneration following myelotoxic therapy, to improve cell production in constitutional and acquired single or multilineage aplasias, and to treat various acquired cytopenias such as anemia in chronic renal failure patients. These pharmacologic

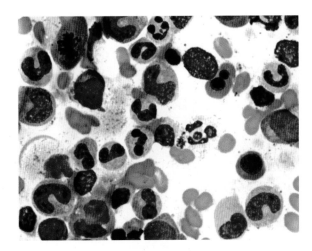

Figure 11-54

**MEGALOBLASTIC CHANGES FOLLOWING
METHOTREXATE THERAPY**

Bone marrow aspirate smear shows megaloblastic changes in the granulocytic cells in a patient on methotrexate (Wright stain). (Courtesy of Dr. C. Sever, Albuquerque, NM.)

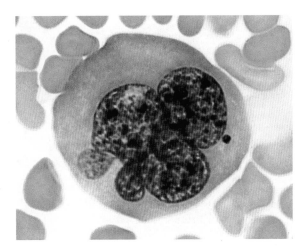

Figure 11-55

VALPROIC ACID-INDUCED DYSERYTHROPOIESIS

Valproic acid-induced dyserythropoiesis is evident on this bone marrow aspirate smear (Wright stain). (Courtesy of Dr. T. Elghetany, Galveston, TX.)

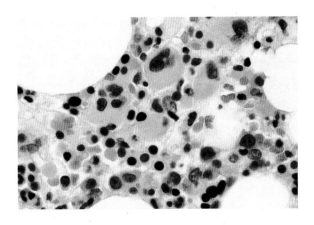

Figure 11-56

**ABNORMAL MEGAKARYOCYTES
FOLLOWING VALPROIC ACID THERAPY**

Megakaryocytes are increased, with clustering and abnormal nuclear lobulation, in the bone marrow of a patient on valproic acid therapy (H&E stain). (Courtesy of Dr. T. Elghetany, Galveston, TX.)

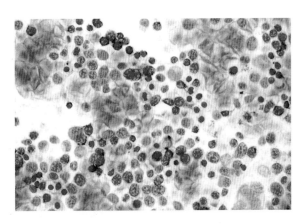

Figure 11-57

SIDEROBLASTIC ANEMIA

Sideroblastic anemia with numerous ringed sideroblasts is evident on this bone marrow aspirate smear. Whether this is due to medication or an acquired red cell disorder is uncertain in this patient (Prussian blue stain). (Courtesy of Dr. C. Sever, Albuquerque, NM.)

agents can produce prominent bone marrow changes. The initial bone marrow response to G-CSF or GM-CSF is an increased number of immature granulocytic/monocytic cells mimicking leukemia (fig. 11-60) (98). After maturation of this initial wave of immature cells, the bone marrow is characterized by lineage-specific hyperplasia based on the type of recombinant cytokine used. In addition to granulocytic hyperplasia, the circulating neutrophils and precursors of patients receiving G-CSF or GM-CSF show toxic changes (figs. 11-61, 11-62). Rare reports describe an atypical monocytosis mimicking acute leukemia in patients receiving recombinant G-CSF therapy (97). Similarly, recombinant therapy thrombopoietin can elicit

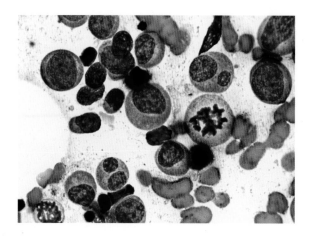

Figure 11-58

COLCHICINE THERAPY

Abnormal mitoses on a bone marrow aspirate smear from a patient on colchicine therapy (Wright stain). (Courtesy of Dr. C. Sever, Albuquerque, NM.)

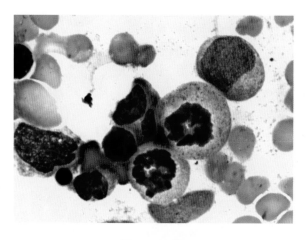

Figure 11-59

COLCHICINE THERAPY

Abnormal mitoses on a bone marrow aspirate smear from a patient on colchicine therapy (Wright stain). (Courtesy of Dr. C. Sever, Albuquerque, NM.)

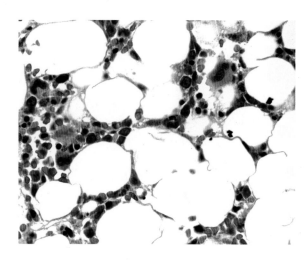

Figure 11-60

GRANULOCYTE COLONY-STIMULATING FACTOR THERAPY

Bone marrow core biopsy from a patient undergoing induction chemotherapy for acute leukemia with concurrent granulocyte–colony-stimulating factor (G-CSF) therapy shows increased immature granulocytic cells without maturation in markedly hypocellular bone marrow (H&E stain).

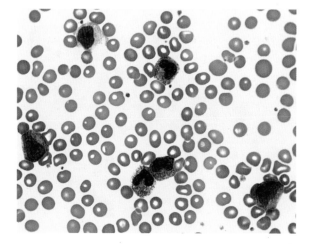

Figure 11-61

GRANULOCYTE COLONY-STIMULATING FACTOR THERAPY

A peripheral blood smear from a patient with carcinoma on G-CSF therapy shows toxic neutrophilia with a left shift (Wright stain).

a bone marrow picture simulating a chronic myeloproliferative disorder, with prominent megakaryocytic hyperplasia, nuclear lobulation defects, and even reticulin fibrosis and osteosclerosis (93).

ASSESSMENT OF PATIENTS WITH SYSTEMIC DISORDERS

Anemia of chronic disease is the most common hematologic abnormality in patients with systemic illnesses, especially chronic inflammatory disorders. Bone marrow examination

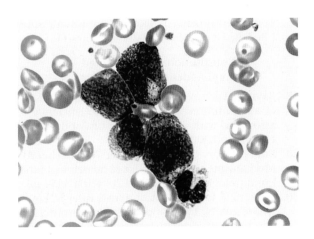

Figure 11-62

**GRANULOCYTE COLONY-
STIMULATING FACTOR THERAPY**

A peripheral blood smear from a patient with carcinoma on G-CSF therapy shows toxic changes and prominent left shift (Wright stain).

may not be necessary in these anemic patients, unless the anemia is more severe than expected or other clinical/hematologic abnormalities warrant assessment of bone marrow.

Bone marrow findings in patients with noninfectious systemic illnesses may be the direct consequence of the systemic disorder such as lymphoid aggregates in patients with collagen vascular (rheumatologic) diseases. In many patients, however, the bone marrow shows findings of secondary complications such as hemophagocytic syndromes in immunodeficient patients or profound bony abnormalities in patients with chronic renal disease. Evaluation of the bone marrow in this patient population should include assessment for changes known to be linked to the primary disorder as well as evaluation for secondary complications, medication toxicities, and other unique post-therapy effects.

REFERENCES

Anemia of Chronic Disease

1. Dallalio G, Law E, Means RT Jr. Hepcidin inhibits in vitro erythroid colony formation at reduced erythropoietin concentrations. Blood 2006;107:2702-4.
2. Delaby C, Pilard N, Goncalves AS, Beaumont C, Canonne-Hergaux F. Presence of the iron exporter ferroportin at the plasma membrane of macrophages is enhanced by iron loading and down-regulated by hepcidin. Blood 2005;106:3979-84.
3. Detivaud L, Nemeth E, Boudjema K, et al. Hepcidin levels in humans are correlated with hepatic iron stores, hemoglobin levels, and hepatic function. Blood 2005;106:746-8.
4. Foucar K. Aplastic and hypoplastic anemias and miscellaneous types of anemia. In: Kjeldsberg C, ed. Practical diagnosis of hematologic disorders, 4th ed. Chicago: ASCP Press; 2006:43-60.
5. Means RT Jr. Hepcidin and anaemia. Blood Rev 2004;18:219-25.
6. Nemeth E, Valore EV, Territo M, Schiller G, Lichtenstein A, Ganz T. Hepcidin, a putative mediator of anemia of inflammation, is a type II acute-phase protein. Blood 2003;101:2461-3.
7. Papadaki HA, Kritikos HD, Valatas V, Boumpas DT, Eliopoulos GD. Anemia of chronic disease in rheumatoid arthritis is associated with increased apoptosis of bone marrow erythroid cells: improvement following anti-tumor necrosis factor-alpha antibody therapy. Blood 2002;100:474-82.
8. Rivera S, Nemeth E, Gabayan V, Lopez MA, Farshidi D, Ganz T. Synthetic hepcidin causes rapid dose-dependent hypoferremia and is concentrated in ferroportin-containing organs. Blood 2005;106:2196-9.
9. Testa U. Apoptotic mechanisms in the control of erythropoiesis. Leukemia 2004;18:1176-99.
10. Weinstein DA, Roy CN, Fleming MD, Loda MF, Wolfsdorf JI, Andrews NC. Inappropriate expression of hepcidin is associated with iron refractory anemia: implications for the anemia of chronic disease. Blood 2002;100:3776-81.
11. Weiss G, Goodnough LT. Anemia of chronic disease. N Engl J Med 2005;352:1011-23.
12. Wians FH Jr, Urban JE, Keffer JH, Kroft SH. Discriminating between iron deficiency anemia and anemia of chronic disease using traditional indices of iron status vs transferrin receptor concentration. Am J Clin Pathol 2001;115:112-8.

Collagen Vascular (Rheumatologic) Disorders

13. Arcasoy MO, Chao NJ. T-cell-mediated pure red-cell aplasia in systemic lupus erythematosus: response to cyclosporin A and mycophenolate mofetil. Am J Hematol 2005;78:161-3.

14. Cimaz R, Spence DL, Hornberger L, Silverman ED. Incidence and spectrum of neonatal lupus erythematosus: a prospective study of infants born to mothers with anti-Ro autoantibodies. J Pediatr 2003;142:678-83.

15. Ekdahl KN, Bengtsson AA, Andersson J, et al. Thrombotic disease in systemic lupus erythematosus is associated with a maintained systemic platelet activation. Br J Haematol 2004;125:74-8.

16. Male C, Foulon D, Hoogendoorn H, et al. Predictive value of persistent versus transient antiphospholipid antibody subtypes for the risk of thrombotic events in pediatric patients with systemic lupus erythematosus. Blood 2005;106:4152-8.

17. Matsuyama W, Yamamoto M, Higashimoto I, et al. TNF-related apoptosis-inducing ligand is involved in neutropenia of systemic lupus erythematosus. Blood 2004;104:184-91.

18. Menke DM, Griesser H, Moder KG, et al. Lymphomas in patients with connective tissue disease. Comparison of p53 protein expression and latent EBV infection in patients immunosuppressed and not immunosuppressed with methotrexate. Am J Clin Pathol 2000;113:212-8.

19. Michel M, Lee K, Piette JC, et al. Platelet autoantibodies and lupus-associated thrombocytopenia. Br J Haematol 2002;119:354-8.

20. Munzert G, Frickhofen N, Bauditz J, Schreiber S, Hermann F. Concomitant manifestation of systemic lupus erythematosus and low-grade non-Hodgkin's lymphoma. Leukemia 1997;11:1324-8.

21. Papadaki HA, Boumpas DT, Gibson FM, et al. Increased apoptosis of bone marrow CD34(+) cells and impaired function of bone marrow stromal cells in patients with systemic lupus erythematosus. Br J Haematol 2001;115:167-74.

22. Papadaki HA, Kritikos HD, Gernetzi C, et al. Bone marrow progenitor cell reserve and function and stromal cell function are defective in rheumatoid arthritis: evidence for a tumor necrosis factor alpha-mediated effect. Blood 2002;99:1610-9.

23. Rajagopalan S, Somers EC, Brook RD, et al. Endothelial cell apoptosis in systemic lupus erythematosus: a common pathway for abnormal vascular function and thrombosis propensity. Blood 2004;103:3677-83.

24. Rosenthal NS, Farhi DC. Bone marrow findings in connective tissue disease. Am J Clin Pathol 1989;92:650-4.

25. Spivak JL. The blood in systemic disorders. Lancet 2000;355:1707-12.

26. Starkebaum G. Chronic neutropenia associated with autoimmune disease. Semin Hematol 2002;39:121-7.

27. Zuppa AA, De Luca D, De Turris P, Cota F, Tortorolo G. Usefulness of rh-G-CSF in early-onset severe neutropenia in neonatal lupus syndrome. J Pediatr Hematol Oncol 2004;26:609-11.

Constitutional and Acquired Immunodeficiency Disorders

28. Bayry J, Lacroix-Desmazes S, Kazatchkine MD, et al. Common variable immunodeficiency is associated with defective functions of dendritic cells. Blood 2004;104:2441-3.

29. Burns S, Cory GO, Vainchenker W, Thrasher AJ. Mechanisms of WASp-mediated hematologic and immunologic disease. Blood 2004;104:3454-62.

30. Canioni D, Jabado N, MacIntyre E, Patey N, Emile JF, Brousse N. Lymphoproliferative disorders in children with primary immunodeficiencies: immunological status may be more predictive of the outcome than other criteria. Histopathology 2001;38:146-59.

31. Foucar K. Bone marrow manifestation of non-infectious systemic diseases. In: Bone marrow pathology, 2nd ed. Chicago: ASCP Press; 2001:640-53.

32. Hong R. The DiGeorge anomaly (CATCH 22, DiGeorge/velocardiofacial syndrome). Semin Hematol 1998;35:282-90.

33. Illoh OC. Current applications of flow cytometry in the diagnosis of primary immunodeficiency diseases. Arch Pathol Lab Med 2004;128:23-31.

34. Janka GE. Hemophagocytic syndromes. Blood Rev 2007;21:245-53.

35. Katano H, Cohen JI. Perforin and lymphohistiocytic proliferative disorders. Br J Haematol 2005;128:739-50.

36. Knowles DM. Immunodeficiency-associated lymphoproliferative disorders. Mod Pathol 1999;12:200-17.

37. Levine S, Smith VV, Malone M, Sebire NJ. Histopathological features of chronic granulomatous disease (CGD) in childhood. Histopathology 2005;47:508-16.

38. Lipton JM, Westra S, Haverty CE, Roberts D, Harris NL. Case records of the Massachusetts General Hospital. Weekly clinicopathological exercises. Case 28-2004. Newborn twins with thrombocytopenia, coagulation defects, and hepatosplenomegaly. N Engl J Med 2004;351:1120-30.

39. Mueller BU, Pizzo PA. Cancer in children with primary or secondary immunodeficiencies. J Pediatr 1995;126:1-10.

40. Muralitharan S, Al Lamki Z, Dennison D, et al. An inframe perforin gene deletion in familial hemophagocytic lymphohistiocytosis is associated with perforin expression. Am J Hematol 2005;78:59-63.

41. Ochs HD. The Wiskott-Aldrich syndrome. Semin Hematol 1998;35:332-45.

42. Paccani SR, Boncristiano M, Patrussi L, et al. Defective Vav expression and impaired F-actin reorganization in a subset of patients with common variable immunodeficiency characterized by T-cell defects. Blood 2005;106:626-34.

43. Puck JM. Primary immunodeficiency diseases. JAMA 1997;278:1835-41.

44. Tardieu M, Lacroix C, Neven B, et al. Progressive neurologic dysfunctions 20 years after allogeneic bone marrow transplantation for Chediak-Higashi syndrome. Blood 2005;106:40-2.

45. Uribe L, Weinberg KI. X-linked SCID and other defects of cytokine pathways. Semin Hematol 1998;35:299-309.

46. van Krieken JH. Lymphoproliferative disease associated with immune deficiency in children. Am J Clin Pathol 2004;122(Suppl):S122-7.

47. Wada T, Schurman SH, Garabedian EK, Yachie A, Candotti E. Analysis of T-cell repertoire diversity in Wiskott-Aldrich syndrome. Blood 2005;106:3895-7.

48. Warnatz K, Denz A, Drager R, et al. Severe deficiency of switched memory B cells (CD27(+)IgM(-)IgD(-)) in subgroups of patients with common variable immunodeficiency: a new approach to classify a heterogeneous disease. Blood 2002;99:1544-51.

Lysosomal Storage Diseases and Other Constitutional Disorders

49. Brunning RD. Morphologic alterations in nucleated blood and marrow cells in genetic disorders. Hum Pathol 1970;1:99-124.

50. Foucar K. Histiocytic disorders involving bone marrow. In: Bone marrow pathology, 2nd ed. Chicago: ASCP Press; 2001:520-41.

51. Hansen HG, Graucob E. Hematologic Cytology of storage diseases. New York: Springer-Verlag; 1985.

52. Knerr I, Metzler M, Niemeyer CM, et al. Hematologic features and clinical course of an infant with Pearson syndrome caused by a novel deletion of mitochondrial DNA. J Pediatr Hematol Oncol 2003;25:948-51.

53. Landas S, Foucar K, Sando GN, Ellefson R, Hamilton HE. Adult Niemann-Pick disease masquerading as sea blue histiocyte syndrome: report of a case confirmed by lipid analysis and enzyme assays. Am J Hematol 1985;20:391-400.

54. Pastores GM, Weinreb NJ, Aerts H, et al. Therapeutic goals in the treatment of Gaucher disease. Semin Hematol 2004;41:4-14.

55. Vellodi A. Lysosomal storage disorders. Br J Haematol 2005;128:413-31.

56. Weinreb NJ, Aggio MC, Andersson HC, et al. Gaucher disease type 1: revised recommendations on evaluations and monitoring for adult patients. Semin Hematol 2004;41:15-22.

Chronic Renal Failure

57. Bennett CL, Luminari S, Nissenson AR, et al. Pure red-cell aplasia and epoetin therapy. N Engl J Med 2004;351:1403-8.

58. Buemi M, Aloisi C, Cavallaro E, et al. Recombinant human erythropoietin (rHuEPO): more than just the correction of uremic anemia. J Nephrol 2002;15:97-103.

59. Casadevall N, Nataf J, Viron B, et al. Pure red-cell aplasia and antierythropoietin antibodies in patients treated with recombinant erythropoietin. N Engl J Med 2002;346:469-75.

60. Clarke BL, Wynne AG, Wilson DM, Fitzpatrick LA. Osteomalacia associated with adult Fanconi's syndrome: clinical and diagnostic features. Clin Endocrinol (Oxf) 1995;43:479-90.

61. Goodnough LT, Skikne B, Brugnara C. Erythropoietin, iron, and erythropoiesis. Blood 2000;96:823-33.

62. Hruska KA, Teitelbaum SL. Renal osteodystrophy. N Engl J Med 1995;333:166-74.

63. Spivak JL. The blood in systemic disorders. Lancet 2000;355:1707-12.

Chronic Alcoholism

64. Ballard HS. Alcohol-associated pancytopenia with hypocellular bone marrow. Am J Clin Pathol 1980;73:830-4.

65. Foucar K. Anemia of chronic disease and normochromic, normocytic nonhemolytic anemias. In: Kjeldsberg C, ed. Practical diagnosis of hematologic disorders, 4th ed, Vol 1. Chicago: ASCP Press; 2006:31-41.

66. Foucar K. Bone marrow manifestation of noninfectious systemic diseases. In: Bone marrow pathology, 2nd ed. Chicago: ASCP Press; 2001:640-53.

67. Latvala J, Parkkila S, Niemela O. Excess alcohol consumption is common in patients with cytopenia: studies in blood and bone marrow cells. Alcohol Clin Exp Res 2004;28:619-24.

68. McCurdy PR, Rath CE. Vacuolated nucleated bone marrow cells in alcoholism. Semin Hematol 1980;17:100-2.

69. Nakao S, Harada M, Kondo K, Mizushima N, Matsuda T. Reversible bone marrow hypoplasia induced by alcohol. Am J Hematol 1991;37:120-3.

70. Spivak JL. The blood in systemic disorders. Lancet 2000;355:1707-12.

Pregnancy-Associated Bone Marrow Disorders

71. Allford SL, Hunt BJ, Rose P, Machin SJ; Haemostasis and Thrombosis Task Force, British Committe for Standards. Guidelines on the diagnosis and management of the thrombotic microangiopathic haemolytic anaemias. Br J Haematol 2003;120:556-73.

72. Baker WF Jr. Iron deficiency in pregnancy, obstetrics, and gynecology. Hematol Oncol Clin North Am 2000;14:1061-77.

73. Bick RL. Syndromes of disseminated intravascular coagulation in obstetrics, pregnancy, and gynecology. Objective criteria for diagnosis and management. Hematol Oncol Clin North Am 2000;14:999-1044.

74. Brenner B. Clinical management of thrombophilia-related placental vascular complications. Blood 2004;103:4003-9.

75. Falkenberry SS. Cancer in pregnancy. Surg Oncol Clin N Am 1998;7:375-97.

76. Foucar K. Pregnancy-related hematologic disorders. In: Bone marrow pathology, 2nd ed. Chicago: ASCP Press; 2001:608-16.

77. Frenkel EP, Yardley DA. Clinical and laboratory features and sequelae of deficiency of folic acid (folate) and vitamin B12 (cobalamin) in pregnancy and gynecology. Hematol Oncol Clin North Am 2000;14:1079-100.

78. Kujovich JL. Hormones and pregnancy: thromboembolic risks for women. Br J Haematol 2004;126:443-54.

79. McCrae KR. Thrombocytopenia in pregnancy: differential diagnosis, pathogenesis, and management. Blood Rev 2003;17:7-14.

80. Michel M, Novoa MV, Bussel JB. Intravenous anti-D as a treatment for immune thrombocytopenic purpura (ITP) during pregnancy. Br J Haematol 2003;123:142-6.

81. Nabhan C, Kwaan HC. Current concepts in the diagnosis and management of thrombotic thrombocytopenic purpura. Hematol Oncol Clin North Am 2003;17:177-99.

82. Oosterkamp HM, Brand A, Kluin-Nelemans JC, Vandenbroucke JP. Pregnancy and severe aplastic anaemia: causal relation or coincidence? Br J Haematol 1998;103:315-6.

83. Peleg D, Ben-Ami M. Lymphoma and leukemia complicating pregnancy. Obstet Gynecol Clin North Am 1998;25:365-83.

84. Webert KE, Mittal R, Sigouin C, Heddle NM, Kelton JG. A retrospective 11-year analysis of obstetric patients with idiopathic thrombocytopenic purpura. Blood 2003;102:4306-11.

Heavy Metal Toxicities

85. Dai J, Weinberg RS, Waxman S, Jing Y. Malignant cells can be sensitized to undergo growth inhibition and apoptosis by arsenic trioxide through modulation of the glutathione redox system. Blood 1999;93:268-77.

86. Feussner JR, Shelburne JD, Bredehoeft S, Cohen HJ. Arsenic-induced bone marrow toxicity: ultrastructural and electron-probe analysis. Blood 1979;53:820-7.

87. Rezuke WN, Anderson C, Pastuszak WT, Conway SR, Firshein SI. Arsenic intoxication presenting as a myelodysplastic syndrome: a case report. Am J Hematol 1991;36:291-3.

88. Salzman MB, Smith EM, Koo C. Excessive oral zinc supplementation. J Pediatr Hematol Oncol 2002;24:582-4.

89. Shen ZX, Chen GQ, Ni JH, et al. Use of arsenic trioxide (As2O3) in the treatment of acute promyelocytic leukemia (APL): II. Clinical efficacy and pharmacokinetics in relapsed patients. Blood 1997;89:3354-60.

90. Summerfield AL, Steinberg FU, Gonzalez JG. Morphologic findings in bone marrow precursor cells in zinc-induced copper deficiency anemia. Am J Clin Pathol 1992;97:665-8.

91. Willis M, Monaghan S, Miller M, et al. Zinc-induced copper deficiency. Am J Clin Pathol 2005;123:125-31.

Unique Post-Therapy Effects In Bone Marrow

92. Adelstein DJ, Hines JD. Bone marrow morphologic changes after combination chemotherapy including VP-16. Cancer 1985;56:467-71.

93. Douglas VK, Tallman MS, Cripe LD, Peterson LC. Thrombopoietin administered during induction chemotherapy to patients with acute myeloid leukemia induces transient morphologic changes that may resemble chronic myeloproliferative disorders. Am J Clin Pathol 2002;117:844-50.

94. Foucar K. Effects of therapy and transplantation, and detection of minimal residual disease. In: Bone marrow pathology, 2nd ed. Chicago: ASCP Press; 2001:654-81.

95. Hoagland HC. Hematologic complications of cancer chemotherapy. Semin Oncol 1982;9:95-102.

96. Lan Q, Zhang L, Li G, et al. Hematotoxicity in workers exposed to low levels of benzene. Science 2004;306:1774-6.

97. Liu CZ, Persad R, Inghirami G, et al. Transient atypical monocytosis mimics acute myelomonocytic leukemia in post-chemotherapy patients receiving G-CSF: report of two cases. Clin Lab Haematol 2004;26:359-62.

98. Schmitz LL, McClure JS, Litz CE, et al. Morphologic and quantitative changes in blood and marrow cells following growth factor therapy. Am J Clin Pathol 1994;101:67-75.

99. So CC, Wong KF. Valproate-associated dysmyelopoiesis in elderly patients. Am J Clin Pathol 2002;118:225-8.

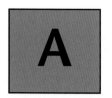

A APPENDIX

Appendix Table 1
AVERAGE NORMAL HEMATOLOGIC VALUES BIRTH TO 1 YEAR[a]

Parameter[b]	Birth (Term)	1 Week	1 Month	6 Months	1 Year
RBC[c] count	5.5	5.0	4.2	3.8	4.2
Hemoglobin	16–18	16.8	14	11.5	12.0
Hematocrit	48–55	50	43	35	36
MCV	108	100	98	90	78
MCHC	32–35	33–35	33	33	33
NRBC	200–400	0–5	0	0	0
Reticulocytes (%)	3–7	0–1	0–1	0–1	0–2
WBC	15–30,000	12,000	11,000	11,000	11,000
ANC	10–25,000	5,000	3,500	3,500	3,500
ALC	4–5,000	5–6,000	6,000	7,500	7,000
Platelets	300,000	300,000	300,000	300,000	300,000

[a]Adapted from references 1, 5, 10, and 12.
[b]In conventional units (cell count per μL).
[c]RBC = red blood cell; MCV = mean corpuscular volume; MCHC = mean corpuscular hemoglobin concentration; NRBC = nucleated red blood cell; WBC = white blood cell; ANC = absolute neutrophil count; ALC = absolute lymphocyte count.

Appendix Table 2
AVERAGE NORMAL HEMATOLOGIC VALUES IN CHILDREN AND ADULTS[a]

Parameter[b]	2-6 Years	6-13 Years	>14 Years (Male)	>14 Years (Female)
RBC[c] count	4.6	4.7	4.5–5.8	3.8–5.2
Hemoglobin	12.5	13.5	14–17	12–16
Hematocrit	37	40	42–52	35–45
MCV	80	86	90	90
MCHC	34	34	34	34
Reticulocytes (%)	1–2	1–2	<1–2	<1–3
WBC	9,000	8,000	7,500	7,500
ANC[d]	3,800	4,400	4,400	4,400
ALC	5,000	3,000	3,000	3,000
Platelets	300,000	250,000	250,000	250,000

[a]Adapted from references 1 and 10.
[b]In conventional units.
[c]RBC = red blood cell; MCV = mean corpuscular volume; MCHC = mean corpuscular hemoglobin concentration; WBC = white blood cell; ANC = absolute neutrophil count; ALC = absolute lymphocyte count.
[d]Absolute neutrophil counts lower in some genetic groups such as blacks.

Appendix Table 3
ABSOLUTE CELL COUNTS FOR CYTOPENIA/CYTOSIS BY PATIENT AGE[a,b]

	Newborn	<1 Year	Child	Adult
Neutrophilia	>28,000	>10,000	>8,000	>7,000
Neutropenia[c]	<7,000	<2,500	<1,500	<1,500
Eosinophilia	>500	>500	>500	>500
Eosinopenia	0	0	0	0
Monocytosis	>3,500	>800	>800	>800
Monocytopenia	<1,000	<200	<200	<200
Basophilia	>100	>100	>100	>100
Basophilopenia	0	0	0	0
Lymphocytosis	>10,000	>9,000	>7,000	>4,000
Lymphopenia	<2,500	<4,000	<2,800	<1,500

[a]Data adapted from references 4, 6, 7, and 13.
[b]Units = cell count per μL.
[c]Absolute neutrophil counts may be physiologically lower in certain ethnic groups such as black populations.

Appendix Table 4

AGE-BASED BONE MARROW DIFFERENTIAL COUNT PERCENTAGES[a]

	Infant	Child	Adult Male	Adult Female
Myeloblasts	2–5	2–4	<2	<2
Promyelocytes	2–4	2–5	1–4	1–4
Myelocytes	4–6	4–6	6–8	6–8
Metamyelocytes	6–8	6–8	8–10	8–10
Bands/Segs	25–30	20–25	15–20	15–20
Erythroid cells	10–25[b]	15–20	15–25	15–25
Lymphocytes	15–45	20–45	5–10	5–10
Eosinophils	2	3	1–3	1–3
Basophils	<1	<1	<1	<1
Monocytes	1	2	1–3	1–3
Plasma cells	<1	<1	1–2	1–2
M:E[c]	>4:1	3:1	3:1	>3:1

[a]Data from references 1 and 16.
[b]Physiologic nadir around 4 months of age associated with low numbers of erythroid cells.
[c]M:E = myeloid to erythroid ratio.

Appendix Table 6

AGE-RELATED LYMPHOID CELLS IN BONE MARROW[a]

	Infant/ Young Child	Child	Adult	Elderly Adult
% lymphoid cells (of total cells)	15–45	15–20	<5–15	<5–15
% B cells (of total cells)	Up to 40[b]	Up to 20[b]	<10	<10
% T cells (of total cells)	<15	<15	<15	<15
H:S ratio[c]	H = S	S > H	S > H	S > H
% NK cells (of total cells)	2–4	2–4	2–4	2–4

[a]Data from references 2, 3, 9, 11, 14, and 16.
[b]Includes a substantial component of hematogones.
[c]H = helper T cells; S = suppressor T cells; NK = natural killer.

Appendix Table 5

AGE-RELATED BONE MARROW HISTOLOGY[a]

Parameter	Newborn	Infant	Child	Adult	Elderly Adult
Cellularity (%)	80–100	70–90	60–80	40–60	25–40
Bone	Active remodeling	Active remodeling	Active remodeling	Inconspicuous osteoblasts, osteoclasts Osteopenia common (females)	Inconspicuous osteoblasts osteoclasts Osteopenia common (females)
Lymphoid cells	Abundant hematogones	Abundant hematogones	Hematogones present	Inconspicuous hematogones	Inconspicuous hematogones
Lymphoid aggregates	Usually absent	Usually absent[b]	Usually absent[b]	Variable	Common
Lipogranulomas	Usually absent	Usually absent	Usually absent	Variable	Common

[a]Adapted from references 8, 15, 17, and 18.
[b]Lymphoid aggregates linked to immune disorders.

Appendix Table 7

SPECIAL TECHNIQUES IN BONE MARROW EVALUATION

Technique	Utility
Cytochemical Stains	
Myeloperoxidase	Primary granules in myeloblasts
Nonspecific esterase	Granules in monocytic cells
Chloroacetate esterase[a]	Secondary granules in maturing neutrophils
Histochemical Stains	
Prussian blue	Iron stores, erythroid iron incorporation
Reticulin	Reticulin fibers
Trichrome	Collagen fibers
PAS[b]/diastase	Fungal organisms
GMS/diastase	Fungal organisms
Acid fast (Fite stain)	Mycobacterial organisms
Brown Bren	Bacteria
Immunohistochemical stains *(selected list)*	
CD20, CD79a	B cells
CD3, CD5; CD4, CD8	T cells; subsets
TIA-1	Cytotoxic granules
CD34	Immature cells (myeloblasts, lymphoblasts)
TdT	Immature cells (lymphoblasts, rare myeloblasts)
Myeloperoxidase	Primary granules in granulocytic cells
Hemoglobin A/glycophorin A	Erythroid cells
CD42b, CD31, factor VIII[c]	Megakaryocytic cells
EBER in situ hybridization	EBV RNA
Parvovirus	Parvoviral inclusions
Flow Cytometric Immunophenotyping	
Myeloid antigen profile	Delineate mature, immature granulocytic cells
Lymphoid antigen profile	Delineate mature, immature B, T, NK populations
Additional lineage profiles	Delineate monocytic, histiocytic, erythroid, and megakaryoblastic populations
Cytogenetics/FISH	
Cytogenetics	Full karyotype of proliferating cells in bone marrow
FISH	Detect specific translocations, inversions, deletions, as well as gain or loss of probe-specific chromosome regions

[a]Chloroacetate esterase works on paraffin-embedded tissue; may be used in a combined esterase stain, although separate cytochemical slide stains are generally preferable.

[b] PAS = periodic acid–Schiff; GMS = Gomori methenamine silver; TIA = T-cell restricted intracellular antigen; TdT = terminal deoxynucleotidyltransferase; EBER = Epstein-Barr encoded RNA; NK = natural killer; EBV = Epstein-Barr virus; RNA = ribosomal nuclei acid; FISH = fluorescence in situ hybridization.

[c]Factor VIII may also stain erythroid cells.

Appendix Table 8

GENERAL GUIDELINES FOR SELECTING DIAGNOSTIC PROCEDURES IN BONE MARROW EVALUATION[a]

Diagnostic Procedure	Acquired Hematologic Disorder	Suspected Congenital Hematologic Disorder	Suspected Infectious Disease (FUO)[b]	Suspected Malignant Hematolymphoid Disorder	Suspected Biochemical/ Metabolic Disorder
Morphology +/– Immunohistochemistry	Required	Required	Required	Required	Required
Flow Cytometry	Possibly required	Possibly useful	Not required	Required	Not required
Special Stains:					
Iron	Required	Required	Required	Required	Required
Organism (PAS/ GMS/acid fast)	Possibly required	Not required	Required	Possibly required (to exclude infectious process)	Not required
NSE/MPO/PAS	Not required	Possibly useful	Not required	Required	Possibly required (for assessing storage disorders)
Reticulin	Possibly required	Not required	Not required	Often required	Not required
Microbial/Viral Cultures	Possibly required	Not required	Required	Not required except to exclude other differential diagnoses	Not required
Cytogenetics/FISH	Possibly required	Possibly required (e.g., Fanconi syndrome)	Not required	Typically required	Not required
Molecular Analysis (PCR)	Possibly required	Possibly required	Possibly required	Frequently required	Possibly useful

[a]This table is a general guide to the use of primary ancillary testing. The choice of additional tests is based on individual case situations; however, if it is suspected that additional studies are needed, extra bone marrow aspirate material should be requested or obtained at the time of the procedure.

[b]FUO = fever of unknown origin; PAS = periodic acid–Schiff; GMS = Gomori methenamine silver; NSE = nonspecific esterase; MPO = myeloperoxidase; FISH = fluorescence in situ hybridization; PCR = polymerase chain reaction.

REFERENCES

1. Brugnara C. Reference values in infancy and childhood. In: Nathan DG, Orkin SH, Ginsburg D, et al., eds. Nathan and Oski's hematology of infancy and childhood, 6th ed, Vol. 2. Philadelphia: Saunders; 2003:1848-51.

2. Clark P, Normansell DE. Phenotype analysis of lymphocyte subsets in normal human bone marrow. Am J Clin Pathol 1990;94:632-6.

3. Clark P, Normansell DE, Innes DJ, et al. Lymphocyte subsets in normal bone marrow. Blood 1986;67:1600-6.

4. Foucar K. Monocytosis. In: Kjeldsberg C, ed. Practical diagnosis of hematologic disorders, 4th ed, Vol. 1. Chicago: ASCP Press; 2006:219-26.

5. Foucar K. Neonatal hematopathology: special considerations. In: Collins R, Swerdlow S, eds. Pediatric hematopathology. New York: Churchill Livingstone; 2001:173-84.

6. Foucar K. Neutropenia. In: Kjeldsberg C, ed. Practical diagnosis of hematologic disorders, 4th ed, Vol 1. Chicago: ASCP Press; 2006:227-37.

7. Foucar K. Neutrophilia In: Kjeldsberg C, ed. Practical diagnosis of hematologic disorders, 4th ed, Vol. 1. Chicago: ASCP Press; 2006:191-202.

8. Friebert SE, Shepardson LB, Shurin SB, et al. Pediatric bone marrow cellularity: are we expecting too much? J Pediatr Hematol Oncol 1998;20:439-43.

9. Horny HP, Wehrmann M, Griesser H, et al. Investigation of bone marrow lymphocyte subsets in normal, reactive, and neoplastic states using paraffin-embedded biopsy specimens. Am J Clin Pathol 1993;99:142-9.

10. Kjeldsberg C. Hematology reference values. Practical diagnosis of hematologic disorders, 4th ed., Vol. 1. Chicago: ASCP Press; 2006:408-13.

11. O'Donnell LR, Alder SL, Balis UJ, et al. Immunohistochemical reference ranges for B lymphocytes in bone marrow biopsy paraffin sections. Am J Clin Pathol 1995;104:517-23.

12. Ozyurek E, Cetintas S, Ceylan T, et al. Complete blood count parameters for healthy, small-for-gestational-age, full-term newborns. Clin Lab Haematol 2006;28:97-104.

13. Peterson LC. Infectious mononucleosis. In: Kjeldsberg CR, ed. Practical diagnosis of hematologic disorders, 4th ed, Vol. 1. Chicago: ASCP Press; 2006:257-70.

14. Rego E, Garcia A, Viana S, et al. Age-related changes of lymphocyte subsets in normal bone marrow biopsies. Cytometry 1998;34:22-9.

15. Rosenthal NS, Farhi DC. Bone marrow findings in connective tissue disease. Am J Clin Pathol 1989;92:650-4.

16. Rosse C, Kraemer MJ, Dillon TL, et al. Bone marrow cell populations of normal infants; the predominance of lymphocytes. J Lab Clin Med 1977;89:1225-40.

17. Salisbury JR, Deverell MH, Cookson MJ. Three-dimensional reconstruction of benign lymphoid aggregates in bone marrow trephines. J Pathol 1996;178:447-50.

18. Thiele J, Zirbes TK, Kvasnicka HM, et al. Focal lymphoid aggregates (nodules) in bone marrow biopsies: differentiation between benign hyperplasia and malignant lymphoma—a practical guideline. J Clin Pathol 1999;52:294-300.

Index*

---

*In a series of numbers, those in boldface indicate the main discussion of the entity.